# AMERICAN ACADEMY OF ORTHOPAEDIC SURGEONS

# EMERGENCY

## CARE AND TRANSPORTATION

### of the Sick and Injured

## Sixth Edition

This textbook is intended solely as a guide to the appropriate procedures to be employed when rendering emergency care to or transporting the sick and injured. It is not intended as a statement of the standards of care required in any particular situation, because circumstances and the patient's physical condition can vary widely from one emergency to another. Nor is it intended that this textbook shall in any way advise emergency personnel concerning legal authority to perform the activities or procedures discussed. Such local determinations should be made only with the aid of legal counsel.

**Notice**
The scenes depicted in the photographs and the patients described in "You are the EMT" throughout this text are fictitious.

## AMERICAN ACADEMY OF ORTHOPAEDIC SURGEONS

# EMERGENCY

## CARE AND TRANSPORTATION
### of the Sick and Injured

editors **Lynn A. Crosby, MD**
**David G. Lewallen, MD**

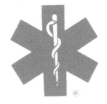
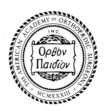

## Sixth Edition

## CREDITS

*Director, Division of Education:* Mark W. Wieting
*Director, Department of Publications:* Marilyn L. Fox, PhD
*Senior Editor:* Lynne Roby Shindoll
*Production Manager:* Loraine Edwalds
*Assistant Production Manager:* Kathy M. Brouillette
*Associate Editor:* Gayle Ekblad
*Production Editor:* Rhoda Sterling
*Graphic Design Coordinator:* Pamela Hutton Erickson
*Editorial Assistants:* Susan Baim, Katy O'Brien
*Secretary:* Brigid Flanagan

*Design:* Proof Positive/Farrowlyne Associates, Inc.
*Illustrators:* Christine Young, Young, McKenna & Associates, Inc.
   Lauren Shavell and Pat Carrico, Medical Imagery
   Joanna Koperski, JAK Graphics
*Photography:* Elizabeth Sawyer
   Susan Steinkamp
   Linda Gheen

# CONTRIBUTORS

Hans-Peter Boksberger, MD
Assistant Director
Surgical Emergency Unit
Kaiser Permanente Medical Center
Los Angeles, California

James C. Cronan, MD, DMD
Associate Professor
Creighton University School of Medicine
Omaha, Nebraska

Alice "Twink" Dalton, BSN, NRPM
Faculty
Prehospital Education Program
Department of Family Practice
Creighton University
Omaha, Nebraska

Maryann DiLibero, OD
Developmental Vision Specialist
Southern California College of Optometry
Harbor City, California

Robert J. DiLibero, JD
Boston, Massachusetts

Hunter A. Hamill, MD
Associate Professor
Department of Obstetrics and Gynecology
Baylor College of Medicine
Houston, Texas

Susan A. Harris, MD
Director of Medical Quality Management
Affiliated Medical Services
Baylor College of Medicine
Houston, Texas

David E. Persse, MD
Assistant Medical Director
Houston Fire Department
Houston, Texas

Joan E. Shook, MD, MBA
Chief, Emergency Medicine Service
Texas Children's Hospital
Houston, Texas

Charles Taylon, MD
Associate Professor
Division of Neurosurgery
Creighton University School of Medicine
Omaha, Nebraska

Bradley H. Walz, MD
Research Fellow
Division of Orthopaedic Surgery
Creighton University School of Medicine
Omaha, Nebraska

Stephen P. Wenger, PharmD
Pharmacist Specialist
Temple City, California

Katherine H. West, BSN, MSEd, CIC
Infection Control Consultant
Infection Control/Emerging Concepts, Inc.
Springfield, Virginia

Brian S. Zachariah, MD, FACEP
Associate Medical Director
City of Houston Emergency Medical Services
Houston, Texas

Robert Zickler, MS, ED
Deputy Chief
Indianapolis Fire Department
Indianapolis, Indiana

# REVIEWERS

Brenda Beasley, RN, BS, EMT-P
EMS Program Director
Southern Union State Community College
Opelika, Alabama

Chip Boehm, RN, EMT-P
Training Coordinator
Maine Emergency Medical Services
Augusta, Maine

Kevin S. Brame, Bachelors of Vocational Education
Fire Battalion Chief
Orange County Fire Department
Orange, California

Alice "Twink" Dalton, BSN, NRPM
Faculty
Prehospital Education Program
Department of Family Practice
Creighton University
Omaha, Nebraska

Michael R. Fleenor, MD
Midway Orthopaedic Associates, PC
Bristol, Tennessee

Charles "Punky" Garoni, BA, EMT-P
Associate Professor
University of Texas Health Science Center
San Antonio, Texas

Donald J. Gordon, PhD, MD
Medical Director, City of San Antonio
    Emergency Medical Services
Professor and Chair
Department of Emergency Medical
    Technology
University of Texas Health Science Center
San Antonio, Texas

Joseph A. Grafft, MS
EMS Specialist
Minnesota State Board of Technical Colleges
F.I.R.E./EMS Center
St. Paul, Minnesota

Carol L. Gupton, REMT-P
Faculty
Prehospital Education Program
Department of Family Practice
Creighton University
Omaha, Nebraska

Coy R. Harris, EMT-P
Coordinator
Kentucky EMS for Children
Russell Springs, Kentucky

George L. Johnson, EMT
Chairman
ASTM Committee on EMS Training
Albany, New York

Christopher Jordan, MD
Clinical Professor
Department of Orthopaedic Surgery
University of Southern California School
    of Medicine
Los Angeles, California

Louis Jordan, PA
Emergency Training Associates
Union Bridge, Maryland

Richard L. Judd, PhD, EMSI
Vice President and Professor of Emergency
    Medical Services
Connecticut State University
New Britain, Connecticut

Mark A. Koenig, RN, BS
Fire Captain, EMS Program Coordinator
California Department of Forestry and
    Fire Protection
Ione, California

Denny Kurogi, NREMT-A
Director
Emergency Medical Science Program
Johnson County Community College
Overland Park, Kansas

Jeffrey T. Mitchell, PhD
Clinical Associate Professor
Emergency Health Services Department
University of Maryland
Catonsville, Maryland

John P. Mullen, MD
San Antonio, Texas

Paul L. Ogburn, Jr, MD
Director Maternal/Fetal Medicine
Head of Obstetrics
Associate Professor
Mayo Medical School
Rochester, Minnesota

Julia A. Rosekrans, MD
Asst. Professor Pediatrics
Mayo Medical School
Rochester, Minnesota

David Schottke, BS, BSN, MPH, REMT-B
Washington, DC

Tom Vines, EMT-D
Training Officer
Carbon County Sheriff's Search and Rescue
Red Lodge, Montana

William C. Wade, EMT-P, AS
Captain
Tampa Fire Department
Tampa, Florida

Richard Withington, MD
North County Orthopaedic Group
Watertown, New York

## TECHNICAL CONSULTATION

American Heart Association
American Lung Association
Anderson Ambulance Service
BCI International
Brimfield Township Fire Department
Center Laboratories
Dolton Fire Department
Downers Grove Fire Department
Dyna Med
Emergency Products and Research
Ericsson GE Mobile Communications, Inc.
Ferno-Washington, Inc.
SpaceLabs Medical
Franklin Park Fire Department
Gibbons/McClincy
Hinsdale Fire Department
Lemont Fire Department
Leon Valley Fire Department
MAB Enterprises, Inc.
Mayo Clinic
New Lenox Fire Department
Oak Lawn Fire Department
Physio-Control Corp.
Rollin Schnieder
Rosemont Department of Public Safety
San Antonio Fire Department
Sheridan Catheter Corp.
SKEDCO, Inc.
Texas Department of Health, Bureau
   of Emergency Management
Times Mirror International Publishers Ltd., UK
University of Texas at Galveston
WesTech

# CONTENTS

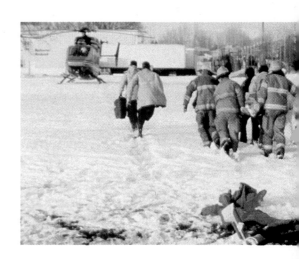

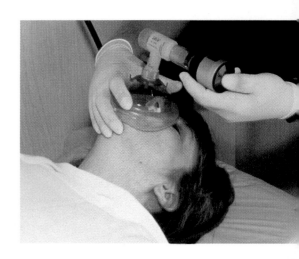

# SECTION 3 PATIENT ASSESSMENT 230

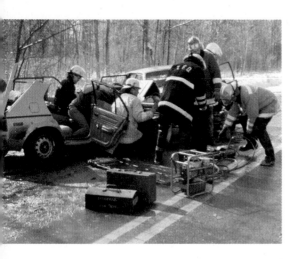

# SECTION 4 MEDICAL EMERGENCIES 304

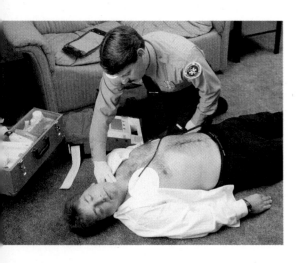

## SECTION 5 TRAUMA 460

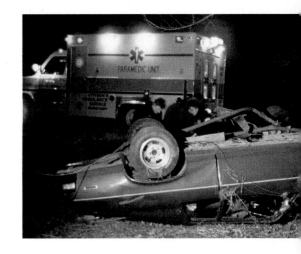

## SECTION 6 INFANTS AND CHILDREN 590

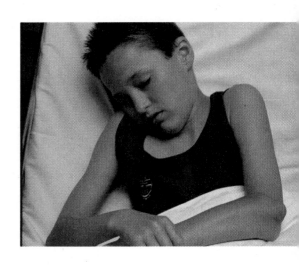

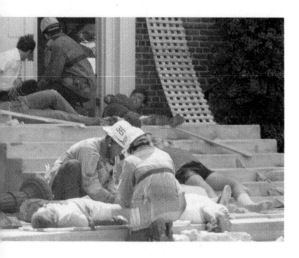
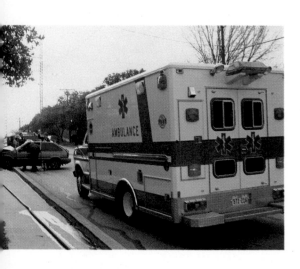

# Preface

In 1994, the U.S. Department of Transportation approved a new 110-hour curriculum for training Emergency Medical Technicians (EMTs). The new designation for EMTs trained in this 110-hour course is EMT-Basic.

The reason for this change is to redirect initial treatment of the sick and injured. The EMT-B learns to base treatment primarily on assessment findings rather than on specific diagnoses. This change has been difficult for some in the field to accept. The Editorial Board for the sixth edition of *Emergency Care and Transportation of the Sick and Injured* has also struggled through many meetings discussing the most optimal way to blend the best features of these two approaches to EMT training. As a result, this sixth edition follows the objectives and outline of EMT-Basic National Standard Curriculum, but also includes scenario-based and additional (FYI) information for further study.

We have also made a conscientious effort in this sixth edition to review and incorporate safeguards that are important to prehospital care providers when they are faced with potentially dangerous or harmful situations. With the nearly epidemic increase in infectious diseases, such as AIDS and hepatitis, and the alarming increase in violence over the past decade, prehospital care providers are now at greater risk than ever before. Thus, we have made sure that safety precautions, such as safety barriers, BSI techniques, and especially scene size-up, have been incorporated into the text so that students are constantly aware of the hazards of this profession.

The sixth edition of *Emergency Care and Transportation of the Sick and Injured* could not have been possible without the commitment of time and energy put forth by the Editorial Board, especially Dr. David Lewallen, Co-Editor-in-Chief. The many weekends away from our families and countless hours after working long days can only be explained by a sincere dedication to improve the care of the sick and injured. To these individuals I give my deepest and most sincere appreciation.

The publications staff of the American Academy of Orthopaedic Surgeons continues to do an outstanding job. Without these people, this project would have been impossible. Their dedication and professionalism are evident on each page of this text. Most of all, I would like to personally thank Lynne Roby Shindoll and Kathy Brouillette for managing all aspects of this project. They have helped the Board get through the highs and lows of this project for the past 2 years. I would also like to thank the Academy's Committee on Publications, specifically Dr. Michael H. McGuire, who had both the confidence and the insight to recommend me for this project. My background as an EMT was important in that selection.

Finally, I am most grateful to my family—Sheila, Shanna, Allison, and Ryan—for never complaining and continuing to give their love and support for the many hours I was away working on this textbook.

Lynn A. Crosby, MD
Omaha, Nebraska

# Foreword

Excellence in education has always been the primary function of the American Academy of Orthopaedic Surgeons, and nowhere is it more clearly expressed than in the field of prehospital care. In the 1960s practicing orthopaedists in many parts of this country sensed the need to enhance the education and training of ambulance drivers. This interest lead to the creation of courses on rescue and first aid techniques taught by orthopaedists and other experts using the educational resources of the Academy. From these courses evolved the first edition of this text in 1971. It was upon that edition that the first U.S. Department of Transportation (DOT) National Standard Curriculum for EMT education was designed. Subsequently, four new editions of "The Orange Book" in 1977, 1981, 1987, and 1991 continued to set the standard for excellence in prehospital care. More than a million of these texts and workbooks have been the foundation for innumerable basic EMT courses both in this country and around the world.

The most recent revision of the basic curriculum was completed last year by the National Highway Traffic and Safety Administration (NHTSA) of the U.S. DOT. This revision is yet another advance in this dynamic and ever-growing field. To continue to provide the best educational resource as a complement to the revised curriculum, the Editorial Board has created this sixth edition. This new work accurately reflects all of the additions and changes in the curriculum and retains the strong emphasis upon medical accuracy that has distinguished every previous edition.

Students will find this text easy to read, clear in its presentation, and certain in its content. It is the distillation of all relevant scientific inquiry in the field combined with, and indeed seasoned by, the tremendous wealth of clinical experience of the members of the Editorial Board—a combination not found in many textbooks. Literally hundreds of experts have contributed to the content of this text. The Academy is extremely appreciative of their efforts.

This textbook has always been special because of the work done on a voluntary basis by the members of the Editorial Board and this edition is no exception. Lead by co-chairmen Lynn Crosby, MD, of Omaha, Nebraska, and David Lewallen, MD, of Rochester, Minnesota, the members of the Editorial Board have given an uncountable number of hours of very hard work to this project. Without their dedication and perseverance, this outstanding work would never have been published. Each member of the Editorial Board, Ralph DiLibero, MD, Ronald Lindsey, MD, Daniel Hankins, MD, Joseph Stothert, MD, PhD, Paul Pepe, MD, Richard Vomacka, REMT-P, Karla Holmes, RN, Mike Smith, REMT-P, and Joseph Ferko III, PhD, is to be congratulated both on his or her individual contributions as well as the team's reliable and unswerving commitment to this most important project. To each one, the Academy says thanks for a job very well done. Just as was true with the previous editions, I am sure that, to all who have contributed, this sixth edition of *Emergency Care and Transportation of the Sick and Injured* will be a source of pride for many years to come.

James D. Heckman, MD
Chairman of the Council on Education

# SECTION 1

# Preparing to Be an EMT-B

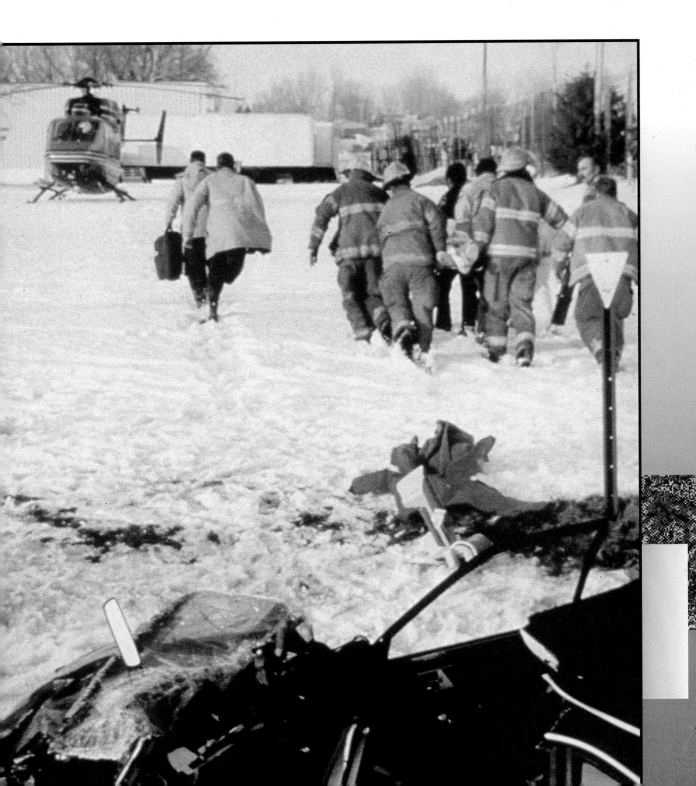

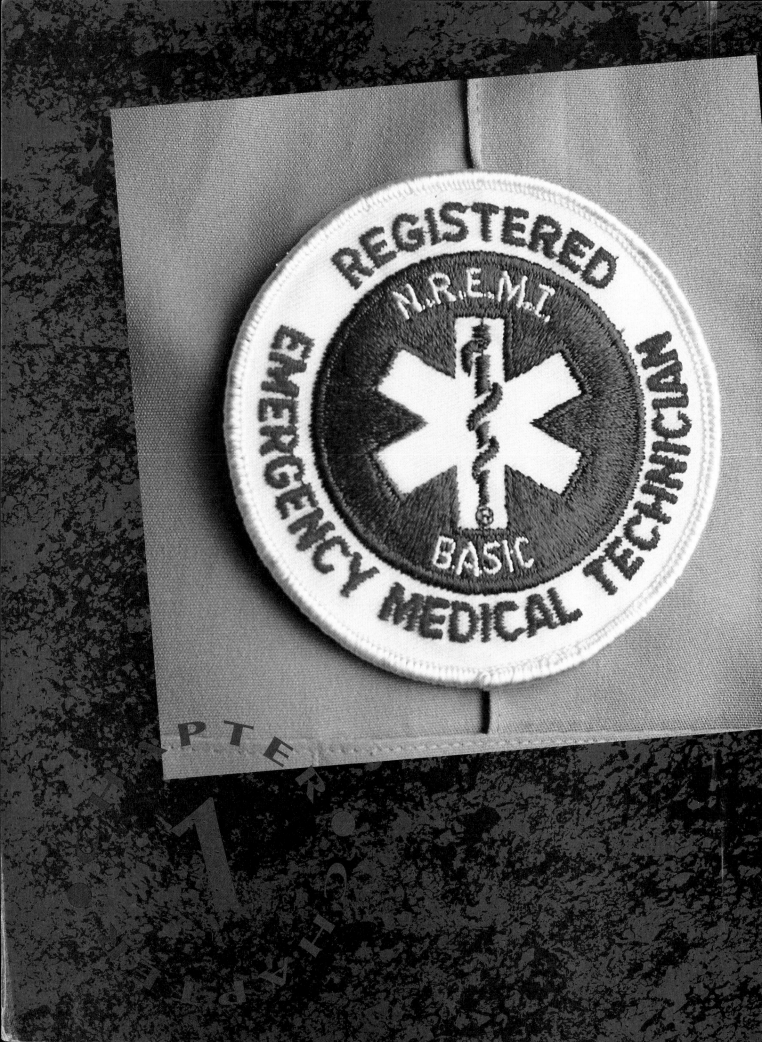

# CHAPTER 1

# Introduction to Emergency Medical Care

## Objectives

After you have read this chapter, you should be able to:

- Define the Emergency Medical Services (EMS) system.
- Differentiate the roles and responsibilities of the EMT-B from other prehospital care providers.
- Discuss the roles and responsibilities of the EMT-B related to personal safety and the safety of the crew, the patient, and bystanders.
- Define quality improvement and discuss the EMT-B's role in the process.
- Define medical direction and discuss the EMT-B's role in the process.

## Overview

Emergency care of the sick and injured was inadequate in many areas of the United States before the 1970s. Through a series of reforms in health care, systems of emergency medical services (EMS) were born. EMS systems are staffed by well-trained, professional emergency medical technicians (EMTs) and other health care professionals. This process continues today. This sixth edition of *Emergency Care and Transportation of the Sick and Injured* follows the 1994

EMT-Basic National Standard Curriculum. The text also conforms to the 1994 National Emergency Medical Services Education and Practice Blueprint.

As with earlier editions, this text provides step-by-step procedures in the actual assessment and care of patients. From the initial assessment through transport issues, this text also answers the "why" questions you may have about a variety of issues. Keep in mind that the goal of your training is to save lives and reduce suffering. To do so, you must learn the procedures and understand the explanations presented in your training. You must learn that incorrect procedures and lack of understanding can prove costly. It is possible to prolong recovery, make the patient's condition worse, or cause permanent injury. Finally, you will learn to combine effective interpersonal relationships with medical knowledge and practical skills.

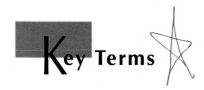

## Key Terms

**Americans with Disabilities Act (ADA)** Comprehensive legislation designed to protect disabled individuals against discrimination.

**Emergency medical services (EMS)** System that represents the combined efforts of several professionals and agencies to provide prehospital emergency care to the sick and injured.

**Emergency medical technician (EMT)** A member of the EMS system who is trained to provide prehospital medical care. EMTs are categorized into three levels of training: basic, intermediate, paramedic.

**First Responder** The first medically trained person to arrive at the scene of sudden illness or injury.

**Medical control** Physician instructions given directly by radio (on-line) or indirectly by protocol/guidelines (off-line) to EMTs in the field.

**Medical director** Physician who authorizes or delegates the authority to perform medical care in the field.

**Paramedic** An EMT who has completed an extensive course of training in ALS. Skills include IV therapy, advanced pharmacology, cardiac monitoring and defibrillation, and advanced airway management.

**Quality improvement** A system of internal and external reviews and audits of all aspects of an EMS system.

# COURSE DESCRIPTION

You have chosen an exciting field of study. You are about to enter the field of emergency medical services. **Emergency medical services** represents the combined efforts of several professionals and agencies to provide prehospital emergency care to the sick and injured. An **emergency medical technician (EMT)** is a member of the EMS system who is trained to provide prehospital medical care. EMTs are categorized into three levels of training: basic, intermediate, and paramedic. Everything that is taught in your class will be important when it comes to saving lives and easing human suffering. You have already completed a course in BLS skills. You are now ready to start your journey to becoming an EMT-B. This course combines theoretical information, practical skills, and common sense. To become an effective EMT-B, you must master the information and the skills. Equally important, though, is the combination of common sense, compassion, and understanding. As with all other skills, you must practice and be patient. The goal of the course is to become an effective EMT-B, not simply pass a test.

The U.S. Department of Transportation's (DOT) 1994 EMT-Basic National Standard Curriculum specifies that training must consist of 110 hours. Your state may require more than 110 hours. Ask your instructor about the requirements of your state. This text includes all the information that must be covered in those 110 hours, and more. The 1994 National EMS Education and Practice Blueprint requires that the EMT-B be taught basic fundamentals of hazardous materials rescue, emergency vehicle operations, and an introduction to infection control issues. *Emergency Care and Transportation of the Sick and Injured* includes these topics, along with a section on extrication essentials.

# TRAINING AND CERTIFICATION REQUIREMENTS

EMT-B training is divided into three main categories. The first and most important category is the care of life-threatening conditions. For such situations, you must know how to do the following:

- establish and maintain an open airway
- provide adequate pulmonary ventilation
- perform cardiopulmonary resuscitation (CPR)
- perform semiautomated external defibrillation (AED)
- control external bleeding
- treat signs and symptoms of shock (hypoperfusion)
- care for cases of poisoning

The second category of training covers conditions that are not life threatening. However, these conditions must be addressed before transport. To handle these situations, you will learn to do the following:

- dress and bandage wounds
- splint injured extremities
- deliver a baby and care for newborn and premature infants
- cope with the psychological stresses on patients, families, colleagues, and yourself

The third category covers important issues related to other aspects of care. You will develop the following skills:

- verbal and written communications
- defensive and emergency driving
- maintenance and use of supplies and equipment
- basic extrication techniques and equipment
- avoiding or coping with medicolegal and ethical problems

Check with your instructor about the requirements for becoming a certified EMT-B in your state. Generally, you must meet the following criteria for certification:

- provide proof of personal immunization as defined in each state
- successfully complete a course that follows the 1994 EMT-Basic National Standard Curriculum
- mentally and physically meet the criteria of safe and effective practice of job functions
- successfully complete a written certification examination
- successfully complete a practical certification examination
- comply with other state and local provisions

## THE AMERICANS WITH DISABILITIES ACT (ADA)

The **Americans with Disabilities Act (ADA)** of 1990 is the most comprehensive legislation in 30 years designed to protect individuals against discrimination. You must be familiar with the ADA, as its requirements affect both you and your patients. Your state EMS agency may have specific information on policies regarding the ADA and employment as an EMT-B.

There are five sections or "titles" of the ADA, as follows:

1. *Title I.* This section prohibits employment discrimination.

2. *Title II.* This section of the ADA affects EMS providers. It states that no one can be denied access to programs and services provided by state or local governments on the basis of his or her disability. As an EMT-B, you must provide equal care to a disabled patient. You must also provide "consistent communication" with a disabled patient. This means that you must make sure that a disabled patient understands his or her medical problem. EMS systems must also be designed to allow access to the disabled.

3. *Title III.* This section applies to businesses and providers of "services." It prohibits employers from failing to provide full and equal employment to the disabled.

4. *Title IV.* This section deals with communications and specifically addresses the responsibilities of telephone companies.

5. *Title V.* This section discusses how the ADA interacts with other laws, and it explains the implementation of the ADA.

Disabled patients may have special needs or problems. Patients who are hearing impaired may have trouble understanding your questions and instructions. Some may be able to read lips. These patients may be able to respond only with sign language or in writing. Patients with impaired vision should be able to talk with you. You must be sure to explain who you are, what is happening, and what you are doing. Most disabled patients are self-reliant, but when disoriented and confused, such as after an accident or when they are ill, they behave like any other patient. Such situations can be avoided by keeping them fully informed.

It is important that you understand the following concepts with regard to the disabled and your responsibility under the ADA:

- disabled patients must receive equal patient care
- disabled patients must have equal access to information about their medical problem(s)

# PROFESSIONAL ORGANIZATIONS

Several professional EMS organizations exist to promote quality care, education, licensure, and certification of EMT-Bs. Among the many professional organizations for EMTs are the following:

- National Council of State EMS Training Coordinators, Inc.
- National Registry of Emergency Medical Technicians
- International Society of Fire Service Instructors
- National Association of Emergency Medical Technicians

# OVERVIEW OF THE EMERGENCY MEDICAL SERVICES SYSTEM

## HISTORY OF EMS SYSTEMS

EMS as we know it today was born in 1966. The Committees on Trauma and Shock of the National Academy of Sciences/ National Research Council jointly published "Accidental Death and Disability: The Neglected Disease of Modern Society." This report revealed to both the public and Congress that prehospital care was seriously inadequate in many areas of the country. Congress mandated that two federal agencies address this issue: 1) The National Highway Traffic Safety Administration (NHTSA) of the Department of Transportation (DOT) through the Highway Safety Act of 1966, and 2) the Department of Health and Human Services (HHS) through the Emergency Medical Act of 1973. These agencies created funding sources to develop and improve systems of prehospital emergency care.

In the 1980s, the focus changed from establishing EMS systems to developing standardized EMT training programs. These programs combined classroom training with hands-on skill sessions. Training programs provided a way for EMTs to be certified, obtain advanced training, and obtain mandatory retraining. Despite these improvements, the demand for EMS was still greater than the supply of EMS providers in many areas of the country.

In the 1990s and in the future, EMTs will find new technology in their practice and rapidly developing systems of care. The responsibilities placed upon you as an EMT-B will continue to grow. Currently, most of the U.S. population is served by paramedics (EMT-Ps). However, modern technology has made it possible for you to perform many skills that were once reserved for paramedics. For example, the automated external defibrillator (AED) makes it possible for you to provide advanced lifesaving care.

## COMPONENTS OF EMS SYSTEMS

The EMS system is made up of various components that work together to provide patients with the best emergency care in the shortest time possible. Thus, access to the EMS system is important. Partners in the EMS systems include dispatchers, EMTs, hospital personnel, poison control centers, physicians, and allied health personnel. Administration is also an important part of the team, including NHTSA and your state and local EMS agencies. As an EMT-B, you will also work with local, state, and federal law enforcement and fire service officials.

## Administration

The way an EMS system works varies widely. Generally, it depends on your geographic area and the population you serve. Regardless of your area, NHTSA is available to evaluate EMS systems. NHTSA's Technical Assistance Program Assessment Standards evaluate EMS systems based on the following 10 criteria:

1. Regulation and policy

2. Resource management

3. Human resources and training

4. Transportation equipment and system

5. Medical and support facilities

6. Communications system

7. Public information and education

8. Medical direction

9. Trauma system and development

10. Evaluation

## Access to the EMS System

In many areas of the country, the EMS system is "activated" by calling 9-1-1. This number, or the local number for EMS, should be widely publicized in your community. It is very important that citizens, including the very young, know how to activate the EMS system in your community. The public should know how and when to request help through the EMS system in your community.

## Levels of Training

There are recognized differences among basic First Aid training, a DOT First Responder training course, and a DOT-approved EMT training course. Basic First Aid and the more advanced first responder training programs teach basic lifesaving measures.

**Basic First Aid**    Ideally, basic First Aid training should begin with children. EMTs should actively participate as instructors in these community training programs. First Aid training should be made available to as many citizens as possible. Individuals who need to know and use emergency medical techniques because of their jobs or recreational interests especially need training. First Aid and First Responder training programs should be under the direction of a physician and may be taught by other health care professionals.

**First Responder**    The First Responder plays an important role in the EMS system. The **First Responder** is the first medically trained person to arrive at the scene of sudden illness or injury before the ambulance. The care given by a First Responder is essential because it is given first. That first person could be a fire fighter, police officer, safety engineer, occupational health or school nurse, coach or trainer, lifeguard, youth leader, or one of many other professionals in public places.

A First Responder should call for additional help and then attempt to gain access to the patient, if possible. The First Responder should then provide necessary, lifesaving care, control external bleeding, comfort the patient, and await arrival of EMS. At times, the patient's position or the scene itself makes it impossible to provide lifesaving care. Only then should the First Responder attempt to move the patient before you arrive with appropriate equipment.

Just as it is essential for the First Responder to do enough for the patient, it is essential for the First Responder not to try to do too much. One of the most serious dangers to patients is improper removal from a vehicle or accident scene. Many other injuries, including permanent paralysis, have been caused by such well-intentioned, but potentially dangerous, actions.

First Responders should be trained using the DOT First Responder Curriculum. This training includes cardiopulmonary resuscitation (CPR). First Responders may have little or no equipment, and in reality, they need none to sustain life until an EMT-B or paramedic arrives on the scene. First Responders can assess the injury or illness, provide air to the lungs, blood to the brain, and control bleeding. In other words, they can provide BLS before the ambulance arrives.

**EMT-Basic** On arrival, you and your partner should assume responsibility for the patient immediately but tactfully. Assess the effectiveness of the care given by the First Responders. Then ask them to continue to help as needed. Give the First Responder credit for what was done. If you see improper care being given, do not criticize the skills or techniques of the First Responder at the scene. Remember that the training of First Responders is a vital link in the EMS chain. You should promote continuing education and evaluation for First Responders and other EMTs. It is possible that the next life the First Responder saves might be your own.

**EMT-Intermediate and EMT-Paramedic** There are two categories of prehospital care providers with advanced training: the EMT-intermediate (EMT-I) and the EMT-paramedic (EMT-P). Some states have established other levels of training between the EMT-B and the EMT-P. The EMT-intermediate (EMT-I) has training in specific aspects of advanced

life support (ALS), such as IV therapy and interpretation of cardiac rhythms. The **paramedic** (EMT-P) has completed an extensive course of training in ALS. Skills include IV therapy, advanced pharmacology, cardiac monitoring and defibrillation, advanced airway maintenance and intubation, and other advanced assessment and treatment skills. How you transfer patient care to other units, such as ALS providers and air medical, is a local responsibility. Your medical director will coordinate these responsibilities.

### The Health Care System

Many EMS systems use specialty centers such as trauma centers, burn centers, pediatric centers, and poison control centers. The way an EMS system functions and the specialty centers it uses can vary, depending on the geographic area and population served.

### Hospital Personnel

One of the best ways to understand how your care influences the extent of the patient's recovery is to watch hospital personnel continue care of the patient. As an observer, you will become familiar with hospital equipment and its use, the functions of staff members, and the policies and procedures in all emergency areas of the hospital. In addition, you will learn about advances in emergency care, as well as the use of new equipment. You will also learn how to interact with hospital personnel. This experience will emphasize the importance and benefits of proper prehospital care and efficient transportation. You will also see the consequences of delay, inadequate care, or poor judgment.

Physicians are rarely at the scene of an accident. They are rarely at the scene when a patient suddenly becomes ill. In most cases, a physician will not be present to give you personal, on-the-spot instructions. However, you may consult with a physician over the radio through established medical control procedures.

A physician may train you in the emergency department by showing you assessment and treatment techniques on actual patients. A physician may also act as an instructor for the medical subjects presented in

YOU ARE THE EMT

## IN THE CLASSROOM

You've just begun to attend class, and read this text, and are on your way to becoming an EMT-Basic (EMT-B). Many of the words, theories, and techniques relative to EMS are probably new to you. However, you must have a working understanding of the fundamental concepts of EMS. These fundamentals will help you to build the foundation on which you will develop your skills to provide quality patient care. Simply put, that is why EMS exists: to provide the best patient care possible.

To help develop your critical thinking skills, you will find special sections such as this one, called **You Are the EMT**, located in each chapter throughout the text. They will present brief scenarios, followed by a pair of **discussion questions.** These are not yes or no, or right or wrong, type questions. The discussion questions are designed to stimulate discussion. These will help you and your classmates to understand more about some of the **ambiguous, or gray, areas** of prehospital medicine. Talk about them with your classmates, your study group, or your instructor. This feature will help you to add depth to the material you are learning. It will help you to take cookbook medicine and make it work, because you will be a thinking cook!

### For Discussion

1. Explain the differences in the roles and responsibilities of an EMT-Basic, a First Responder, an EMT-Intermediate, and a paramedic.

2. List some of the potential problems that might be associated with an EMT-B having a "bad" attitude, or an EMT-B who displays unprofessional conduct.

your training program. With such instruction, you become more comfortable using medical terms. You will become better able to interpret signs and symptoms of injury and disease. You will also develop needed patient management skills. Face-to-face communication with physicians and other hospital personnel early in your training improves radio communication later.

Hospital staffs are usually eager and willing to help you improve your skills and efficiency, not only during initial training, but throughout your career. Some physicians and nurses may have completed the EMT curriculum as part of their formal medical education. A close rapport among all emergency care providers results in the best patient care. It also affords you and the hospital staff the opportunity to discuss your mutual problems, benefit from each other's experiences, and better fulfill your roles as members of the emergency medical care team.

### Public Safety Workers

Public safety workers, such as fire service personnel, are often cross trained in EMS. As an EMT-B, you must know the roles and responsibilities of all the agencies that will be interacting with you and your team. Cooperation among agencies is necessary to provide the best, most efficient patient care possible. Remember that personnel from certain agencies may be better prepared than you to perform certain tasks. For example, the power company is much better suited than you and your partner to control downed power lines. Similarly, law enforcement is better suited to handle violent scenes and traffic control. You and your partner are trained to provide emergency medical care. Working together, recognizing that each person has talent and a special job to do at the scene, will result in effective scene and patient management.

# ROLES AND RESPONSIBILITIES OF THE EMT

The cornerstone of the EMS system is the emergency medical technician. As an EMT-B, you have an extraordinary opportunity to relieve human suffering and provide life-saving care. As a valued member of the pre-hospital emergency medical care team, you must be responsible for all of the following:

- your own safety at the scene
- the safety of your partners, the patient, and bystanders at the scene
- thorough, accurate patient assessment
- prompt, efficient patient care based on assessment findings
- safe, efficient lifting and moving of patients
- safe, efficient transport and transfer of patient care
- record keeping and report writing
- the rights of the patient

*Remember that your first responsibility is your safety and the safety of others at the scene.*

## PROFESSIONAL APPEARANCE

You have to earn the respect and recognition of the community in which you live and work. You must be viewed as a responsible member of the emergency medical care team. As such, your attitude and behavior must be professional at all times. Your attitude and behavior must reflect a sincere dedication to serve humanity. Your moral and ethical standards must also be of the highest order. Aiming for excellence in job performance is very important.

However, you must also recognize your personal limitations and be able to accept and benefit from constructive criticism and advice.

As a professional, you must take pride in your personal appearance and hygiene, as well as in your technical knowledge and skills (Figure 1-1). A professional appearance and manner put the patient at ease. However, to keep your knowledge and skills up-to-date, you must actively seek continuing education.

## FIGURE 1-1

Maintain a professional appearance.

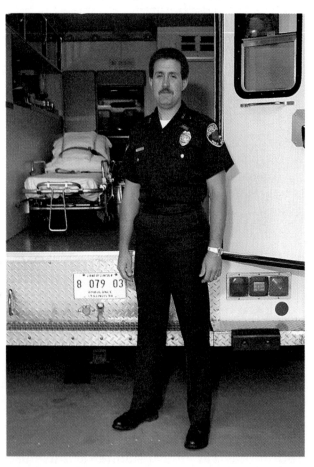

## CONTINUING EDUCATION

Procedures for licensing, certification, re-certification, and continuing education vary from state to state. The 1994 EMT-Basic National Standard Curriculum represents a step toward establishing a national educational standard. However, it is important for you to understand and conform to local requirements. EMT training is not a one-time effort. To maintain, update, and expand your knowledge and skills, you must continue to study. You are responsible for continuing education whether you are a member of a full-time paid ambulance service or a volunteer in a rural rescue squad. In fact, volunteers probably have a greater need for continuing education. There are not as many opportunities to refresh your knowledge and skills in actual patient situations if you are not working as a full-time EMT-B.

## PROFESSIONAL CONDUCT

As an EMT-B, you will be expected to perform under pressure with composure and self-confidence. You must control and suppress your emotions at the scene through self-discipline. Patients and families under stress need to be handled with understanding and sympathy. Dealing with death is an unfortunate, yet routine, part of your job. Remember that it is not routine for the deceased patient's family and friends. Therefore, you must not allow "sick humor" or any callousness to enter into your interactions. Your job is to ensure the health, survival, safety, comfort, and confidence of your team, your patients, and their families from the time you arrive on the scene until you transfer patient care to other medical professionals.

You will often see trauma. At times, you may be in the middle of extremely tense and sometimes dangerous situations. No matter what the situation, you have a moral obligation to provide the best emergency medical care possible to your patient. You are relieved of this responsibility only when an equally or more highly trained person at the scene or at the hospital takes over.

# QUALITY IMPROVEMENT

Medical care improves only when measures for quality control, or quality improvement, are included as part of an on-going evaluation of your EMS system. **Quality improvement** is a system of internal and external reviews and audits of all aspects of an EMS system. These reviews and audits identify where improvements may be needed.

Data collection is essential to the development of these reviews and audits. Data collection begins with you, the EMT-B. New technology makes documenting all aspects of an EMS event relatively easy. This data may then be used to review and audit the EMS system performance. It also provides records of skill performance and results of medical intervention. Unified data allows EMTs, paramedics, law enforcement and fire officials, and hospital personnel to speak the same language. This common language provides many opportunities for different people in the system to improve their own performance, as well as system performance. A system that collects data in an organized manner will permit medical research to be safely and effectively conducted. This, in turn, will improve the quality of care your EMS system can provide to your community.

# MEDICAL DIRECTION

The medical director plays an extremely important role in your EMS system. The **medical director** is a physician who authorizes or delegates the privilege to perform medical care in the field. As prehospital medical care is examined more closely, it is important for your medical director to actively supervise and support you and your team.

The medical director is responsible for coordinating and ensuring that appropriate, consistent care is provided. The medical director authorizes on-line and off-line medical direction, commonly called **medical control.** On-line medical control is delivered by a physician or a health care professional designated by the medical director. Medical control communicates orders directly to you in person, by radio, or by telephone. Off-line medical control is delivered by standing orders, protocols, or standard medical operating procedures (SMOPs). These orders are written down, authorized, and delegated in writing by the medical director. Thus, you can follow these standing orders in the absence of direct on-line medical control.

The medical director is also responsible for the following:

- ensuring appropriate EMT education and continuing training
- providing a system of quality improvement for the EMS system
- providing liaison with the medical community
- ensuring that appropriate standards are met by EMS personnel

The medical director is your primary medical support, because it is through his or her medical authority that you can provide

# SURVIVE Study Technique

Your EMT-B course includes a great deal of information and many, many skills to learn. You are responsible for a lot of information. To master this information and these skills, you must be able to study effectively. To help you successfully complete this course, you may want to use a study technique called **SURVIVE.** The purpose of SURVIVE is to help you retain more from your reading assignments and classroom activities. Take a few minutes to review this study technique.

### S - Skim
Read the chapter overview and objectives. Briefly **skim** the chapter. Look at all the headings, pictures, charts, and diagrams.

### U - Underline
**Underline** or highlight any words or medical terms that you do not recognize. Do not underline long sentences or passages. The purpose of underlining is to allow you to quickly locate key information.

### R - Read
**Read** the objectives at the beginning of the chapter again. Read the questions in your workbook and student review manual. This type of review directs reading toward the objectives listed at the beginning of each. Now, read the chapter.

### V - Verbalize
Answer the questions from the workbook and the student review manual

out loud **(verbalize).** This will help you to remember in two ways. First, it allows you to hear the written words. At the same time, it holds the answer in your brain long enough to transfer it to long-term memory.

### I - Integrate
**Integrate** the new material with information you have already learned. Using new material helps you understand it better. And, it is an excellent way to help you retain it in your memory.

### V - Vary
**Vary** your activity. Take a break from studying. Let the new information sink in. Stop frequently to review the material you have just covered.

### E - Evaluate
**Evaluate** the new material. Does it agree with information that you previously studied? Were all of your questions answered? If not, ask your instructor to clarify any questions you might have.

The SURVIVE format gives you a structure to sharpen your study skills. Remember that education never ends, even after you have successfully completed your EMT-B course and passed your exams. To be the best EMT-B you can, make sure your learning process never ends. Eagerly pursue continuing education as your schedule allows.

medical care. You are not licensed to practice medicine. You function under the license of the physician. The medical director coordinates your interactions with all levels of health care professionals. Medical problems, including possible liability and infectious disease exposures, need to be immediately brought to the attention of the medical director.

Most states have laws that require an EMS system providing BLS and/or ALS services to have a licensed physician as medical director. The state EMS law usually defines the duties and responsibilities of the medical director. The medical director is in a unique position because the director understands and supervises your day-to-day operations. All EMS systems should have a medical director who sets the standard of care. He or she should also act as a mentor and role model for you as you learn the practice of prehospital emergency medicine.

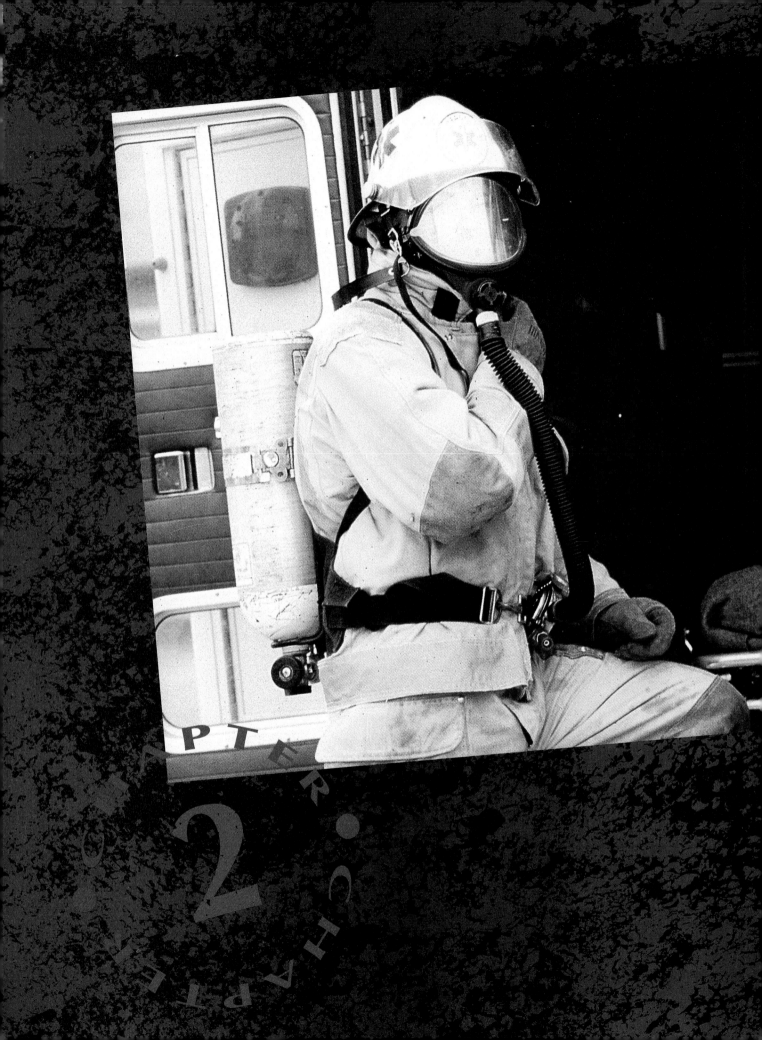

CHAPTER 2:

# The Well-Being
## of the EMT-B

## Objectives

After you have read this chapter, you should be able to:

- List possible reactions that the EMT-B may experience when faced with trauma, illness, death, and dying.
- Discuss the possible reactions that a family member may exhibit when confronted with death and dying.
- State the steps in the EMT-B's approach to the family confronted with death and dying.
- State the possible reactions that the family of the EMT-B may exhibit due to their outside involvement in EMS.
- Recognize the signs and symptoms of critical incident stress.
- State possible steps that the EMT-B may take to help reduce or alleviate stress.
- Explain the need to determine scene safety.
- Discuss the importance of body substance isolation (BSI), and the steps taken for personal protection from airborne and bloodborne pathogens.
- List the personal protective equipment necessary for each of the following situations:
  - Hazardous materials
  - Rescue operations
  - Violent scenes
  - Crime scenes
  - Exposure to bloodborne and airborne pathogens

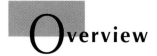

# Overview

The personal safety and well-being of all EMTs is vital to EMS operations. As a part of your training, you will begin to recognize and protect yourself from possible hazards. These hazards vary greatly, ranging from personal neglect to environmental and man-made threats to your safety. You will also learn about the mental and physical stress that you must cope with as a result of dealing with the sick and injured. Death and dying challenge you to deal with the realities of human weaknesses and the emotions of the survivors.

It is important that you remain calm and perform effectively when confronted with horrifying events, life-threatening illness, or injury. A special kind of self-control is needed to respond effectively to the suffering of others. This self-control is developed through the following:

- proper training
- on-going experience in dealing with all types of physical and mental distress
- a dedication to serve humanity

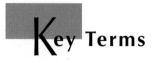

# Key Terms

**Body substance isolation (BSI)** An infection control concept and practice that assumes all body fluids as being potentially infectious.

**Burnout** A condition of chronic fatigue and frustration that results from mounting stress over time.

**Critical Incident Stress Debriefing (CISD)** A confidential group discussion of a highly traumatic incident that usually occurs within 24 to 72 hours of the incident.

**OSHA** Occupational Safety and Health Administration. Develops and publishes guidelines concerning safety in the workplace.

## EMOTIONAL ASPECTS OF EMERGENCY CARE

At times, even the most experienced care providers have difficulty overcoming personal reactions and proceeding without hesitation. Patients need to be removed from life-threatening situations. Life support measures need to be given to patients who are severely injured. You may also be called to recover remains from highway accidents, aircraft disasters, or explosions (Figure 2-1). In all of these situations, you must be calm and act responsibly as a member of the emergency medical care team. You must also realize that while your personal reactions must be kept under control, these are normal feelings. Every EMT-B who must deal with such situations has these feelings. This struggle for the need to remain calm in the face of horrible circumstances contributes to the emotional stress of your job.

## FIGURE 2-1

Scene of an airline crash with mass casualties

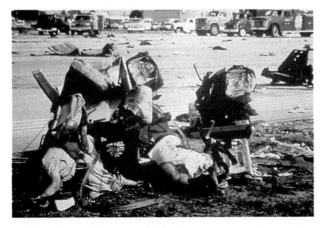

*Photo courtesy of Captain William Peterson, Woodbury County Sheriff's Department, Sioux City, Iowa*

## DEATH AND DYING

The death of a human being is one of the most difficult events for another human being to accept. And if the survivor is a relative or close friend of the deceased, it is even more difficult. Emotional responses to the losses of loved ones and friends are appropriate and should be expected. In fact, it is expected that you will feel emotional about the death of a patient. Feelings and emotions are part of the grieving process. All of us experience these feelings after a stressful situation that causes us personal pain. The grieving process has been described in the following five stages:

1. Denial
2. Anger
3. Bargaining
4. Depression
5. Acceptance

These same stages of grieving are experienced by a patient who is close to death. Even though the event (death) has not yet happened, the patient knows it will happen. The patient has no control over this process. The patient will die regardless of whether or not he is ready to die. You may encounter situations where the patient is close to death. You may have to help the patient with this process.

### Dealing with the Patient and Family Members

Many patients will be rational and cooperative. Their concerns will usually be relieved by your calm, efficient care. You should also explain what you are doing and why you are doing it. Often, you will realize that the patient's condition is not a true medical emergency. However, to the patient it might seem truly serious. Your actions and words, even a simple touch, can communicate caring. While you must treat all patients with respect and dignity, use special care with dying patients and their families. Be concerned with their privacy and their wishes. You must let the patient know that you take his or her concerns seriously. However, do not give patients and their families false hope. Be honest with patients and their families.

## STRESSFUL SITUATIONS

Many situations, such as automobile accidents involving serious trauma, abuse situations, amputations, and death, will be stressful for everyone involved. During these situations, you must exercise extreme care in both your words and your actions. Be careful about what you say at the scene. Words that do not seem important, or that are said jokingly, may hurt someone. Conversations at the scene must be professional. You should not say, "Everything will be all right," or "There is nothing to worry about." A person who is trapped in a wrecked car, hurting from head to foot, and worrying about a loved one, knows that all is not well. What will reassure the patient is that you are there to help. Briefly explain what you are going to do, that you are there to help, and that you need the patient's help too.

How a patient reacts to injury or illness may be influenced by certain personality traits. Some patients may become highly emotional over what may seem to be a minor problem. Others may show little or no emotion, even after a serious injury or illness. Many other factors influence how a patient reacts to the stress of an EMS incident. Among these factors are the following:

- socioeconomic background
- fear of medical personnel
- alcohol or substance abuse

- mental disorders
- reaction to medication
- nutritional status
- history of chronic disease
- feelings of guilt

You are not expected to always know why a patient is having an unusual emotional response. However, you can quickly and calmly assess the actions of the patient, family members, and bystanders. This assessment will help you to gain the confidence and cooperation of everyone at the scene. In addition, you should show courtesy, a professional tone of voice, along with sincere concern and efficient action. These simple considerations will go far to relieve worry, fear, and insecurity. Calm reassurance will inspire confidence and cooperation. Compassion is important, but you must be careful. Your professional judgment takes priority over compassion. For example, a screaming child with no obvious life-threatening injuries is covered with another patient's blood. This frightened child appeals to your compassion and thus gets your attention. In the meantime, an unconscious, nonbreathing adult nearby could die from lack of care.

Patients must be given the opportunity to express their fears and concerns. You can easily relieve many of these concerns at the scene. Usually, patients are concerned about the safety or well-being of others involved in the accident and for the damage or loss of personal property. Your responses must be discreet and diplomatic, giving reassurance when appropriate. In the event that a loved one is killed or critically injured, you should wait, if possible, until clergy or emergency department staff can give the patient the news. They can then provide the psychological support the patient may need.

Some patients, especially children and the elderly, may be terrified or feel rejected when separated from family members.

Other patients may not want family members to share their stress or see their injury or pain. It is usually best if parents go with their children, and relatives accompany confused elderly patients (Figure 2-2).

Religious customs or needs of the patient must also be respected. Many people have strong convictions against being given drugs, blood, and blood products. Some people will cling to religious medals or amulets, especially if an attempt is made to remove them. Others will express a strong desire for religious counsel, baptism, or last rites if death is near at the scene. You must try to accommodate these requests.

In the event of a death, you must handle the body with respect and dignity. It must be exposed as little as possible. Learn your local regulations about moving the body or changing its position, especially if you are at a possible crime scene. Even in these situations, CPR and appropriate treatment must be given unless there are obvious signs of death. These signs include rigor mortis, decapitation, or other massive injuries in which the patient obviously did not survive. More information on your responsibilities in these situations is presented in chapter 3, Medicolegal and Ethical Issues.

**Uncertain Situations**

There will be times when you are unsure whether a true medical emergency exists. If you are unsure, contact medical control about the need to transport. If you cannot reach medical control, it is always best to transport the patient. For both ethical and medicolegal reasons, a physician must examine all patients transported and judge the degree of medical need.

You must also realize that the most minor symptoms may be early signs of severe illness or injury. Symptoms of many illnesses can be similar to those of substance abuse, hysteria, or other conditions. You must accept the patient's complaints and provide appropriate care until you are able to transfer the care of the patient to a hospital or physician. Your local protocols will direct your actions in these uncertain situations.

## STRESS WARNING SIGNS AND THE WORK ENVIRONMENT

Supporting patients in emergency situations is difficult. It is stressful for them, but also for you. You are vulnerable to all the stresses that go with your profession. It is critical that you recognize the signs of stress, so that it does not interfere with your work or life away from work, including your family life. The signs and symptoms of chronic stress may not be obvious at first. They may be subtle and not present all the time. Be aware of the following warning signs of stress:

- irritability to co-workers, family, and friends
- inability to concentrate

## FIGURE 2-2

Parents should accompany children during transport

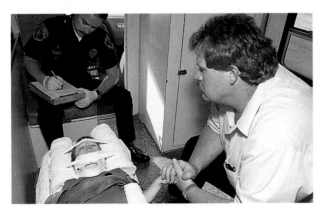

- difficulty sleeping and nightmares
- anxiety
- indecisiveness
- guilt
- loss of appetite
- loss of interest in sexual activities
- isolation
- loss of interest in work
- increased use of alcohol

The sections presented below provide some suggestions for you on how to better cope with stress. Some suggestions may be useful in helping you to prevent problems from developing. Others may simply try to help you to solve problems should they develop.

## LIFESTYLE CHANGES

Your well-being is of primary importance to effective EMS operations. The effectiveness and efficiency with which you do your job depends on your ability to stay in shape and to avoid the risk of personal injury. **Burnout** is a condition of chronic fatigue and frustration that results from mounting stress over time. To avoid burnout, you need to be in good physical and mental health. Be aware of the potential hazards in rescue and emergency medical care. You must also learn how to avoid or prevent personal injury or illness.

### Nutrition

To perform efficiently, you must eat nutritious food. Food is the fuel that makes the body run. The physical exertion and stress that are a part of your job require a high energy output. If you do not have a ready source of fuel, your performance may be less than satisfactory. This can be dangerous for you, your partner, and your patient.

Therefore, it is important for you to learn about and follow the rules of good nutrition.

Candy and soft drinks contain sugar. These foods are quickly absorbed and converted to fuel by the body. But simple sugars also stimulate the body's production of insulin, which reduces blood sugar levels. For some people, eating a lot of sugar can actually result in lower energy levels.

Complex carbohydrates rank next to simple sugars in their ability to produce energy. Complex carbohydrates such as pasta, rice, and vegetables, are among the safest, most reliable sources for long-term energy production. However, some carbohydrates take hours to be converted into usable body fuel.

Fats are also easily converted to energy, but eating too much fat can lead to obesity, cardiac disease, and other long-term health problems. The proteins in meat, fish, chicken, beans, and cheese take several hours to convert to energy.

Carry an individual supply of high-energy food to help you maintain your energy levels (Figure 2-3). Try eating several small meals throughout the day to keep your energy resources at constant high levels. Remember, however, that overeating may reduce your physical and mental performance. After a large meal, the blood needed for the digestive process is not available for other activities.

You must also make sure that you maintain an adequate fluid intake. Hydration is important for proper functioning. Fluids can be easily replenished by drinking any nonalcoholic, noncaffeinated fluid. Water is generally the best fluid available. It is absorbed by the body faster than any other fluid. Avoid fluids that contain high levels of sugar. These can actually slow the rate of fluid absorption by the body, and they can cause abdominal discomfort as well. One indication of adequate hydration is frequent urination. Infrequent urination or urine that has a deep yellow color indicates dehydration. Thus, keep your fluid intake at a level that maintains adequate hydration.

### Exercise

A regular program of exercise will enhance the benefits of maintaining good nutrition and adequate hydration. When you are in good physical condition, you can handle job stress more easily. A regular program of aerobic exercise will increase your strength and endurance.

### Balancing Work, Family, and Health

As an EMT-B, you will often be called to assist the sick and injured any time of the day or night. Unfortunately, there is no rhyme or reason to the timing of illness and injury. Volunteer EMT-Bs may often be called away from family or friends during social activities. Shift workers may be required to be apart from loved ones for long periods of time. You should never let the job interfere excessively with your own needs. Find a balance between work and family. You owe it to yourself and your family. Make sure that you have the time that you need to relax with family and friends.

When possible, rotate your schedule to give yourself time off. If your EMS system allows you to move from station to station, rotate to reduce or vary your call volume. Take vacations to provide for your good health, so that you will be able to respond the next time you are needed. If at any point you feel that the stress of work is more than you can handle, seek help. You may want to discuss your stress informally with your family or co-workers. Help from more experienced team members can be invaluable. You may also wish to get help from peer counselors or other professionals. Seeking this help does not make you "weak" in the eyes of others. Rather, it shows that you are in control of your life.

## FIGURE 2-3

Nutritious foods and fluids are essential to maintain performance

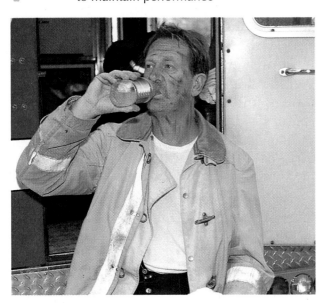

## CRITICAL INCIDENT STRESS DEBRIEFING (CISD)

You may be called to a situation so horrible that you find it difficult to respond as you were trained. You may have an immediate or delayed negative response to the incident. Do not be ashamed of such feelings, as almost all responders have had the same reaction at one time or another. If you feel overwhelmed, step back and call for help. Sometimes, simply knowing that help is on the way can help you overcome your fear or anxiety and enable you to respond to the situation. Remember that if you have these feelings from time to time, your partner and other members of the team may have them too. Keep an eye on other members of your team. See that they are under control and act appropriately during a major disaster.

After a stressful run or a disaster, there is often an emotional letdown. This "letdown" is often overlooked. However, it may be more important to deal with than the initial contact response. Critical Incident Stress Debriefing is a way to deal with this emotional letdown phase. **Critical Incident Stress Debriefing (CISD)** is a program in which severe stressful job-related incidents are discussed. These discussions are conducted in strict confidence with other emergency workers trained in CISD. The purpose of CISD is to relieve personal and group anxieties and stress. Never be ashamed to report your feelings, because such a debriefing can be vital to your emotional well-being. It should not be dismissed as trivial or nonessential.

CISD teams consist of peer counselors and mental health professionals who help you deal with critical incident stress. Usually, CISD meetings are held within 24 to 72 hours of a major incident. CISD meetings may also have to be repeated at a later time. A "critical incident" is any event which causes anxiety and mental stress to emergency workers. A CISD meeting is not an investigation or an interrogation. It is an opportunity to discuss your feelings, fears, and reactions to the event. All information discussed in the meeting should remain confidential. The CISD leaders and mental health professionals will help you by listening and then offering suggestions on how to overcome the stress. These meetings are helpful to all rescuers involved in an incident, regardless of whether or not they think they were "stressed." A CISD meeting provides a means to quickly vent feelings in a nonthreatening atmosphere.

A comprehensive Critical Incident Stress Management (CISM) system includes the following 10 components:

1. Preincident stress education
2. On-scene peer support
3. One-on-one support
4. Disaster support services
5. Defusings
6. CISD
7. Follow-up services
8. Spouse and family support
9. Community outreach programs
10. Other health and welfare programs, such as wellness

## SCENE SAFETY AND PERSONAL PROTECTION

The personal safety of all those involved in an emergency situation is very important. In fact, it is so important that the steps you take to preserve personal safety must become automatic. A second accident at the scene or an injury to you or your partner creates more problems, delays emergency medical care for patients, increases the burden on the other EMT-Bs, and may result in unnecessary death.

You should begin protecting yourself as soon as you are dispatched. Before you leave for the scene, begin preparing yourself both mentally and physically. Make sure you wear seat belts and shoulder harnesses en route to the scene. Wear seat belts and shoulder harnesses at all times, unless patient care makes it impossible. Many EMS units have mandatory seat belt policies for the driver at all times, for all EMT-Bs during transit to the scene, and for anyone riding with a patient.

Protecting yourself at the scene is also very important. A second accident may damage the ambulance and may result in additional injury to you, your partner, or the patient. The scene must be well marked (Figure 2-4). If law enforcement has not already done so, you should make sure that proper warning devices are placed at a sufficient distance from the scene. This will alert motorists coming from both directions that an accident has occurred. You should park the ambulance at a safe, yet convenient, distance from the scene. Before attempting to access patients trapped in vehicles, check the vehicle's stability. Then, take any necessary measures to secure it. Do not rock or push on a vehicle to see if it will move. This can overturn the vehicle or send it crashing into a ditch. A step-by-step explanation of gaining access is presented in chapter 28, Scene Techniques.

When working at night, you must have plenty of light. Poor lighting increases the risk of further injury to both you and the patient. It also results in poor emergency medical care. Proper lighting is included in the equipment requirements for ambulances. Reflective emblems or clothing help make you more visible at night and decrease your risk of injury (Figure 2-5).

## BODY SUBSTANCE ISOLATION

You should always follow body substance isolation techniques to protect yourself and your patient. **Body substance isolation (BSI)** is an infection control concept and practice designed to approach all body fluids as being potentially infectious. Modes of transmission include the following:

- blood splash
- surface contamination
- needle stick exposure
- oral contamination due to lack of or improper handwashing

### Handwashing

Handwashing is perhaps one of the simplest, yet most effective ways to control disease transmission. You should always wash your hands before and after contact with a patient, regardless of whether you wear

## FIGURE 2-4

Accident scene marked for safety

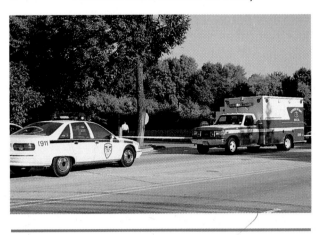

## FIGURE 2-5

Reflective emblems/strips improve safety in the dark

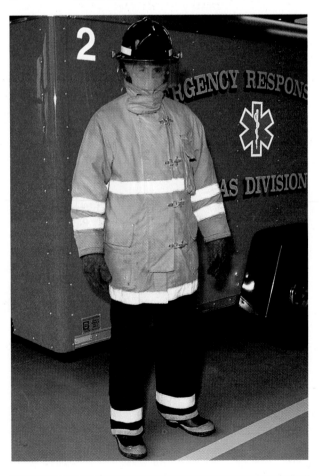

gloves. You should wash your hands before performing a procedure, after glove removal, and between patients. If there is no running water available, you may use waterless handwashing substitutes (Figure 2-6). If you use a waterless substitute in the field, make sure you wash your hands once you arrive at the hospital. The proper procedure for handwashing is as follows:

- use soap and water
- rub your hands together for at least 10 to 15 seconds to work up a lather
- rinse your hands and dry them with a paper towel
- use the paper towel to turn off the faucet

### Gloves and Eye Protection

Gloves and eye protection are the minimum standard for all patient care if there is any possibility for exposure to blood or body fluids. Both vinyl and latex gloves provide adequate protection. Your department may prefer one type of glove over the other, or you may choose yourself. You may wish to select a particular type of glove for

a particular patient care task. Wear double gloves if there is massive bleeding. You may also wear double gloves if you will be exposed to large volumes of other body fluids. Also, be sure to change gloves as you move from patient to patient. For cleaning and disinfecting the unit, you should use heavy-duty utility gloves (Figure 2-7). *You should never use lightweight latex or vinyl gloves for cleaning!*

Eye protection is important in the event blood splatters into your eye (Figure 2-8). If this is a possibility, wearing goggles is your best protection. However, you need not wear goggles if you wear prescription glasses. Prescription glasses are acceptable as eye protection, but you must add removable side shields when on duty.

### Mask and Cover Gowns

Occasionally, you may need to wear a mask and gown. A mask and gown provide protection from extensive blood splatter. As such, gowns may be worn in situations such as field delivery of a baby or major trauma. However, wearing a gown may not be practical in many situations. In fact, in

### FIGURE 2-6

Use of waterless handwashing solution in the unit

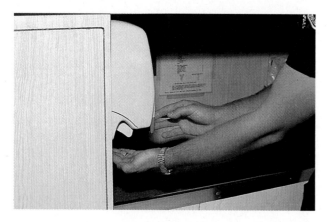

### FIGURE 2-7

Heavy-duty gloves are to be used to clean the unit

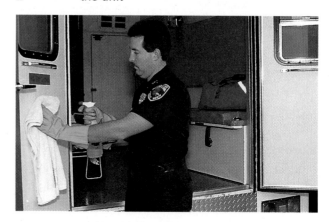

## FIGURE 2-8

Wearing protective eyewear prevents splatter of blood or other fluids

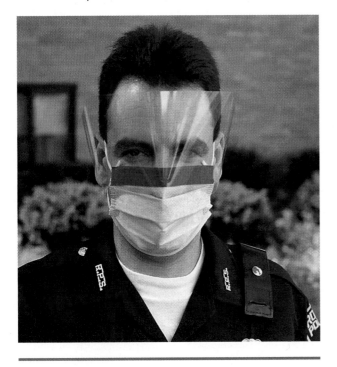

some instances a gown may pose a risk for injury. Your department will likely have a policy regarding gowns. Be sure you know your local policy.

The use of a mask is becoming a very complex issue in prehospital care. If blood splatter is a real possibility, you should wear a standard surgical mask. If you suspect that a patient has an airborne disease, you should place a surgical mask on the patient. If you suspect that the patient has tuberculosis, you should place a surgical mask on the patient. In addition, you should wear a High-Efficiency Particulate Air (HEPA) respirator (Figure 2-9). You should not place a HEPA respirator on a patient.

Remember that the outside surfaces of these items are considered contaminated after they have been exposed to the patient. You must make sure that gloves, masks, gowns, and all other items exposed to infectious processes or blood are properly disposed of according to local guidelines. OSHA requires

## FIGURE 2-9

HEPA respirators, disposable (right) and reusable (left)

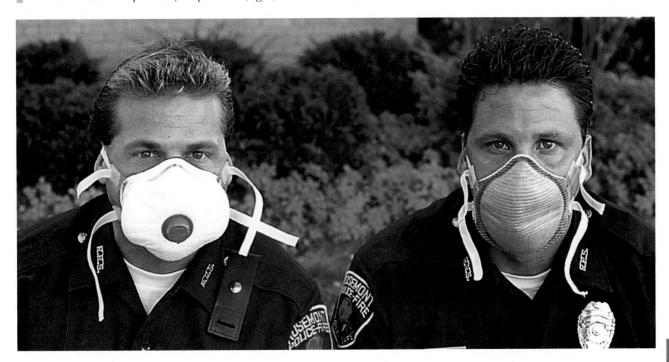

all EMT-Bs to be trained in the handling of bloodborne pathogens. **OSHA** is the Occupational Safety and Health Administration. This agency develops and publishes guidelines concerning safety in the workplace. In the event that you are stuck by a needle, get blood in your eye, or have any body fluid contact with the patient, immediately report this incident to your supervisor. Infection control is covered in detail in appendix B.

## HAZARDS

In the course of your career, you will be exposed to many hazards. Some situations will be dangerous. Some will be life threatening. In these cases, you must be properly protected, or you must avoid the hazard completely.

### Hazardous Materials

Your safety is the most important consideration at a hazardous materials incident. A more detailed introduction to hazardous materials is presented in chapter 28, Scene Techniques. Upon your arrival, you should first try to read labels and identification numbers. All hazardous materials should be marked with safety placards. However, this is not always the case. These placards are marked with multi-colored diamond-shaped labels (Figure 2-10). Although it is

## DEALING WITH DEATH

You are dispatched to a nearby address for an "unknown emergency." About 3 minutes later, you and your partner arrive at a small apartment complex. Law enforcement officers are already on the scene. They are trying to manage the six to eight neighbors and family members that are gathered outside the first floor apartment. One police officer tells you that the patient is in the bathroom. You enter to find a 23-year-old woman hanging in the shower. Even though there appears to be little chance of saving the patient, you and your partner cut the rope and lower the body to the bathroom floor. As you are attempting to perform an initial assessment, the patient's mother starts yelling at you and your partner, demanding to know why it took you so long to respond.

### For Discussion

1. Why do professional caregivers, such as those in EMS, often neglect to take care of themselves?

2. Maintaining control of the scene is an important part of your job. Is it appropriate to give that control back to family members? When?

YOU ARE THE EMT

## FIGURE 2-10

Hazardous materials placards

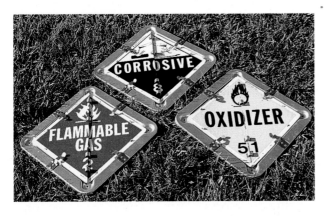

important for you to obtain information from the placards, you should never approach any object marked with a placard. A specially trained and equipped hazardous materials team will be called to handle disposal of materials and removal of patients. You should not begin caring for patients until either they have been moved away from the scene or the scene is safe for you to enter. However, it is useful for you to carry binoculars in the ambulance so that you can read the placards from a safe distance.

The DOT's *Hazardous Materials: The Emergency Response Book* is an important resource. It lists most hazardous materials and the proper procedures for scene control and emergency care of patients. Several similar resources are available. Some state and local government agencies may also have information about the hazardous materials in their areas. A copy of the *Response Book* and other information relevant to your area should be available in your unit or at the dispatch center. Thus, you should be able to begin proper emergency management as soon as the hazardous material is identified. Again, do not go into an area and risk exposure to yourself. Do not enter the area unless you are absolutely sure that no hazardous spill has occurred.

## TABLE 2-1 TOXICITY LEVELS OF HAZARDOUS MATERIALS

| Level | Health Hazard | Protection Needed |
|-------|---------------|-------------------|
| 0 | Little to no hazard | None |
| 1 | Slightly hazardous | SCBA only |
| 2 | Slightly hazardous | SCBA only |
| 3 | Extremely hazardous | Full protection, with no exposed skin |
| 4 | Minimal exposure causes death | Special HazMat gear |

If there is no HazMat team and you must enter the area, be sure you are wearing the proper protective equipment. Hazardous materials are classified according to toxicity levels and according to protection levels. Toxicity levels—0, 1, 2, 3, 4,—measure the risk the substance poses to an individual. The higher the number the greater toxicity and the greater protection needed (Table 2-1). It is important for you to remember that you are at great risk in hazardous materials situations. Do not enter the scene if a HazMat team is en route. If your area does not have such a team and you have to enter, make sure you are wearing the proper protective gear.

### Electricity

Electrical shock can be produced by man-made or natural sources. No matter what the source, you must evaluate the risk to you and to the patient before you begin patient care.

**Power Lines**   The amount of current involved greatly affects the level of risk for injury. Your local power company can help you by providing training to evaluate the risks in electrical emergencies. They can also teach you how to deal with power lines once the risks have been established. *You should NOT touch downed power lines.* Dealing with power lines is beyond the scope of EMT-B training. However, you should mark off a danger zone around the downed lines.

Energized or "live" power lines, especially high-voltage lines, behave in unpredictable ways. You need in-depth training to be able to handle the equipment used in an electrical emergency. The equipment also has specific storage needs and requires careful cleaning. Dirt or other contaminants can make this equipment useless or dangerous.

At the scene of an automobile accident, aboveground and below-grade power lines may become hazards. Disrupted overhead wires are usually a visible hazard. You must be careful even if you do not see sparks coming from the lines. Visible sparks are not always present in charged wires. The area around downed power lines is always a danger zone. This danger zone extends well beyond the immediate accident scene.

Use the utility poles as landmarks for establishing the perimeter of the danger zone (Figure 2-11). The danger zone must be a

**FIGURE 2-11**

Use of utility poles to mark perimeter of danger zone

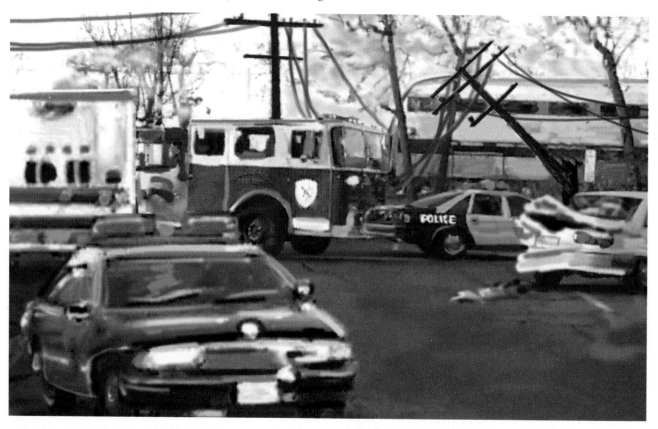

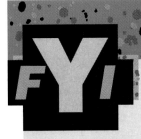

## Cold Weather Clothing

When dressing for cold weather, you should wear several layers of clothing. Many layers provide much better protection than a single thick cover. You have more flexibility to control your body temperature by adding or removing a layer. Cold weather protection should consist of at least three layers, as follows:

1. Wear a thin inner layer (sometimes called the transport layer) next to your skin. This layer pulls moisture away from your skin, keeping you dry and warm. Underwear made from polypropylene or polyester material works well.

2. Wear a thermal middle layer of bulkier material for insulation. Wool has been the material of choice for warmth, but newer materials, such as polyester pile, are also commonly used.

3. Wear an outer layer that will resist chilling winds and wet conditions, such as rain, sleet, or snow. The two top layers should have zippers to allow you to vent some body heat should you become too warm.

When choosing clothing to protect yourself from the weather, you should pay attention to the type of material used. Cotton should be avoided in cold, wet environments. Cotton tends to absorb moisture, causing chilling from wetness. For example, if you wear cotton trousers and walk through wet grass, the cotton soaks up the moisture from the grass. This will chill you in cold weather. However, cotton is appropriate in warm, dry weather because it absorbs moisture and pulls heat away from the body.

As an outer layer in cold weather, you might consider plastic-coated nylon, as it provides good waterproof protection. However, it can also hold in body heat and perspiration, which makes you wet both inside and out. Newer, less airtight materials allow perspiration and some heat to escape while the material retains its water resistance. Avoid flammable or meltable synthetic material anytime there is any possibility of fire.

restricted area. Only emergency personnel, equipment, and vehicles are allowed inside this area.

In these situations, you should always wear a helmet with chin strap and face shield. The shell of the helmet should be made of a certified electrical nonconductor. The chin strap should not stretch. In fact, it should fasten securely so that the helmet stays in place if you are knocked down or a power line hits your head. You should also be able to lock the face shield on the helmet. This will protect your face and eyes from power lines and flying sparks.

Turnout gear or a bunker jacket provides minimal protection from electrical shock.

## FIGURE 2-12

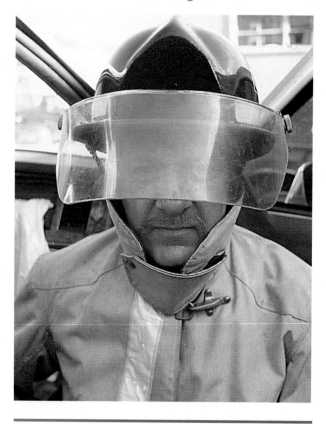

EMT wearing nonconductor helmet and bunker gear

But it does protect you from heat, fire, possible flashovers, and flying sparks. The front opening of the jacket should be fastened and the jacket worn with the collar up and closed in front to protect your neck and upper chest (Figure 2-12). Proper fit is important so you can move freely.

**Lightning**   Lightning is a complex natural phenomenon. You are unwise to think that "lightning never strikes in the same place twice." If the right conditions remain, a repeat strike in the same area can occur.

Lightning is a threat in two ways: 1) through a direct hit, and 2) through ground current. After the lightning bolt strikes, the current drains along the earth following the most conductive pathway.

To avoid being injured by a ground current, stay away from drainage ditches, moist areas, small depressions, and wet ropes. If you are involved in a rescue operation, you may need to delay it until the storm has passed. Recognize the warning signs just before a strike. As your surroundings become charged, you may feel a slight tingling sensation on your skin or your hair may even stand on end. In this situation, a strike may be imminent. Move immediately to the lowest possible area.

If you are caught in an open area, try to make yourself the smallest possible target for a direct hit or for ground current. To keep from being hit by the initial strike, stay away from projections from the ground such as a single tree. Drop all equipment, particularly metal objects, that project above your body. Avoid fences and other metal objects. These can transmit current from the initial strike over a long distance. Try to stand in a low crouch. This position exposes only your feet to the ground current. If you sit, both your feet and your buttocks are exposed. Place an object made of nonconductive material, such as a blanket, under your feet. Get inside a car or your unit, if possible, as vehicles will protect you from lightning.

## FIRE

You will often be called to the scene of a fire. Therefore, you should understand some basic information about fire, if you do not know it already. There are five common hazards in a fire, as follows:

1. Smoke
2. Oxygen deficiency
3. High ambient temperatures
4. Toxic gases
5. Building collapse

Smoke is made up of particles of tar and carbon. These particles irritate the respira-

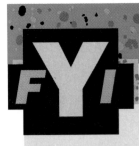

## More About Fire

As an EMT-B, your first priority is the treatment of your patients. However, you should never let this priority override your common sense. Use extreme caution in and around a burning building, or where a fire has just been put out. You can quickly become a victim of a fire. You need special training and equipment to deal with a fire. Fire fighters have this training. Always look to trained fire fighters when rescue decisions must be made at a fire.

Temperatures in a fire can exceed 1,500°F. Most combustible materials burn at temperatures ranging from 400 to 1,400°F. Remember, an uncontrolled fire can change rapidly. These changes can create several possible hazards, including flashover, backdraft, and building collapse.

A **flashover** occurs when all the flammable items in a fire suddenly burst into flame. A flashover is a violent reaction similar to an explosion. If you are exposed to a flashover without protective clothing and equipment, you will probably die. If you are wearing protective equipment when a flashover occurs, you are still at great risk for severe injuries or even death. Even the best fire-fighting clothing cannot withstand these very high temperatures.

When a fire is smoldering, this means that there is a lack of oxygen and that the fire is burning slowly. Without oxygen, burning is incomplete. When oxygen is added to a smoldering fire, the flames begin to rekindle. This creates the ideal conditions for a **backdraft.** In a backdraft, the fire produces gases. These gases mix with the additional oxygen and the result is an explosion. A backdraft may occur if any of the following signs are present:

- little, if any, fire seen outside of the building

- hot exterior doors and windows

- grayish-yellow puffs of smoke coming from the building

- air or smoke forcefully reentering the burning building

- sounds such as whistling or moaning coming from the burning building

The third hazard is the danger of a **building collapse** during and after a fire. There are usually no warning signs. You risk serious injury or even death in a building collapse. Once inside the building, you are in an unfriendly environment. It cannot be stressed heavily enough that a fire is a hazardous environment, where you can quickly become a victim. This is why you should always look to fire fighters to direct rescue decisions.

tory system on contact. Most smoke particles are trapped in the upper respiratory system, but many smaller particles enter the lungs. Some smoke particles not only irritate the airway but may be deadly. You must be trained in the use of appropriate airway protection, such as a self-contained breathing apparatus (SCBA) or a disposable short-term device, and have it available at all fire scenes.

Fire consumes oxygen. Particularly in a closed space, such as a room, fire may consume most of the available oxygen. This will make breathing difficult for anyone in that space. The high ambient temperatures in a fire can result in thermal burns and damage to the respiratory system. Breathing air that is heated above 120°F can damage the respiratory system.

There are a number of toxic gases in a typical building fire, including carbon monoxide and carbon dioxide. Carbon monoxide is a colorless, odorless gas that is responsible for more fire deaths each year than any other by-product of combustion. Carbon monoxide combines with the hemoglobin in your red blood cells about 200 times more rapidly than oxygen does. It blocks the ability of the hemoglobin to transport oxygen to your body tissues. Carbon dioxide is also a colorless, odorless gas. Exposure causes increased respirations, dizziness, and sweating. Breathing concentrations of carbon dioxide above 10% to 12% will result in death within a few minutes.

During and after a fire, there is always a possibility that all or part of the burned structure will collapse. Often, there are no warning signs. Therefore, you should never run into a burning building. Your hasty entry into a burning structure may result in serious injury and possibly death. Once inside the burning building, you are subject to an uncontrolled, hostile environment. Fires are not selective about their victims. You must be extremely cautious whenever

you are near a burning structure or one in which a fire has just been put out. Trained fire fighters will be at the scene. Follow their instructions at the scene of any fire.

Fuel and fuel systems of vehicles involved in accidents are also a hazard. Although vehicle fires rarely happen, any fuel may ignite under the right conditions. If you see or smell a known fuel leak, or if people are trapped in the vehicle, you must coordinate appropriate fire protection.

Make sure that you are properly protected if there is or has been a fire in the vehicle. Wear appropriate respiratory protection and thermal protection, as the smoke from a vehicle fire contains many toxic by-products. The use of full protective gear at an accident scene can reduce your risk of injury. Avoid using oxygen in or near a vehicle that is smoking, smoldering, or leaking fuel.

### Explosions

Scene safety should be your primary concern if you are at the scene where an explosion has occurred. If one explosion has occurred, chances are great that a second explosion may occur as well. Law enforcement and/or fire officials will determine whether the explosion was deliberately set. Therefore, do not enter the area until it has been cleared as safe.

## PROTECTIVE CLOTHING

Wearing protective clothing and other appropriate gear is critical to your personal safety. Become familiar with the protective equipment available to you. Then you will know what clothing and gear are needed for the job. You will also be able to adapt or change items as the situation and environment change. Remember that protective clothing and gear are safe only when they are in good condition. It is your responsibility to inspect your clothing and gear. Learn to recognize how wear and tear can make your equipment unsafe. Be sure to inspect equipment before you use it, even if you must do so at the scene.

Clothing worn for rescue must be appropriate for the activity and the environmental conditions in which the activity will take place. For example, bunker gear worn for fire fighting is usually too restrictive for working in a confined space. But in every situation involving blood and/or other body fluids, be sure to follow BSI techniques. Thus, you must protect yourself and the patient by wearing gloves and eye protection, along with increasingly more protective clothing as needed.

## TURNOUT GEAR

Turnout or bunker gear is a fire service term for protective clothing, designed for use in structural fire-fighting environments. Turnout gear provides head to toe protection. It uses different layers of fabric/material to provide protection from the heat of fire, to reduce trauma from impact or cuts, and to keep water away from the body. As with most protective clothing, turnout gear adds weight and reduces range of motion to some degree.

The exterior fabrics used provide increased protection from cuts and abrasions. They also act as a barrier to high external temperatures. In cold weather, an insulated thermal inner layer of material that helps retain body heat is recommended.

## GLOVES

You must wear latex or vinyl gloves any time you may be exposed to blood or other body fluids. In many EMS rescue operations you must also protect your hands

and wrists from injury. Fire-fighting gloves will provide the best protection from heat, cold, and cuts (Figure 2-13). Yet these gloves reduce manual dexterity. In addition, fire-fighting gloves will not protect you from electrical hazards. In rescue situations, you must be able to use your hands freely in order to operate rescue tools, provide patient care, and perform other duties. You may wear puncture-proof leather gloves, with latex gloves underneath. This combination will allow you free use of your hands with added protection from blood and body fluids. Remember that latex or vinyl gloves are considered medical waste and must be disposed of properly.

### FIGURE 2-13

Puncture-proof leather gloves

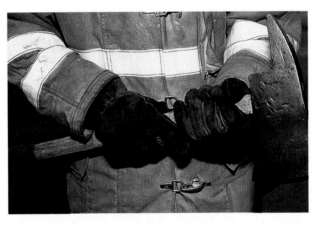

## HELMETS

You should wear a helmet any time you are working in a fall zone. A fall zone is an area where you are most likely to encounter falling objects. The helmet should provide top and side impact protection. It should also have a secure chin strap (Figure 2-14). Objects will often fall one after another. If the strap is not secure, the first falling object may knock off your hel-

**FIGURE 2-14**

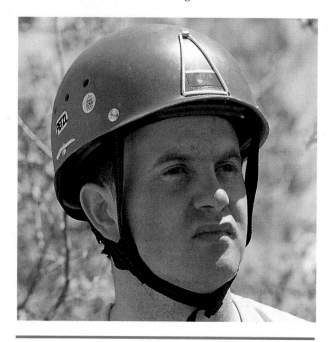

Helmet for working in a fall zone

met. This leaves your head unprotected as the remaining objects fall.

Construction-type helmets are not well suited for rescue situations. They offer minimal impact protection and have inadequate chin straps. Modern fire helmets offer impact protection. However, the projecting brim at the back of the neck may get in your way in a rescue situation. In cold weather, you can lose a good bit of body heat if you are not wearing a hat or helmet. An insulated hat made from wool or a synthetic material can be pulled down over the face and the base of the skull to reduce heat loss in extremely cold weather.

## BOOTS

Boots should protect your feet. They should be water resistant, fit well, and be flexible so you can walk long distances comfortably. If you will be working outdoors, you should choose boots that cover and protect your

ankles, keeping out stones, debris, and snow. In colder weather, your boots must also protect you from the cold. Leather is one of the best materials for boots. However, other materials, such as Gore-Tex water-repellent fabric, are also very good. The soles of your boots must provide traction. Lug-type soles may grip well in snow, but they become very slippery when caked with mud.

The fit of boots and shoes is extremely important, because a minor annoyance can develop into a disabling injury. You may develop painful blisters if your feet slip around inside your boots. However, make sure you have enough room to wiggle your toes.

Boots should be puncture resistant, protect the toes, and provide foot support. It may be difficult to obtain a good fit on firefighting boots, so shoe inserts or sock layering may be needed for a comfortable fit. Make sure the tops of your boots are sealed off to keep rain, snow, glass, or other materials from getting into your boots.

Socks will keep your feet warm and provide some cushioning for you as you walk. In cold weather, two pairs of socks are generally preferable to one thick pair. A thin sock next to the foot helps to wick perspiration away to a thicker, outer sock. This tends to keep your feet warmer, drier, and generally more comfortable. When you purchase new shoes or boots, keep these points in mind.

## EYE PROTECTION

The human eye is very fragile. Permanent loss of sight can occur from very minor injuries. You need to protect your eyes from blood and other body fluids, foreign objects, plants, insects, and debris from extrication. You may wear eyeglasses with side shields during routine patient care. However, when tools are being used during extrication, you must wear a face shield and goggles. In these instances, prescription eyeglasses do not provide adequate protection. In snow or white sand, particularly at higher altitudes, you must protect your eyes from ultraviolet (UV) exposure. This can be provided by specially designed glasses or goggles. In addition, your eye protection must be adaptable to the weather and the physical demands of the task. It is critical that you have clear vision at all times.

## EAR PROTECTION

Exposure to loud noises for long periods of time can cause permanent hearing loss. Certain equipment, such as helicopters, some extrication tools, and sirens produce high noise levels. Wearing soft foam industrial-type ear plugs usually provides adequate protection.

## SKIN PROTECTION

Your skin needs protection against sunburn while you are working outdoors. Long-term exposure to the sun increases the possibility of skin cancer. It might be considered simply an annoyance, but sunburn is a type of thermal burn. In reflective areas such as sand, water, and snow, your risk of sunburn is increased. Protect your skin by applying a sunscreen with a minimum rating of SPF 15. It may also be necessary to wear masks and gowns when treating certain patients. Wearing them will protect both you and the patient. Remember that masks and gowns are considered medical waste and must be disposed of properly.

# VIOLENT SITUATIONS

The safety of you and your team is of primary concern. Civil disturbances, domestic disputes, and crime scenes, especially involving gangs can create many hazards for EMS personnel. Large gatherings of hostile or potentially hostile people are also dangerous. Several agencies will respond to large civil disturbances. In these instances, it is important for you to know who is in command and will be issuing orders. However, you and your partner may be on your own when a group of people seems to grow larger and become increasingly hostile. In these cases, you should call law enforcement immediately, if they are not already at the scene. You may need to wait for law enforcement to arrive before you can treat the patient.

Remember that you and your partner must be protected from the dangers at the scene before you can provide patient care. Law enforcement must make sure the scene is safe before you and your partner enter.

In some areas, EMS personnel wear body armor (bulletproof vests) if a scene has the potential to turn violent. Several types of body armor are available. They range from extremely lightweight and flexible to heavy and bulky. The lighter vests do not stop large-caliber bullets. However, they offer more flexibility and are preferred by most law enforcement personnel. Lighter vests are commonly worn under a uniform shirt or jacket. The larger, heavier vests are worn on the outside of your uniform. Remember, your personal safety is of utmost importance. You must thoroughly understand the risks of each environment you enter.

Whenever you are in doubt about your safety, do not put yourself at risk. Never enter an unstable environment, such as a shooting, a brawl, a hostage situation, or a riot. Thus, as part of your scene size-up, evaluate the potential for violence. If it is a possibility, call for additional help. Failure to do so may put you and your partner at serious risk. Rely on the advice of law enforce-

## IS THE SCENE MEAN?

You are returning to quarters from a call, when you see a young man drive his bike into traffic and get hit by a car. He is thrown approximately 20' from the point of impact, and lands on his head. He is not wearing a helmet. Your partner gets out, and immediately evaluates the patient's responsiveness, opens the airway, and manually immobilizes the cervical spine, while you park the ambulance. The patient is unconscious, and unresponsive to any stimuli. There is extensive soft tissue damage, especially to the face, shoulders, and both arms. You see fluids coming from the nose and left ear. If that isn't enough, several bystanders are starting to get loud and verbal about the care that is being provided. A friend of the patient, who was riding with him, tells you that his friend has been abusing amphetamines for the last 6 months.

### For Discussion

1. What are the advantages and disadvantages of bystanders?

2. What are some of the concepts of universal precautions?

---

ment as they have more experience and expertise in handling these situations.

You may be called to provide care at a crime scene. If you believe that an event is a crime scene, remember to maintain the chain of evidence. This issue is discussed in detail in chapter 3, Medicolegal and Ethical Issues. Briefly, make sure you do not disturb the scene, unless it is absolutely necessary to care for the patient.

## IMMUNIZATIONS

As an EMT-B, you are at risk for acquiring an infectious or communicable disease. This

risk can be minimized by using basic protective measures. You are responsible for protecting yourself.

Prevention begins by maintaining your personal health. Regular annual health examinations should be required for all personnel. A history of all your childhood infectious diseases should be recorded and kept on file. Childhood infectious diseases include chickenpox, mumps, measles, and whooping cough. If you have not had one of these diseases, you must be immunized.

The Centers for Disease Control and Prevention (CDC) and OSHA have developed requirements for protection from bloodborne pathogens such as hepatitis B and human immunodeficiency viruses. An immunization program should be in place in your EMS system. Immunizations should be kept up to date and recorded in your file. Recommended immunizations include the following:

- tetanus-diphtheria boosters
- measles vaccine
- rubella (German measles) vaccine
- mumps vaccine
- influenza vaccine (yearly)
- hepatitis B vaccine

You should also have a skin test for tuberculosis (PPD) before you begin working as an EMT-B. The purpose of the test is to identify anyone who has been exposed to tuberculosis in the past. PPD testing should be repeated every year.

If you know that you will be transporting a patient with a communicable disease, you have a definite advantage. This is when your health record will be valuable. If you have already had the disease or been vaccinated, you are not at risk. However, you will not always know if a patient has a communicable disease. Thus, you should always follow BSI techniques if there is possible exposure to blood or other body fluids.

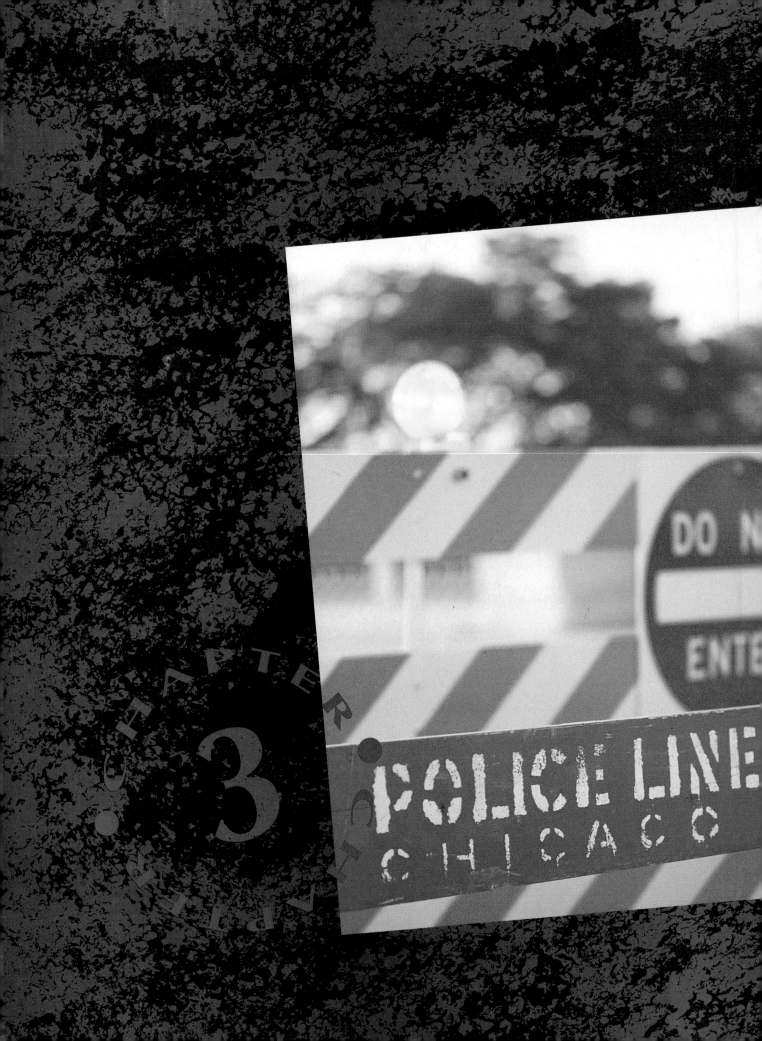

CHAPTER 3

# Medicolegal and
# Ethical Issues

## Objectives

After you have read this chapter, you should be able to:

- Define the EMT-B scope of practice.
- Discuss the importance of do not resuscitate (DNR) orders, advance directives, and local or state provisions regarding EMS application.
- Define consent and discuss the methods of obtaining consent.
- Differentiate between expressed and implied consent.
- Explain the role of consent of minors in providing care.
- Discuss the implications to the EMT-B in patient refusal of transport.
- Discuss the issues of abandonment, negligence, and battery, and their implications to the EMT-B.
- State the conditions necessary for the EMT-B to have a duty to act.
- Explain the importance, necessity, and legality of patient confidentiality.
- Discuss the considerations of the EMT-B in issues of organ retrieval.
- Differentiate the actions that an EMT-B should take to assist in the preservation of a crime scene.
- State the conditions that require an EMT-B to notify local law enforcement officials.

# Overview

Like other health care professionals, special legal requirements and responsibilities come with your special training. This chapter acts as an introduction to some of the basic legal terms and concepts you need to know as an EMT-B. The first section discusses your scope of practice and ethical responsibilities. The very important concepts of expressed consent and implied consent are explained in detail. Other important medicolegal concepts, such as negligence, abandonment, duty to act, and assault and battery are presented as well. The chapter concludes with a discussion of reporting requirements.

# Key Terms

**Abandonment**  Failure to continue treatment.

**Advance directive**  Written documentation that a competent patient uses to specify medical treatment should he or she become unable to make decisions. Also called a living will.

**Assault**  Unlawfully placing a patient in fear of bodily harm.

**Battery**  Touching a patient or providing emergency care without consent.

**Competent**  Able to make rational decisions about personal well-being.

**DNR orders**  Written documentation that gives medical personnel permission not to attempt resuscitation in the event of cardiac arrest.

**Expressed consent**  Type of consent in which a patient expressly authorizes you to provide care or transport.

**Implied consent**  Type of consent in which a patient who needs immediate emergency medical care to prevent death or permanent physical impairment is given treatment under the legal assumption that he or she would want treatment.

**Informed consent**  Permission to be treated given by a competent patient who has had the potential risks, benefits, and alternatives to treatment explained.

**Negligence**  Consists of four elements: duty, breach of that duty, physical or psychological injury, and cause.

## SCOPE OF PRACTICE

The care you provide to a patient is outlined in your scope of practice. This scope of practice is most commonly defined by state law. Your medical director develops protocols and standing orders to further define your scope of practice. Legally, your medical director authorizes or delegates to you the privilege to provide patient care. This is done through telephone or radio communication (on-line) or standing orders and protocols (off-line). Your director must also make sure that you and other EMS personnel provide proper, consistent patient care. You must report problems, such as possible liability, exposure to airborne or bloodborne pathogens or infectious disease, to the director immediately.

### ETHICAL RESPONSIBILITIES

In addition to legal duties, you also have certain ethical responsibilities to the public. You must meet your legal responsibilities, and at the same time, make the physical and emotional needs of the patient a priority. Patient needs vary depending on the situation. As such, you must practice and maintain your skills to the point of mastery. In other words, you must strive to be at your best at all times.

From time to time, you should review your performance. Assess your techniques, your response times, and patient outcomes. Think about ways you can improve your performance. Through hands-on experience and critical review, you can maintain and improve your skills. Another way to maintain your skills is by taking continuing education classes and refresher programs.

Another ethical responsibility is honest reporting. Absolute honesty in reporting is essential. You must provide a complete account of the events and the details of all patient care and professional duties. Accurate records are also important for quality improvement activities.

## ADVANCE DIRECTIVES

Occasionally you and your partner may respond to a call in which a patient is dying from some illness. When you arrive at the scene, you find that family members present do not want you to try to resuscitate the patient. Without written documentation from a physician, such as an advance directive or a do not resuscitate (DNR) order, this type of request places you in a very difficult position. An **advance directive** is a written document that specifies medical treatment for a competent patient should he or she become unable to make decisions. In this situation, a **competent** patient is able to make rational decisions about his or her well-being. An advance directive is also commonly called a living will. **DNR orders** give you permission *not* to attempt resuscitation in the event of cardiac arrest.

Unfortunately, you may be faced with this situation often, due to terminal nursing home placement, hospice, and home health programs. Your ambulance service, under the direction of your medical director and legal counsel, must develop a protocol for these situations. While specific guidelines vary from state to state, the following four statements may be considered general guidelines:

1. Patients have the right to refuse treatment, including resuscitative efforts, if they can communicate their wishes.

2. In a health care facility, a written physician's order is required for DNR orders to be valid.

3. You should periodically review state and local protocols and legislation regarding advance directives.

4. When in doubt, resuscitate.

In most states, EMT-Bs do not have the authority to pronounce a patient dead. If there is any chance that the patient is still alive or can be resuscitated, you must make every effort to save the patient—both at the scene and during transport. At times, death is obvious, such as in the following instances:

- rigor mortis, which is stiffening of the body after death

- dependent lividity, which is a discoloration of the body due to pooling of the blood

- decomposition of the body

- separation or obvious destruction of major body parts, such as the brain or heart

In these instances, there is no urgent reason to move the body. Your responsibility in this situation is to cover the body and prevent anyone or anything from disturbing it. Local rules and protocols from the medical examiner or coroner will outline your responsibilities in these situations.

Of all the situations you will encounter as an EMT-B, dealing with the deceased is one of the hardest. Family and friends, if at the scene, will be anxious and upset with the situation and possibly with you. Thus, how you handle the body and communicate with the family is of the utmost importance. Laws and guidelines for dealing with this situation will vary by state and by area. Your medical director, often along with legal counsel, will create standard procedures for dealing with the deceased. Make sure you know the guidelines specific to your area.

## CONSENT

As an EMT-B, you must understand the laws of consent. Consent is a long-established legal right. A person cannot be intentionally touched by another person without his or her permission or consent.

### EXPRESSED CONSENT

**Expressed consent** occurs when a patient expressly authorizes you to provide care or transport. Expressed consent may take the form of words, a nod of agreement, or other expression of approval or consent. You should try to obtain expressed consent whenever possible.

For expressed consent to be valid, the patient must be of legal age and able to make a rational decision to give consent. Verbal consent is valid and binding, although it may be difficult to prove.

### IMPLIED CONSENT

The law assumes that a patient who needs immediate emergency medical care to prevent death or permanent physical impairment would consent to care and transport to a medical facility. This is called **implied consent**. However, implied consent is limited to true emergency situations. This type of consent is appropriate when you find a patient unconscious, delusional, unresponsive due to drugs or alcohol, or otherwise physically incapable of giving expressed consent.

When a patient is unable to give expressed consent, but another responsible person or relative is present, you should try to obtain permission from that person. In most instances, the law allows the right of a spouse, close relative, or next of kin to give consent for injured persons who are unable to give consent themselves.

## MINORS AND CONSENT

The law recognizes that a minor may not have the wisdom, maturity, or judgment to give valid consent. Therefore, parents or individuals who are close to the minor much like parents must give consent. Despite this rule, in some cases a minor can give valid consent, depending on the minor's age and maturity. For example, a 17-year-old girl is more likely to give valid consent than a 4-year-old child. Many states have laws that permit minors to give binding consent to receive medical care. Many states also allow emancipated, married, or pregnant minors to be treated as adults for the purposes of consenting to medical treatment.

The laws and principles related to consent of minors merely determine who has the right to give consent—not whether consent is needed. If a true emergency exists, the consent to treat the minor is implied, just as with an adult. However, you should obtain parents' consent, if possible.

### CONSENT OF THE MENTALLY INCOMPETENT

An adult patient who is mentally incompetent is not capable of giving informed consent. **Informed consent** is permission to be treated given by a competent patient who has had the potential risks, benefits, and alternatives to treatment explained. If a patient has been declared legally incompetent, another individual, such as a guardian or conservator, usually has the right to give consent on behalf of the patient.

In many situations, you will care for patients who may appear confused or in mental distress. You should consider these factors in deciding whether the patient can give valid consent. When a true emergency situation exists, you can assume implied consent applies.

## ASSAULT AND BATTERY

Serious legal problems may arise in situations where a patient has not given consent for treatment. **Assault** is unlawfully placing a patient in fear of bodily harm. Touching a patient or providing emergency care without consent is called **battery**. If you do so, the patient may have grounds to sue you for assault, battery, or both. To protect yourself from these charges, make sure that you obtain expressed consent or that the situation allows for implied consent. Consult your medical director if you have questions or doubt about a specific situation.

## THE RIGHT TO REFUSE TREATMENT

Mentally competent adults have the right to refuse treatment or withdraw from treatment at any time. However, these patients present you with a dilemma. Should you provide care against their will and risk being accused of battery? Do you leave them alone? If you do, you risk the possibility that their condition becomes worse, in which case you can be accused of negligence or abandonment.

If a patient refuses treatment or transport, you must make sure that he or she understands, or is informed about, the potential risks, benefits, treatments and alternatives to treatment. The patient must also be fully informed about the consequences of refusing treatment and be encouraged to ask questions. Remember that competent adults who refuse specific kinds of treatment for religious reasons generally have a legal right to do so.

When a patient refuses treatment, you must assess whether the patient's mental condition is impaired. Thus, if the patient refusing treatment is delusional or confused, you cannot assume that the refusal is an informed refusal. When in doubt, it is always best to proceed with treatment. This is the best course of action because providing treatment is a much more defensible position than failing to treat a patient. Failure to treat a patient is considered abandonment, which is discussed in the next section.

You may also be faced with a situation in which a parent refuses to permit treatment of an ill or injured child. In this situa-tion, you must consider the emotional impact of the emergency on the parent's judgment. In this, and virtually all cases of refusal, you can usually resolve the situa-tion with patience and calm persuasion. You may also need the help of others, such as law enforcement.

There will be times when you are not able to persuade the patient, guardian, con-servator, or parent of a minor or mentally incompetent patient to proceed with treat-ment. If this is the case, you must obtain their signature on an official release form

## OFF TO LEGAL LAND

You no sooner sit down for a quick lunch when your pager goes off. It's back out to the ambulance. Dispatch informs you of a request for EMS for a "woman down" at a home in the country. About 8 minutes later, you pull up in front of a small farm house. A couple of loud knocks on the door produce no response. You try again, but still no reply, so you decide to see if the door is open. It is, so you enter and shout, "Anybody home?" In the middle of the floor you see an elderly woman. Her bluish appearance immediately suggests cardiac arrest. Just as your partner is bending over to assess her level of consciousness and to open her airway, a voice booms out, "If you touch my mom, I'll kill you."

Obviously startled, you and your partner turn quickly to see a virtual mountain of a man sitting in a chair behind you. He also tells you he thinks his mom has a living will, but he has not ever seen it.

### For Discussion

1. In this case, you and your partner believe that the son might make good on his threat. You have him sign a patient refusal and leave the scene. What are some of the legal, personal, and moral issues in this situation?

2. Describe the difference in implied and expressed consent.

that acknowledges refusal. You must also obtain a signature from a witness to the refusal. You should then keep the refusal with the run report and the medical incident report. In addition to the release form itself, you should write a note about the refusal on the medical incident report and the run report as well. If the patient refuses to sign the release form, the best you can do is inform medical control and thoroughly document the situation and the refusal. Make sure your department keeps a copy of the record for future reference.

## ABANDONMENT

Once you begin to provide care, you must follow through with all necessary and appropriate treatment. You must continue to provide care until responsibility for patient care is transferred to another medical professional of an appropriate level of training, or until the patient is transferred to a medical facility. This is to be a person of equal or higher level of skill. Failure to continue the treatment is known as **abandonment**. Abandonment is legally and ethically the most serious act you can commit.

## NEGLIGENCE

**Negligence** consists of four elements: duty, breach of that duty, physical or psychological injury, and cause. Once you have been called to the scene to provide care, you have a *duty* to act to help the patient. Your failure to do so, or to give care in a manner that is not consistent with the level of care that other similarly trained EMT-Bs would give, is a *breach of duty*. If *physical or*

*psychological harm* is *caused* by doing something or failure to do something to the patient, then you have acted in a negligent manner. If this is the case, you may be liable to the patient for the harm you have caused. All four elements must be present for the legal doctrine of negligence to apply.

Examples of negligence include the following:

- failure to provide care to a patient once you have arrived at the scene

- failure to perform important or necessary techniques

- providing care in a manner not consistent with the skill that other similarly trained EMT-Bs would give under similar circumstances

If your actions are judged to be the same or similar as another EMT-B would or might respond, you would not be negligent. However, if your actions or performance was judged reckless, careless, or lacking in skill, you would have violated the standard of care. In this instance, you might be found negligent. As a result, you may be held responsible for making the patient's condition worse due to your performance.

## DUTY TO ACT

Once a unit responds to a call, it has a duty to act. In some situations, there may be no legal duty for an ambulance to respond, such as if it is off duty or the call is out of its jurisdiction. If you are off duty and happen upon the scene of an accident, you are not legally obligated to stop and assist the victims. However, if you come upon an accident, you have a moral and ethical duty to act due to your special training and expertise.

# CONFIDENTIALITY

Communication between you and the patient is considered confidential. Examples of confidential information include the patient history, assessment findings, and the treatment you give. Generally, this information cannot be disclosed without permission from the patient or a court order. You cannot disclose information regarding a patient's diagnosis, treatment, or mental or physical condition. If you disclose this information without consent, you may find yourself liable for a breach of confidentiality.

In certain situations you may release confidential information to designated individuals. In most states, records may be released when a legal subpoena is presented. You may also obtain a written release signed by the patient. However, the patient must be mentally competent and must fully understand the nature of the release. A third legal means for disclosing information is with an automatic release. This type of release does not require a written form. It allows you to share information with other health care providers so that they may continue the patient's care. In many states, you do not need a written release to report information about cases of rape or abuse to the proper authorities. Third party payment billing forms may also be completed without written consent.

# SPECIAL SITUATIONS

## ORGAN DONORS

Although it rarely happens, you may be called to a scene involving a potential organ donor. If this is the case, you should inform medical control immediately. An individual who has expressed his or her wishes to donate organs is a potential organ donor. Consent to organ donation must be voluntary and knowing. This consent is evidenced by either a donor card or a driver's license that indicates the individual's desire to be a donor.

Once a patient has been identified as a potential donor, you must treat him or her in the same way as you would any other patient who needs treatment. The mere fact that a patient is a possible donor does not mean that you should not use all means necessary to keep him or her alive. Patients will often donate organs such as a kidney, heart, or liver that require oxygen at all times. Thus, the possible donor must be given oxygen, or the organs would be damaged and would become useless. Remember, even in this situation, your priority is saving the patient's life. However, if it seems that saving the patient is not possible, you should still provide the necessary care to make sure the organs remain viable. This generally means providing adequate ventilation as needed until arrival at the hospital.

You may encounter potential organ donor situations at a multiple-casualty incident. Remember the potential organ donor should be triaged with other patients and assigned a category. In some cases, potential organ donors may be a lower priority than less severely injured patients.

The guidelines given above are general. Your area may have a specific protocol regarding these situations.

## MEDICAL IDENTIFICATION INSIGNIA

Many patients will carry important medical identification and information that can help you. This identification is often in the form of a bracelet, necklace, or may be a separate card found in the patient's pocket or in a

# CONSTRUCTION CRUNCH

A bricklayer slips and falls from a two-story scaffold, and the foreman calls 9-1-1. He meets you at the front gate of the construction project and leads you to where the man has fallen. You find a 28-year-old man who has severe pain in his left leg. He is alert and oriented, denies any loss of consciousness, and can remember the entire accident. His vital signs are stable. In spite of the potential seriousness of the fall, other than some minor abrasions, he appears only to have broken his left leg. As you are applying the traction splint, your partner, who was applying manual traction, inadvertently drops the patient's leg. The patient screams. A bone end is now visible where it has protruded through the skin.

## For Discussion

1. When is it appropriate to discuss the specific details of an emergency call?

2. What are some of the things that you can do to defend yourself should you be sued?

---

wallet. The information identifies whether the patient has allergies, diabetes, epilepsy, or some other serious medical condition. This information could change the way you treat the patient. Failure to take this information into account could result in harm to the patient.

## POTENTIAL CRIME SCENE

If you suspect that a crime may have been committed at the scene, you must notify the dispatcher so that law enforcement can be informed. Dispatch may also inform you that you are en route to a potential crime scene. The possibility that a crime has been committed should not affect your care of the patient. However, you must consider the following two questions:

1. Is the scene safe to enter, or is a crime still in progress?

2. Is there evidence that must be preserved?

Thus, as you provide care, make sure you do not disturb the scene any more than absolutely necessary. Observe and document anything unusual at the scene. If possible, do not cut through holes in clothes from weapons or gunshot wounds. You should make drawings and record the patient's position. You should also note the presence and position of any weapon or other objects that may be valuable to law enforcement. However, remember that patient care is your priority at the scene. Thus, you should discuss with local authorities exactly what you and your partner can do to be helpful to them at the scene of a possible crime. It is best if these guidelines can be established by protocol.

## RECORDS AND REPORTS

Most states require you to complete a written report of all incidents. Specific reporting requirements vary from state to state. However, a complete, accurate record is one of your most important safeguards against legal problems. The absence of a written record, or an incomplete record, may mean serious problems for you should you need to go to court. Should you have to testify in court, you will have to rely on memory alone. Relying on your memory can be inadequate and embarrassing.

The courts consider the following two rules of thumb regarding reports:

1. In a court of law, if it wasn't documented, it wasn't done.

2. An incomplete or untidy report is evidence of incomplete or inexpert medical care.

You can avoid these potential problems by completing and maintaining accurate reports and records of all events and patients. Specific information about writing reports and correcting errors is presented in chapter 13, Communications and Documentation.

### ABUSE OF CHILDREN, ELDERLY, AND OTHERS

All states have laws that protect abused children. Some states have extended protection to the elderly, mentally incompetent, and spouses who may be at special risk for physical or sexual abuse. Most states require certain individuals to report abuse situations. These individuals may range from a physician to "any citizen." Learn the requirements of the law in your state and local protocols.

These laws often grant immunity from liability for libel, slander, or defamation of character to the individual who makes the report, if the report is made in good faith. This is especially true when the report is made as part of a person's professional responsibilities, such as your patient care report.

### INJURY DURING THE COMMISSION OF A FELONY

Many states require EMS personnel to report injuries likely to have occurred as a result of a crime or sexual assault. Specific injuries such as gunshot or knife wounds and poisonings are often included in these requirements. Again, you must know the requirements of your state. In some instances, drug-related injuries must be reported. The U.S. Supreme Court has ruled that drug addiction, as opposed to drug possession or sale, is an illness, not a crime. Therefore, an injury as a result of a drug overdose may not be within the definition of an injury resulting from a crime.

### CHILDBIRTH

Many states require that anyone in attendance at a live birth in any place other than a licensed medical facility report the birth.

As before, you must be familiar with the laws in your state and local protocols.

## OTHER REPORTING REQUIREMENTS

Other special reporting requirements may include attempted suicides, dog bites, certain communicable diseases, assaults, rapes, or sexual assaults. These situations are discussed in detail in their appropriate chapters. Most EMS agencies require that all exposures to infectious disease be reported. In some instances, you may be asked to transport patients in restraints. You must report these instances as well. Each of these situations can present significant legal problems. Learn your local protocols regarding these situations.

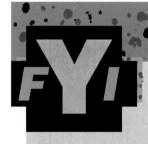

## Good Samaritan Laws and Immunity

Good Samaritan laws are designed to protect individuals who voluntarily give emergency medical care in good faith to accident victims or persons who are suddenly ill. Someone who voluntarily helps an injured or suddenly ill person is not legally liable for errors or omissions in giving good faith emergency care. However, Good Samaritan laws do not provide immunity for gross negligence or willful misconduct that results in further injury.

Another group of laws, which vary from state to state, grants immunity from liability to official emergency medical care providers, such as EMT-Bs. As with Good Samaritan laws, these state laws do not provide immunity when injury or damage is caused by gross negligence or willful misconduct.

Most states have also adopted specific laws that grant special privileges to EMS personnel. These laws most often authorize EMS personnel to perform certain medical procedures. Many also grant a partial immunity to EMTs and the physicians and nurses who give emergency instructions to EMS personnel via radio or other forms of communication. Consult your medical director for more information about the laws in your area.

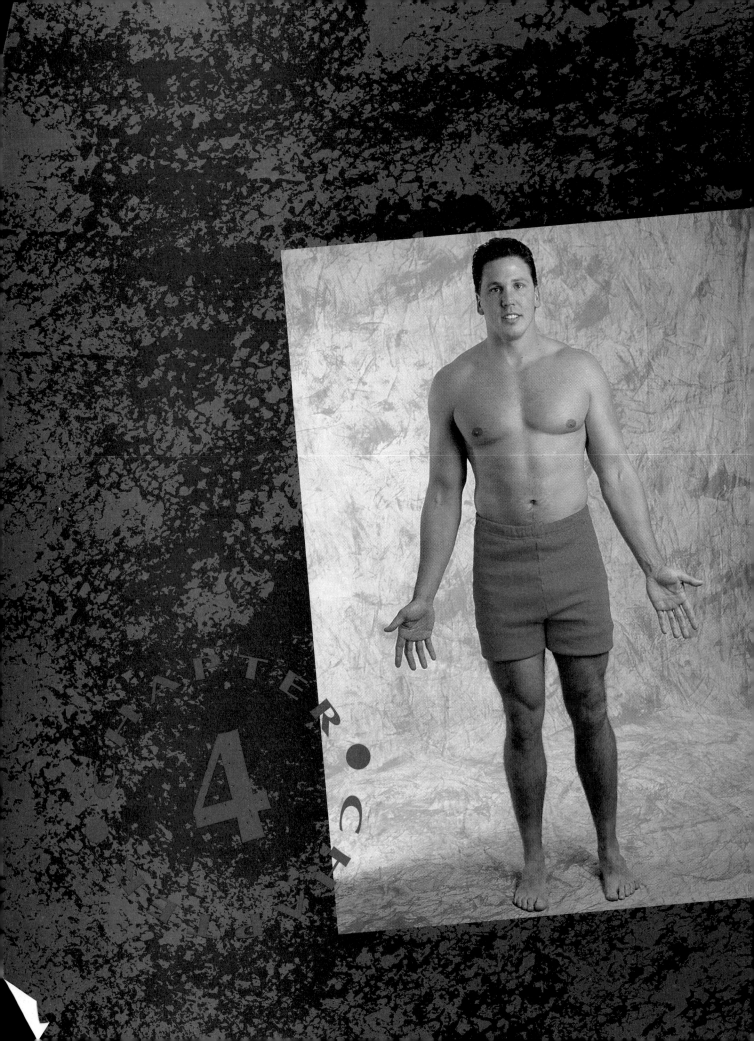

# The Human Body

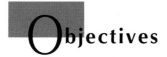

## Objectives

After you have read this chapter, you should be able to:

- Identify and locate on the body the following topographic terms: medial, lateral, proximal, distal, superior, inferior, anterior, posterior, midline, right and left, midclavicular, bilateral, and midaxillary.
- Describe the anatomy and function of the following major body systems: respiratory, circulatory, musculoskeletal, nervous, and endocrine.

## Overview

A working knowledge of human anatomy is important for you as an EMT-B. Even though you will not make diagnoses, you can help hospital personnel by communicating information using the correct medical terms. All EMT-Bs must be familiar with the language of topographic anatomy. By using the proper medical terms, you will be able to communicate correct information with the least possible confusion.

Using topographic anatomy is actually like using a road map. The terms introduced in this chapter will help you identify the topographic (on the surface) landmarks of the body. These landmarks are used as guides to locate the internal structures that lie under them. These terms also refer to the names of the major regions of the body and the way the locations of these regions are described in relationship to one another.

# Key Terms

**Anatomic position**  Position of reference with the patient standing, facing you, arms at the side, with the palms of the hands forward.

**Anterior**  The front surface of the body, the side facing you.

**Circulatory system**  Complex arrangement of connected tubes, including the arteries, arterioles, capillaries, venules, and veins. System moves blood, oxygen, nutrients, carbon dioxide, and cellular waste throughout the body.

**Distal**  Structures that are nearer to the free end of the extremity.

**Endocrine system**  Complex message and control system that integrates many body functions, including the release of hormones.

**Inferior**  The part of the body, or any body part nearer to the feet.

**Lateral**  Parts of the body that lie at some distance from the midline. Also called outer structures.

**Medial**  Parts of the body that lie closer to the midline. Also called inner structures.

**Midaxillary line**  Imaginary vertical line drawn through the middle of the axilla (armpit), parallel to the midline.

**Midclavicular line**  Imaginary vertical line drawn through the middle portion of the clavicle and parallel to the midline.

**Midline**  Imaginary vertical line drawn from the middle of the forehead through the nose and the umbilicus (navel) to the floor.

**Musculoskeletal system**  The bones and voluntary muscles of the body.

**Nervous system**  System that controls virtually all activities of the body, both voluntary and involuntary activities.

**Posterior**  The back surface of the body, the side away from you.

**Proximal**  Structures that are closer to the trunk.

**Respiratory system**  All the structures of the body that contribute to the process of breathing, consisting of the upper and lower airways.

**Skeleton**  Framework for the attachment of muscles. Also designed to allow motion of the body and protection of vital organs.

**Superior**  The part of the body, or any body part nearer to the head.

**Topographic anatomy**  The superficial landmarks of the body that serve as guides to the structures that lie beneath them.

# THE LANGUAGE OF TOPOGRAPHIC ANATOMY

The surface of the body has many definite visible features. These serve as guides or landmarks to the structures that lie beneath them. You must be able to identify the superficial landmarks of the body—its **topographic anatomy**—in order to perform an accurate assessment. Understanding this language is also important so that you can describe patient findings correctly to your team, ALS personnel, and hospital personnel.

Learning the terms introduced in this chapter will make your job as an EMT-B easier. You will be able to correctly identify structures as you complete and report your assessment findings. Hospital personnel will use these terms to ask you questions about a patient. Therefore, you must learn what these terms mean and how to use them.

The terms used to describe the topographic anatomy are applied to the body when it is in the **anatomic position.** This is a position of reference with the patient standing, facing you, arms at the side, with the palms of the hands forward (Figure 4-1). The terms right and left refer to the *patient's* right and left sides.

## FIGURE 4-1

Standard anatomic position

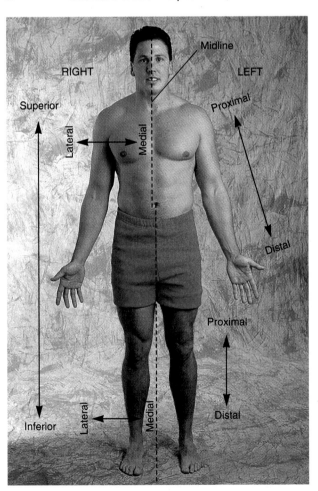

## THE PLANES OF THE BODY

The front surface of the body, the side facing you, is called the **anterior** surface. The term ventral also refers to the anterior surface of the body. The back surface of the patient, the side away from you, is called the **posterior** surface. The term dorsal also refers to the posterior surface of the body. This includes the back of the hand. The front region of the hand is referred to as the palm or palmar surface. The bottom of the foot is referred to as the plantar surface.

An imaginary vertical line drawn from the middle of the forehead through the nose and the umbilicus (navel) to the floor is called the **midline** of the body. This imaginary line divides the body into two halves that are mirror images. The nose, chin, umbilicus (navel), and spine are examples of midline structures. The term **midclavicular line** identifies an imaginary line drawn vertically through the middle portion of the clavicle and parallel to the midline. For example, the nipples of the breasts are in the midclavicular line on either side of the body (Figure 4-2). The term **midaxillary line** is an imaginary vertical line drawn through the middle of the axilla (armpit).

## FIGURE 4-2

The midclavicular lines of the body

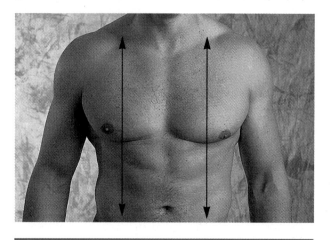

This line is also in the middle of the anterior and posterior surfaces of the body.

## DIRECTIONAL TERMS

The terms above are used to identify the different planes of the body. In this section, terms that indicate direction are introduced. These terms indicate distance and direction from the midline. Parts of the body that lie at some distance from the midline are called **lateral** (outer) structures. The parts that lie closer to the midline are called **medial** (inner) structures. For example, the knee has medial (inner) and lateral (outer) aspects. The **superior** part of the body, or any body part, is that portion nearer to the head. The part nearer to the feet is the **inferior** portion. We also use these terms to describe the relationship of one structure to another. For example, the nose is superior to the mouth and inferior to the forehead.

The terms proximal and distal are used to describe the relationship of any two structures on a limb. **Proximal** describes structures that are closer to the trunk. **Distal** describes structures that are nearer to the free end of the extremity. For example, the elbow is distal to the shoulder. Yet, it is proximal to the wrist and hand. The term superficial

means closer to or on the skin while the term deep means further inside the body and away from the skin.

Apices (apex for one) refer to the tip or the topmost portion of a structure. For example, the tips of the shoulder are the apices of the shoulder. The most superior portions of the lungs are the apices of the lungs.

Many structures of the body occur bilaterally. A bilateral structure is a body part that appears on either side of the midline. For example the eyes, ears, hands, and feet are bilateral structures. This is also true for structures inside the body, such as the lungs and kidneys. Structures on only one side of the body are said to occur unilaterally. For example, the spleen is on the left side of the body only and the liver is on the right side.

It is important to learn all of these terms so that you can describe the location of any injury or assessment findings. These terms are summarized in Tables 4-1 and 4-2. When

## TABLE 4-1    THE PLANES OF THE BODY

| Term | Definition |
| --- | --- |
| Anterior | Front |
| Posterior | Back |
| Midline | Line drawn through nose and umbilicus |
| Midclavicular | In the middle of the clavicle, parallel to the midline |
| Midaxillary | In the middle of the armpit, parallel to the midline |

you use these terms properly, any other medical personnel caring for the patient will know immediately where to look and what to expect.

## ANATOMIC POSITIONS

Prone and supine are terms used to describe the position of the body. A prone position is when the body is lying facedown. A supine position is when the body is lying faceup. A patient who is sitting up with the knees bent is in Fowler's position. In Trendelenburg's position, the body is supine with the head lower than the feet. This helps to increase blood flow to the brain.

**TABLE 4-2    DIRECTIONAL TERMS**

| Term | Definition |
|------|------------|
| Lateral | Farther from midline |
| Medial | Closer to midline |
| Superior | Closer to the head, higher |
| Inferior | Farther from the head, lower |
| Proximal | Closer to the midline (in an extremity, closer to the trunk) |
| Distal | Farther from the midline (in an extremity, closer to the free end) |

# THE SKELETAL SYSTEM

The **skeleton** gives us our recognizable human form and protects our vital internal organs. The brain lies within the skull. The heart, lungs, and great vessels are protected by the thorax. Much of the liver and spleen is protected by the lower ribs. The spinal cord is contained within and protected by a bony spinal canal formed by the vertebrae.

The approximately 206 bones of the skeleton provide a framework for the attachment of muscles. The skeleton is also designed to allow motion of the body. Bones come in contact with one another at joints where, with the help of muscles, we are able to bend and move (Figure 4-3).

The major functions of the skeleton are to:

- give us form
- allow us to move
- protect our vital internal organs
- produce red blood cells
- serve as a reservoir for calcium, phosphorus, and other important body chemicals

## THE SKULL

### Cranium

The skull has two major parts: the cranium and the face (Figure 4-4). The cranium is composed of a number of thick bones that fuse together to form a shell that protects the brain. The cranium holds the brain. The brain connects to the spinal cord through a large opening at the base of the skull. The

# FIGURE 4-3

The human skeleton

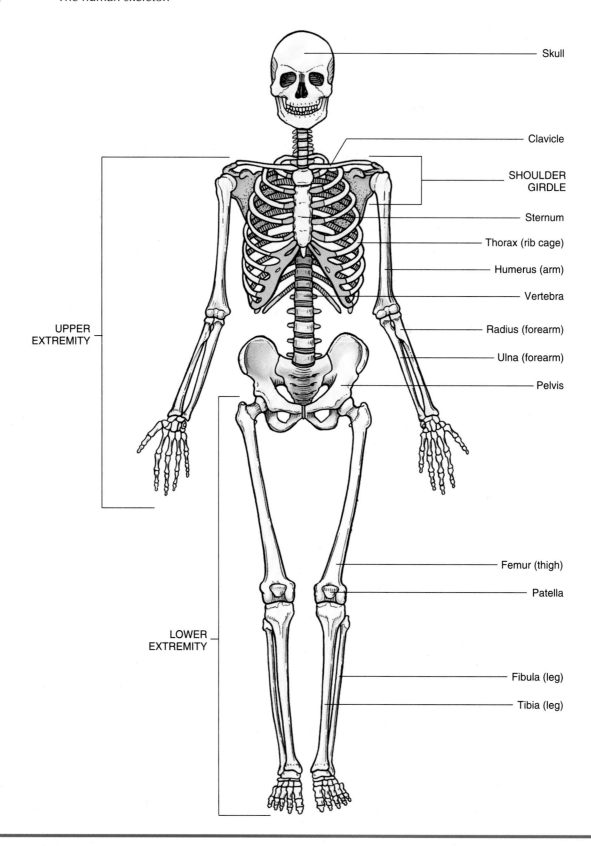

Skull

Clavicle

SHOULDER GIRDLE

Sternum

Thorax (rib cage)

Humerus (arm)

Vertebra

Radius (forearm)

Ulna (forearm)

Pelvis

UPPER EXTREMITY

Femur (thigh)

Patella

LOWER EXTREMITY

Fibula (leg)

Tibia (leg)

**FIGURE 4-4**

The cranium and face

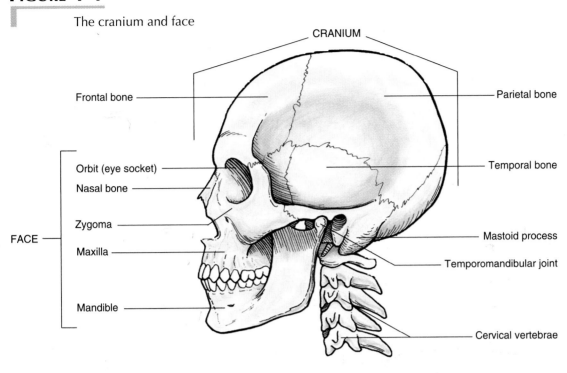

CRANIUM

Frontal bone

Parietal bone

Orbit (eye socket)

Temporal bone

Nasal bone

FACE

Zygoma

Maxilla

Mastoid process

Temporomandibular joint

Mandible

Cervical vertebrae

spinal cord is composed of virtually all the nerves that carry messages between the brain and the rest of the body.

The most posterior portion of the cranium is called the occiput. On each side of the cranium, the lateral portions are called the temples or temporal regions. Between the temporal regions and the occiput lie the parietal regions. The forehead is called the frontal region. Just anterior to the ear, in the temporal region, you can feel the pulse of the superficial temporal artery. The thick skin covering the cranium and usually bearing hair is called the scalp.

### Face

The face is composed of the eyes, ears, nose, mouth, and cheeks. Six bones—the nasal bone, the two maxillae (upper jaw bones), the two zygomas (cheek bones), and the mandible (lower jaw bone)—are the major bones of the face.

The orbit (eye socket) is made up of two facial bones—the maxilla and the zygoma. The orbit also includes the frontal bone of the cranium. Together, these bones form a solid bony rim that protrudes around the eye to protect it. If you look at the face from the side, you can see that the eyeball sits back within the orbit. The nasal bone is very short, because most of the nose is made of flexible cartilage. In fact, only the proximal one third of the nose, the bridge, is formed by bone. Unlike the nose, the exposed portion of the ear is made up entirely of cartilage that is covered by skin. The visible part of the ear is called the pinna. The earlobes are the fleshy parts at the bottom of each ear. About 1" posterior to the external opening of the ear is a prominent bony mass at the base of the skull called the mastoid process.

The maxilla contains the upper teeth and forms the hard palate (roof of the mouth). The mandible is the only movable facial bone that has a joint (temporomandibular

FIGURE 4-5

The sections of the spinal column

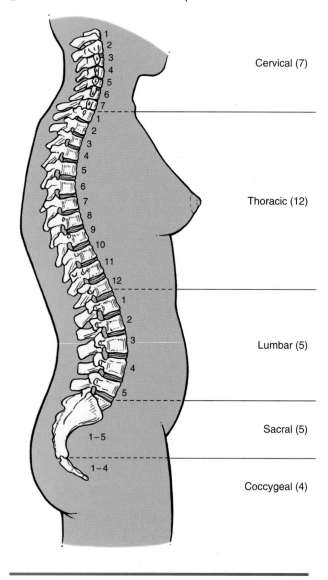

Cervical (7)

Thoracic (12)

Lumbar (5)

Sacral (5)

Coccygeal (4)

joint). This joint meets with the cranium just in front of each ear.

## THE SPINAL COLUMN

The spinal column is the central supporting structure of the body. It is composed of 33 bones, each called a vertebra. From the top down, the spine is divided into five sections:

- cervical (neck)
- thoracic (upper back)
- lumbar (lower back)
- sacral (part of pelvis)
- coccygeal (coccyx or tail bone)

The vertebrae are named according to the section of the spine in which they lie and are numbered from top to bottom (Figure 4-5). The first seven vertebrae form the cervical spine (C1 through C7). The skull rests on the first cervical vertebra and articulates with it. The next 12 vertebrae make up the thoracic spine. One pair of ribs is attached to each of the thoracic vertebrae. The next five vertebrae form the lumbar spine. The five sacral vertebrae are fused together to form one bone called the sacrum. The sacrum is joined to the iliac bones of the pelvis with strong ligaments at the sacroiliac joints to form the pelvis. The last three or four vertebrae form the coccyx.

The front part of each vertebra consists of a round, solid block of bone—the body. The back part of each vertebra forms a bony arch. This series of arches from one vertebra to the next forms a tunnel that runs the length of the spine. This is called the spinal canal. The bones of the spinal canal encase and protect the spinal cord (Figure 4-6). Nerves branch from the spinal cord and exit from the spinal canal between each two vertebrae to form the motor and sensory nerves of the body (Figure 4-7).

The vertebrae are connected by ligaments, and between each two vertebrae is a cushion called the intervertebral disk. These ligaments and disks allow some motion so that the trunk can bend forward and back. However, they also act to limit motion of the vertebrae so that the spinal cord will not be injured. When a spinal injury occurs, the spinal cord and its nerves may be damaged as they may not be protected by the vertebrae. Until the injury is stabilized, you must use extreme caution in caring for the patient to prevent injury to the spinal cord.

The spinal column itself is virtually surrounded by muscles. However, the posterior

**FIGURE 4-6**

The spinal cord protected by the spinal column

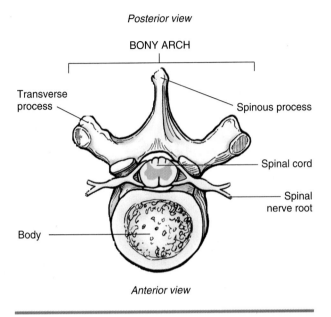

*Posterior view*

BONY ARCH

Transverse process

Spinous process

Spinal cord

Spinal nerve root

Body

*Anterior view*

**FIGURE 4-7**

Peripheral nerves exiting the spinal canal

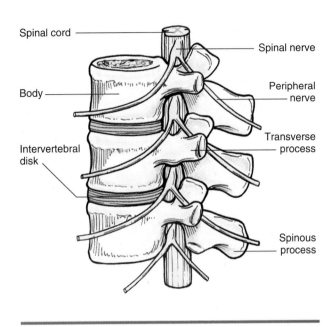

Spinal cord

Spinal nerve

Body

Peripheral nerve

Intervertebral disk

Transverse process

Spinous process

spinous process of each vertebra can be felt as it lies just under the skin in the midline of the back. The most prominent and most easily palpable spinous process is that of the seventh cervical vertebra at the base of the neck (Figure 4-8).

## THE THORAX

The thorax (rib cage) is made up of the ribs, the 12 thoracic vertebrae, and the sternum (breast bone) (Figure 4-9). The thorax also contains the heart, lungs, esophagus, and the great vessels (the aorta and two venae cavae). There are 12 pairs of ribs, which are long, slender, curved bones. Each rib forms a joint with its respective thoracic vertebra and then curves around to form the rib cage. At the front of the rib cage, ribs 1 through 10 connect with the sternum through a bridge of cartilage. For the lower five ribs, this bridge is called the costal arch.

The sternum forms the middle part of the front of the thoracic cage. In the adult, this

**FIGURE 4-8**

Palpating the C7 spinous process

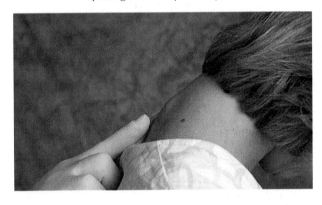

bone is approximately 7" long and 2" wide. The sternum has three parts: the manubrium (upper part), the body, and the xiphoid process. The junction of the manubrium and the body of the sternum is located at the level of the second ribs. Here there is a consistent bony prominence, the angle of Louis, that can be palpated on all patients. The xiphoid process projects from the lower part

**FIGURE 4-9**

The thorax (rib cage)

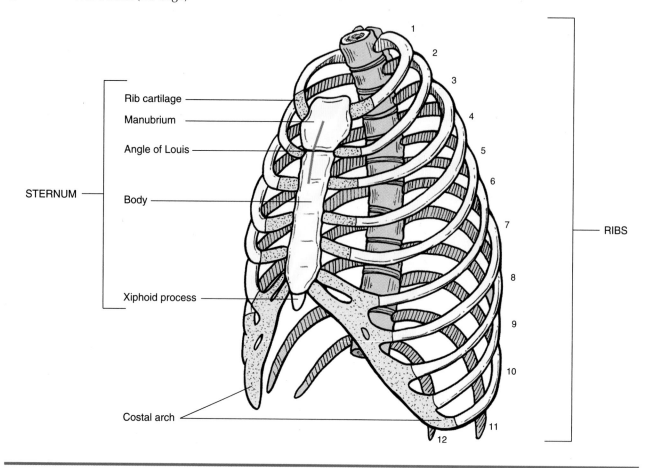

of the sternum. It is made of cartilage and is very tender to palpation.

## THE PELVIS

The pelvis is a closed bony ring that consists of three bones: the sacrum and the two pelvic bones. Much like the skull, each pelvic bone is formed by the fusion of three separate bones. In the pelvis, these three bones are called the ilium, the ischium, and the pubis (Figure 4-10). The prominent anterior bony landmarks of the pelvis are the symphysis pubis in the midline and the anterior superior iliac spines. The inguinal ligament attaches to these two bony promi-

nences and can be palpated in a thin person. Just distal to the midpoint of the inguinal ligament, the femoral artery can be palpated as it enters the thigh. From the anterior superior iliac spine, the ilium extends laterally and posteriorly to form the rim of the pelvis. This bony ridge is called the iliac crest.

Posteriorly, the pelvis appears flat, and in the middle third, the firm bony sacrum can be palpated. Just lateral to the sacrum on either side is a joint with the iliac portion of the pelvic bone (the sacroiliac joint). In the sitting position a bony prominence is easily felt below the middle of each buttock. These prominences are the ischial tuberosities. The sciatic nerve—the major

## FIGURE 4-10

The bony pelvis

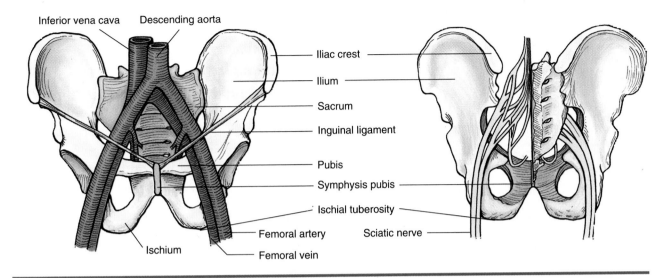

Inferior vena cava · Descending aorta · Iliac crest · Ilium · Sacrum · Inguinal ligament · Pubis · Symphysis pubis · Ischial tuberosity · Femoral artery · Sciatic nerve · Ischium · Femoral vein

nerve to the lower extremity—lies just lateral to the tuberosity as it enters the thigh.

The sacrum and the two pelvic bones meet at three joints: the two posterior sacroiliac joints and the anterior midline symphysis pubis. All three joints allow very little motion, as they are firmly held together by strong ligaments. Thus, the pelvic ring is strong and stable. The pelvic ring is designed to support the body weight and protect the structures within the pelvic cavity (the bladder, the rectum, and the female reproductive organs). On the lateral side of each pelvic bone—where the three component bones join—is the socket for the hip joint. This depression, in which the femoral head fits very snugly, is called the acetabulum.

## THE LOWER EXTREMITY

The main parts of the lower extremity are the thigh, the leg, and the foot (Figure 4-11). Three joints connect the parts of the lower extremity. The joint between the thigh and pelvis is called the hip. The joint between the thigh and the leg is the knee, and the joint between the leg and the foot is the ankle.

### Thigh

On the proximal lateral side of the thigh, just below the hip joint, is a bony prominence called the greater trochanter. This prominence is sometimes called the "hip bone." During patient assessment, you should always compare the position of the greater trochanter with that on the opposite side as a guide to injury or deformity of the hip.

The femur (thigh bone) is the longest and one of the strongest bones in the body. The femoral head (at the top of the femur) forms the hip joint with the acetabulum of the pelvis. This ball-and-socket joint allows for flexion, extension, and motion toward (adduction) and away (abduction) from the midline. It also allows for internal and external rotation of the entire lower extremity. The shaft of the femur is surrounded by large muscles (the quadriceps in front and the hamstrings in back). Just above the knee, the medial and lateral femoral condyles can be palpated.

### Knee

Between the thigh and the leg is the largest joint in the body—the knee. The knee is essentially a hinge joint, allowing only

**FIGURE 4-11**

Bones of the lower extremity

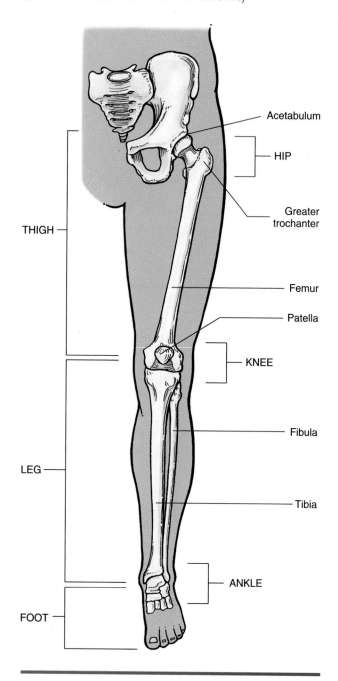

THIGH

Acetabulum

HIP

Greater trochanter

Femur

Patella

KNEE

Fibula

LEG

Tibia

ANKLE

FOOT

(knee cap). It lies within the tendon of the quadriceps muscle and protects the front of the knee from injury.

### Leg

Between the knee and the ankle joint lies the leg (Figure 4-12). It contains two bones: the tibia and the fibula. The tibia (shin) is the larger bone and lies in the front of the leg. The entire length of the tibia can be palpated on the anterior surface of the leg just under the skin. The fibula lies on the lateral side of the leg. Its head can be palpated on the lateral aspect of the knee joint. Its distal end forms the lateral malleolus of the ankle joint.

### Ankle and Foot

The ankle is also a hinge joint that allows flexion and extension of the foot on the leg. The end of the tibia forms the medial malleolus. The end of the fibula forms the lateral malleolus. These two bony prominences form the socket of the ankle joint (Figure 4-13). Both are surface landmarks of the ankle joint and are easily palpated. The talus is one of seven tarsal bones. The calcaneus (heel bone) is the other large tarsal bone. It forms the prominence of the heel. The Achilles tendon inserts into the back of the calcaneus. The talus and the calcaneus, along with the five other bones, make up the rear portion of the foot. Five metatarsal bones form the substance of the foot. The five toes are formed by 14 phalanges—two in the great toe and three in each of the smaller toes.

flexion and extension between the distal femur and the proximal tibia. Adduction, abduction, and rotation of the knee are resisted by complex ligaments that are quite susceptible to injury. Anterior to the knee is a specialized bone called the patella

### THE UPPER EXTREMITY

The upper extremity extends from the shoulder girdle to the fingertips. It is composed of the arm, elbow, forearm, wrist, hand, and fingers. The arm extends from the shoulder to the elbow.

## FIGURE 4-12

Anterior and lateral aspects of the leg

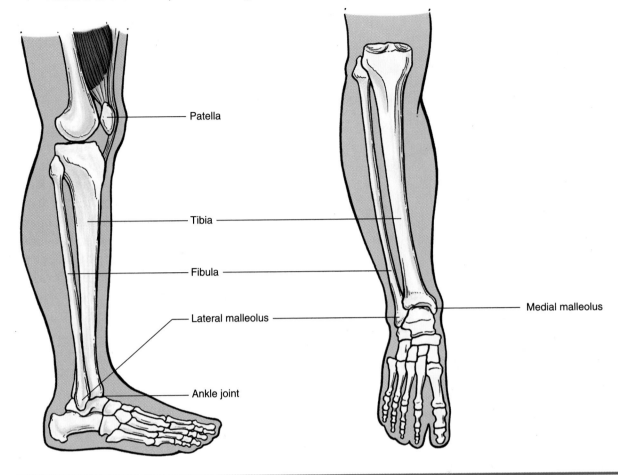

- Patella
- Tibia
- Fibula
- Lateral malleolus
- Ankle joint
- Medial malleolus

## FIGURE 4-13

Bones of the ankle and foot

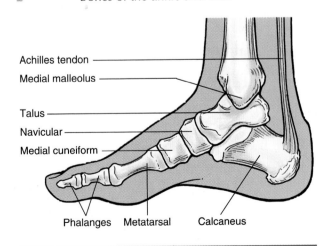

- Achilles tendon
- Medial malleolus
- Talus
- Navicular
- Medial cuneiform
- Phalanges
- Metatarsal
- Calcaneus

## Shoulder Girdle

The proximal portion of the upper extremity is called the shoulder girdle. It consists of three bones: the clavicle, the scapula, and the humerus (Figure 4-14). The shoulder girdle is where the upper extremity attaches to the trunk. The upper extremity can move through a wide range of motion, allowing the hand to be placed in almost any position. This motion occurs at three joints within the shoulder girdle: the sternoclavicular joint, the acromioclavicular (A/C) joint, and the glenohumeral joint. Only slight motion occurs normally at the sternoclavicular and acromioclavicular (A/C) joints. The ball-and-socket arrangement of

**FIGURE 4-14**

Bones of the shoulder girdle

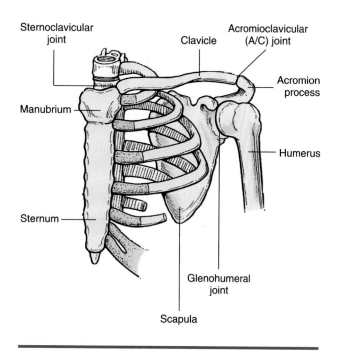

the glenohumeral joint allows great freedom of motion in almost any direction.

The clavicle (collar bone) is a long, slender bone that lies just under the skin and provides support for the upper extremity. The clavicle is palpable though its entire length from the sternum to its attachment to the scapula. Its medial end is attached by very strong ligaments to the manubrium of the sternum to form the sternoclavicular joint. Its lateral end forms a joint with the acromion process of the scapula to create the A/C joint.

The scapula (shoulder blade) is a large, flat, triangular bone that overlies the posterior wall of the thorax and is surrounded by large muscles. Because of these muscles, only small parts of this bone are palpable. The scapula has two specially named regions that form joints with the clavicle and the humerus. The acromion process in the front forms part of the A/C joint. The glenoid fossa joins with the humeral head to form the glenohumeral

joint. The spine and medial border of the scapula can be seen and palpated posteriorly. The acromion process forms the rounded edge of the shoulder girdle. You can feel this if you slowly move your finger along the clavicle and across the A/C joint.

### Arm

The supporting bone of the arm is the humerus. Its long, straight shaft serves as an effective lever for heavy lifting. Just like the thigh, there are few bony landmarks in the arm because it is covered by large muscles—the biceps in the front and the triceps in the back. The head of the humerus is covered by muscles that form the rounded prominence of the shoulder girdle laterally. The distal end articulates with both the radius and ulna at the elbow joint (Figure 4-15).

The humerus joins with the radius and ulna to form a relatively simple hinge joint, the elbow. You can easily see and feel three prominences on the back of the elbow. These are the medial and lateral condyles of the humerus and the olecranon process of the ulna.

### Forearm

The forearm is composed of two bones: the radius and the ulna. The ulna is larger in the proximal forearm, and the radius is larger in the distal forearm. The olecranon process of the ulna forms most of the elbow joint. The entire ulna shaft from the tip of the olecranon process distally can be palpated, because it lies just under the skin on the back of the forearm. The radius is covered by muscles and cannot be palpated except in the lower third of the forearm, where it enlarges to form a major portion of the wrist joint. The radius rotates about the ulna, which allows the palm of the hand to turn up or down. At the wrist, the ends of the radius and ulna (the styloid processes) lie directly under the skin and can be easily palpated. The radial styloid is slightly

**FIGURE 4-15**

Bones of the arm and forearm

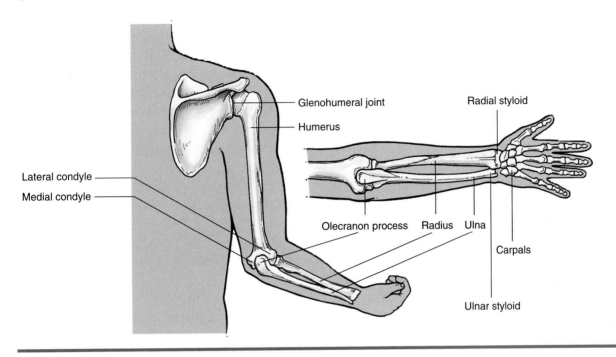

**FIGURE 4-16**

Bones of the wrist and hand

longer than the ulnar styloid. The radius lies on the lateral, or thumb, side of the forearm, and the ulna is on the medial or little finger side.

### Wrist and Hand

The wrist is a modified ball-and-socket joint formed by the ends of the radius and ulna and several small wrist bones. There are eight bones in the wrist called the carpal bones. Extending from the carpal bones are five metacarpals, which serve as a base for each of the five fingers or digits. The carpometacarpal (thumb joint) is a modified ball-and-socket joint that allows the thumb to rotate as well as to flex and extend. The other joints in the hand are simple hinge joints. In the thumb, there are two bones beyond the metacarpal: the proximal and distal phalanges. The remaining four digits of the hand are named in order: the index, the middle, the ring, and the little finger. Each of these contains three phalanges (Figure 4-16).

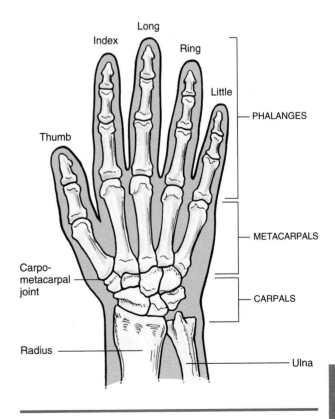

# THE RESPIRATORY SYSTEM

The **respiratory system** consists of all the structures of the body that contribute to the process of breathing. The system consists of the upper and lower airways (Figure 4-17).

## THE UPPER AIRWAY

The structures of the upper airway are located anteriorly and at the midline. The upper airway includes the nose, mouth, and throat. The nostrils lead to the nasopharynx (above the roof of the mouth). The lining of the nasopharynx gives off watery secretions and helps to moisten the air as we breathe. Air enters through the mouth more rapidly and directly. As a result, it is less moist than air that enters through the nose. The nose and mouth lead to the pharynx (throat). Two passageways are located at the bottom of the pharynx—the esophagus behind and the trachea (windpipe) in front. Food and liquids enter the pharynx and pass into the esophagus, which carries them to the stomach. Air and other gases enter the trachea and go to the lungs.

Protecting the opening of the trachea is a thin, leaf-shaped valve called the epiglottis. This valve allows air to pass into the trachea but prevents food or liquid from entering the airway under normal circumstances. Air moves past the epiglottis into the larynx and the trachea.

## THE LOWER AIRWAY

The first part of the lower airway is the larynx (voice box), a rather complex arrangement of tiny bones, cartilage, muscles, and the two vocal cords. The larynx does not tolerate any foreign solid or liquid material. A violent episode of coughing and spasm of the vocal cords will result from contact with solids or liquids.

The Adam's apple, or thyroid cartilage, is easily seen in the middle of the front of the neck. The thyroid cartilage is actually the front part of the larynx. Tiny muscles open and close the vocal cords and control tension on them. Sounds are created as air is forced past the vocal cords, making them vibrate. These vibrations make the sound. The pitch of the sound changes as the cords open and close. You can feel the vibrations if you place your fingers lightly on the larynx as you speak or sing. The vibrations of air are shaped by the tongue and muscles of the mouth to form understandable speech.

Immediately below the thyroid cartilage is the palpable cricoid cartilage. Between these two prominences lies the cricothyroid membrane, which can be felt as a depression in the midline of the neck just inferior to the thyroid cartilage. Below the cricoid cartilage is the trachea. The trachea is approximately 5" long and is a semirigid, enclosed air tube made up of rings of cartilage that are open in the back. This enables food to pass through the esophagus, which lies right behind the trachea. The rings of cartilage keep the trachea from collapsing when air moves in and out of the lungs. The trachea ends at the carina and divides into smaller tubes. These tubes are the right and left main bronchi, which enter the lungs. Each main bronchus immediately branches within the lung into smaller and smaller airways. Within the right lung, three major bronchi are formed. Within the left, there are only two. Each bronchus supplies air to one lobe of the lung.

## THE LUNGS

The lungs are held in place within the chest by the trachea, the arteries and veins that run to and from the heart, and the pulmonary ligaments. Each lung is divided

**FIGURE 4-17**

Upper and lower airways

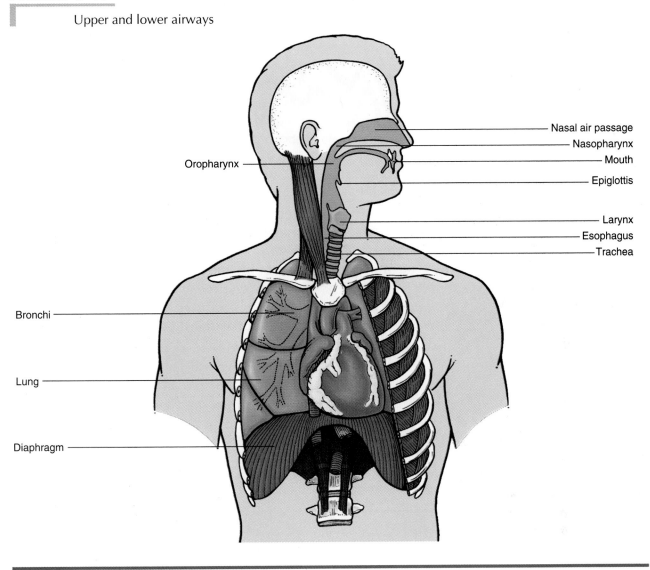

Oropharynx

Nasal air passage
Nasopharynx
Mouth
Epiglottis
Larynx
Esophagus
Trachea

Bronchi

Lung

Diaphragm

into lobes. The right lung has three lobes: the upper, middle, and lower lobes. The left lung has an upper lobe and a lower lobe. Each lobe is divided further into segments. Also within each lung, the main bronchi divide until they end in very fine airways called bronchioles. The bronchioles end in about 700 million tiny grape-like sacs called alveoli (Figure 4-18). If you spread the alveoli from each lung on a flat surface, you would cover about one half of a tennis court (Figure 4-19). The exchange of oxygen and carbon dioxide occurs within these alveoli. The walls of the alveoli contain a network of tiny blood vessels (pulmonary capillaries) that carry the carbon dioxide from the body to the lungs and the oxygen from the lungs to the body (Figure 4-20). A detailed discussion of oxygen exchange in the lungs, and the general mechanics of breathing is presented in chapter 7, The Mechanics of Breathing.

FIGURE 4-18

Alveoli of the lung

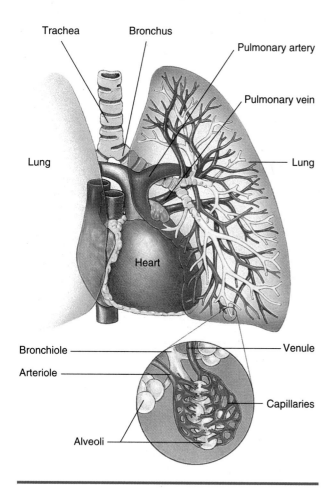

THE DIAPHRAGM

The diaphragm is a dome-shaped muscle that divides the thorax from the abdomen. It is pierced by the great vessels and the esophagus (Figure 4-21). The diaphragm is special because it acts like both a voluntary muscle and an involuntary muscle. It acts like a voluntary muscle whenever we take a deep breath, cough, or hold our breath. We control these variations in the way we breathe. However, unlike other skeletal or voluntary muscles, the diaphragm performs an automatic function. Breathing continues while we sleep and at all other times. Even though we can hold our breath or temporarily breathe faster or slower, we cannot con-

tinue these variations in breathing pattern indefinitely.

During inhalation, the diaphragm and intercostal muscles contract. When the diaphragm contracts, it moves down slightly and enlarges the thoracic cage from top to bottom. When the intercostal muscles contract, they raise the ribs up and out. These actions combine to enlarge the chest cavity in all dimensions. Pressure within the cavity falls, and air rushes into the lungs.

During exhalation, the diaphragm and the intercostal muscles relax. Unlike inhalation, exhalation does not normally require muscular effort. As these muscles relax, all dimensions of the thorax decrease, and the ribs and muscles assume a normal resting position. When the volume of the chest cavity decreases, air in the lungs is compressed into a smaller space. Pressure is increased, and air is pushed out through the trachea.

FIGURE 4-19

The surface area of the alveoli equals ½ of a tennis court

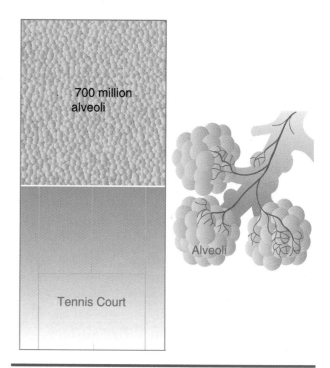

## FIGURE 4-20

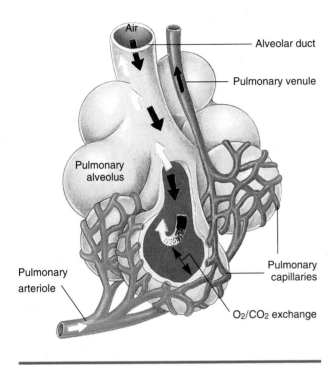

Enlarged view of an alveolus

Air

Alveolar duct

Pulmonary venule

Pulmonary alveolus

Pulmonary arteriole

Pulmonary capillaries

$O_2/CO_2$ exchange

## FIGURE 4-21

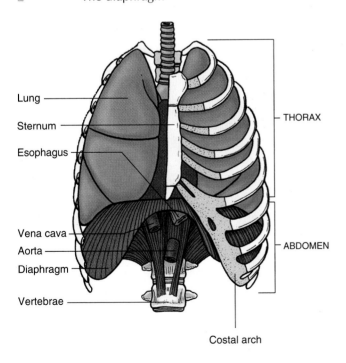

The diaphragm

Lung

Sternum

Esophagus

Vena cava

Aorta

Diaphragm

Vertebrae

THORAX

ABDOMEN

Costal arch

A detailed explanation of respiratory physiology and breathing patterns is described in chapter 7, The Mechanics of Breathing.

### PEDIATRIC ANATOMY CONSIDERATIONS— RESPIRATORY SYSTEM

A child's nose and mouth are much smaller than that of an adult. The larynx, cricoid cartilage, and trachea are smaller and softer as well. This makes the mechanics of breathing much more delicate. A child's pharynx is also smaller and less deeply curved. The tongue takes up proportionally more space in a child's mouth than in an adult's mouth. Infants younger than 1 month do not know how to breathe through the mouth. Therefore, as you assess an infant or a child, you must carefully consider these differences.

The respiratory system of children is proportionally smaller and less rigid than that of an adult. These differences are important for your assessment. For example, the smaller larynx of a child becomes obstructed more easily. The chest wall in children is softer. Therefore, they depend more heavily on the diaphragm for breathing. You will notice the abdomen moves in and out considerably with each breath, especially in an infant.

# THE CIRCULATORY SYSTEM

The **circulatory system** is a complex arrangement of connected tubes, including the arteries, arterioles, capillaries, venules, and veins. The circulatory system is entirely closed, with capillaries connecting arterioles and venules. There are two circuits in the body—the systemic circulation and the pulmonary circulation. The systemic circulation, the circuit in the body, carries oxygen-rich blood from the left ventricle through the body and back to the right atrium. In the systemic circulation, as blood passes through the tissues and organs it gives up oxygen and nutrients and absorbs cellular wastes and carbon dioxide. The cellular wastes are eliminated in passages through the liver and the kidneys. The pulmonary circulation, the circuit in the lungs, carries oxygen-poor blood from the right ventricle through the lungs and back to the left atrium. In the pulmonary circulation, as blood passes through the lungs, it is refreshed with oxygen and gives up carbon dioxide.

At the center of the system, and providing its driving force, is the heart. Blood circulates through the body under pressure generated by the two sides of the heart.

## THE HEART

The heart is a hollow muscular organ about the size of a clenched fist. It is an involuntary muscle made of a special tissue called cardiac muscle or myocardium. As such, it is under the control of the autonomic nervous system. However, the heart has its own internal regulatory system. It will continue to function even if our external nerve impulses stop working.

The heart differs from skeletal or smooth muscle in that it needs a continuous supply of oxygen and nutrients. The heart can tolerate a serious interruption of its blood supply for only a very few seconds before the signs of a heart attack develop. Thus, its blood supply is as rich and well distributed as possible. It receives the first blood distribution from the aorta (Figure 4-22). The two main coronary arteries have their open-

## FIGURE 4-22

The coronary arteries

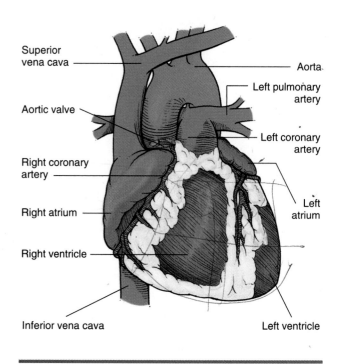

Superior vena cava

Aortic valve

Right coronary artery

Right atrium

Right ventricle

Inferior vena cava

Aorta

Left pulmonary artery

Left coronary artery

Left atrium

Left ventricle

ing immediately above the aortic valve at the beginning of the aorta.

The heart is always working. Because it works continuously, the heart has a number of special features other muscles do not.

First, the heart works as two paired pumps. The heart is divided down the middle into two sides by a wall called the septum. Each side of the heart has an upper chamber (atrium) and a lower chamber (ventricle). Blood leaves each chamber of the heart through a one-way valve. These valves keep the blood moving through the circulatory system in the proper direction by preventing backflow of blood. Normally, blood moves in only one direction through the entire system (Figure 4-23).

The right side of the heart receives oxygen-poor (deoxygenated) blood from the veins of the body. Blood enters into the

## FIGURE 4-23

The circulatory system

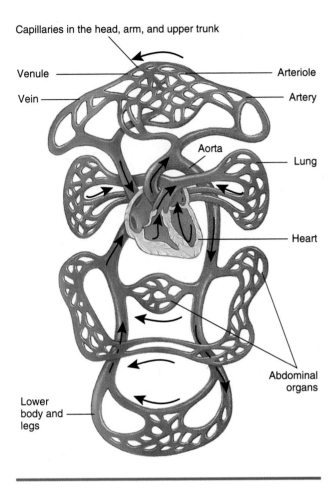

Capillaries in the head, arm, and upper trunk

Venule — Arteriole
Vein — Artery
Aorta
Lung
Heart
Abdominal organs
Lower body and legs

---

side of the heart is more muscular than the other because it must pump blood into the aorta and then to the arteries (Figure 4-25).

### The Electrical System of the Heart

A network of specialized tissue capable of conducting electrical current runs throughout the heart. The flow of electrical current through this network causes smooth, coordinated contractions of the heart. These contractions produce the pumping action of the heart (Figure 4-26, Table 4-3). The heart's electrical system becomes disturbed if part of the heart is oxygen deficient, injured, or dies. As a result, the heart may not continue to beat properly. Blood pressure decreases and a patient may lose consciousness.

The body acts as a conductor of electrical current. Any two points on the body may be connected with electrical "leads" to record the electrical activity of the heart. The tracing produced by the electrical activity of the

## FIGURE 4-24

The right side of the heart

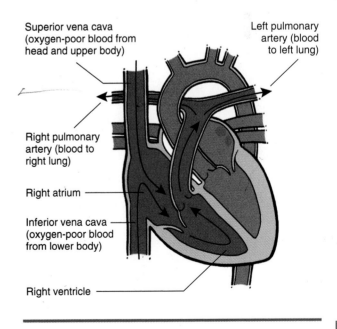

Superior vena cava (oxygen-poor blood from head and upper body)

Left pulmonary artery (blood to left lung)

Right pulmonary artery (blood to right lung)

Right atrium

Inferior vena cava (oxygen-poor blood from lower body)

Right ventricle

---

right atrium from the vena cava, then fills the right ventricle. As blood moves from the right atrium to the right ventricle, it passes through a one-way valve that immediately closes to prevent backflow after the right atrium contracts. After contraction of the right ventricle, blood flows into the pulmonary artery and the pulmonary circulation (Figure 4-24).

The left side of the heart receives oxygen-rich (oxygenated) blood from the lungs through the pulmonary veins. Blood enters into the left atrium then passes through a one-way valve into the left ventricle. This

## FIGURE 4-25

The left side of the heart

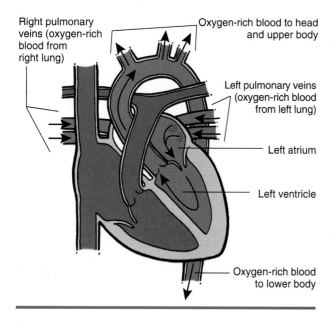

Right pulmonary veins (oxygen-rich blood from right lung)

Oxygen-rich blood to head and upper body

Left pulmonary veins (oxygen-rich blood from left lung)

Left atrium

Left ventricle

Oxygen-rich blood to lower body

## FIGURE 4-26

The electrical conduction system of the heart

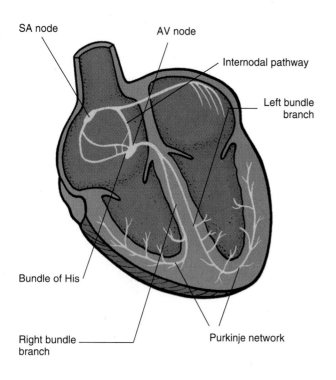

SA node

AV node

Internodal pathway

Left bundle branch

Bundle of His

Right bundle branch

Purkinje network

heart, as it depolarizes and repolarizes, forms a series of impulses and complexes that are separated by regularly occurring intervals on the screen of the ECG monitor. The waves or deflections of the ECG are called the P-wave, the QRS complex, and the T-wave. Depolarization of the atria produces the P-wave. Depolarization of the ventricles and repolarization of the atria produces the QRS complex. This is when the main mechanical contraction of the heart occurs. When the ventricles repolarize, the T-wave is formed (Figure 4-27).

## THE BLOOD VESSELS

### Arteries

The arteries carry blood from the heart to all body tissues. They branch into smaller arteries and then into arterioles. The arterioles, in turn, branch into smaller vessels until they connect to the vast network of capillaries. The walls of an artery

### TABLE 4-3    NORMAL HEART RATES

| Adults | 60 to 100 beats per minute |
|---|---|
| Children | 80 to 100 beats per minute |
| Toddlers | 100 to 120 beats per minute |
| Newborns | 120 to 140 beats per minute |

To obtain a heart rate in most patients, count the number of beats over a 30-second period and multiply by two.

**FIGURE 4-27**

ECG tracing of a normal cardiac rhythm

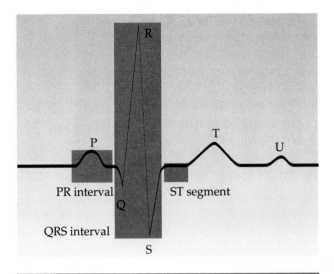

are made of fine, circular muscle tissue. Some arteries even have elastic tissue.

Arteries contract to accommodate for loss of blood volume and also to increase blood pressure. Blood is supplied to tissues as they need it. For example, the digestive system is supplied with more blood after you eat a meal. The leg muscles are supplied as you are jogging. Some tissues need a constant blood supply, especially the heart, the kidneys, and the brain. Other tissues, such as the muscles in the extremities, the skin, and the intestines, can function with less blood when at rest.

The aorta is the major artery that leaves the left side of the heart. It carries fresh, oxygen-rich blood to the body. The aorta is found just in front of the spine in the chest and abdominal cavities. It has many branches that supply the heart, the head and neck, the arms, and many of the vital organs before it ends in the middle of the abdomen. The aorta divides at the level of the umbilicus into the two common iliac arteries that lead to the lower extremities (Figure 4-28).

The pulmonary artery begins at the right side of the heart and carries oxygen-poor blood to the lungs. It divides into finer and finer branches until it meets with the pulmonary capillary system located in the thin walls of the alveoli.

The carotid artery is the major artery that supplies blood to the head and brain. The carotid arteries are located on both sides of the neck. You can easily feel the carotid pulse if you place your fingers at the anterior lateral part of your neck. Since the carotid artery is rather close to the heart, you can feel its pulse even after the pulse in the distal extremities is too weak to feel.

The femoral artery is the major artery that supplies blood to the lower extremities. It is palpable in the groin. It divides at the level of the knee and supplies blood to the leg. At the ankle, two of these branches are palpable. You can feel a pulse at the posterior tibial artery, which is behind the medial prominence of the ankle (medial malleolus). You can also feel a pulse at the dorsalis pedis artery on the anterior surface of the foot (dorsum of foot).

In the upper extremity, the brachial artery is the major vessel that supplies blood to the arm. It divides into two major branches just below the elbow. The radial artery is palpable at the wrist on the thumb side (radial side). The ulnar artery is also palpable at the wrist on the opposite side (ulnar side), although the pulse is not as strong. Both arteries supply blood to the hand. The nail bed under the finger nail appears pink because the capillaries are located close to the surface. If the nail bed is pink, the blood supply to the hand is adequate.

### The Capillaries

The capillaries are the fine-channel network where oxygen and nutrients reach the cells and carbon dioxide is removed. It is at this level that each individual cell in our body lives. In our bodies, we have billions of cells and billions of capillaries. The capillaries are a network of very fine vessels where the arteries meet the veins. Capillaries con-

## HEAVE HO, AWAY WE GO!

You are working a call where you and your partner have to carry a 280-lb patient up 10 stairs leading out of a basement apartment. There are no bystanders around, and there is no other crew available to help. It looks like it's just the two of you. As you reach the top of the stairs, there is a small step that causes you to stumble and almost fall. You struggle to control the stretcher, and manage to get control before you drop the patient. However, you feel a sharp pain in your lower back. A couple of hours after the call, your back is so stiff and painful that you can't get off the couch at quarters without your partner's help.

### For Discussion

1. Why is prompt care of a back injury so important?
2. What is the purpose of pain?

nect directly at one end with the flow-regulating arterioles and at the other end with the venules. In this vast network, the cells of the body tissues make contact with the plasma and the red blood cells. Oxygen and other nutrients pass from the blood cells and plasma to individual tissue cells through the very thin walls of the capillaries (Figure 4-29). Carbon dioxide and other metabolic waste products pass from the tissue cells to the blood to be carried away. Capillary perfusion is the process in which oxygen and nutrients are brought to every cell. With capillary perfusion, waste and carbon dioxide are also removed at the cellular level.

Perfusion is the flow of fluid through an organ or tissue. Through perfusion, our tissues and cells receive the oxygen and nourishment they need to work properly. Perfusion works much like a delivery and collection service. When perfusion is working as it should, the blood delivers nutrients and oxygen to all body cells. At the same time, it picks up waste products and carbon dioxide from the cells. Perfusion of the whole body by blood keeps its cells alive and healthy. No part of the body can exist without adequate perfusion for an indefinite period of time. Perfusion of an organ can fail for a number of reasons: 1) when the blood vessels are injured; 2) when shock (hypoperfusion) develops; and 3) when the heart is injured. Shock occurs with inadequate circulation of blood through tissue or an organ. Without adequate perfusion, cells and tissues eventually die.

### The Veins

Once blood passes through the network of capillaries, it returns to the heart

**FIGURE 4-28**

Major arteries of the body

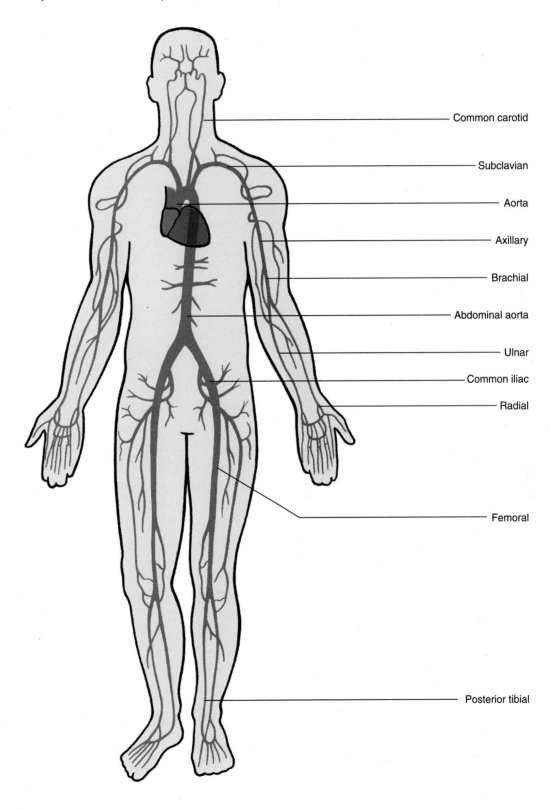

Common carotid

Subclavian

Aorta

Axillary

Brachial

Abdominal aorta

Ulnar

Common iliac

Radial

Femoral

Posterior tibial

## FIGURE 4-29

Oxygen and carbon dioxide exchange

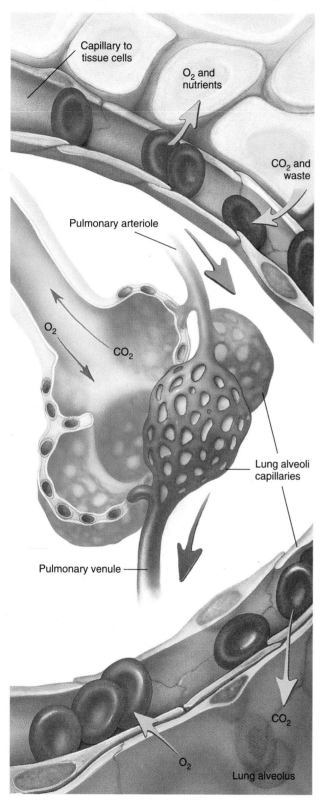

Capillary to tissue cells

$O_2$ and nutrients

$CO_2$ and waste

Pulmonary arteriole

$O_2$

$CO_2$

Lung alveoli capillaries

Pulmonary venule

$CO_2$

$O_2$

Lung alveolus

through the veins. Capillaries empty into small venules that join to form veins. The veins become larger and larger and ultimately form two major vessels—the superior and inferior venae cavae (Figure 4-30). Veins have much thinner walls than arteries and are generally larger in diameter (Figure 4-31).

Veins in the arms and legs have one-way valves that allow blood to flow in a central direction, but prevent backflow. Varicose veins in the legs develop when the veins become dilated and eventually fail due to excessive back pressure. Veins in the thorax, abdomen, head, and neck have no such valves.

The venae cavae channel blood from the body and collect it just before it enters the heart. These two major vessels, part of the great vessels, are located in the midline, just to the left of the spine. Blood from the head, neck, shoulders, and upper extremities passes through the superior vena cava. Blood from the abdomen, pelvis, and lower extremities passes through the inferior vena cava. The superior and inferior venae cavae join at the right atrium of the heart. The right ventricle receives blood from the right atrium and pumps it through the pulmonary arteries into the lungs.

Blood is pumped from the right side of the heart through the pulmonary artery into the lungs. It divides into right and left pulmonary arteries. The arteries divide until they finally connect to the pulmonary capillary system. The exchange of oxygen and carbon dioxide between air in the lungs and blood in the capillaries is rapid and completed before the blood reaches the end of the capillaries. The newly oxygenated blood is then collected in a network of combining veins and enters the four pulmonary veins that unite at the left atrium. It then passes into the left ventricle and is pumped to the body to be distributed by the arterial circulation.

**FIGURE 4-30**

Major veins of the body

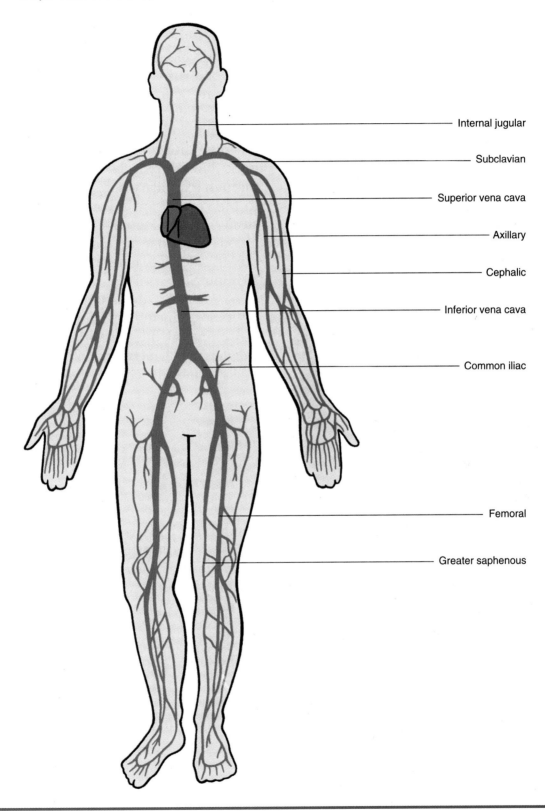

Internal jugular

Subclavian

Superior vena cava

Axillary

Cephalic

Inferior vena cava

Common iliac

Femoral

Greater saphenous

## FIGURE 4-31

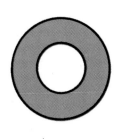

Cross section of a vein (right) and an artery (left)

## FIGURE 4-32

Red blood cells, white blood cells, platelets

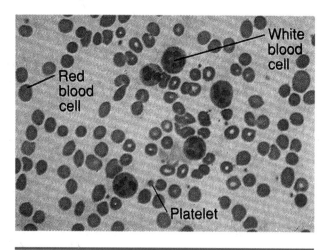

White blood cell

Red blood cell

Platelet

## COMPONENTS OF BLOOD

Blood is a complex, thick, red fluid composed of plasma, erythrocytes (red blood cells), leukocytes (white blood cells), and platelets. Plasma is a sticky, yellow fluid that carries the blood cells and nutrients. It also transports cellular waste material to the organs of excretion. Plasma contains most of the compounds needed to produce a blood clot. The hemoglobin molecules in red blood cells contain iron, give color to the blood, and carry oxygen. White cells

play a role in helping the body to fight infection. Platelets are tiny, disk-shaped elements that are much smaller than the red blood cells. Platelets are essential in the initial formation of a blood clot—the mechanism that stops bleeding (Figure 4-32).

Blood in arteries is characteristically bright red, because its hemoglobin is rich in oxygen. Blood from an artery is under pressure and will gush or spurt intermittently when an artery is cut. Blood in the veins is dark bluish red, because it has passed through a capillary bed, giving up its oxygen to the cells. From a vein, blood flows in a steady stream (Figure 4-33). From capillaries, blood will ooze at many tiny individual points. Clotting normally takes from 6 to 10 minutes.

A detailed explanation of circulatory physiology, including information about the pulse and blood pressure, is presented in chapter 5, Vital Signs and Patient History.

# THE MUSCULOSKELETAL SYSTEM

The human body is a well-designed system whose form, upright posture, and movement are provided by the **musculoskeletal system.** As its combination form suggests, the term musculoskeletal refers to the bones and voluntary muscles of the body. The musculoskeletal system also protects the vital internal organs of the body.

## MUSCLES

Muscles are a form of tissue that allow the body to move. There are more than 600 muscles in the musculoskeletal system. They are generally divided into three types: skeletal, smooth, and cardiac.

**FIGURE 4-33**

Venous, arterial, capillary bleeding

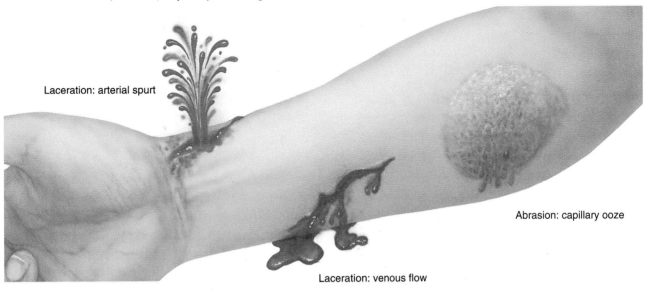

Laceration: arterial spurt

Abrasion: capillary ooze

Laceration: venous flow

## Skeletal Muscle

Skeletal muscle, so named because it attaches to the bones of the skeleton, forms the major muscle mass of the body. It is also called voluntary muscle, because all skeletal muscle is under direct voluntary control of the brain and can contract or relax at will. Skeletal muscle is also called striated muscle, because when viewed under the microscope it has characteristic stripes (striations). All bodily movement results from contraction or relaxation of skeletal muscle. Usually, a specific movement is the result of several muscles contracting and relaxing at the same time.

All skeletal muscles are supplied with arteries, veins, and nerves. Arterial blood brings oxygen and nutrients to the muscles, and the veins carry away carbon dioxide and water. Muscles cannot function without an on-going supply of oxygen and nutrients and removal of waste products. Muscle cramps result without adequate oxygen or nutrients or when acidic waste products are not carried away (Figure 4-34).

Skeletal muscle is under direct control of the nervous system and responds to a command from the brain to move a specific body part. Specific nerves pass directly from the brain to the spinal cord. There they connect with other nerves that exit from the spinal cord and pass to each skeletal muscle. Electrical impulses are carried from the cells in the brain and spinal cord along the peripheral nerves to each muscle, signaling it to contract. When this normal nerve supply is lost through injury to the brain, spinal cord, or peripheral nerves, the voluntary control of the muscle is lost and the muscle becomes paralyzed.

Most skeletal muscles attach directly to bone by tough, rope-like cords of fibrous tissue called tendons. Tendons continue the fascia that covers the skeletal muscles. The fascia is much like the skin of a sausage in that it surrounds the muscle tissue. At either end of the muscle, the fascia extends beyond the muscle to attach to a bone. This muscle-tendon unit crosses a joint and is responsible for the motion of that joint.

## FIGURE 4-34

Venous, arterial, nerve supply to skeletal muscle

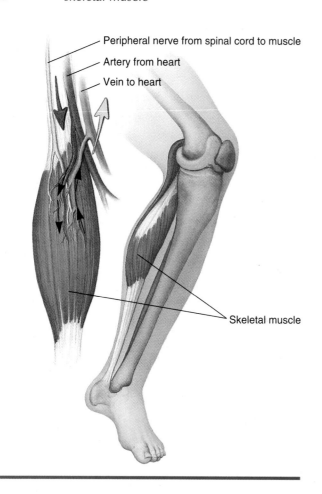

— Peripheral nerve from spinal cord to muscle
— Artery from heart
— Vein to heart

Skeletal muscle

can change the diameter of the vessel to control the amount of blood flowing through it (Figure 4-35).

Smooth muscle responds only to primitive stimuli such as stretching, heat, or the need to relieve waste. Generally speaking, you cannot control the motion of this type of muscle.

### Cardiac Muscle

As described earlier, the heart is a specialized muscle composed of a pair of pumps of unequal force—one of lower and one of higher pressure. The heart is always working, from the time we are born until the time we die. It is an especially adapted involuntary muscle with its own very rich blood supply and its own regulatory system. Microscopically, it looks different from both skeletal and smooth muscle. Cardiac muscle can tolerate an interruption of its blood supply for only a few seconds. It requires a continuous supply of oxygen and glucose to work properly. Because of its special structure and function, cardiac muscle is placed in a separate category.

### Smooth Muscle

Smooth muscle carries out much of the automatic work of the body. Therefore, it is also called involuntary muscle. Smooth muscle is found in the walls of most tubular structures of the body, such as the gastrointestinal tract, the urinary system, the blood vessels, and the bronchi of the lungs. Contraction and relaxation of smooth muscle propels or controls the flow of the contents of these structures along their course. For example, the rhythmic contraction and relaxation of the smooth muscles of the wall of the intestine propel ingested food through it. Smooth muscle in the walls of a blood vessel

## FIGURE 4-35

Contraction (bottom) and relaxation (top) of smooth muscle

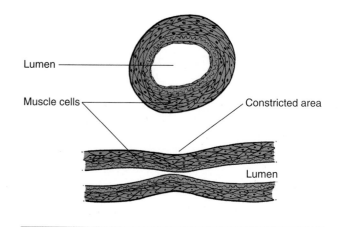

Lumen

Muscle cells

Constricted area

Lumen

# THE NERVOUS SYSTEM

The **nervous system** controls virtually all activities of the body, both voluntary and involuntary activities. The nervous system can be divided functionally into somatic (voluntary) and autonomic (involuntary) components, and anatomically into the central and peripheral nervous systems.

## FUNCTIONAL COMPONENTS

The part of the nervous system that regulates voluntary activities, such as walking, talking, and writing, is called the somatic nervous system. However, many activities occur without voluntary control. These activities are under the control of the autonomic, or in-voluntary, nervous system. The autonomic nervous system controls automatic body functions. These include all involuntary actions necessary for basic body functions, such as digestion, dilation and constriction of blood vessels, and sweating. Some of the cells that form the autonomic nervous system are inside the central nervous system. Others lie alongside the spinal column in the cervical and lumbar regions.

## ANATOMIC COMPONENTS

The nervous system is divided into two anatomic parts: the central nervous system and the peripheral nervous system. The central nervous system (CNS) is made up of the brain and the spinal cord. Many of the cells in the CNS have long fibers. These

## EMT

### CIRCULATION SITUATION

It's been a slow Friday night on shift when the radio crackles to life: "Rescue 5 respond to the East End Machine Works for an explosion." En route, the dispatcher radios to tell you that a piece of machinery has exploded, injuring the operator. On arrival, you make your way inside and past the crowd of co-workers. You find a 27-year-old man lying by a smoking machine. He is conscious and answering questions, but is very anxious. There is blood spurting from a 4" laceration on the inside of his upper arm. He also has several small cuts on his face and chest.

### For Discussion

1. Why is it difficult to stop arterial bleeding?
2. How important is it to be able to accurately estimate blood loss?

**YOU ARE THE EMT**

## FIGURE 4-36

Anatomic regions of the brain

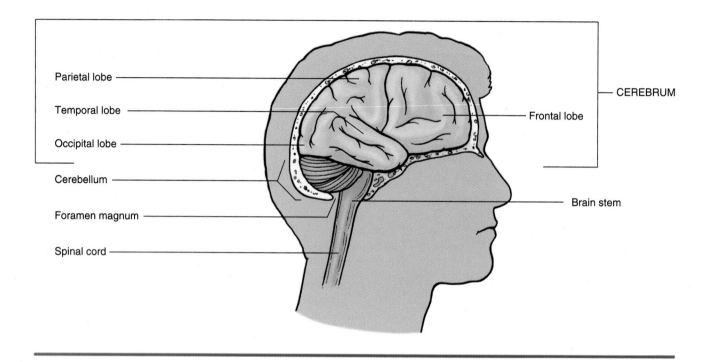

Parietal lobe

Temporal lobe

Occipital lobe

Cerebellum

Foramen magnum

Spinal cord

CEREBRUM

Frontal lobe

Brain stem

---

fibers extend out from the cell body through openings in the bony covering. The fibers then form a cable of nerve fibers that link the CNS to the various organs of the body. These cables of nerve fibers make up the peripheral nervous system. In the peripheral nervous system, there are two major types of nerves—sensory and motor nerve fibers. The sensory nerves carry information from the body to the central nervous system. The motor nerves carry information from the central nervous system to the muscles of the body.

### The Central Nervous System

The CNS is the part of the nervous system that is covered and protected by bones. The brain is covered by the skull, and the spinal cord is covered by the spinal column. The major parts of most nerve cells (the nucleus and the cell body) lie within the CNS. It is here that the majority of the nerve cells reside and connect to the peripheral areas of the body through the long nerve fibers.

**The brain** The brain is responsible for all voluntary body activities, the perception of our surroundings, and the control of our reactions to the environment. The brain also enables us to experience all the fine shadings of thought and feeling that make us individuals. It receives a vast amount of information from the environment, sorts it all out, and directs the body to respond appropriately. The brain is divided into several areas, all of which have specific functions. The three major divisions of the brain are the cerebrum, the cerebellum, and the brain stem.

The largest part of the brain is the cerebrum, which is sometimes called the "gray matter." The cerebrum makes up about 75% of the volume of the brain and is composed of several lobes: frontal, parietal, temporal, and occipital (Figure 4-36). The cerebrum on one side of the brain controls activities on the opposite side of the body. You may have heard the phrases "left brain" and "right brain." The cerebrum on the left side of the brain controls activities on the right side of the body.

Each lobe of the cerebrum is responsible for a specific function. For example, one group of brain cells in the frontal lobe is responsible for the activity of all the voluntary muscles of the body. Brain cells in this area create impulses that are sent along nerve fibers that extend from each cell into the spinal cord. Another area in the parietal lobe has cells that receive sensory impulses from the peripheral nerves of the body. Other parts of the cerebrum are responsible for other body functions. For instance, the occipital region, on the back of the cerebrum, receives visual impulses for the eyes, and other areas control hearing, balance, and speech. Still other parts of the cerebrum are responsible for emotions and other characteristics of our personality.

Underneath the great mass of cerebral tissue lies the cerebellum, sometimes called the "little brain." The major function of this area is to coordinate the various activities of the brain, particularly body movements. Without the cerebellum, very specialized muscular activities such as writing or sewing would be impossible.

**The brain stem**    The brain stem is so called because the brain appears to be sitting on this portion of the CNS as a plant sits on its stem. The brain stem is the most primitive part of the central nervous system. It lies deep within the cranium and is the best protected part of the CNS. The brain stem is the controlling center for virtually all body functions that are absolutely necessary for life. Cells in this part of the brain control cardiac, respiratory, and other basic body functions.

**The spinal cord**    The spinal cord is the other major portion of the central nervous system. Like the brain, the spinal cord contains nerve cell bodies, but the major portion of the spinal cord is made up of nerve fibers that extend from the cells of the brain (Figure 4-37). These nerve fibers transmit information to and from the brain. All the fibers join together just below the brain stem to form the spinal cord. The spinal cord exits through a large opening at the base of the skull called the foramen magnum. It is contained within the spinal canal down to the level of the second lumbar vertebra. The spinal canal is created by the vertebrae, stacked one on the other. Each vertebra surrounds the cord to form the bony spinal canal.

The spinal cord transmits messages between the brain and the body. These messages are passed along the nerve fibers as electrical impulses, just as messages are

## FIGURE 4-37

The spinal cord

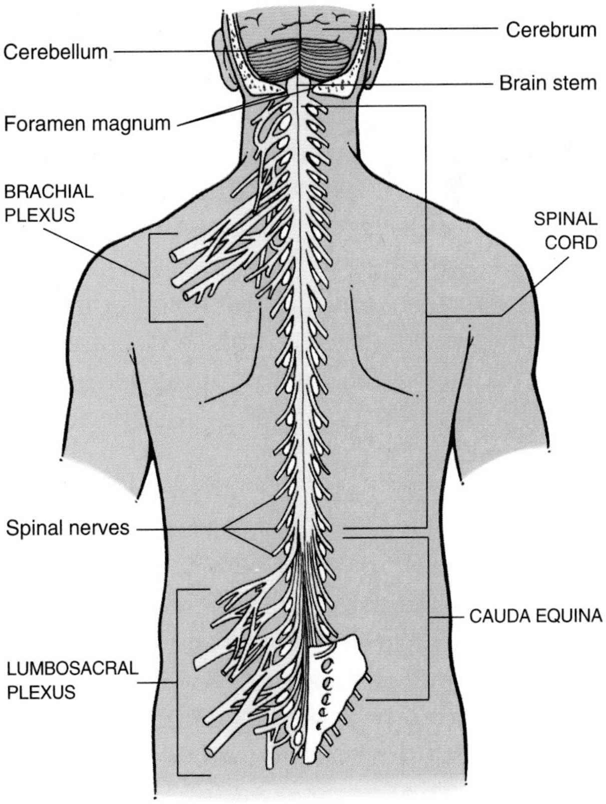

passed along a telephone cable. The nerve fibers are arranged in specific bundles within the spinal cord to carry the messages from one specific area of the body to the brain and back.

### The Peripheral Nervous System

The peripheral nervous system is composed of 31 pairs of spinal nerves and 12 pairs of cranial nerves. At each vertebral level, on each side of the spinal cord, a spinal nerve exits the spinal cord and passes through an opening in the bony canal (Figure 4-38).

The spinal nerves are composed of nerve fibers from nerve cells that originate within the spinal cord. These nerve fibers conduct sensory impulses from the skin and other organs to the spinal cord. They also conduct motor impulses from the spinal cord to the muscles that are present in that part of the body. For example, the spinal nerve between the seventh and eighth ribs carries sensory fibers from the skin between those two ribs. This nerve also has motor nerve fibers to innervate the intercostal muscle between the seventh and eighth ribs (Figure 4-39).

This specific arrangement of nerve fibers becomes more complex in the cervical and lumbar regions. This is due to the large number of muscles in the arms and legs that must be supplied with nerve fibers. The spinal nerves combine to form complex nerve networks (plexi) in these two areas—the brachial plexus for the upper extremity and the lumbosacral plexus for the lower extremity.

There are 12 pairs of cranial nerves that exit the brain through holes in the skull. For the most part, they are very specialized nerves designed to provide specific functions in the head and face. For example, the facial (seventh cranial) nerves send motor impulses to many of the facial muscles.

There are three categories of peripheral nerves: sensory nerves, motor nerves, and connecting nerves.

## FIGURE 4-38

Spinal nerves exiting the vertebral canal

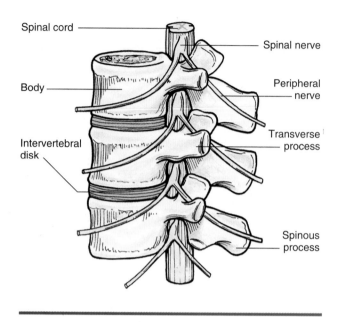

**Sensory nerves**    Sensory nerves are quite complex, and there are many different types in the nervous system. One type forms the retina of the eye; others are responsible for the hearing and balancing mechanisms in the ear. Still other sensory cells are located within the skin, muscles, joints, lungs, and other organs of the body. When a sensory cell is stimulated, it transmits its own special message to the brain. There are special sensory nerves to detect heat, cold, position, motion, pressure, pain, balance, light, taste, and smell, as well as other sensations. Specialized nerve endings are adapted for each cell so that it perceives only one type of sensation and it transmits only that message.

Sensory impulses constantly provide information to the brain about what the different parts of our body are doing in relation to our surroundings. Thus, the brain is continuously made aware of its surroundings. The cranial nerves supply sensations directly to the brain. What we see reaches the brain directly by way of the optic nerve in each eye. The nerve cells and sensory

## FIGURE 4-39

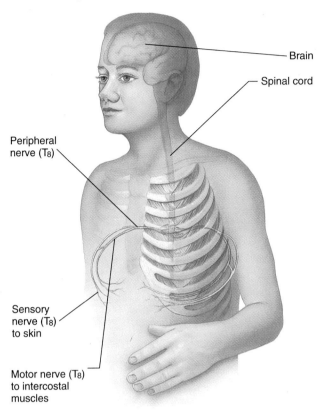

Spinal nerves innervating intercostal muscles

Brain

Spinal cord

Peripheral nerve (T8)

Sensory nerve (T8) to skin

Motor nerve (T8) to intercostal muscles

endings of the optic nerve lie in the retina of the eye. The sensory endings are stimulated by light. The impulses are then carried along the optic nerve, which passes through a hole in the back of the eye socket and carries impulses to the occipital portion of the brain.

When sensory nerve endings in the extremities are stimulated, the impulses are transmitted along a peripheral nerve to the spinal cord. The cell body of the peripheral nerve lies in the spinal cord. The impulse is then transmitted from that cell body to another nerve ending in the spinal cord. The impulse is then sent up the spinal cord to the sensory area in the parietal lobe of the brain, where the sensory information can be interpreted and acted on by the brain (Figure 4-40).

**Motor nerves**     Each muscle in the body has its own motor nerve. The cell body for each motor nerve lies in the spinal cord, and a fiber from the cell body extends as part of the peripheral nerve to its specific muscle. Electrical impulses produced by the cell body in the spinal cord are transmitted along the motor nerve to the muscle and cause it to

## FIGURE 4-40

Central and peripheral nervous systems

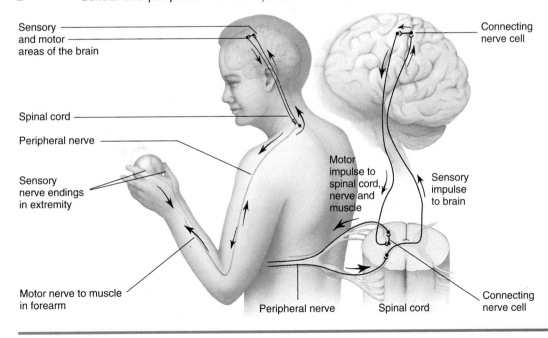

Sensory and motor areas of the brain

Spinal cord

Peripheral nerve

Sensory nerve endings in extremity

Motor nerve to muscle in forearm

Peripheral nerve

Spinal cord

Connecting nerve cell

Motor impulse to spinal cord, nerve and muscle

Sensory impulse to brain

Connecting nerve cell

**FIGURE 4-41**

Reflex arc

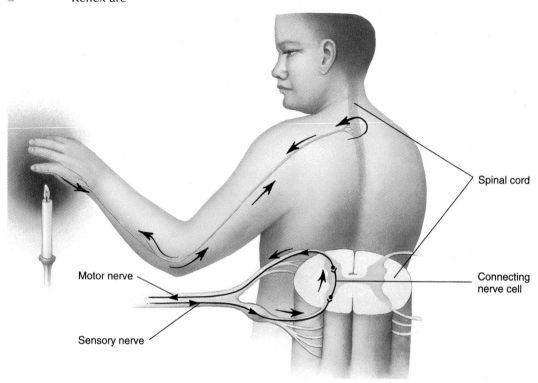

Spinal cord

Motor nerve

Connecting
nerve cell

Sensory nerve

contract. The cell body in the spinal cord is stimulated by an impulse produced in the motor strip of the cerebral cortex. This impulse is transmitted along the spinal cord to the cell body of the motor nerve.

**Connecting nerves**     Within the brain and the spinal cord are cells with short fibers that connect the sensory nerves with the motor nerves. In the spinal cord, they connect the sensory and motor nerves directly, bypassing the brain. These connecting nerves allow sensory and motor impulses to be transmitted from one nerve to another within the central nervous system.

The connecting nerves in the spinal cord complete a reflex arc between the sensory and motor nerves of the limbs. An irritating stimulus to the sensory nerve, such as heat, will be transmitted from the sensory nerve along the connecting nerve directly to the

motor nerve. This will stimulate the sensory nerve (Figure 4-41). The muscle responds promptly, withdrawing the limb from the irritating stimulus even before this information can be transmitted to the brain. When a physician taps your knee with a rubber hammer, he or she is testing to see whether your reflex arc is intact.

# THE SKIN

The skin is the largest single organ in the body. The skin has three major functions, as follows:

1.  To protect the body in the environment
2.  To regulate the temperature of the body
3.  To transmit information from the environment to the brain

## FUNCTIONS OF THE SKIN

Our skin protects us in many ways. Over 70% of the body is composed of water. This water contains a delicate balance of chemical substances in solution. The skin is watertight and serves to keep this balanced internal solution intact. The skin also protects the body from the invasion of infectious organisms—bacteria, viruses, and fungi. These organisms are everywhere and are routinely found lying on the skin surface and deep in its grooves and glands. However, they never penetrate intact skin. Germs cannot pass through the skin unless it is broken by injury or disease. Thus, the skin provides us with constant protection against outside invaders.

The skin also regulates body temperature. Energy in the body is derived from metabolism (chemical reaction) that must take place within a very narrow temperature range. If our body temperature is too low, these reactions cannot proceed, metabolism ceases, and the body dies. If our body temperature becomes too high, the rate of metabolism increases. Dangerously high temperatures producing too high a metabolic rate can result in permanent tissue damage and death.

Blood vessels in the skin constrict when the body is in a cold environment and dilate when the body is in a warm environment. In a cold environment, constriction of the blood vessels diverts blood away from the skin. This decreases the amount of heat radiated from the body surface. When the environment is hot, the blood vessels dilate, and the skin becomes flushed or red. As a result, heat radiates from the body surface.

Also, in a hot environment, sweat is secreted to the skin surface from the sweat glands. Evaporation of the sweat requires energy. This energy, as body heat, is taken from the body during the evaporation process, which causes the body temperature to fall. Sweating alone will not reduce body temperature; evaporation of the sweat must also occur.

Our skin also transmits information from the environment to the brain. This is done through a rich supply of sensory nerves that originate in the skin. Nerve endings that lie in the skin are adapted to perceive and transmit information about heat, cold, external pressure, pain, and the position of the body in space. The skin recognizes any changes in the environment. The skin also reacts to pressure, pain, and pleasurable stimuli.

## ANATOMY OF THE SKIN

The skin is divided into two parts: the superficial epidermis and the deeper dermis. The superficial epidermis contains several layers of cells. The deeper dermis contains the specialized skin structures. Below the skin lies the subcutaneous layer of fat (Figure 4-42). The cells of the epidermis are sealed to form a watertight protective covering for the body.

The epidermis is composed of several layers of cells. At the base of the epidermis is the germinal layer. This part of the skin continuously produces new cells that gradually rise to the surface. On the way to the surface, these cells die and form the watertight covering. The cells of the epidermis are held together securely by an oily substance called sebum. Sebum is secreted by the sebaceous (oil) glands of the dermis. The outermost cells of the epidermis are constantly rubbed away and replaced by new cells produced by the germinal layer. The deeper cells in the germinal layer also contain pigment granules that (along with the blood vessels lying in the dermis) produce skin color.

The epidermis varies in thickness in different areas of the body. It is quite thick on the soles of the feet, the back, the palm of the hand, and the scalp. However, in some

## FIGURE 4-42

Layers of the skin

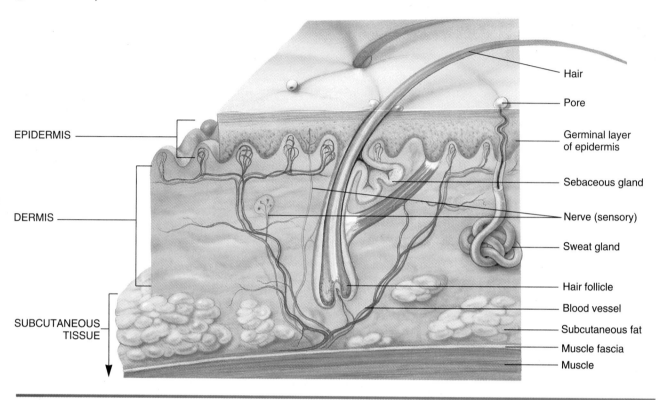

EPIDERMIS

DERMIS

SUBCUTANEOUS TISSUE

Hair

Pore

Germinal layer of epidermis

Sebaceous gland

Nerve (sensory)

Sweat gland

Hair follicle

Blood vessel

Subcutaneous fat

Muscle fascia

Muscle

areas of the body, such as the lips, the epidermis is only two or three cell layers in thickness. The watertight seal provided by the epidermis prevents the invasion of bacteria and other organisms.

The deeper part of the skin, the dermis, is separated from the epidermis by a layer of germinal cells. Within the dermis lie many of the special structures of the skin, such as sweat glands, sebaceous glands, hair follicles, blood vessels, and specialized nerve endings.

### Specialized Structures

**Glands**    Glands are special structures that produce substances to the skin, membranes, or circulation. Several glands produce sweat for cooling the body. Sweat is discharged onto the surface of the skin through small pores, or ducts, that pass through the epidermis onto the skin surface. The sebaceous glands lie next to hair follicles and secrete sebum along the hair follicle to the skin surface. In addition to providing waterproofing for the skin, sebum keeps the skin supple so that it does not crack.

**Hair follicles**    Hair follicles are small organs that produce hair. There is one follicle for each hair connected with a sebaceous gland and also with a tiny muscle. The muscle serves to pull the hair into an erect position when the individual is cold or frightened. All hair grows continuously and is either cut off or worn away by clothing.

**Blood vessels**    Blood vessels provide nutrients and oxygen to the skin. The blood

## THE LANGUAGE OF MEDICINE

You've just finished transporting a 10-year-old boy who fell out of his grandfather's apple tree to Saint Mary's Hospital. You give your report to the triage nurse, and the emergency department staff begins to work him up. Even though he fell approximately 15' out of the tree, in what certainly could have been a very dangerous fall, he appeared to have only minor injuries, even though he bumped and scraped a fair amount of his body. You pour yourself a cup of coffee and sit down to write up the run report.

### For Discussion

1. What could happen if patient care information is not accurately communicated either during the radio report or on the run report?

2. Ineffective written or verbal communication with the emergency physician or nursing staff could have what impact?

---

vessels lie in the dermis. Small branches extend up to the germinal layer. There are no blood vessels in the epidermis. A complex array of nerve endings also lie in the dermis. These specialized nerve endings are sensitive to environmental stimuli. These nerve endings respond to the stimuli and send impulses along the nerves to the brain.

**Subcutaneous tissue**     Beneath the skin, immediately under but attached to the dermis, lies the subcutaneous tissue. The subcutaneous tissue is composed largely of fat cells. Fat serves as insulation for the body and as a reservoir to store energy. The amount of subcutaneous tissue varies greatly from per-

son to person. Beneath the subcutaneous tissue lie the muscles and the skeleton.

**Mucous membranes**     Skin covers all external surfaces of the body. However, various openings to the body, including the mouth, nose, anus, and vagina, are not covered by skin. These openings are lined with mucous membranes. A mucous membrane also lines the entire gastrointestinal tract from the mouth to the anus. Mucous membranes are quite similar to skin in that they provide a protective barrier against bacterial invasion. However, they differ from skin in that they secrete mucus, a watery substance that lubricates the openings. Thus, mucous membranes are moist whereas the skin is dry.

**TABLE 4-4**     ENDOCRINE GLANDS

| Endocrine Gland | Location | Function | Hormones Produced |
|---|---|---|---|
| Pituitary | Base of skull | Regulate all other endocrine glands | Multiple, very important hormones |
| Thyroid | Neck (over the larynx) | Regulate metabolism | Thyroxin and others |
| Parathyroid | Neck (behind the thyroid) (3–5 glands) | Regulate serum calcium | Parathormone |
| Adrenal | Abdomen | Regulate salt, sugar, and sexual function | Adrenalin and others |
| Ovary | Female pelvis (2 glands) | Regulate sexual function, characteristics, and reproduction | Estrogen and others |
| Testes | Male scrotum (2 glands) | Regulate sexual function, characteristics, and reproduction | Testosterone and others |
| Pancreas | Abdomen | Regulate sugar metabolism and other functions | Insulin and other hormones |

# THE ENDOCRINE SYSTEM

The brain controls the body through both the nervous system and the endocrine system. The **endocrine system** is a complex message and control system that integrates many body functions. It releases substances called hormones, either by target organs or released directly. Adrenaline and insulin are examples of hormones (Table 4-4). Each endocrine gland produces one or more hormones. Each hormone has a specific effect on some organ, tissue, or process. The brain controls the release of hormones by the endocrine glands with other (stimulating or inhibiting) hormones.

The final effect influences the endocrine gland and the brain. As a result, we have a tightly controlled system with primary and secondary feedback loops to keep body systems in balance. For example, when we are frightened, the brain stimulates the adrenal gland through a hormone to release adrenaline from the adrenal gland. Release of adrenaline increases our blood pressure and heart rate. The resulting increase in blood pressure and heart rate decreases the amount of hormone released by the adrenal gland. The brain then reduces the amount of stimulation to the adrenal gland. Thus, a new steady state is achieved at a heightened level of alertness. Insulin is another hormone intimately involved in the control of the blood sugar and metabolism of food.

Excesses or deficiencies in hormones cause various diseases. With endocrine diseases, specific bodily functions are increased, decreased, or absent. Diabetes mellitus is a common problem. Because production of the hormone insulin is deficient, the body is unable to use sugar normally. This disease also damages the small blood vessels in the body. The tissue damage that results is as much a part of diabetes as is the difficulty in regulating the amount of sugar in the blood. A more detailed explanation of diabetes is presented in chapter 17, Diabetic Emergencies.

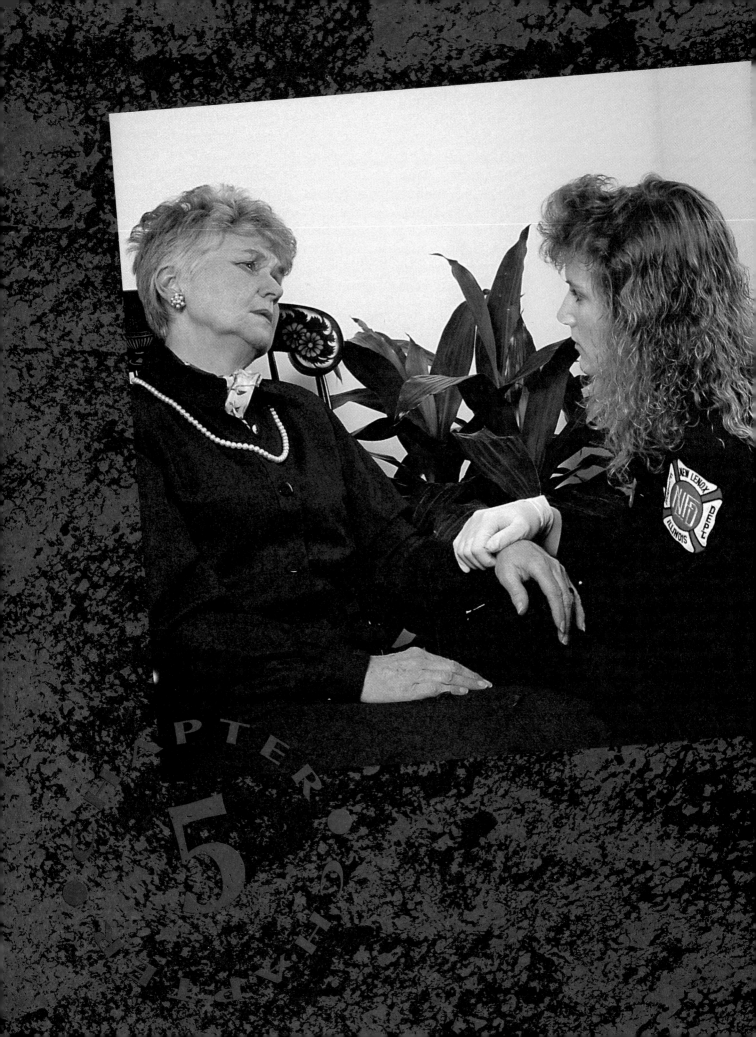

# Vital Signs and Patient History

After you have read this chapter, you should be able to:

- Describe the methods to obtain a breathing rate and differentiate between shallow, labored, and noisy breathing.
- Describe the methods to obtain a pulse rate and differentiate between a strong, weak, regular, and irregular pulse.
- Identify normal and abnormal skin colors, temperatures, and conditions.
- Identify normal and abnormal pupils.
- Identify normal and abnormal capillary refill in infants and children.
- Explain how to use auscultation or palpation to obtain a blood pressure.
- Discuss the need to accurately report, record, and reassess the baseline vital signs.
- List the components of a SAMPLE history.
- Discuss the need to search for additional medical information.

## Overview

As an EMT-B, you will be using your eyes, ears, nose, hands, and a few simple instruments to obtain a great deal of information about your patient. As you begin your assessment, you will be gathering and recording a variety of information on the patient. You need to know the patient's chief complaint, age, sex, race, and most importantly, baseline vital signs. This information will help you to identify and treat any life-threatening conditions first, and then assess the patient carefully for other complaints or findings.

There are five basic vital signs: respirations, pulse, perfusion, pupils, and blood pressure. These signs are considered "vital" because they measure very important functions of the respiratory, cardiovascular, and central nervous systems. By accurately measuring and recording vital signs over a period of time, you will be able to note trends in the patient's condition.

## Key Terms

**Auscultation**   Listening to sounds within the organs, usually with a stethoscope; a method of taking a patient's blood pressure.

**Blood pressure**   The pressure of the circulating blood against the walls of the arteries.

**Chief complaint**   The patient's response to a general question such as "What's wrong?" or "What happened?"

**Palpation**   Examination by touch.

**Perfusion**   Circulation of blood within an organ or tissue in adequate amounts to meet the cells' current needs.

**Pulse**   The pressure wave that is felt with the expansion and contraction of an artery, consistent with the beat of the heart. It may be felt with a finger.

**SAMPLE history**   A patient's history consisting of **S**igns/ symptoms, **A**llergies, **M**edications, **P**ertinent past history, **L**ast oral intake, and **E**vents leading to the illness/injury.

**Sign**   A condition displayed by the patient that you observe, such as bleeding or a contusion.

**Symptom**   A condition that the patient tells you about, such as "I feel dizzy."

# GENERAL INFORMATION

When you arrive at the scene, begin to assess the patient and the environment. You may have already received some general information from the dispatcher. This may include the patient's age, sex, race, and why the patient called for help. This is known as the **chief complaint.** From here, you can proceed to assessing the patient's baseline vital signs.

# BASELINE VITAL SIGNS

## RESPIRATIONS

Normal breathing occurs easily, without pain, noise, or effort. The rate of respirations is usually between 12 and 20 breaths per minute for an adult (Table 5-1). However, the respiration rate can vary widely. A patient who is a well-trained athlete may breathe only 6 to 8 times per minute. You should begin a record of the rate and type of respirations when you first see a patient, and observe and record any changes that occur.

| **TABLE 5-1** | **NORMAL RESPIRATION RATE RANGES** |
|---|---|
| Adults | 12 to 20 breaths per minute |
| Children | 15 to 30 breaths per minute |
| Infants | 25 to 50 breaths per minute |

To obtain the breathing rate in a patient, count the number of breaths in a 30-second period and multiply by two. Avoid letting the patient know that you are counting to prevent influencing the rate.

Breathing is assessed by observing the patient's chest rise and fall. Breathing is assessed both in rate and quality. The rate is determined by counting the number of breaths in a 30-second period and multiplying by 2. Make sure the patient does not know that you are counting respirations. This will avoid influencing the rate.

The quality of breathing can be determined while assessing the rate. Quality can be described in one of four of the following ways:

1. *Normal.* There is average chest wall motion, with no use of accessory muscles. Breathing is neither shallow nor deep.

2. *Shallow.* There is slight chest or abdominal wall motion.

3. *Labored.* There is increased breathing effort, grunting, and use of accessory muscles. Nasal flaring is present, along with possible gasping, and supraclavicular and intercostal retractions in infants and children.

4. *Noisy.* There is an increase in the sound of breathing, which may include snoring, wheezing, gurgling, stridor, and crowing.

While you are counting respirations, make a note of the breathing rhythm. Normal breathing is fairly regular, but certain illnesses and injuries may produce irregular or abnormal breathing patterns.

Rapid, shallow respirations are often associated with shock. Very deep, rapid respirations in an unconscious patient with head trauma point to signs of severe injury. Deep, gasping, labored, and noisy breathing may indicate a partial airway obstruction, respiratory failure, or chronic lung disease. With respiratory depression or arrest, there is little or no movement of the chest and abdomen. There is also little or no airflow felt or heard at the nose and mouth. Choking can be identified by the patient's inability to cough or talk. You can

FIGURE 5-1

The universal gesture for choking

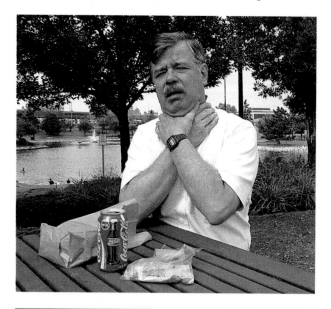

also identify a choking victim by the instinctive, nearly universal, gesture of a patient clutching the throat (Figure 5-1).

Sputum is matter that is coughed from the lungs. An injury to the chest may cause a patient to cough up blood or frothy (foam-like) sputum. Congestive heart failure can also cause the production of a frothy pink sputum. Patients with pneumonia and bronchitis may cough up thick sputum of various colors. You should note the volume, color, and other characteristics of any sputum that is produced. Coughing up red blood is a critical emergency.

## PULSE

The **pulse** is the pressure wave that is felt as the heart contracts and propels blood through the arteries. It is a useful indicator of the condition of the heart, the blood vessels, and the blood itself. You measure a pulse by palpating (feeling) an artery at a pulse point, which is where an artery lies close to the surface of the skin.

Although a pulse can be palpated at any of several pulse points, the most common place is in the wrist, along the path of the radial artery (Figure 5-2a). A radial pulse should be assessed in all patients 1 year or older. In patients younger than 1 year, a brachial pulse should be assessed. If a pulse is present, the rate and quality should be assessed.

If a radial pulse cannot be palpated at either wrist, you should attempt to find it in the neck along the path of the carotid artery (Figure 5-2b). The carotid pulse is easier to feel in an emergency situation, particularly when the blood pressure is low. First, make sure that the patient is in a lying or sitting

**FIGURE 5-2**

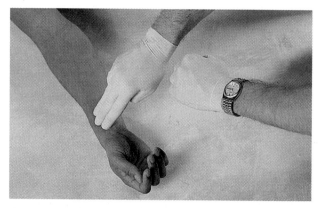

**A**  Palpating the radial pulse

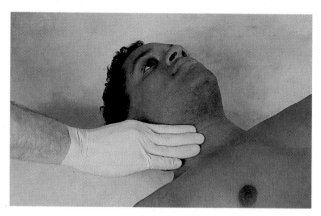

**B**  Palpating the carotid pulse

position. Palpate for the pulse in the neck under the anterior edge of the sternocleidomastoid muscle. Use caution and avoid excess pressure when assessing the carotid pulse in an elderly patient. Never try to feel both carotid pulses at the same time because excessive pressure on the two arteries might cut off circulation to the brain.

### Taking a Pulse

Taking a pulse consists of assessing the rate, volume, and regularity of the pulse. The normal pulse rate is the number of beats per minute and is a reflection of the heart rate. The average adult's pulse rate ranges from 60 to 100 beats per minute. In a child, the normal rate is 80 to 100 beats per minute. In toddlers, it is 100 to 120 beats per minute and in newborn infants, normal rates range from 120 to 140 beats per minute (Table 5-2). The pulse rate is usually obtained by counting the number of beats that occur over a 30-second period and multiplying that number by 2. However, if the pulse is slower than 70 beats/min or is irregular, the rate should be counted for a full minute to more accurately measure the pulse rate.

The pulse volume is a rough indicator of the strength of the heart's contractions. After palpating the pulse in many patients, you will develop a sense of the pulse volume. A rapid, "thready," weak pulse can indicate shock from loss of blood. A "bounding" pulse can be present in fright or with high blood pressure. If you cannot feel a pulse, it may mean that the artery being palpated is blocked from disease or injury, or that the heart is weak or has stopped beating.

The third important characteristic of the pulse is the regularity of its rhythm. The frequency of beats should be regular. When beats are absent (skipped beats) or irregular, this usually signals a heart rhythm problem. The pulse is an instant indicator of the condition of the patient. This means it should be taken and recorded (rate, volume, and regularity) frequently during any emergency call. The frequency of recording the pulse and other vital signs should be governed by medical control or local protocol.

The pulse is one of the vital signs that you can monitor continuously in most emergency situations, including in the back of a moving ambulance. For conscious patients, the hands-on contact with the radial pulse by a caring EMT-B is a very reassuring gesture that has a medically useful function as well.

| **TABLE 5-2** | **AVERAGE PULSE RATE RANGES** |
|---|---|
| Adults | 60 to 100 beats per minute |
| Children | 80 to 100 beats per minute |
| Toddlers | 100 to 120 beats per minute |
| Newborns | 120 to 140 beats per minute |

To obtain a pulse rate from most patients, count the number of beats over a 30-second period and multiply by two.

## SKIN CHARACTERISTICS

To continue your vital signs assessment, you need to look at the skin color to determine perfusion. **Perfusion** means that blood enters an organ or tissue through the arteries and leaves through the veins. Nutrients and oxygen are delivered and waste products are removed. With inadequate perfusion, cells and tissue die. Skin color depends primarily on the presence of this circulating blood in the vessels of the skin and on the amount and kind of pigment present in the skin.

## GETTING AN AMPLE SAMPLE

A call for help from a private residence results in your unit being dispatched. On arrival, you find a 65-year-old man complaining that he is "dizzy and weak all over." He looks angry and demands to know why it took so long for you to respond. He's alert and oriented and tells you he's felt this way for the past 3 weeks. He appears quite agitated as he waves his arms and gestures as he is relating his history. He denies any allergies and tells you that he's been taking one aspirin a day for the last 15 years to "keep his blood thin." He has a blood pressure of 154/88 mm Hg, a pulse of 90/min, and respirations of 16/min. He has clear lungs, warm, dry skin, and equal, reactive pupils. As you are finishing the detailed physical exam, the patient states that he's been having trouble eating for the past 6 months. He thinks that food today has too many preservatives. However, he tells you that he did eat some toast this morning without any problems. Finally, he tells you that he hasn't seen a doctor in 10 years, but that maybe today is the day.

### For Discussion

1. Why is it important to obtain a SAMPLE history when assessing a patient?

2. Based on the patient's history, list at least three possibilities in regard to this patient's needs.

### Color

To assess a patient's skin color, look at the nail beds, oral mucosa, and the lining of the eyelids (conjunctivae). In infants and children, the palms of the hands and soles of the feet should be assessed. The normal skin color is pink. Abnormal colors include the following:

- flushed (red)
- pale (white, ashen, or grayish)
- cyanotic (blue-gray)
- jaundice (yellow)

Skin pigment may hide changes in skin color that result from illness or injury. In patients with deeply pigmented skin, changes in color may be apparent in several areas. These areas include the fingernail beds, in the sclera (whites) of the eye, or the membranes inside the mouth. In lightly pigmented patients where changes are seen more easily, the skin colors of medical importance are red, white, and blue (Figure 5-3).

A red color may be present with high blood pressure, fever, late stages of carbon monoxide poisoning, alcohol intoxication, or heatstroke. A patient who has severe high blood pressure may sometimes be plethoric. This is a dark, reddish-purple skin color that occurs due to filling of all visible blood vessels. A patient who has carbon monoxide poisoning may, in later stages, have cherry red lips.

## FIGURE 5-3

Flushed hand and cyanotic feet

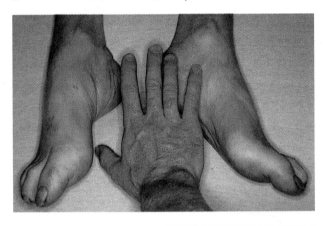

Pale, white, ashen, or gray skin indicates insufficient circulation. This is seen in patients who are in shock, in certain stages of fright, or suffering from cold exposure. In these circumstances, there is literally not enough blood circulating in the skin.

A bluish color results from poor oxygenation of the circulating blood. Blood is blue when it is oxygen poor. When fully saturated with oxygen, blood is red. Thus, cyanotic blood in the vessels makes them blue. Cyanosis always indicates a significant lack of oxygen and calls for a rapid correction of the underlying respiratory problems. Cyanosis is usually first seen in the fingertips and the lips.

Chronic illness may also produce color changes such as the jaundice (yellow color) seen in liver disease. In this condition, bile pigments that are normally present in the liver and the gastrointestinal tract are deposited in the patient's skin (Figure 5-4). Patients with dangerous infectious hepatitis are often jaundiced. The presence of jaundice should alert you to follow BSI techniques.

Assessment of the patient's color can lead to an immediate decision about the need for treatment. Oxygen may be necessary, you may need to control bleeding or begin full resuscitation. Sometimes a glance at the patient is all you need to identify treatment priorities.

## FIGURE 5-4

Jaundiced skin

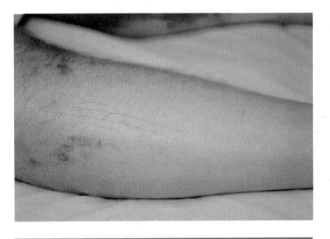

### Temperature

Measurement of the patient's temperature is classically a part of taking vital signs. In the field, however, it will usually be sufficient to simply estimate the patient's temperature by placing the back of your hand on the patient's skin. There are times, however, when a temperature is relevant to the patient's chief complaint. It should then be measured accurately with a thermometer. A normal temperature is warm (98.6°F, 37.0°C). Skin temperatures that are hot, cool, or cold are considered abnormal.

The skin is largely responsible for regulation of the body temperature, by radiating heat from the skin's blood vessels and the evaporation of sweat. Illness or injury can bring about changes in skin temperature. A cool, damp (clammy) skin indicates a general response of the involuntary (sympathetic) nervous system to an insult, such as blood loss (shock) or heat exhaustion. As a result of nervous stimulation, sweat glands are hyperactive and skin blood vessels contract, resulting in cold, pale, wet, or clammy skin. These signs are often the first indication of shock or severe pain. Exposure to cold will produce a cool, dry skin. Dry, hot skin may be caused by fever or by a reaction to excessive heat, such as in heatstroke.

A patient's temperature is usually taken by mouth, with the bulb of the thermometer placed under the tongue. The thermometer should be left in place with the patient's mouth closed for 3 minutes. In a child or an uncooperative patient, the thermometer can be placed in the axilla (armpit), keeping the patient's arm at the side. Axillary temperatures are known to be inaccurate, take a long time to register (10 minutes), and should be used only as a last resort. A special thermometer can also be placed in the ear. Rectal temperatures are very accurate and are usually taken, if necessary, in the emergency department. A rectal temperature is routinely ½ to 1 degree above an oral temperature and is taken with a rectal thermometer left in place for 1 minute (Figure 5-5).

## FIGURE 5-5

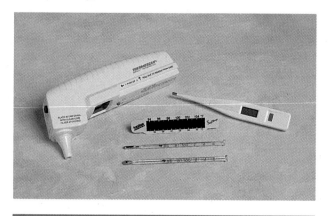

Types of thermometers

### Moisture

When checking the patient's temperature, you need to assess the condition of the skin. A sign to look for is the amount of moisture, such as excessive sweating. Normal skin is dry. Abnormal skin is wet, moist, or excessively dry and hot. Skin may also "tent up" when pinched lightly due to severe dehydration.

### Capillary Refill

Capillary refill is the ability of the circulatory system to restore blood to the capillary blood vessels after it has been squeezed out by the examiner. Generally, the capillary bed under the fingernails is the most reliable area to test. Capillary refill should be both prompt and pink. The normal pink color underneath the nail bed should return within 2 seconds after gentle compression is released. It may be delayed or completely absent. If the returning color is blue, this test is not valid. The blue color may indicate that the capillaries are refilling from the veins, rather than with fresh, oxygenated blood from the arteries (Figure 5-6).

When assessing capillary refill in infants and children, a normal capillary refill is less

## FIGURE 5-6

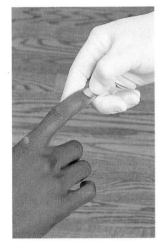

**A** Press the fingernail until it blanches

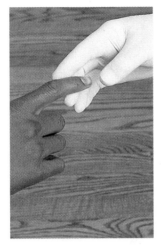

**B** Release the pressure

than 2 seconds. An abnormal capillary refill is greater than 2 seconds. Keep in mind that this test may not be accurate if the patient has been exposed to a cold environment.

## PUPILS

The pupils of normal eyes are regular in outline and usually about the same size. Changes and variation in the size of one or both pupils are important signs in emergency medical care. To assess the pupils, briefly shine a light into the patient's eyes and determine the pupils' size and reactivity. Pupils are described using the following terms:

- dilated (very large), normal, or constricted (small)
- equal or unequal to each other
- reactivity

1. reactive (pupils change when exposed to light)
2. nonreactive (pupils do not change when exposed to light)
3. equally or unequally reactive

In a small percentage of healthy, uninjured persons, anisocoria (unequal pupil size) is found (Figure 5-7). Anisocoria may be the result of a birth abnormality, dilation of the pupil with eye drops, or a previous eye injury. This condition is considered so rare, however, that in the injured and unconscious patient, variation in pupil size is regarded as a reliable sign of possible brain damage.

Constricted pupils are often present in a narcotic drug addict or a patient with a central nervous system disease (Figure 5-8).

## FIGURE 5-7

Unequal pupils (anisocoria)

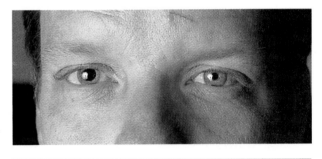

## FIGURE 5-8

Constricted pupils

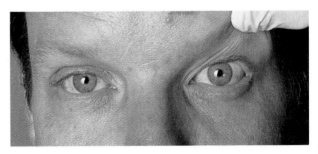

## FIGURE 5-9

Dilated pupils

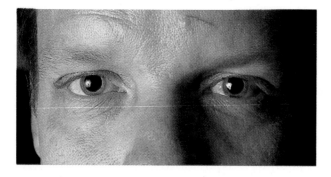

Unequal pupil size may be seen in patients with head injuries or stroke. Dilation of both pupils may indicate a relaxed or unconscious state (Figure 5-9). Such dilation of the pupils usually occurs rapidly (within 30 seconds) after cardiac arrest. Head injury or previous drug use, however, may cause both pupils to remain constricted, even in patients in cardiac arrest.

Ordinarily, the pupils constrict equally and promptly when a bright light shines into either eye. This is a normal protective reaction of the eye. Failure of the pupils to constrict when a light shines into the eye occurs in disease, poisoning, drug overdose, and injury. In death, the pupils are widely dilated and fail to respond to light.

The state of the pupils, especially any progressive change, is a rapid reflection of central nervous system injury or disease. Note all such changes. Report and record them early in your examination of all patients.

## BLOOD PRESSURE

As you continue your assessment of vital signs, you should measure a patient's blood pressure. Blood pressure should be measured in all patients older than 3 years of age. When evaluating infants and children under the age of 3, a general assessment, such as a sick appearance, respiratory distress, or unresponsiveness, is more valuable than vital sign numbers.

**Blood pressure** is the pressure of the circulating blood against the walls of the arteries. In an uninjured, healthy person, the arterial system is a closed system attached to the heart and completely filled with blood. Changes in the blood pressure may indicate changes in the blood volume, capacity of the vessels to contain the blood, or ability of the heart to pump the blood. Changes in the blood pressure can occur rapidly, but usually not as rapidly as changes in pulse occur. This is because the body attempts to maintain a normal blood flow to critical organs by first increasing the pulse rate. Thus, a falling blood pressure is a late and dangerous sign in injury or disease.

Blood pressure can fall greatly after severe bleeding, following a heart attack, or in other states of shock. Low blood pressure means there is not enough pressure in the arterial system to supply blood to all the organs of the body. As a consequence, organs may be severely damaged. The causes of low blood pressure must be identified promptly and treated aggressively. The treatment of low blood pressure that is caused by severe bleeding requires emergency control of the source of the bleeding.

If the blood pressure is abnormally high, damage to or rupture of the vessels in the arterial circuit may occur. It is equally important that the cause of elevated blood pressure be found and treated. Some patients may know their usual blood pressure level. Thus, if the patient is alert and oriented, ask about his or her usual blood pressure. This will provide more information for hospital staff.

Blood pressure can change rapidly during transport of a patient to the hospital. It is important that emergency department personnel be notified of the status of your patient's blood pressure as soon as possible. They should also be made aware of any changes before arrival at the hospital. For this reason, you should check and record the blood pressure at frequent intervals, along with the time it was taken.

## Systolic and Diastolic Pressures

Blood pressure is recorded at systolic and diastolic levels. Systolic pressure is a measurement of the pressure exerted against the walls of the arteries during contraction of the heart. Diastolic pressure represents the pressure exerted against the walls of the arteries while the left ventricle is at rest. Systolic pressure is the maximum pressure to which the arteries are subjected, and diastolic pressure represents the minimum amount of pressure that is always present in the arteries.

## FIGURE 5-10

Blood pressure cuff

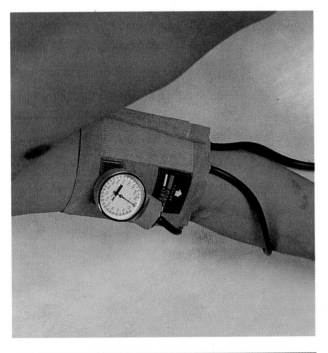

With most diseases or injuries, these pressures change in a parallel fashion—in other words, both rise or both fall. Three exceptions to this rule occur: brain injury, cardiac tamponade, and tension pneumothorax. Brain injury can cause a rise in the systolic pressure with a stable or falling diastolic pressure. A fall in systolic pressure, accompanied by a rising diastolic pressure, occurs in cardiac tamponade and in tension pneumothorax. In cardiac tamponade, blood fills the sac around the heart, impeding its filling and pumping. In tension pneumothorax, air under abnormal pressure in the chest obstructs the filling of the right heart, thereby limiting its output. Both conditions cause the systolic and diastolic pressures to approach each other. This condition is called a narrow pulse pressure.

## Measuring Blood Pressure

Blood pressure is measured by one of two methods or a combination of the two. Both methods require the use of a blood pressure cuff, called a sphygmomanometer (Figure 5-10). It is important to select a cuff that is the appropriate size for the patient. The sphygmomanometer has a rubber bladder inside of it. This bladder should be long enough to encircle the patient's arm completely. The width of the bladder should be at least 20% greater than the diameter of the arm (Figure 5-11a).

Narrow cuffs are made for taking children's blood pressure, and extra-large cuffs are made for obese adults (Figure 5-11b). Cuffs that are too small may give falsely high readings, and cuffs that are too large may give falsely low readings. The blood pressure may also be taken in the thigh, using the extra-large cuff.

Wrap the cuff snugly around the patient's upper arm, with the lower edge of the cuff about 1" above the inside of the patient's elbow (Figure 5-12). The center of the

**FIGURE 5-11**

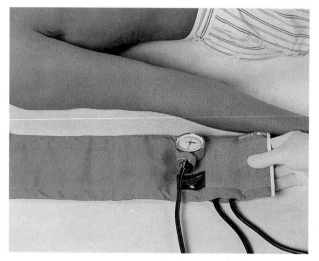

**A**   Use of a proper-sized blood pressure cuff

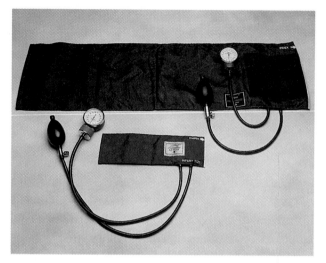

**B**   Extra-large (top) and pediatric (bottom) cuffs

inflatable bladder, usually marked with an arrow on the cuff, should cover the patient's brachial artery along the medial aspect of the lower arm at the elbow.

**Palpation**   You may take the blood pressure by **palpation**. This is done by finding the patient's radial pulse. Then, with your other hand, inflate the blood pressure cuff until the pulse is no longer felt, and then for another 30 mm of mercury (mm Hg) on the gauge of the blood pressure cuff. Deflate the cuff slowly until the pulse returns (Figure 5-13). The reading on the gauge when the pulse returns is the patient's systolic blood pressure, by palpation. Because a blood pressure determined by palpation is less accurate than if determined by auscultation, it should be recorded with the word "palpation" written beside it. Only the systolic pressure can be measured using the palpation method.

**Auscultation**   You may also take the blood pressure by auscultation. **Auscultation** is the method of listening to sounds within the

organs, usually with a stethoscope. Reinflate the cuff to the same point as before—about 30 mm Hg above the systolic blood pressure as determined by palpation. Place the stethoscope in the patient's antecubital fossa, located at the anterior aspect of the elbow over the brachial artery (Figure 5-14).

**FIGURE 5-12**

Proper placement of a cuff on the arm

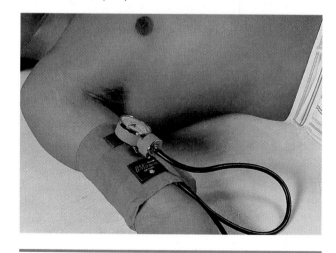

## FIGURE 5-13

Blood pressure by palpation

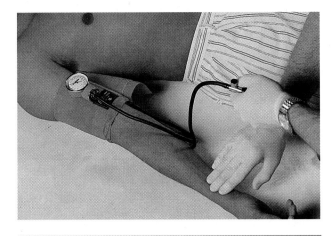

Gradually deflate the cuff while you listen for the sound of the pulse "tapping" in the artery. Record the sound first heard as the systolic pressure. Continue to deflate the cuff until the "tapping" sounds disappear. The pressure at which the sounds disappear is the second reading, or the dia-stolic pressure. Record the blood pressure in the form systolic/diastolic, for example, 120/80 mm Hg. Also record the position of the patient (sitting, standing, or lying) and the extremity in which the pressure is taken.

Blood pressure levels vary with age and sex. One useful rule of thumb for estimating the normal systolic pressure in a male is to add 100 to the age of the patient, up to 150 mm Hg. Normal dia-stolic pressure in adult males ranges between 65 and 90 mm Hg. Both pressures are about 10 mm Hg lower in adult fe-males. Sounds at the elbow are, at times, impossible to hear in a moving ambulance. You must then rely on measuring the blood pressure by palpation during transport. Occasionally, the blood pressure sounds do not disappear as you decrease the cuff pressure. This indicates continued turbu-lence in the artery after the pressure of the cuff has been released. The pressure is then reported as the systolic pressure and "all the way down." For example, you would write, "120 over all the way down."

## FIGURE 5-14

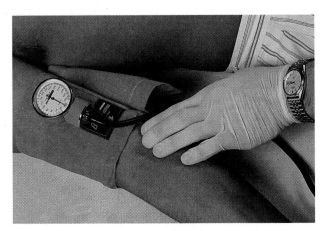

**A**  Palpation of the brachial pulse for placement of a stethoscope

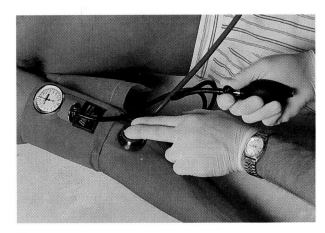

**B**  Blood pressure by auscultation

You will obtain blood pressure readings in the arm in almost all situations. Only rarely will you take a patient's blood pressure in the thigh. If you must, make sure to use an extra-large cuff and palpate the pulse in the posterior tibial artery.

## REASSESSMENT OF VITAL SIGNS

Once you have completed and accurately recorded the baseline vital signs, you must periodically monitor the patient's vital signs. In a stable patient, you should reassess and record vital signs at least every 15 minutes. In an unstable patient, you should reassess and record vital signs at least every 5 minutes. You should also reassess and record vital signs following all medical interventions.

You should make a careful recording of all findings and treatments. Repeat assessments should always be documented. The progression of vital signs is especially important to hospital personnel and should be carefully recorded. Care is not complete until the case is completely recorded.

## STEPS AT THE SCENE

☐ Ask the patient or an informed bystander about the events leading up to the current episode.

☐ Assess the patient for **S**igns and **S**ymptoms.

☐ Check for a medical identification tag.

☐ Obtain information about **A**llergies to medication, food, and the environment.

☐ Ask about all prescription and over-the-counter **M**edications the patient is currently taking or has been recently taking.

## OBTAINING A SAMPLE HISTORY

☐ Obtain **P**ertinent past history about medical, surgical, or trauma occurrences.

☐ Ask the patient when his or her **L**ast oral intake was, how much was consumed, and whether it was solid or liquid.

☐ Ask the patient about **E**vents leading to the injury or illness.

# SAMPLE HISTORY

If time permits, you should attempt to learn the patient's **SAMPLE history.** To do this you should ask the patient or an informed bystander about the events leading up to the current episode. Ask questions that will shed light on the patient's current problem as it relates to the patient's overall medical state. It is important for you to know about the following:

- any major medical problems such as diabetes or heart disease
- medications the patient takes
- any allergies the patient may have
- when the patient last ate or drank
- the events that led up to the current illness or injury

This information can be easily remembered through the use of the word SAMPLE:

**S** Signs/Symptoms: A **sign** is any medical or trauma condition displayed by the patient and identifiable by you (hearing = respiratory distress, seeing = bleeding, feeling = skin temperature). A **symptom** is any condition described by the patient (shortness of breath).

**A** Allergies: Obtain information about all medication, food, and environmental allergies. Consider the medical identification tag.

**M** Medications: Ask about all prescription medications the patient is currently taking or has been recently taking. Make sure to include birth control pills. Ask about all over-the-counter (OTC) drugs the patient is currently taking or has been recently taking. Again consider the medical identification tag.

**P** Pertinent past history: Obtain information about medical, surgical, or trauma occurrences. Consider the medical identification tag.

**L** Last oral intake: Ask the patient when he or she last ate or drank, how much was consumed, and whether it was solid or liquid.

**E** Events leading to the injury or illness: Find out what happened before EMS was summoned. For example: chest pain with exertion, chest pain while at rest.

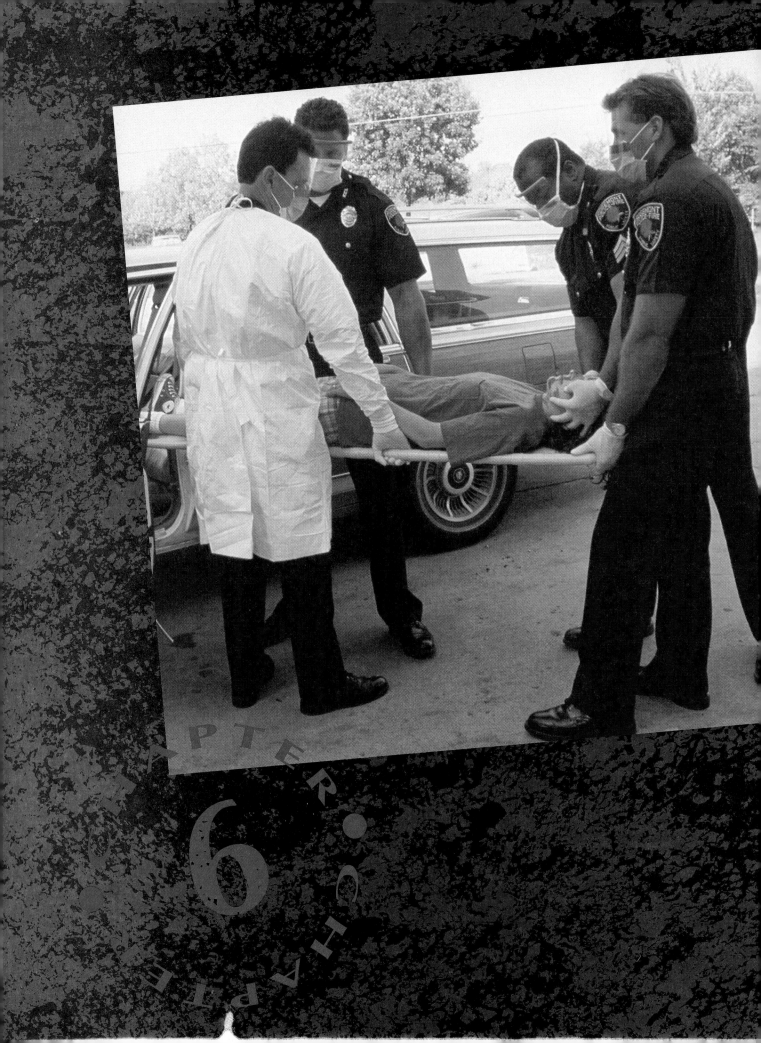

CHAPTER

6

# Lifting and Moving Patients

## Objectives

After you have read this chapter, you should be able to:

- Define body mechanics and why they are important to the EMT-B.
- Discuss the guidelines and safety precautions that need to be followed when lifting a patient.
- Describe the safe lifting of cots and stretchers.
- Describe the guidelines and safety precautions for carrying patients and/or equipment.
- Discuss one-handed carrying techniques.
- Describe correct and safe carrying procedures on stairs.
- State the guidelines for reaching and their application.
- Describe correct reaching for logrolls.
- State the guidelines for pushing and pulling.
- Discuss the general considerations of moving patients.
- State three situations that may require the use of an emergency move.
- Identify the following patient carrying devices: wheeled ambulance stretcher, portable stretcher, stair chair, scoop stretcher, long spine board, basket stretcher, and flexible stretcher.

# Overview

The safe handling of patients, whether they are found on the street or highway, at home or at work, presents a wide variety of challenges—not the least of which is to protect yourself and your partners from injury. When it comes to lifting and moving, patients fall into two general categories as follows:

1. Those found in easily accessible locations
2. Those who must be extricated from locations difficult to access

In both types of locations, there is always possible danger to you, your partner, the patient, and others at the scene.

Patients in the first group—no matter how serious their injuries—can be moved rather routinely. With this group, you must be concerned with proper lifting techniques and body mechanics. Do not try to lift too much and try to avoid injuring yourself in any way while supporting the patient's weight. Many prehospital care providers are injured every year, some with career-ending disabilities, because they lift patients improperly.

With the patients in the second group, the injuries may or may not be serious. However, moving them may require special rescue techniques and extrication. These techniques are typically taught in formal rescue programs and are not part of the 1994 EMT-Basic National Standard Curriculum. An introduction to basic extrication is presented in appendix C, Fundamentals of Extrication.

# Key Terms

**Backboard** Device used to provide support to patients suspected of having a hip, pelvic, spinal, or lower extremity injury. Also called a spine board.

**Basket stretcher** Device commonly used in technical rescues and water rescues. Also called a Stokes litter.

**Direct ground lift** Lifting technique used for patients with no suspected spinal injury who are found lying supine on the ground.

**Extremity lift** Lifting technique that may be used for patients with no suspected extremity or spinal injuries who are supine or in a sitting position.

**Flexible stretcher** Device that can be folded or rolled when not in use. A rigid carrying device when secured around a patient.

**Packaging** The positioning, covering, and securing of an ill or injured patient for transportation.

**Portable stretcher** Lightweight folding device without undercarriage and wheels.

**Power grip** Technique that allows you to get maximum force from your hands.

**Power lift** Posture that is safe and helpful for EMT-Bs when they are lifting. Also called squat lift.

**Rapid Extrication** Technique developed to quickly move a patient from sitting in a vehicle to supine on a long spine board in less than 1 minute.

**Scoop stretcher** Designed to be split into two or four sections that can be fitted around a patient who is lying on the ground or other relatively flat surface. Also called a split litter.

**Stair chair** A lightweight folding device used to carry a seated patient, especially up or down stairs.

**Wheeled ambulance stretcher** A specially designed stretcher that can be rolled along the ground. It has a collapsible undercarriage so that it can be loaded into an ambulance.

## BODY MECHANICS

To move a patient from one place to another, you need a definite plan. Just as you mentally organize for work each day, you need a strategy for packaging and transporting a patient. **Packaging** is the positioning, covering, and securing of a patient for transportation. Part of this planning includes knowing your limitations, as well as knowing what other resources are available and how to access them. Use equipment such as stretchers, blankets, straps, and splints whenever possible. You should be able to move a patient without unnecessary risk of injury.

*Dead or injured EMT-Bs cannot save lives.* The four factors you need to consider when you plan to package and transfer a patient are as follows:

1. The patient's problem, including the actual and possible threats to the patient's health and safety

2. The environmental risks and limitations that may compromise the safety of the patient, you, or your partners

3. The availability of equipment and/or other emergency personnel at the scene

4. Your own physical and technical capabilities and limitations, as well as those of your partners.

## PRINCIPLES OF SAFE LIFTING

You should follow two basic principles of body mechanics and lifting when you perform a patient transfer. First, use the longest and strongest available muscle groups (biceps, quadriceps, and gluteals) to move patients. Maximum efficiency of contraction occurs when the muscle smoothly contracts at a moderate rate. *Using your legs, not your back, to lift is an important safety point.* Second, keep your arms and legs close to your body so that your center of gravity is not out of alignment. Keeping the weight as close to you as possible will help prevent your muscles from being overstressed.

Evaluate every situation to make sure that you and your partners are able to lift a patient's weight and to negotiate any unusual circumstances. For example, if the stretcher or cot cannot be moved right next to the patient, you will have to support the patient's weight while you move the patient. Plan in advance and assemble the needed resources to make the move a success. Knowing and being realistic about your physical limitations is essential.

For a long, healthy career without a disabling back injury, follow these basic principles of good body mechanics when lifting. When you lift, your body works very much like a mechanical crane. There is a footing or base, and an amount of energy available for overcoming the resting weight of the object (person) to be lifted. Even the largest crane must have a secure base and must obey the laws of physics in order to work efficiently. Your body is no different.

### Guidelines for Safe Lifting

1. Only lift weights that you can comfortably handle. The maximum amount of weight you can lift is based on your age, sex, muscle mass, and conditioning.

2. Use equipment whenever it is available. Make sure you use equipment properly, and that it is in good working order.

3. Place both feet flat on the ground, with one foot slightly in front of the other, to establish a firm support base.

4. Distribute the patient's weight evenly over both of your feet.

5. When working below knuckle height, bend your body at the knees and hips and keep your back straight. Avoid bending at the waist to lift.

6. Keep your head up. Move in a smooth, coordinated manner. Sudden, jerky movements tend to overstress muscles, resulting in injury.

7. Hold your abdomen firm as you lift and tuck in the buttocks, keeping your shoulders aligned over the spine and pelvis.

8. Straighten your knees as you lift to make sure that the major lifting forces are provided by the thigh and buttocks muscles.

9. Use pivoting movements rather than rotating or twisting actions when changing direction. Keep your shoulders square over your pelvis.

10. Walk slowly, using coordinated movements. Steps should not be longer or wider than shoulder width when you carry a patient or a stretcher.

11. Whenever possible, move forward rather than backward to facilitate normal balance and smoothness of movement.

12. When lowering a stretcher or backboard, reverse the above steps to maintain a safe posture and lifting advantage.

13. Communicate with your partners clearly and often during the move. This will maintain coordination and help to alert each other to uneven ground or other obstacles.

When you are lifting a patient on a stretcher or cot, remember that you are also lifting the added weight of the stretcher. A normally equipped wheeled stretcher adds over 70 lb to the weight you will lift. You must also add the weight of any extra equipment, such as oxygen cylinders, that is being carried with the patient. Cots and stretchers also do not always maneuver around corners as well as people do. This can add physical stress to an otherwise uncomplicated move.

When you have a choice, select the lightest, smallest appropriate device to limit your physical stress. For example, using a stair chair when moving down flights of stairs is much easier than carrying a full wheeled stretcher or even a backboard. In fact, use a stair chair when a patient can be in a sitting position and needs to be carried over rough ground.

## Power Lift Position

The **power lift** or squat lift position is a useful posture for lifting, especially if you have weak knees or thighs. This position helps to keep your back locked in a normal curvature and avoids injury. To lift in this position, spread your feet a comfortable distance apart, with your abdominal muscles tensed to lock your back into a slight inward curve. Straddle the end of the backboard or cot with your feet flat on the floor. Distribute your weight to the balls of your feet or just behind them. Stand up by locking your back in and raising your upper body before your hips begin to rise (Figure 6-1).

## Power Grip

A technique known as the **power grip** is used to obtain the most force from your hands. Place your palm and all your fingers in complete contact with the object being lifted. Make sure that all your fingers are bent at the same angle. Place your hands about 10" apart (Figure 6-2).

**FIGURE 6-1**

The power lift

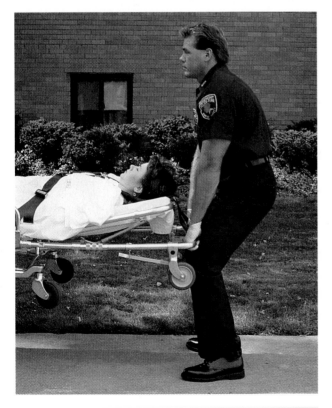

**FIGURE 6-2**

The power grip

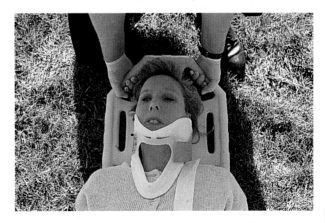

## PRINCIPLES OF SAFE CARRYING

When a patient must be carried some distance, you can use other techniques to help avoid injury. First, try to avoid having to actually carry the patient. Instead, use a wheeled stretcher or other device that can be rolled along the ground.

### Guidelines for Safe Carrying

1. Determine the approximate weight that must be lifted.
2. Compare the weight to be lifted to the lifting and carrying limitations of you and your team.
3. Work in a coordinated manner and communicate clearly and often with your team.
4. Use the safe lifting techniques described earlier, including keeping the weight as close to your body as possible, keeping your back "locked in," and avoiding twisting whenever possible.
5. Bend at the knees, not at the waist. Do not lean backward from the waist.
6. Work with a partner of similar height and strength to carry a patient or heavy object, whenever possible.

When four or more EMT-Bs are carrying a stretcher, each usually uses only one hand to support the stretcher. This is so they can face forward as they are walking. While this makes walking easier, it reduces the amount of strength that each person brings to the carry. It is important to begin such a carry by first lifting the stretcher or object face on and with both hands (Figure 6-3a). Once the object has been lifted to carrying height, you and your partners can turn in the direction you will be walking and switch to using only one hand (Figure 6-3b). If you find that you tend to lean away from the load you are carrying, or are drawn in

**FIGURE 6-3**

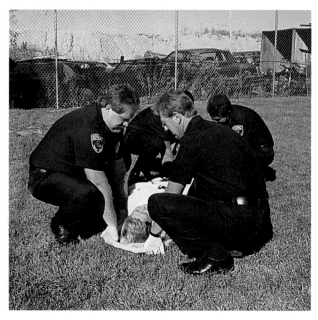

**A**    Lift the stretcher straight-on using both hands

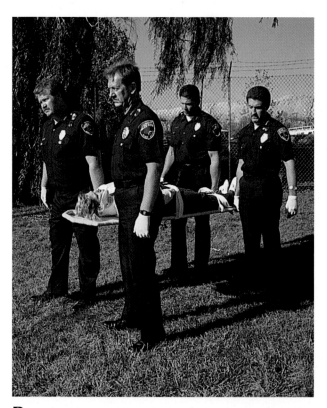

**B**    Face the direction in which you will walk

toward it, the weight probably exceeds your limitations. At this point, you and your partners should add helpers or reevaluate the carry before going on and possibly injuring yourselves or dropping the patient.

## PRINCIPLES OF SAFE REACHING AND PULLING

Most EMT-Bs think of lifting and carrying as the most common strenuous prehospital activities. However, reaching, pulling, and pushing are three other common maneuvers in which you may be injured or experience trouble. As with lifting, keep your back locked in and avoid twisting when you are reaching. In addition, avoid hyperextending your back when reaching overhead. Avoid reaching out in front of you more than 15" to 20" to support any sizable load. You should also avoid having to provide strenuous support for more than a minute or so at a time.

When you reach forward to log roll a patient onto his or her side, remember to keep your back straight while leaning over the patient. Lean from your hips and use your shoulder muscles to help roll the patient.

Making a conscious effort to push a stretcher or object—rather than to pull it—will also help to protect your back. If you must pull, keep your back locked in and keep the line of pull as close to the center of your body as possible. Bend your knees and keep the load close to your body. Keep your elbows bent and your arms close to your sides.

When you push, exert the force from the area between your waist and your shoulders. Do not push with your arms alone. If the load is above you, try repositioning yourself before you attempt to push or pull a weight that is overhead. When the object to be moved is below the

level of your waist, begin in a kneeling position to avoid bending over and risking injury to your back.

## GENERAL CONSIDERATIONS IN MOVING PATIENTS

Moving a patient should be done in an orderly, planned, and unhurried fashion, except in situations in which your life or your patient's life is in danger. This approach will protect both you and the patient from further injury. It will also reduce the risk of making the patient's condition worse. Usually, you and your team will be moving a patient from a bed, a chair or other sitting position, or the floor or the ground to an ambulance stretcher. Two EMT-Bs are needed to complete a move. Bystanders are used only if absolutely necessary. If you use bystanders, you must give them simple but detailed instructions about their roles before the patient is actually moved. If a move is not done correctly, you, your team, and the patient may experience discomfort and possible injury.

The stretcher or carrying device should be placed as close as possible to the patient before the transfer to reduce the distance needed to move the patient. Consider placing an injured or seriously ill patient on a long spine board or scoop stretcher first. This will often allow the easiest transfer to an ambulance stretcher, an emergency department stretcher, or an X-ray table, with minimal movement or risk of making the patient's condition worse. However, for nonemergency transfers and patients who are not seriously ill, rigid backboards and stretchers can be extremely uncomfortable. Using them may even make the patient's condition worse. Studies have shown that even healthy, uninjured persons who are immobilized to rigid backboards are extremely uncomfortable in a short period of time.

As you plan a move, make sure to consider the number of times you actually must lift, move, and carry a patient. One of your main goals should be to eliminate or reduce the need for additional movement of the patient after the transfer is completed. For example, a trauma patient should be placed on a long spine board with a pneumatic antishock garment (PASG) in place, ready to be applied (Figure 6-4).

## FIGURE 6-4

A long spine board with a PASG in place

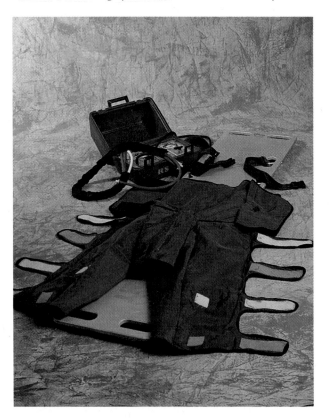

The only time a patient should be moved before initial assessment, care, and stabilization is when the patient's or your life is in danger. An immediate emergency move is performed without any attempt to first provide treatment or otherwise stabilize the patient. An emergency move is done in dangerous situations, such as fire, explosives, hazardous materials, or other dangers at the scene. Emergency moves are also done if you are unable to administer needed emergency medical care due to the location or position of the patient. For example, a patient in full cardiac arrest is found sitting in a chair. CPR cannot be done effectively with the patient sitting in the chair. Therefore, you must first move the patient to a supine position on the floor before you try to open the airway or provide ventilation. Another example is when you have to move one patient who is not critically injured or in immediate danger in order to gain access to a second patient who needs immediate lifesaving care.

You may also have to move other patients on an urgent basis. For example, patients with serious but not desperately critical conditions may have to be moved before you can complete a full assessment. In these situations, you may not know the extent of the patient's injuries and problems. Conditions, such as weather extremes, unconsciousness, inadequate ventilation, and shock (hypoperfusion) might also make an urgent move necessary.

When performing an emergency move, one of your primary concerns is the danger of aggravating an existing spinal injury. If you follow basic guidelines, you can usually move a patient from a life-threatening situation without causing further injury to the patient. If you have to pull the patient, you should pull along the long axis of the patient's body. This will help keep the spinal column in line as much as possible. You can

*Rapid exctrication*

**FIGURE 6-5**

Clothes drag

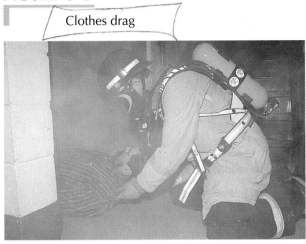

**FIGURE 6-6**

Blanket drag

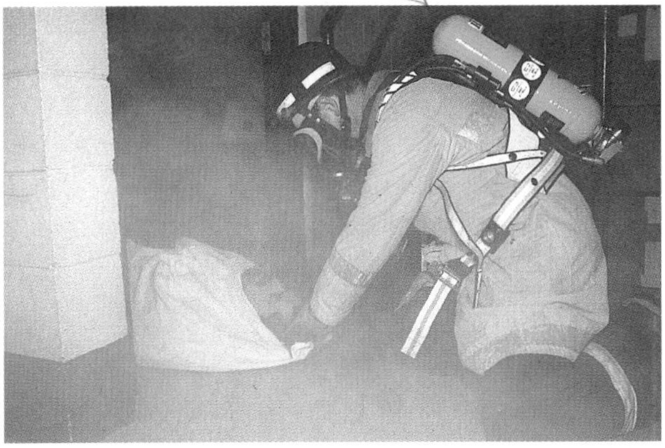

**FIGURE 6-7**

Fire fighter's drag

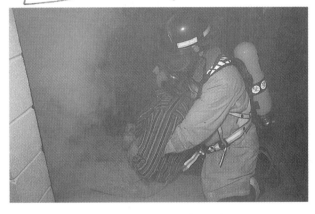

move a patient along the floor or the ground using one of the following techniques:

- pulling on the patient's clothing in the neck and shoulder area (Figure 6-5)

- placing the patient on a blanket or coat or other item, then dragging the blanket rather than directly pulling on the patient (Figure 6-6)

- placing your hands under the patient's armpits, grasping the forearms, and dragging the patient backward (this is done only if you can get behind the patient) (Figure 6-7)

You should resort to one-person techniques only when the patient must be moved immediately due to a life-threatening hazard and you are alone. For example, you might have to act alone to remove a patient from a fire, a smoke-filled or contaminated area, or a building in danger of collapse. *Remember that these are emergency transfer methods only.* These techniques are difficult and should not be used if you can get help immediately. Also remember to protect yourself in dangerous environments. Hazardous environments such as a smoke-filled area require protective equipment, including a self-contained breathing apparatus (SCBA). You should not attempt any hazardous-environment rescue that poses a danger to yourself without proper training. For these situations, you must know and be trained in the use of an SCBA and other protective equipment. Moreover, the scene of an accident is not the time or place for such training. Some additional drags, carries, and lifts for one-person rescue are presented on the following pages (Figures 6-8 to 6-10). Again, you and your team must practice these techniques *before* they are needed!

## FIGURE 6-8

Fire fighter's carry

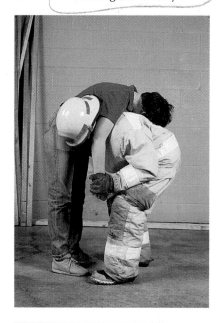
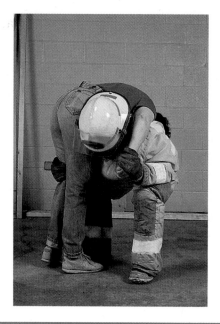
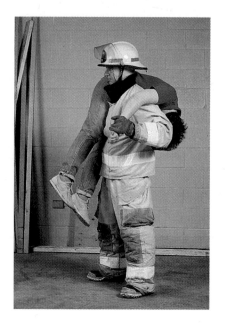

## URGENT MOVES

### Rapid Extrication Technique

In some cases, patients must be quickly moved from dangerous situations. Some patients need immediate lifesaving care, but they are trapped sitting in an automobile. The extra minutes you need to apply a spinal immobilization device could mean the difference between life and death. A technique called **Rapid Extrication** has been developed for just such cases. With Rapid Extrication, the time needed to move a patient from sitting in an automobile to supine on a long spine board is less than 1 minute, not the usual 6 to 8 minutes. Ideally, the Rapid Extrication technique requires a team of three EMT-Bs who have practiced the procedure often.

This technique should be used only in two general instances. First, you should use the technique when a patient's injuries require that he or she be removed from a sitting position so that you can perform lifesaving care. Second, it should be used when the scene is so dangerous for both you and the patient that an immediate move is needed. If the patient does not need to be removed immediately, you should take the time to apply traditional devices, such as vest-type or half-board immobilization devices. The Rapid Extrication technique provides some support to the patient's spine, but not as much as a spinal immobilization device.

You and your team will not become instant experts at this technique with only a few minutes of practice during class. Once you have learned the steps, you should practice with a variety of "victims" and vehicles until you can perform the technique quickly and accurately. You should also switch positions, so that each member of the team has practiced each position.

## Rapid Extrication Technique

1. EMT-B #1 applies manual in-line support of the patient's head and cervical spine from behind (Figure 6-11a). Support may be applied from the side, if necessary, by reaching through the driver's side doorway.

2. EMT-B #2 serves as team leader and, as such, gives the commands until the patient is supine on the backboard. EMT-B #2 must be physically capable of moving the patient, as he or she lifts and turns the patient's torso. EMT-B #2 works from the driver's side doorway. If EMT-B #1 is also working from that doorway, EMT-B #2 should stand closer to the door hinges toward the front of the vehicle.

3. EMT-B #2 provides continuous support of the patient's torso until the patient is supine on the backboard. Once EMT-B #2 takes control of the torso, usually in the form of a body hug, he or she should not let go of the patient for any reason (Figure 6-11b). A critically injured patient is too weak to support himself or herself in any way. Thus, the body hug is the appropriate way to hold the patient. You cannot simply extend your arms and reach into the car to grab the patient. This will only twist the patient's torso, not rotate the patient as a unit.

### FIGURE 6-9

Front cradle

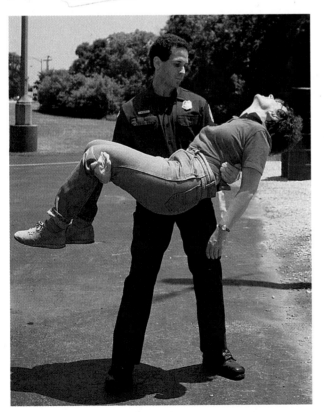

### FIGURE 6-10

One-person walking assist

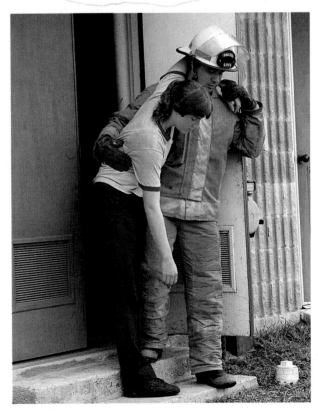

**FIGURE 6-11**

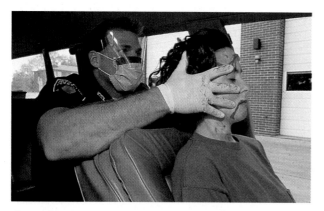

**A** EMT-B #1 applies manual in-line support to the cervical spine

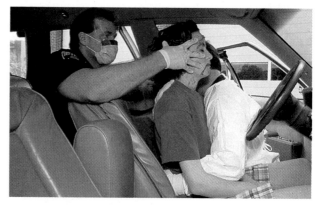

**B** EMT-B #2 supports the patient's torso with a body hug

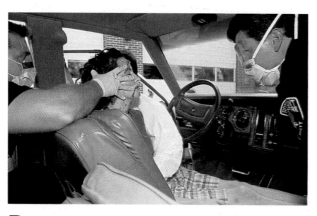

**D** EMT-B #2 directs quick turns and lower extremities are extended on the seat

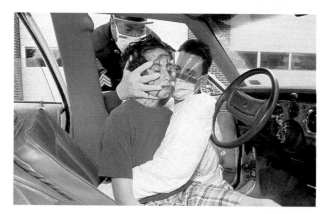

**E** EMT-B #3 supports the head, EMT-B #1 gets out of the vehicle

Some type of cross-chest shoulder hug usually works well, but you will have to decide what method works best for you on any given patient.

4. EMT-B #3 works from the front passenger's seat and is responsible for rotating the patient's legs and feet as the torso is turned. If necessary, this position can be filled by an on-scene recruit, such as a fire fighter or law enforcement official. EMT-B #3 should first move the patient's nearer leg laterally (Figure 6-11c). This should be done with care and without rotating the patient's pelvis and lower spine. The pelvis and lower spine

rotate only as EMT-B #3 moves the second leg during the next step. Moving the nearer leg early makes moving the second leg in concert with the rest of the body much easier. After EMT-B #3 moves the legs together, they should be moved as a unit together.

*The first four steps of the Rapid Extrication technique direct the team to their starting positions and responsibilities. EMT-B #1 applies in-line support of the cervical spine. EMT-B #2 gives orders and supports the torso. EMT-B #3 moves the patient's nearer leg laterally to prepare for rotation. The team is now ready to move the patient.*

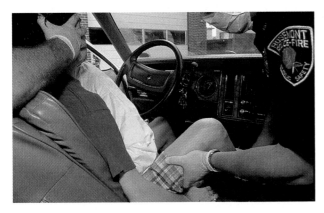

**C** EMT-B #3 moves the patient's nearest leg laterally

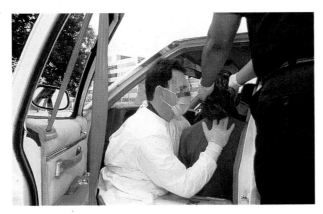

**F** EMT-B #1 places the backboard into a ready position

5. The patient is rotated 90° so that his or her back is facing out the driver's door and the feet are on the front passenger's seat. This movement is done in three or four short, quick "eighth turns" (Figure 6-11d). EMT-B #2 directs each quick turn by saying, "Ready, turn," or "Ready, move." Hand position changes should be made between moves.

6. In most cases EMT-B #1 will be working from a back seat. At some point, EMT-B #1 will be unable to reach far enough to follow the torso rotation—either due to the door post or simply due to distance. At that time, EMT-B #3 provides

temporary support of the head and neck as EMT-B #1 gets out of the vehicle. EMT-B #1 then regains control of the head from outside the vehicle. If a fourth EMT-B is present, EMT-B #4 stands next to EMT-B #2. EMT-B #4 takes control of the head and neck from outside the vehicle without involving EMT-B #3 (Figure 6-11e). As soon as the change has been made, the rotation can continue.

7. Once the patient has been fully rotated, the backboard should be placed against the patient's buttocks on the seat. Do not try to wedge the backboard under the patient. Do not try to place the backboard behind the patient before the torso is fully rotated. The EMT-Bs working in the driver's open doorway need the space to work. With only three EMT-Bs, place the backboard within arm's reach of the driver's door before the move. That way the board can be pulled into place when needed. In such cases, the far end of the board can be left on the ground. When a fourth EMT-B is available, EMT-B #1 places the backboard against the patient's buttocks and then maintains pressure in toward the vehicle from the far end of the board (Figure 6-11f).

8. As soon as the backboard is in place, EMT-B #2 and EMT-B #4 lower the patient onto the board as quickly as possible. EMT-B #1 holds the backboard until the patient is secured. The longer it takes to lower the patient, the more likely that the patient's spine will "sag" (Figure 6-11g).

9. Next, EMT-B #3 must move across the front seat to be in position at the patient's hips. If EMT-B #3 stays at the patient's knees or feet, he or she will be ineffective in helping to move the body's weight. The knees and feet follow the hips. The hips will not necessarily move when

**FIGURE 6-11** *continued*

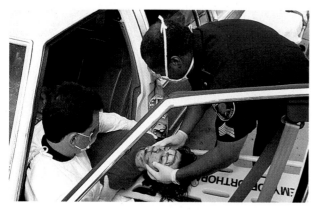

**G** The patient is lowered onto the backboard

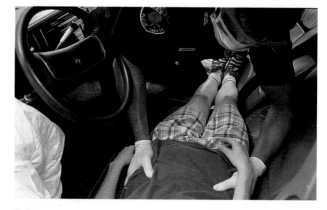

**H** EMT-B #3 in the proper position to move the patient

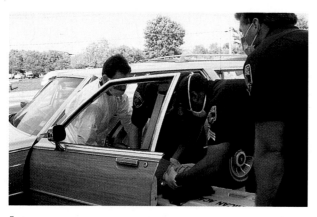

**I** EMT-B #3 takes control at the shoulders, EMT-B #2 takes the hips

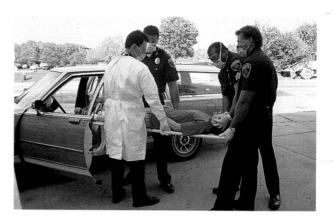

**J** EMT-B #4 maintains manual in-line support of the cervical spine, the patient is moved away from the vehicle

pressure is exerted at the knees or feet (Figure 6-11h).

10. EMT-B #4 maintains manual in-line support at the cervical spine and now takes over giving the commands. EMT-B #2 stands with his or her back to the door, facing the rear of the vehicle. The backboard should be immediately in front of EMT-B #2. EMT-B #2 grasps the patient's shoulders or armpits. Then, on command, EMT-B #2 and EMT-B #3 slide the patient 8" to 12" along the backboard. This slide is repeated until the patient's hips are firmly on the backboard. At that time, EMT-B #3 gets out of the vehicle and moves to the opposite side of the backboard, across from EMT-B #2. EMT-B #3 now takes control at the shoulders and EMT-B #2 moves back to take control of the hips (Figure 6-11i). On command, these two EMT-Bs move the patient along the board in 8" to 12" slides until the patient is fully on the board.

11. EMT-B #4 continues to maintain manual in-line support. EMT-B #2 and EMT-B #3 now grasp their side of the board, and then carry it and the patient away from the vehicle (Figure 6-11j).

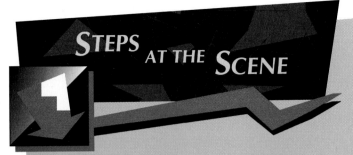

## DIRECT GROUND LIFT

☐ Line up on one side of the patient. EMT-B #1 is at the patient's head. EMT-B #2 is at the patient's knees. EMT-B #3, if available, is at the patient's waist.

☐ All EMT-Bs kneel on one knee, preferably the same knee.

☐ Place the patient's arms on his or her chest, if possible.

☐ EMT-B #1 places one arm under the patient's neck and shoulder and cradles the patient's head. EMT-B #1 then places the other arm under the patient's lower back.

☐ EMT-B #2 places one arm under the patient's knees and one arm above the buttocks.

☐ EMT-B #3, if available, places both arms under the patient's waist. The other two EMT-Bs should slide their arms either up to the middle back or down to the buttocks, as appropriate.

☐ On signal, the team lifts the patient up to knee level. Next, the team rolls the patient in toward their chests.

☐ On signal, the team stands and carries the patient to the stretcher.

☐ The steps are reversed to lower the patient.

Once the patient has been removed from the vehicle, you and your team should immediately lower the patient to the ground or into an *immediately* accessible ambulance. You should then begin lifesaving treatment immediately. If Rapid Extrication was used because the scene was dangerous, you and your team should immediately move away from the scene before you assess or treat the patient.

The steps of the Rapid Extrication technique must be considered a general procedure to be adapted as needed. Two-door cars differ from four-door models. Cars differ from small pickup trucks and from full-size, four-wheel drive vehicles. You will handle a large, heavy adult differently than a small adult or child. Every situation will be different—a different car, a different patient, and a different crew. Your resourcefulness and ability to adapt are necessary elements to successful Rapid Extrication.

## NONURGENT MOVES

When both the scene and the patient are stable, you should carefully plan how to move the patient. Any patient move that is rushed or not well planned—and occasionally even rehearsed on site—may result in discomfort to the patient and injury to you and your team. Before any move is attempted, the team leader has to make sure of the following:

- that there is enough manpower
- that obstacles have been identified or removed

- that the best equipment is available
- that the procedure and path to be followed have been clearly discussed

In nonurgent situations, you and your team may choose one of several methods for lifting and carrying a patient. Three general methods for moving patients are presented below. These methods may serve as a basis for your plan. You can adapt these procedures to meet your needs on a case-by-case basis.

### Direct Ground Lift

The **direct ground lift** is used for patients with no suspected spinal injury who are found lying supine on the ground. This lift is used when the patient has to be carried some distance in order to be placed on the stretcher. In most cases, you and your team lift the patient a few inches so that a long spine board can be slid under the patient. However, there will be times when the patient's location will make the use of a long spine board impossible until the patient is carried to the stretcher. Ideally, the direct ground lift will require two or three EMT-Bs who have practiced the procedure often.

1. Line up on one side of the patient. EMT-B #1 is at the patient's head. EMT-B #2 is at the patient's knees. EMT-B #3, if available, is at the patient's waist (Figure 6-12a). All EMT-Bs kneel on one knee, preferably the same knee.

2. Place the patient's arms on his or her chest, if possible.

3. EMT-B #1 places one arm under the patient's neck and shoulders and cradles the patient's head. EMT-B #1 then places the other arm under the patient's lower back.

4. EMT-B #2 places one arm under the patient's knees and one arm above the buttocks.

FIGURE 6-12

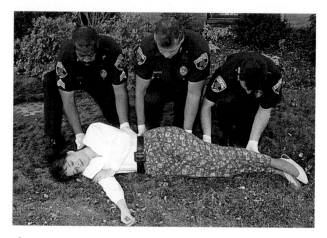

**A** The team in the proper position for a direct ground lift

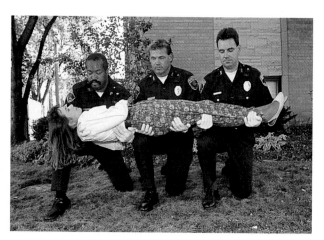

**B** Raise the patient to chest level

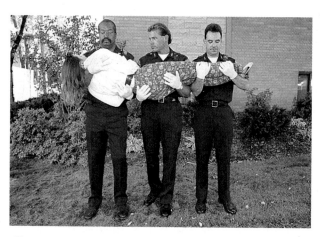

**C** Completed lift

5. EMT-B #3, if available, places both arms under the patient's waist. The other two EMT-Bs should slide their arms either up to the middle back or down to the buttocks, as appropriate.

6. On signal, the team lifts the patient up to knee level (Figure 6-12b). Next, the team rolls the patient in toward their chests (Figure 6-12c).

7. On signal, the team stands and carries the patient to the stretcher.

8. The steps are reversed to lower the patient.

### Extremity Lift

The **extremity lift** may be used with patients with no suspected extremity or spinal injuries who are supine or in a sitting position. The extremity lift may be especially helpful when the space is very narrow. It is also useful when there is not enough room for the patient and a team of two EMT-Bs to stand side by side. The key to success with this lift is direct communication. You and your partner must coordinate your movements through direct verbal commands.

1. EMT-B #1 kneels at the patient's head. EMT-B #2 kneels at the patient's side by his or her knees.

2. Cross the patient's hands over his or her chest (Figure 6-13a).

3. EMT-B #1 places one hand under each of the patient's armpits. EMT-B #2 grasps the patient's wrists.

4. EMT-B #1 reaches forward and grasps the patient's wrists.

5. EMT-B #2 stands between the patient's legs, facing in the same direction as the patient. EMT-B #2 then slips his or her hands under the patient's knees.

6. Both EMT-Bs move up to a crouching position, as soon as they are balanced and have a good grip on the patient.

**FIGURE 6-13**

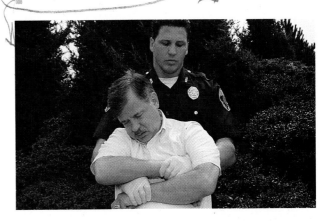

**A** Proper hand position for an extremity lift

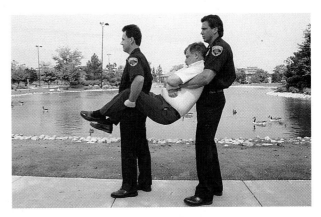

**B** Completed lift

7. Both EMT-Bs then stand fully upright and move the patient to a stretcher (Figure 6-13b).

You will be less likely to injure yourself if you bend at the hips and knees and use your legs for lifting. Remember that the patient may be uncomfortable in this position. This lift and carry increases pressure on the patient's chest, as the abdominal organs are pressing against the diaphragm.

### Supine Transfer

Sliding a patient from a bed to the ambulance stretcher is usually done in one of two ways. One way is to directly lift and then carry the patient a short distance to the bed or stretcher. Another way is to place the stretcher next to the bed. You can then use the bed sheets to slide the patient from the bed to the stretcher. Both methods are acceptable (Figures 6-14 to 6-15). You and your team will have to choose the way that is most appropriate for your situation. Factors involved in this decision include the following:

- the size and weight of the patient
- the number of EMT-Bs and helpers available
- the amount of space around the patient's bed

# PATIENT HANDLING EQUIPMENT

## STRETCHERS

**Wheeled Stretchers**

The **wheeled ambulance stretcher** is the most commonly used device for moving patients, as it makes moving patients easy. A wheeled ambulance stretcher has a number of standard features. The stretcher can be adjusted to a number of different heights and commonly has handles for lifting and rolling. Side bars and restraint straps should be used to secure the patient while moving. The mattress on an ambulance stretcher must not absorb any type of fluid—water, blood, or other body fluids. Fluid-resistant mattresses are necessary so that infectious materials are not absorbed into them. However, stretchers are heavy (about 70 lb) and large, which makes them difficult to maneuver over rough ground.

In most instances, the best way to move a wheeled stretcher is to pull it from the

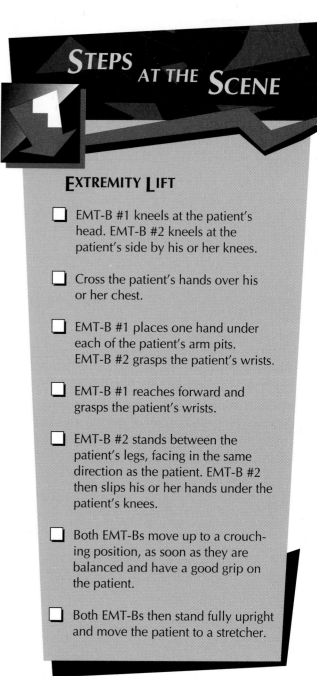

## STEPS AT THE SCENE

### EXTREMITY LIFT

- [ ] EMT-B #1 kneels at the patient's head. EMT-B #2 kneels at the patient's side by his or her knees.

- [ ] Cross the patient's hands over his or her chest.

- [ ] EMT-B #1 places one hand under each of the patient's arm pits. EMT-B #2 grasps the patient's wrists.

- [ ] EMT-B #1 reaches forward and grasps the patient's wrists.

- [ ] EMT-B #2 stands between the patient's legs, facing in the same direction as the patient. EMT-B #2 then slips his or her hands under the patient's knees.

- [ ] Both EMT-Bs move up to a crouching position, as soon as they are balanced and have a good grip on the patient.

- [ ] Both EMT-Bs then stand fully upright and move the patient to a stretcher.

foot end while your partner guides it from the head end. The stretcher can be top-heavy if you have to move a heavy patient and the stretcher is elevated. Therefore, you must turn and roll the stretcher with care to avoid tipping it over. When the stretcher must be carried, it is best to have four EMT-Bs available for the carry. If only two EMT-Bs are present, or if only two EMT-Bs can carry the stretcher due to limited space, there is considerable risk that the stretcher

PREPARING TO BE AN EMT-B

FIGURE 6-14

FIGURE 6-15

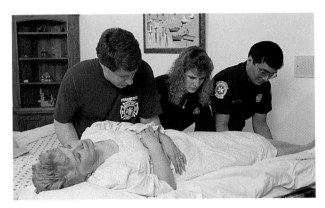

**A** Move and secure the stretcher parallel to the bed and lift the patient on command

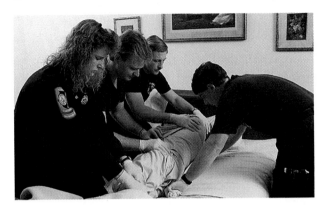

**A** Log roll the patient onto a bed sheet

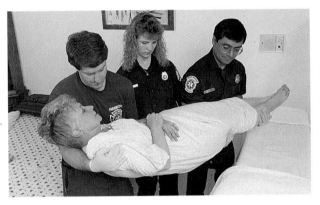

**B** "Walk" the patient around and position over the bed

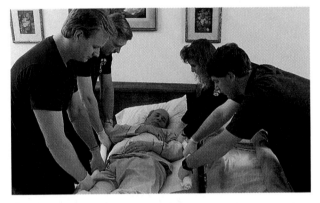

**B** Move and secure the stretcher parallel to the bed

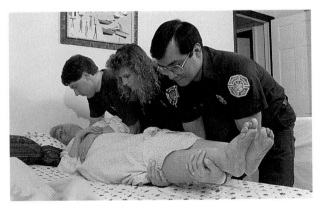

**C** Completed transfer

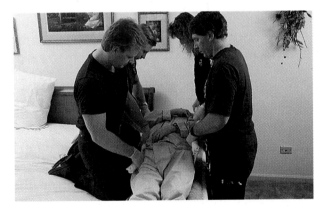

**C** Transfer the patient to a stretcher

will become unbalanced. If two EMT-Bs must carry the stretcher, one should stand at the head end facing the other at the foot end. This type of carry means that one EMT-B will be walking backward.

With a four-person carry, there is much more stability, and the carry requires less strength. With this type of carry, one EMT-B should be positioned at each corner to provide an even lift. This carry is much safer when the stretcher must be moved over rough ground.

Use of a scoop stretcher as an interim device to move a patient onto a wheeled stretcher is presented in Figure 6-16. Use of a blanket lift to move a patient to the stretcher is shown in Figure 6-17. A chair-to-wheelchair transfer is shown in Figure 6-18. The proper methods of lifting, moving, and loading stretchers are shown in Figures 6-19 to 6-22. Because you will use many types of stretchers, it is impossible to describe each type and variation in procedure here. But, remember the following three guidelines when loading a stretcher into an ambulance:

1. Make sure there is sufficient lifting power.

2. Follow the manufacturer's directions for safe and proper use of the stretcher.

3. Make sure that all stretchers and patients are fully secured before moving the ambulance.

### Portable Stretchers

**Portable stretchers** may be used to move patients from difficult areas where the wheeled stretcher cannot reach, or may be placed on the squad bench in the ambulance when two patients must be transported.

Portable stretchers are also available in a wide variety of designs and configurations. One of the most common has an aluminum frame with canvas or some type of fabric stretched within the frame. Typically,

## FIGURE 6-16

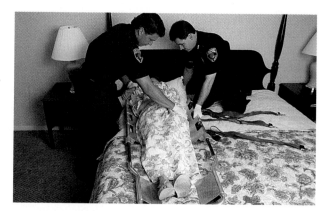

**A**    Place scoop stretcher around the patient

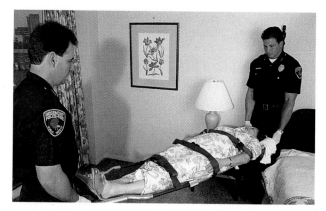

**B**    Lock scoop stretcher and transfer the patient

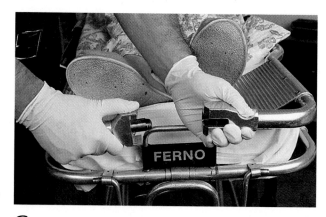

**C**    Unlock and remove the scoop stretcher

the frame is hinged at the sides to allow easy storage (Figure 6-23). The portable stretcher weighs much less than the wheeled

## FIGURE 6-17

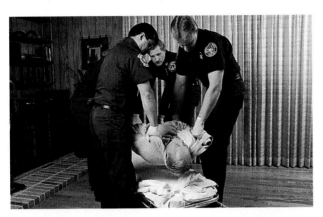

**A** Log roll the patient onto a blanket

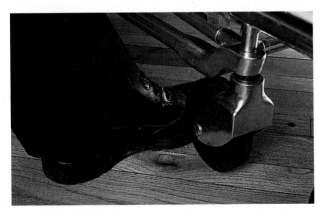

**B** Lift the patient from the floor to the stretcher

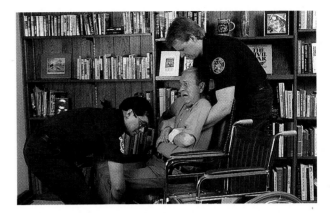

*(stretcher image C)*

**C** Secure the stretcher so it does not roll during transfer

stretcher. A portable stretcher does not have the bulky undercarriage of a wheeled

## FIGURE 6-18

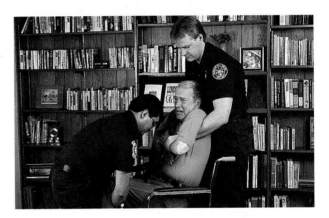

**A** The proper position for lifting a patient from a chair

*(wheelchair image B)*

**B** Lower the patient into the wheelchair

stretcher. There is a trade-off, however. A portable stretcher has no wheels. Therefore, you and your team must support all of the patient's weight and any equipment along with the weight of the stretcher.

A **stair chair** is used to transport patients up and down stairways. Stair chairs typically have extended handles behind the patient's shoulders and handles or a grab bar below the patient's feet. These extended handles behind the shoulders and below the feet make this difficult task much easier and safer (Figure 6-24). Once you have moved down the stairs or past some other obstacle, you typically transfer the patient to a more conventional stretcher.

## FIGURE 6-19

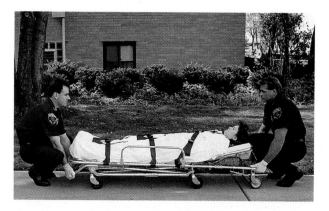

**A** The proper position for lifting a stretcher

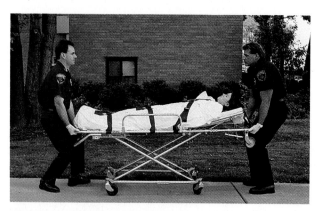

**B** Proper lifting mechanics

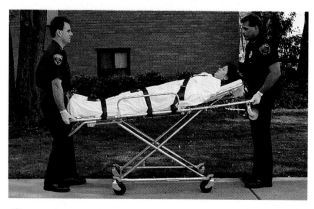

**C** Completed lift

## FIGURE 6-20

Navigating stairs with a loaded stretcher

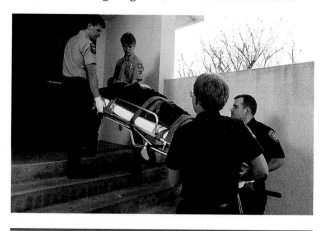

## FIGURE 6-21

Moving a stretcher over an obstacle

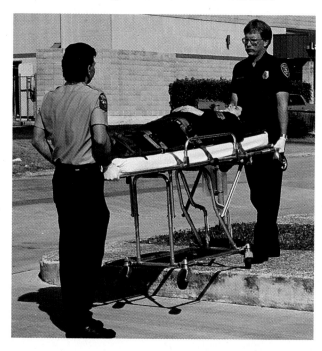

### Scoop Stretchers

The **scoop stretcher** or split litter is a unique piece of equipment designed to be split into two or four pieces. These sections are fitted around a patient who is lying on the ground or other relatively flat surface. The parts are then reconnected and the patient can be lifted for placement on a long spine board or stretcher. A classic use of the scoop stretcher is for patients who have been struck by a motor vehicle (Figure 6-25).

## FIGURE 6-22

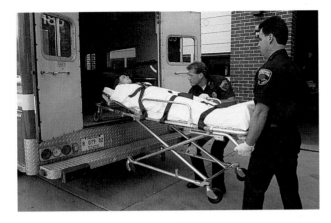

Loading a stretcher into the unit

## FIGURE 6-24

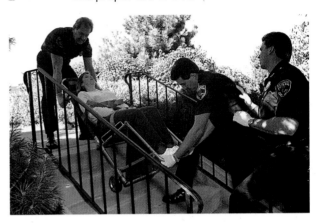

The proper use of a stair chair

## FIGURE 6-23

Portable stretcher

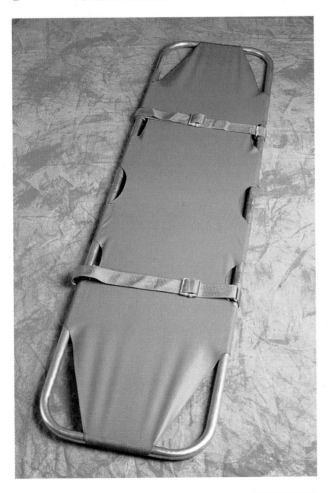

Although efficient, the scoop stretcher requires that both sides of the patient be accessible. "Scooping" a patient also requires special attention to the closure area beneath the patient. The stretcher may trap clothing, skin, or other objects. As with the long spine board, you must fully stabilize and secure the patient before you move him or her. However, unlike a long spine board, the scoop stretcher cannot be slipped under the long axis of the body. Scoop stretchers are narrow, well constructed, compact for storage, and have excellent body support features. They are not adequate when used alone for standard immobilization of a spinal injury. You and your team should practice often with a scoop stretcher so that in a patient situation you will be ready.

### Basket Stretchers

The **basket stretcher** or Stokes litter is commonly used in technical rescues and water rescues. It surrounds and supports the patient, yet has holes in the bottom to allow water to drain through them. Basket stretchers are usually made of plastic or wire (Figure 6-26). Older models include a woven wire basket constructed with a frame and carrying rails of metal tubing.

**FIGURE 6-25**

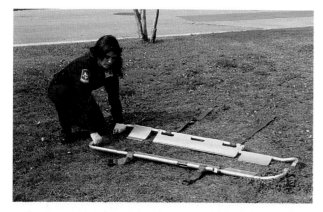

**A**  Separate the scoop stretcher lengthwise

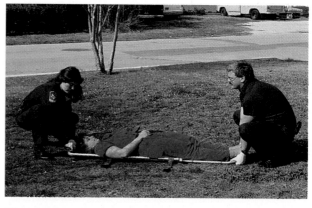

**B**  Slide the stretcher under the patient from each side

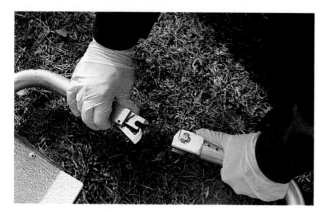

**C**  Lock the brackets

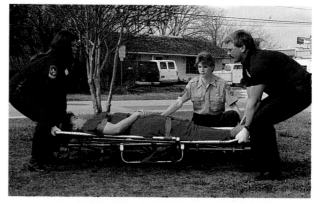

**D**  Load the patient with the appropriate lift

The wire basket Stokes is very uncomfortable for the patient unless the wire is padded. Unpadded woven wire has sharp ends that snag clothing, damage equipment, and may pierce the skin of the patient. Line the bottom of the basket with a waterproof material. Newer types of Stokes litters are made of plastic riveted to a large-diameter aluminum carrying rail. These newer models easily fit a full backboard.

### Flexible Stretchers

The **flexible stretcher**, often called a Reeves, Navy, or SKED stretcher, is the most uncomfortable of all the various devices for the patient. It does, however, pro-vide excellent support and immobilization. Flexible stretchers have two basic designs. A common characteristic to both designs is that while they can be folded or rolled when not in use, they become rigid carrying devices when secured around a patient.

Some flexible stretchers have rigid wooden slats sewn between two canvas sheets. These slats provide complete support along the long axis of the patient's body (Figure 6-27). When the stretcher is wrapped around the patient and the straps are secured, the patient is completely immobilized. The stretcher can then be lowered by rope or slid down a flight of stairs by resting it on the front edge of each step.

## FIGURE 6-26

Basket stretcher

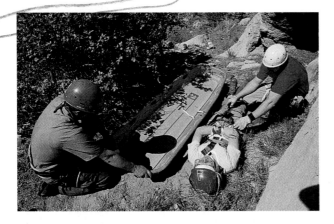

## FIGURE 6-28

Types of short spine boards

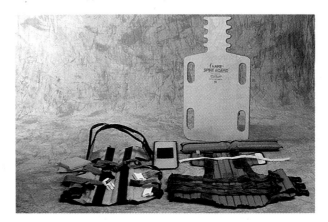

## FIGURE 6-27

Flexible stretcher

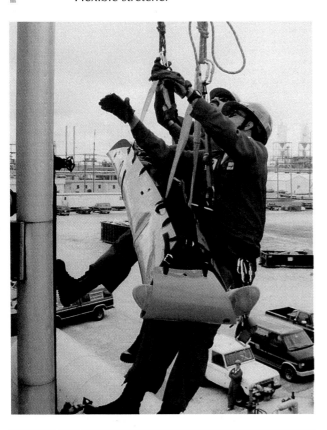

## BACKBOARDS

Long **backboards**, or spine boards, are used primarily for patients with suspected spinal injuries. They are 6' to 7' long and commonly used for patients who are found lying down. Backboards usually have a variety of handholds and strap holes—the more and the larger the better. Backboards were traditionally made of wood. More recent models are made of plastic materials that will not absorb blood or other infectious substances. Backboards can also be used to help move patients out of awkward places.

Short backboards are 3' to 4' long and typically used for patients who are found in a sitting position. The original short wooden backboard has largely been replaced with vest-type devices. These are specifically designed for immobilizing the head and torso of patients with possible spinal injuries (Figure 6-28).

# *IT'S TECHNIQUE, NOT TECHNOLOGY*

You've been off work for the past 3 weeks as a result of the back injury you suffered while carrying a very large patient out of a basement. Since your incident, the Education Specialist for your ambulance service has decided that the focus of this month's continuing education class will be on lifting and moving patients. It's a little late to keep you from getting injured, but it may be helpful for your co-workers. Who knows, you may even be used as a visual aid during the presentation.

## For Discussion

1. What are some of the things you should consider before you lift and move a patient?

2. Why is it important to know and practice a variety of lifting and moving techniques?

## PATIENT HANDLING AND POSITIONING

Every time you have to move a patient, you must be sure that you, your team, and the patient are not injured. Patient packaging and handling are technical skills that you will learn and perfect through practice and training.

Training and practice are required to use all the equipment described in this chapter. You must master the skills necessary for their use and understand the advantages and limitations of each device. Practice each technique with your team often so that when you must move a patient, you can perform the move quickly, safely, and efficiently. After each patient transfer, you and your team should evaluate the appropriate-ness of the technique used, as well as your technical skill in completing the transfer. Also make sure you maintain your equipment according to the manufacturer's instructions. Using clean, well-maintained equipment is but one part of providing quality patient care.

After you deliver the patient to the emergency department, you and your team must begin preparing for your next call. Review the positive points about the transport. Discuss changes that would improve the next run. This process of review and evaluation identifies the following:

- procedures that need more practice

- equipment that needs to be cleaned or repaired

- skills that you need to review or acquire

Most important, a critical review helps you and your team become more confident and better skilled EMT-Bs.

Certain patient conditions, such as head injury, shock, spinal injury, and pregnancy call for special lifting and moving. Patients with chest pain or difficulty breathing should sit in a position of comfort, as long as they are not hypotensive.

Patients with suspected spinal injuries must be immobilized on a long spine board. Patients in shock should be packaged and moved with their legs elevated 8" to 12". Pregnant patients should be positioned and transported on their left sides. These special packaging and transport considerations are fully explained in their corresponding chapters.

# SECTION 2

# Airway

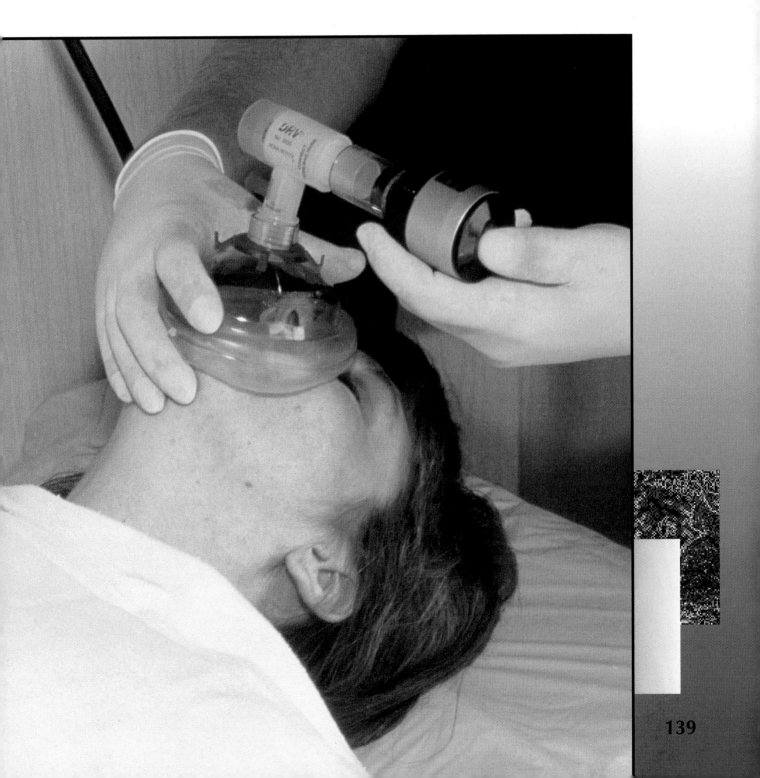

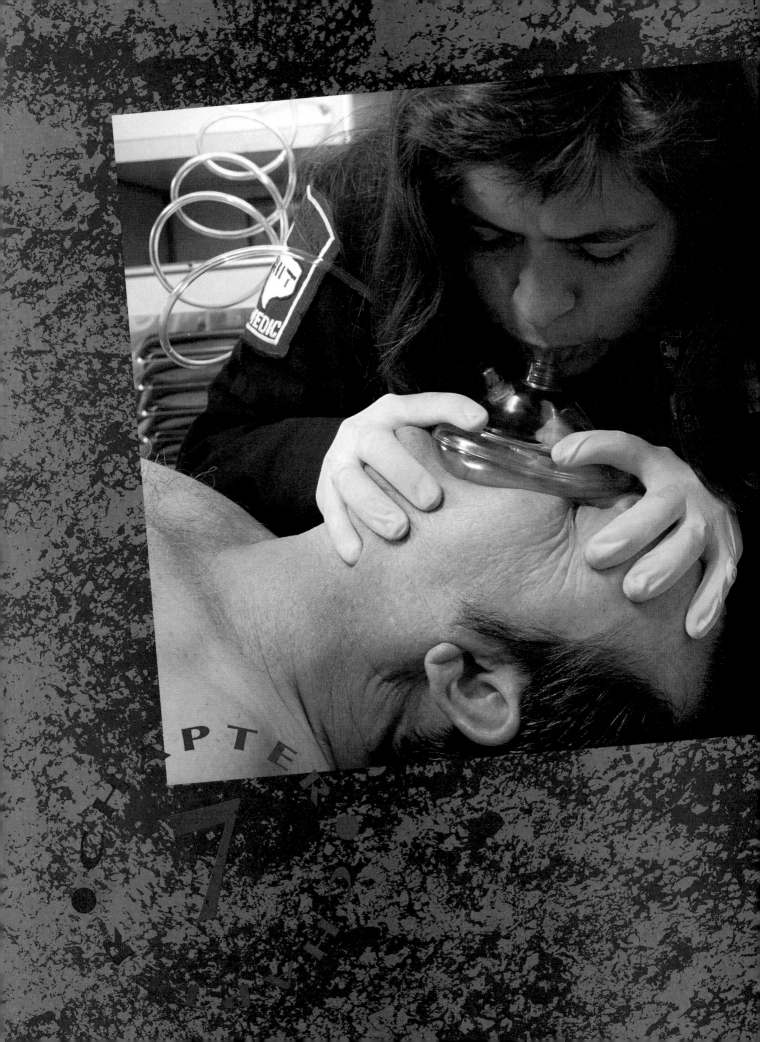

PTE

# The Mechanics of Breathing

## Objectives

After you have read this chapter, you should be able to:

- Name and label the major structures of the respiratory system on a diagram.
- List the signs of adequate breathing.
- List the signs of inadequate breathing.
- Explain the rationale for BLS artificial ventilation and airway protective skills taking priority over most other basic life support skills.

## Overview

The respiratory system is a very important part of the body. It delivers oxygen to the lungs and allows carbon dioxide to be removed. Our tissues and cells need a constant supply of this oxygen to survive. If the airway becomes blocked, or we have trouble breathing, oxygen will not reach the brain as it should. These problems can quickly lead to other, more serious problems with the heart or the brain. Within seconds after being deprived of oxygen, the heart will not beat normally. After as few as 4 to 6 minutes without oxygen, the brain may be severely and permanently damaged.

Oxygen reaches our body's tissues and cells in two ways: breathing and circulation. As we breathe, oxygen moves from the atmosphere into our lungs. The oxygen then passes from the air sacs in the lungs to the capillaries to oxygenate the blood. The blood, enriched with oxygen, travels through the body by the pumping action of the heart. At the same time, carbon dioxide produced by cells moves from the blood into the air sacs. The carbon dioxide then leaves our bodies as we exhale.

The purpose of this chapter is to explain how we breathe and how oxygen is delivered to every part of the body. For you to provide the lifesaving treatment needed when a patient is not breathing effectively, you must be able to locate the parts of the airway and understand how they work.

# Key Terms

**Agonal respirations**   Occasional, gasping breaths that occur after the heart has stopped. The respiratory center in the brain continues to send signals to the breathing muscles.

**Airway**   Refers to the upper airway tract or the passage above the larynx (voice box).

**Basic life support (BLS)**   A series of emergency lifesaving procedures that focus on the patient's airway, breathing, and circulation.

**Diffusion**   A process in which molecules move from an area with higher concentration of molecules to an area of lower concentration.

**Exhalation**   Part of the breathing process in which the diaphragm and the intercostal muscles relax. As these muscles relax, all dimensions of the thorax decrease, and the ribs and muscles assume a normal resting position.

**Inhalation**   The active muscular part of breathing that occurs as we inhale.

**Labored breathing**   Breathing that requires effort, in which the person may be breathing either much slower or much faster than normal.

# BREATHING AND THE BODY

## ANATOMY REVIEW—ADULTS

The respiratory system consists of all the structures in the body that help us breathe (normal respiration) (Figure 7-1). In this text, **airway** usually refers to the upper airway or the passage above the larynx (voice box). It includes the nose, mouth, and throat. The lower airway includes the larynx, trachea, main bronchi, and other air passages within the lungs. The respiratory system also includes the diaphragm, the muscles of the chest wall, and the accessory muscles of breathing. The diaphragm and muscles of the chest wall are responsible for the regular rise and fall of the chest that accompanies normal breathing.

## FIGURE 7-1

The upper and lower airways

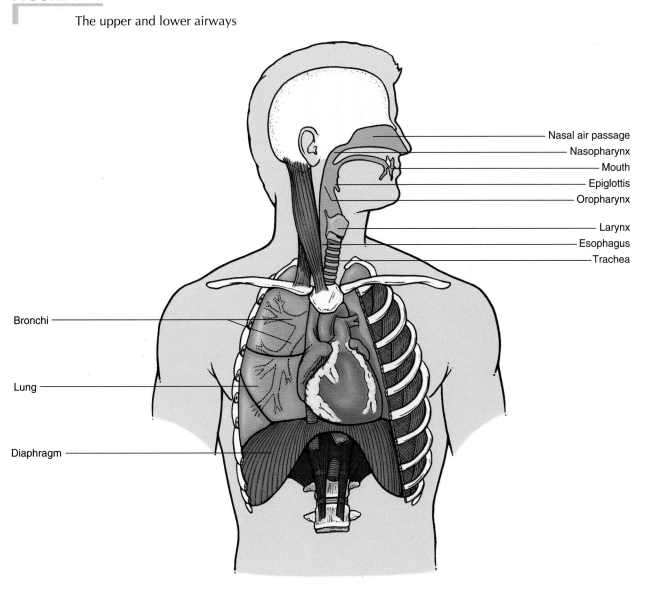

- Nasal air passage
- Nasopharynx
- Mouth
- Epiglottis
- Oropharynx
- Larynx
- Esophagus
- Trachea
- Bronchi
- Lung
- Diaphragm

The chest (thorax) contains the lungs—one in each half, or hemithorax. The lungs hang freely within the chest cavity. Between the lungs, in a space called the mediastinum, lie the heart, the great vessels, the esophagus, the trachea, the major bronchi, and many nerves. The boundaries of the thorax are the rib cage anteriorly, superiorly, and posteriorly, and the diaphragm inferiorly.

The diaphragm is one of the specialized muscles of the body. It is a skeletal muscle in that it is attached to the costal arch and the vertebrae (Figure 7-2). Like all other skeletal muscle, the diaphragm is striated, or marked by streaks or lines when seen under a microscope.

## FIGURE 7-2

The diaphragm

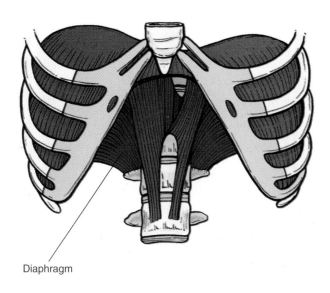

Diaphragm

The diaphragm is special because it can function both like a voluntary muscle and like an involuntary muscle. It acts like a voluntary muscle whenever we take a deep breath, cough, or hold our breath. We control these variations in the way we breathe. However, unlike other skeletal or voluntary muscles, the diaphragm performs an automatic function. Breathing continues while we sleep and at all other times. Even though we can hold our breath or temporarily breathe faster or slower, we cannot continue these variations in breathing pattern indefinitely. When the concentration of carbon dioxide rises, automatic regulation of breathing resumes. Although the diaphragm can act like a voluntary muscle and is attached to the skeleton, most of the time it acts like an involuntary muscle.

## HOW WE BREATHE

The lungs have no muscle tissue and, as a result, cannot move on their own. The lungs need the help of other structures to expand and contract as we inhale and exhale. These structures include the thorax, the thoracic cage (chest), the diaphragm, the intercostal muscles, and the accessory muscles of breathing. The thoracic cage is a semirigid muscular and bony frame enclosed by skin. Through movement of the thoracic cage and the diaphragm, air enters the lungs through the trachea and passes into the alveoli.

### Inhalation

The active muscular part of breathing occurs as we inhale **(inhalation)**. As we inhale, air enters the body through the trachea. It travels to and from the lungs, filling and emptying the alveoli. During inhalation, the diaphragm and intercostal muscles contract. When the diaphragm contracts, it moves down slightly and enlarges the thoracic cage from top to bottom. When the intercostal muscles contract, they raise the ribs up and out. As we inhale, the combined actions of these structures enlarge the thorax in all dimensions. Because the lungs are attached to these structures, the lungs follow the motion of the chest wall exactly. Take a deep breath to see how your chest expands.

The air pressure outside the body (called the atmospheric pressure) is normally higher than the air pressure within the thorax.

## FIGURE 7-3

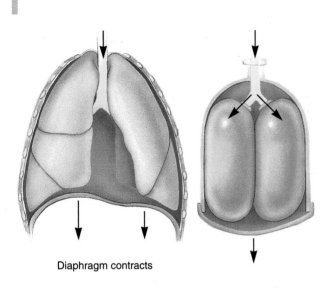

Diaphragm contracts

**A** Inhalation and chest expansion, anatomic (left), and bell jar (right)

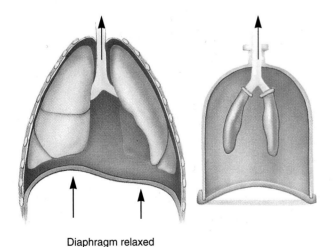

Diaphragm relaxed

**B** Exhalation and chest contraction, anatomic (left), and bell jar (right)

As we inhale and the thoracic cage expands, the air pressure within the thorax decreases a bit more, creating a slight vacuum. This drives air in through the trachea and fills the lungs. When the air pressure outside equals the air pressure inside, air stops moving. Gases, like oxygen, will move from an area of high pressure to an area of lower pressure until the pressures are equal. When the pressures are equal, the air stops moving. At this point, we stop inhaling.

A simple way to visualize how we breathe is to think of the thoracic cage as a bell jar in which balloons are suspended. In this example, the balloons are the lungs. The base of the jar is the diaphragm, which moves up and down slightly with each breath. The ribs, which are the sides of the jar, maintain the shape of the chest. The only opening into the jar is a small tube at the top, similar to the trachea. During inhalation, the bottom of the jar moves down slightly and decreases pressure in the jar, creating a slight vacuum. As a result, the balloons fill with air (Figure 7-3a).

**Exhalation**

Unlike inhalation, **exhalation** does not normally require muscular effort. During exhalation, the diaphragm and the intercostal muscles relax. As these muscles relax, all dimensions of the thorax decrease, and the ribs and muscles assume a normal resting position. When the size of the thoracic cavity decreases, air in the lungs is compressed into a smaller space. The air pressure within the thorax then becomes higher than the pressure outside, and air is pushed out through the trachea (Figure 7-3b).

Let's return to the example of the bell jar. During exhalation, the bottom of the jar (the diaphragm) moves up, returning to its normal resting position. This movement increases air pressure within the jar. With this increase in pressure, the sides of the jar contract, and the balloons empty.

Remember that air will only reach the lungs if it travels through the trachea. Air may readily pass into the chest cavity through another opening, but it will not reach the alveoli. That is why "clearing the airway" and "maintaining the airway" are so important. Clearing the airway means removing obstructing material or tissue from the nose, mouth, or throat (Figure 7-4). "Maintaining the airway" means to keep the airway open so that air can enter and leave the lungs freely.

## FIGURE 7-4

Movement of air in a clear airway

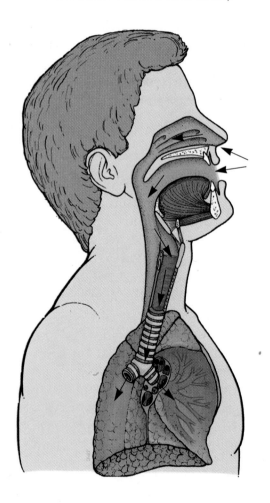

Treating airway problems in children presents special problems, due to key differences in their anatomy. A child's head, in proportion to the rest of the body, is larger than an adult's head. A child's larynx is higher and more anterior than an adult's larynx. The diameter of the airway at all levels is smaller in a child. This means that an object that may cause a partial airway obstruction in an adult would completely obstruct a child's airway. A child's tongue is also relatively large for body size. This means that a child's tongue can cause an airway obstruction more easily than an adult's tongue (Figure 7-5). An illness or injury that causes the tongue or other areas of the airway to swell would affect a child much more seriously than an adult. For example, a condition called epiglottitis, in which the epiglottis becomes swollen, occurs in both adults and children. This condition is rarely serious in adults, but is commonly life threatening in children. All of the supporting cartilages of the larynx, cricoid, and trachea are less rigid in children than adults. As a result, only a moderate amount of external pressure will close off a child's airway. The same pressure would not affect adults or would affect them minimally. It is important for you to remember that a child's airway is much more at risk for obstruction than an adult's airway and may be more difficult to establish and maintain.

# RESPIRATORY PHYSIOLOGY

Each living cell in the body requires a regular supply of oxygen. Some cells need a constant supply of oxygen to survive. For example, cells in the heart may be damaged

## FIGURE 7-5

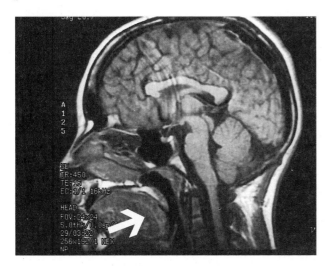

**A**   MRI image of the head and neck of an adult, and tongue size in relation to the airway

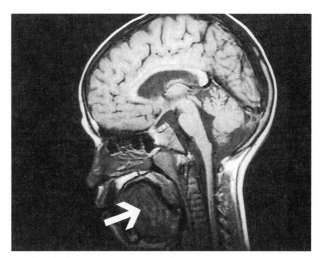

**B**   MRI image of the head and neck of a child—larger tongue in relation to the airway

if the oxygen supply is interrupted for more than a few seconds. Brain cells and cells in the nervous system may die after as few as 4 to 6 minutes without oxygen (Figure 7-6). Dead cells can never be replaced. Permanent changes in the body, such as brain damage, result from the damage caused by a lack of oxygen. Other cells in the body are not as vitally dependent on a constant oxygen supply. They can tolerate short periods without oxygen and still survive.

Normally, the air that we breathe contains 21% oxygen and 78% nitrogen. Small amounts of other gases make up the final 1%.

## THE EXCHANGE OF OXYGEN AND CARBON DIOXIDE

As blood travels through the body, it gives its oxygen and nutrients to various tissues and cells. Oxygen passes from the blood through the capillaries to tissue cells. In the reverse process, carbon dioxide and cell waste passes from tissue cells through capillaries to the blood.

Each time we take a breath, the alveoli receive a supply of oxygen-rich air. The oxygen then passes into a fine network of pulmonary capillaries, which are in close contact with the alveoli. In fact, the capillaries in the lungs are located in the walls of the alveoli. The walls of the capillaries and the alveoli are extremely thin. Thus, the air in

## FIGURE 7-6

Time is critical for the brain to receive oxygen

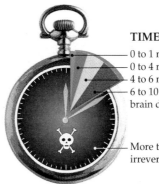

**TIME IS CRITICAL!**
0 to 1 minute: cardiac irritability
0 to 4 minutes: brain damage not likely
4 to 6 minutes: brain damage possible
6 to 10 minutes:
brain damage very likely

More than 10 minutes:
irreversible brain damage

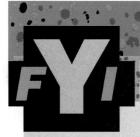

## How the Lungs Breathe

The lungs have no muscle and hang freely in the chest. Thus, they cannot expand or contract on their own. The lungs expand and contract as the chest moves. The lungs move with the chest because of the *pleura*. There are two layers of pleura. The first layer, the visceral pleura, is smooth, glistening tissue that covers each lung. The second layer, called the parietal pleura, lines the inside of the chest cavity. Between the two layers is the *pleural space*. This space contains a thin film of lubricating pleural fluid. As the chest wall expands, the lungs are pulled along with it. The lungs are made to expand by the force exerted through these closely applied pleural surfaces.

As we inhale and exhale, the diaphragm and intercostal muscles move as well. As these muscles contract, the thoracic cage expands in three directions—anteroposterior, transverse, and inferosuperior. The muscles are attached to the pleural surfaces. This enables the lungs to follow the motion of the chest wall exactly.

the alveoli and the blood in the capillaries are separated by two very thin layers of tissue.

Oxygen and carbon dioxide pass rapidly across these thin tissue layers through **diffusion.** Diffusion is a passive process in which molecules move from an area with higher concentration of molecules to an area of lower concentration. For example, a gas such as hydrogen sulfide (the odor of rotten eggs) moves from an area of high concentration near the egg, by spontaneous movement of the gas molecules, until the odor fills the room (Figure 7-7). There are more oxygen molecules in the alveoli than in the blood. Therefore, the oxygen molecules move from the alveoli into the blood. Because there are more carbon dioxide molecules in the blood than in the inhaled air, carbon dioxide moves from the blood into the alveoli (Figure 7-8).

## FIGURE 7-7

Diffusion of odors

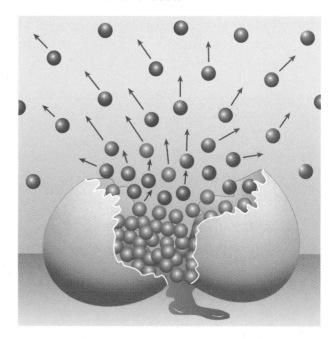

## FIGURE 7-8

Tissue diffusion

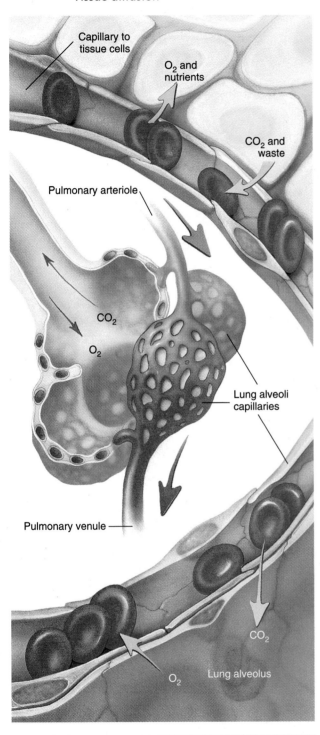

Capillary to tissue cells

O$_2$ and nutrients

CO$_2$ and waste

Pulmonary arteriole

CO$_2$

O$_2$

Lung alveoli capillaries

Pulmonary venule

CO$_2$

O$_2$

Lung alveolus

The blood does not use all the inhaled oxygen as it passes through the body. Exhaled air contains 16% oxygen and 3% to 5% carbon dioxide. The rest is nitrogen (Figure 7-9). This 16% concentration of oxygen is adequate to support artificial ventilation. So, as you provide artificial ventilations to a patient who is not breathing, that patient is receiving 16% concentration of oxygen with each exhaled breath.

## THE CONTROL OF BREATHING

The brain, or more specifically, an area of the brain stem, controls breathing. This area is in one of the best-protected parts of the nervous system—deep within the skull. The nerves in this area act as sensors of the level of carbon dioxide in the blood. The brain automatically controls breathing if the levels of carbon dioxide or oxygen in the arterial blood are too high or too low. In fact, adjustments can be made in just one breath. For these reasons, you cannot hold your breath indefinitely or breathe rapidly and deeply indefinitely.

When the level of carbon dioxide becomes too high, the brain stem sends nerve impulses down the spinal cord that cause the diaphragm and the intercostal muscles to contract. This increases our breathing, or respiratory rate. The higher the level of carbon dioxide in the blood, the stronger the impulses to cause breathing. Once the carbon dioxide levels return to an acceptable level, the strength and frequency of respiration decrease.

We also have a "backup system" to control respiration. It is called the hypoxic drive. When oxygen levels fall, this system will also stimulate breathing. There are nerves in the brain, the walls of the aorta, and the carotid arteries that act as oxygen sensors. These sensors are easily satisfied by minimal levels of oxygen in the arterial blood. Therefore, our backup system, the hypoxic drive, is much less sensitive and less powerful than the carbon dioxide sensors in the brain stem.

FIGURE 7-9

The components of exhaled air

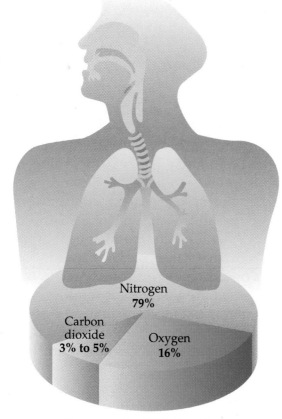

**Components of Exhaled Air**

## CHARACTERISTICS OF NORMAL BREATHING

Earlier in this chapter, breathing was compared to an expandable bell jar with a movable bottom. You can also think of a "normal" breathing pattern as a bellows system. Normal breathing should appear easy, not "labored." As with a bellows used to move air to start a fire, breathing should be a smooth flow of air moving in and out of the lungs. Normal breathing has the following characteristics:

- a normal rate and depth
- a regular pattern of inhalation and exhalation
- good audible breath sounds on both sides of the chest
- regular rise and fall movement on both sides of the chest
- movement of the abdomen

## BREATHING PATTERNS IN ADULTS

An adult who is awake, alert, and talking to you has no *immediate* airway or breathing problems. However, you should keep supplemental oxygen on hand to assist with breathing if it should become necessary. An adult who is not breathing well will appear to be working hard to breathe. This type of breathing pattern is called **labored breathing.** Labored breathing requires effort and may involve the accessory muscles. The person may also be breathing either much slower (less than 8) or much faster (more than 24) than normal. An adult who is breathing normally will have respirations of 12 to 20 breaths per minute (Table 7-1).

With a normal breathing pattern, the accessory muscles are not being used. With inadequate breathing, a person, especially a child, may use the accessory muscles of the chest, neck, and abdomen. Other signs that a person is not breathing normally include the following:

- muscle retractions above the clavicles, between the ribs, and below the rib cage, especially in children
- pale or cyanotic (blue) skin
- cool, damp (clammy) skin

A patient may also appear to be breathing after the heart has stopped. These occasional, gasping breaths are called **agonal respirations.** Agonal respirations occur when the respiratory center in the brain continues to send signals to the breathing muscles. These respirations are not adequate, since they are slow and generally shallow. You should assist ventilations of patients with agonal respirations.

## BREATHING PATTERNS IN INFANTS AND CHILDREN

"Normal" breathing patterns in infants and children are essentially the same as those in adults. However, infants and children breathe faster than adults. An infant who is breathing normally will have respirations of 25 to 50 breaths per minute. A child will

**TABLE 7-1**   NORMAL RESPIRATION RATE RANGES

| | |
|---|---|
| Adults | 12 to 20 breaths per minute |
| Children | 15 to 30 breaths per minute |
| Infants | 25 to 50 breaths per minute |

To obtain the breathing rate in a patient, count the number of breaths in a 30-second period and multiply by two. Avoid letting the patient know that you are counting to prevent influencing the rate.

## HURRY, COME QUICK!

YOU ARE THE EMT

Dispatch receives a call from a frantic caller who says, "Hurry, come quick!" You are sent to a local hardware store for a woman who has quit breathing. Fortunately, your unit is in the area when the call comes in, so you are on the scene within 2 minutes. On arrival, you find a 75-year-old woman lying supine on the floor. The patient is unconscious and unresponsive to any stimuli. A store employee is providing mouth-to-mouth ventilation. You see good rise and fall of the chest with each breath. However, the patient's skin is still slightly cyanotic, warm, and moist. You tell the employee to stop so that you can reassess the patient. You find that she still is not breathing, but she has a regular pulse of 130/min.

### For Discussion

1. How is it possible that a patient can have a pulse, but is not breathing? Give at least two examples of situations where this might occur.

2. Why is timely airway management with this patient such a priority issue?

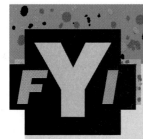

## Metabolism

All living cells need energy to survive. Cells take energy from nutrients through a series of chemical processes. The name given to the sum of these processes is **metabolism.** In the process of metabolism, each cell combines nutrients and oxygen and produces energy and waste products (primarily water and carbon dioxide). This basic metabolic chemical reaction occurs in all cells:

$$C_6H_{12}O_6 + 6O_2 \rightarrow 6CO_2 + 6H_2O + Energy$$

(Glucose)  (Oxygen)   (Carbon Dioxide)   (Water)

have respirations of 15 to 30 breaths per minute. Like adults, infants and children who are breathing normally will have smooth, regular inhalation and exhalation, equal breath sounds, and regular rise and fall movement on both sides of the chest.

Breathing problems in infants and children often appear the same as breathing problems in adults. Signs such as a faster respiratory rate, an irregular breathing pattern, unequal breath sounds, and unequal chest expansion indicate breathing problems in both adults and children. Other signs that an infant or child is not breathing normally include the following:

- muscle retractions, in which the muscles of the chest and neck are working extra hard in breathing

- nasal flaring in children, in which the nostrils flare out as the child breathes

- see-saw respirations in infants, in which the chest and abdominal muscles alternately contract to look like a see-saw

Exhalation becomes active when infants and children have trouble breathing. Nor-

mally, inhalation alone is the active, muscular part of breathing, as described earlier. However, with labored breathing, both inhalation and exhalation are hard work. With labored breathing, exhalation is not passive. Instead, air is forced out of the lungs during exhalation, and the child will often begin to wheeze. This type of labored breathing involves the use of the accessory muscles of breathing.

## HANDLING BREATHING PROBLEMS

Patients with airway and breathing problems need immediate care. As described earlier in the chapter, after as few as 4 to 6 minutes without oxygen, the brain may be severely and permanently damaged. Your first step will be to begin basic life support measures. **Basic life support (BLS)** is a series of emergency lifesaving procedures that focus on the patient's airway, breathing, and circulation. Please refer to appendix A for a review of BLS procedures, including basic principles of CPR.

Starting BLS measures should always be your first steps in caring for any patient with breathing problems. Ideally, only seconds should pass between the time you see that BLS is needed and the start of treatment. Therefore, you must quickly assess the patient for airway, breathing, and/or circulation problems right away. The outstanding advantage of BLS is that it permits the earliest possible treatment of airway obstruction, respiratory arrest, or cardiac arrest without the initial need for specialized equipment or material.

If a patient has trouble breathing or is not breathing at all, you may only need to open or clear the airway and the patient will be able to breathe. You may have to begin artificial ventilation. If a patient stops breathing before the heart stops, there will be enough oxygen in the lungs to maintain life for several minutes. Your efforts at artificial ventilation are successful if you see the following occur:

- the regular rise and fall of the chest with each ventilation

- a regular rate of ventilations, appropriate for the age of the patient

- a resumption of the regular heart rate

If the patient's heart rate does not return to normal, you must begin full CPR, as described in appendix A.

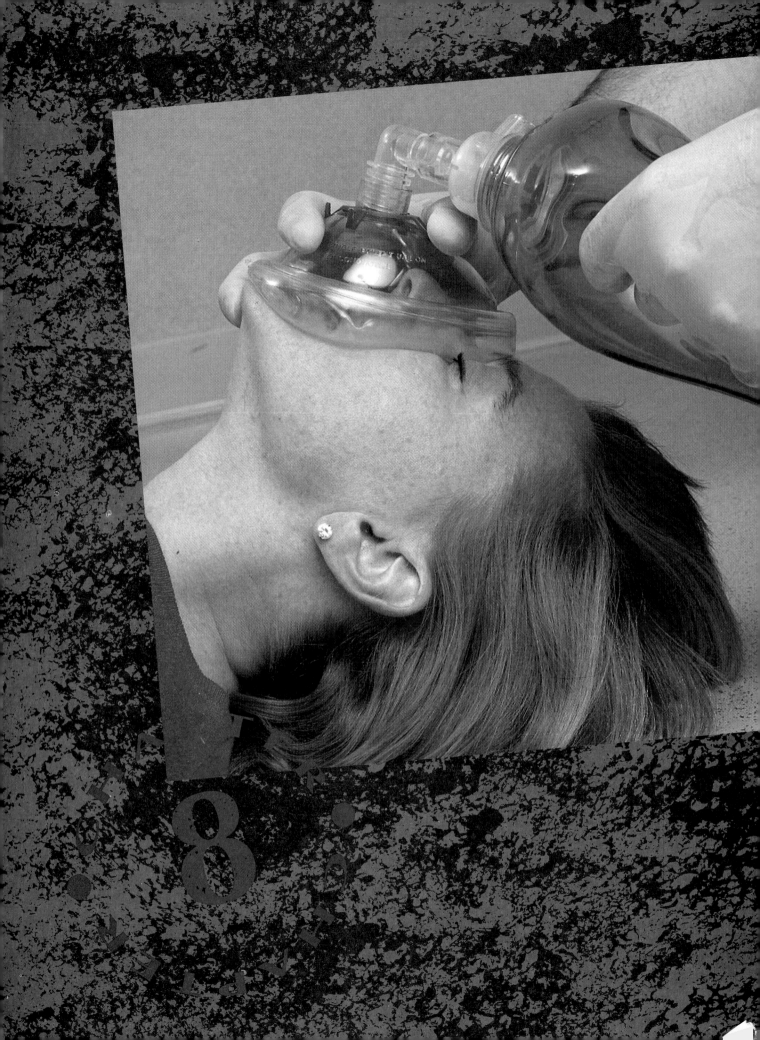

# Airway and Ventilation

## Objectives

After you have read this chapter, you should be able to:

- Describe the steps in the four techniques of opening the airway.
- Relate mechanism of injury to opening the airway.
- State the importance of having a suction unit ready for immediate use when providing emergency care.
- Describe the importance of suctioning.
- Describe how to artificially ventilate patients using various ventilation devices.
- List the parts of a bag-valve-mask device.
- Describe the signs of both adequate and inadequate artificial ventilation using the bag-valve-mask device.
- List the proper steps in performing mouth-to-mouth (or mask) and mouth-to-stoma artificial ventilation.

## Overview

The single most important step in caring for any patient is to make sure that the patient can breathe. As you continue with your training, you will hear and see "establish the airway," "maintain the airway," or "clear the airway" time and again. Without an open airway, the patient will not receive any oxygen.

This chapter describes several ways in which you can open a patient's airway so that the patient can start breathing

155

again or so that you can provide artificial ventilation. The patient's condition—conscious or unconscious, with or without possible head or spinal injury—will dictate the way you open the airway. Similarly, you will use specific techniques to remove foreign objects that block the airway. In all cases, you must clear a patient's airway as quickly and carefully as possible.

The chapter begins by explaining how to properly position patients in order to open the airway. The second section briefly reviews basic techniques for opening the airway. The third section describes the proper technique for suctioning. The fourth section reviews how to provide artificial ventilation and clear foreign body obstructions in adults. This section also describes ventilation techniques for patients with stomas and tracheostomy tubes. The chapter concludes with a discussion of how to manage the airway of patients with special needs.

## Key Terms

**Bag-valve-mask device** Device with face mask attached to a bag with a reservoir and connected to oxygen. Delivers more than 90% supplemental oxygen to the patient.

**Barrier device** A protective item, such as a valved pocket mask, that limits your exposure to the patient's body fluids.

**Gastric distention** Condition in which air fills the stomach as a result of high volume and pressure during artificial ventilation.

**Head-tilt/chin-lift maneuver** Combination of two movements to open the airway in which the forehead is tilted back and the chin lifted.

**Head-tilt maneuver** Technique to open the airway by tilting the patient's head backward.

**Jaw-thrust maneuver** Technique to open the airway by placing the fingers behind the angle of the jaw and bringing the jaw forward.

**Partial airway obstruction** Condition in which a patient is able to exchange air in the lungs, but has some degree of respiratory distress.

**Recovery position** Position used to help maintain a clear airway in a patient who has not had traumatic injuries and is breathing on his or her own.

**Stoma** An opening in the neck that connects the trachea directly to the skin.

**Tonsil tip** Type of suction tip best for suctioning the pharynx. Tonsil tips have a large diameter and are somewhat rigid to prevent collapse.

# POSITIONING THE PATIENT

Because of the urgent need to start BLS, your initial assessment of a patient must be done quickly and carefully. During this assessment, you quickly evaluate the adequacy of the patient's airway, the quality of breathing and circulation, and the level of consciousness. Level of consciousness is often a good guide to the extent of BLS the patient may need. For example, a patient who is alert and oriented does not need BLS. However, patients who are not fully conscious often need some degree of BLS, such as airway and ventilation support. Not all unconscious patients need all parts of BLS. For instance, they may not need circulatory support. However, all patients who are in need of *full* BLS (airway, breathing, and circulatory support) are unconscious.

For an unconscious patient who needs CPR, try to find out what happened to the patient. Was the patient hit in the head? Does the patient have a spinal injury? If you believe a patient may have had such an injury, you must take care during CPR to protect the spinal cord from injury. However, the presence of a head or spinal injury should not keep you from starting BLS. It simply means that you should perform BLS within certain specific physical limits and with extra care. These extra careful measures help to protect and maintain the spine from further damage.

As you learned in your BLS training, for CPR to be effective, you must make sure that the patient is lying down, faceup (supine) on a firm, flat surface. There must also be enough clear space around the patient to allow two rescuers to perform CPR. If the patient is lying facedown, you must quickly and carefully reposition the patient. A supine position is the best for clearing and maintaining the airway. The few seconds spent in positioning the patient properly will greatly improve the delivery of CPR.

The **recovery position** is used to help maintain a clear airway in a patient who has not had traumatic injuries and is breathing on his or her own. The patient is rolled onto the right or left side so that the head, shoulders, and torso move at the same time without twisting. The patient's hands are then placed under the cheek (Figure 8-1).

## FIGURE 8-1

The recovery position

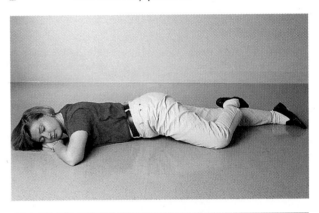

This position is used to help maintain spontaneous breathing. It also helps excretions, such as vomitus, to drain out of the mouth. A patient should be placed in the recovery position after initial resuscitation has restored spontaneous breathing.

However, if you suspect that a patient has had a traumatic spinal or head injury, you and your partner must use considerable caution when repositioning. The patient's head, neck, and back must be log rolled as a single unit.

You should reposition an unconscious adult patient for airway management in the following way: *(Again, always be aware of the possibility of a cervical spine injury!)*

1. Kneel beside the patient. You and your partner must be far enough away so that when rolled toward you, the patient does not come to rest in your lap (Figure 8-2a). For patients with no

spinal injury, use of the recovery position is very important to prevent aspiration of vomitus.

2. Rapidly straighten the patient's legs and move the nearer arm above the head (Figure 8-2b).

3. Place your hands behind the back of the head and neck of the patient to maintain the cervical spine. Your partner should place his or her hands on the distant shoulder and the hip (Figure 8-2c).

4. Turn the patient toward you by pulling on the distant shoulder and the hip. The head and neck should be controlled so that they move as a unit with the rest of the torso. In this way, the head and neck stay in the same vertical plane as the back. This single motion will minimize aggravation of any spinal injury. At this point, apply a cervical collar.

5. Replace the patient's farther arm back at the side once the patient is supine.

## FIGURE 8-2

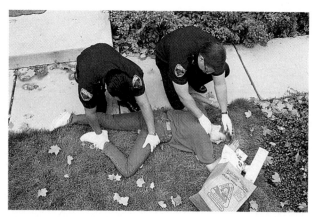

**A**  Place the patient in the recovery position

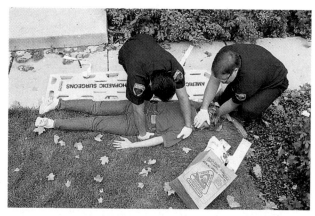

**B**  Reposition the patient's arms and legs

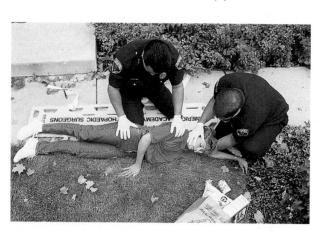

**C**  Protect the head and neck as you log roll the patient onto the backboard

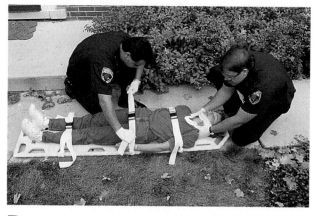

**D**  Secure the patient to the backboard

The patient should be log rolled onto a long spine board, when possible (Figure 8-2d). This device will provide support during transport and emergency department care. Once the patient is properly positioned, you can easily assess the patient's airway, breathing, and circulation, and BLS can be started if necessary.

# OPENING THE AIRWAY

Successful CPR is dependent on your ability to immediately open a patient's airway. Without an open airway, the patient will not get any oxygen during artificial ventilation. In an unconscious patient, the most common cause of airway obstruction usually occurs when the muscles of the throat and tongue relax. The tongue then falls back into the throat and obstructs the airway (Figure 8-3). In this case, the airway's own

## FIGURE 8-3

The tongue obstructing the airway

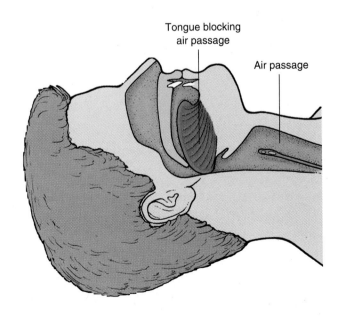

Tongue blocking
air passage

Air passage

tissues cause a blockage. Dentures (false teeth), blood, vomitus, mucus, food, or other foreign objects may also create a blockage. Therefore, you should always have a suction device available to help open and maintain the airway.

Patients with severe facial injuries may also have airway problems. Because the blood supply in the face is so rich, blunt injuries to the face could result in severe tissue swelling and bleeding into the airway. Airway obstruction due to an aspirated foreign body is reviewed later in the chapter and discussed in detail in appendix A, BLS Review. In your BLS course, you learned some basic techniques for opening the airway. These techniques are briefly reviewed here.

## BASIC TECHNIQUES FOR OPENING THE AIRWAY

### Head-Tilt/Chin-Lift Maneuver

Opening the airway can often be done quickly and easily by simply tilting the patient's head backward. This procedure is known as the **head-tilt maneuver**. Sometimes this simple maneuver is all that is needed for the patient to begin breathing on his or her own. The head tilt is the first and most important general step in opening the airway.

You should perform the head-tilt maneuver in an adult in the following way:

1. Make sure the patient is supine. Kneel close beside the patient.

2. Place one hand on the patient's forehead, and apply firm backward pressure with your palm. Move the patient's head as far back as possible (Figure 8-4).

This extension of the neck will move the tongue forward, away from the back of the throat. This movement will clear the airway, if the tongue is blocking it. However, you may have difficulty achieving an effective

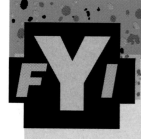

# What is Hypoxia?

Hypoxia is a condition that occurs when the cells in our bodies do not get enough oxygen. It is extremely dangerous and can result in death. Hypoxia develops quickly in the vital organs in patients who are not breathing. The patient will die in a matter of minutes if the hypoxia is not reversed. Patients who are able to breathe but unable to move enough air into the lungs with each breath will show varying signs of hypoxia. These signs may include apprehension, the use of accessory muscles for breathing, difficulty breathing, cyanosis, and even chest pain. The onset and the degree of tissue damage will depend on the quality of the respirations.

Early signs of hypoxia include tachycardia (fast heart rate), nervousness, irritability, apprehension, and fear. Conscious patients will complain of shortness of breath and may not be able to talk in complete sentences. Cyanosis develops later. The best time to give a patient oxygen is before any symptoms appear and whenever you suspect tissue damage. Some conditions that are commonly associated with hypoxia include the following:

1. Heart attack (myocardial infarction). Hypoxia from myocardial infarction occurs when there is inadequate circulation of oxygen-carrying blood to the tissues. This occurs because the heart is not working properly.

2. Pulmonary edema. Fluid accumulates in the lungs. This fluid makes the transfer of oxygen to the blood from the alveoli less efficient.

3. Acute drug overdose. Respirations may become infrequent and shallow.

4. Inhalation of smoke and toxic fumes. These substances cause pulmonary edema and destroy lung tissue, causing problems with gas exchange.

5. Stroke. The cause of hypoxia in a stroke patient is poor control of respiration and heart rhythms by the brain.

6. Chest injury. Pain prevents full chest wall expansion. Lung damage prevents efficient gas exchange.

7. Shock. Shock often occurs as a result of injuries where much blood is lost. With the loss of red blood cells' hemoglobin, not enough oxygen is available to the tissues.

8. Chronic obstructive pulmonary disease (COPD)(emphysema). Chronic irritation of the lungs and air passages produces alveolar damage and poor gas exchange.

All patients who are hypoxic, from whatever cause, should be treated with supplemental oxygen. The method of oxygen delivery will vary, depending on the cause and the severity of the hypoxia.

**FIGURE 8-4**

The head-tilt maneuver

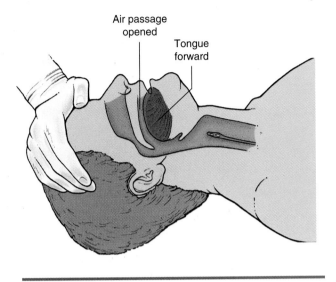

Air passage opened

Tongue forward

head tilt with only one hand on the forehead. You may need to perform a chin lift as well. The **head-tilt/chin-lift maneuver** combines two movements to open the airway. *Remember that neither the head-tilt maneuver nor the head-tilt/chin-lift maneuver should be used in cases of possible spinal injury.*

You should perform the head-tilt/chin-lift maneuver in an adult in the following way:

1. Perform the head-tilt maneuver, as described above, with one hand.

2. Place the tips of the fingers of your other hand under the bony part of the chin.

3. Lift the chin forward, bringing the entire lower jaw with it, helping to tilt the head back (Figure 8-5).

You must be sure that your fingers do not compress the soft tissue under the chin. This would block the airway. Continue to hold the forehead to maintain the backward tilt of the head. You should lift the chin so that the teeth are nearly brought together. However, you should avoid closing the mouth completely.

Loose dentures can be held in place with the chin lift, making obstruction by the lips less likely. Performing mouth-to-mouth ventilation is much easier when dentures are in place. However, dentures that do not stay in place should be removed. Partial dentures (plates) may come loose following an accident or as you are providing care. Check patients with partial dentures periodically to make sure their plates are firmly in place. Performing mouth-to-mask ventilation is much easier if loose dentures are removed.

**Jaw-Thrust Maneuver**

The two methods described above are effective for opening the airway of most patients. In some cases, forward movement of the lower jaw, the jaw-thrust maneuver, may be needed. The **jaw-thrust maneuver** is a technique to open the airway by placing the fingers behind the angle of the jaw and bringing the head forward.

You should perform the jaw-thrust maneuver in an adult in the following way:

1. Kneel above the patient's head. Place your fingers behind the angles of the patient's lower jaw and forcefully move the jaw forward.

2. Tilt the head backward without significantly extending the cervical spine.

3. Use your thumbs to pull the patient's lower jaw down, to allow breathing through the mouth as well as the nose (Figure 8-6).

If you suspect a cervical spine injury, you can modify this maneuver to keep the head in a neutral position as you move the jaw forward and open the mouth. However, only an unconscious patient will tolerate the maneuver. A mask can be used easily with both hands doing the jaw thrust while at the same time you seal the mask around the mouth. The nose may also be sealed with your thumbs using the modified jaw-thrust maneuver. Use your index and long fingers to thrust the jaw anteriorly while the thumbs compress the nose (Figure 8-7).

Once the airway has been opened by one of these techniques, the patient may start to breathe on his or her own. To assess whether breathing has returned, bend over and place your ear about 1" above the patient's nose and mouth. Listen carefully for sounds of breathing (Figure 8-8). Can you feel and hear movement of air? Turn your head to watch the patient's chest and abdomen. If you can see the patient's chest and abdomen move with each breath, breathing has returned. However, feeling and hearing the actual movement of air are more important than seeing the chest and abdomen move.

With complete airway obstruction, it is possible that there will be no movement of air. However, you may see the chest and abdomen rise and fall considerably with the patient's frantic attempts to breathe. Observing chest and abdominal movement often is difficult with a fully clothed patient. You may see little, if any, chest movement, even with normal breathing. This is particularly true in some patients with chronic lung disease. But when you use the three-part approach—look, listen, and feel—and discover that there is no movement of air, you must begin artificial ventilation immediately.

## PEDIATRIC CONSIDERATIONS

BLS principles are essentially the same for infants, children, and adults. The differences relate to the underlying causes of emergencies and the smaller size of infants and children. In most instances, full cardiopulmonary arrest in infants and children results from respiratory arrest. In adults, cardiac arrest usually occurs first. If not corrected, respiratory arrest in infants and children will lead to cardiac arrest and death.

Respiratory arrest in infants and children can occur for many reasons. First, the entire airway of a child, from nose to bronchi, is smaller than that of an adult. Therefore, the airway is much more easily obstructed. In addition, a child's tongue takes up more of the mouth. A child's trachea is smaller and collapses more easily. This also makes it more vulnerable to

**FIGURE 8-5**

The head-tilt/chin-lift maneuver

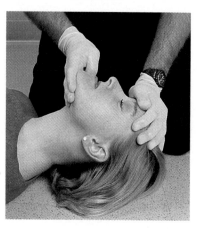

**FIGURE 8-6**

The jaw-thrust maneuver

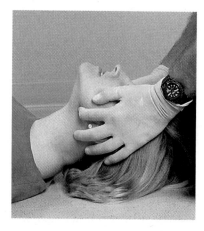

**FIGURE 8-7**

The modified jaw-thrust maneuver

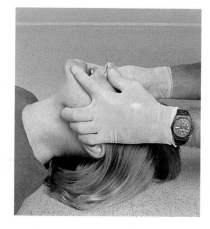

# *A Matter of Life and Breath*

A request for medical aid is received from a local grade school, where an 8-year-old girl is having "difficulty breathing." On arrival, you find her in the school nurse's office with her teacher. The teacher explains that the kids were at recess, playing volleyball, when the little girl chased a ball out of bounds. The ball struck her throat when she ran into a support rope for one of the end poles of the net. The teacher said that the child did not lose consciousness, and that she immediately brought her to the nurse's office, who applied an ice pack to the injured area. You assess the girl and note a red, swollen area on the anterior surface of the throat. She is seated, but is leaning slightly forward, and is breathing at a rate of 38 times a minute.

## For Discussion

1. Why do you need background knowledge of respiratory anatomy and physiology in order to provide high-quality prehospital care?

2. How does, or will, the respiratory system work to support cellular metabolism in harmony with other body systems?

---

obstruction. Other causes of respiratory arrest include the following:

- aspiration of foreign objects, such as peanuts, candy, and small toys
- poisonings and drug overdose
- airway infections
- near drowning or electrocution
- Sudden infant death syndrome (SIDS)

In children and infants, you must first always open the airway, if obstructed, and then provide artificial ventilation. As you learned in your BLS training, if a child is not breathing or struggling to breathe, you should first provide 1 minute of CPR. You should then

## FIGURE 8-8

Look, listen, and feel for respirations

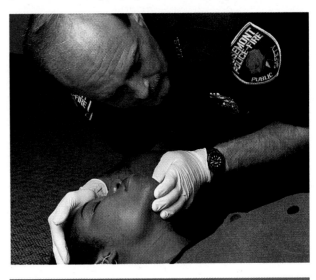

contact dispatch to speed the arrival of ALS. However, in many instances, you may only need to open the airway and provide simple rescue breathing to help a child begin breathing on his or her own.

After the initial assessment, you will have established whether the infant or child is unresponsive, is in respiratory distress, or is cyanotic. The next step is to open the airway. The preferred technique of opening the airway in children is the chin-lift maneuver with a modest head tilt. Place one hand on the forehead and gently tilt the head back into a neutral or slightly extended position. Then place the fingers (but not the thumb) under the chin and lift the mandible up and out (Figure 8-9). Remember that in an infant or a child, the airway tissues are less rigid than in an adult. If you push hard under the chin or close the mouth, you may obstruct the airway further.

## FIGURE 8-9

The chin-lift maneuver on a child

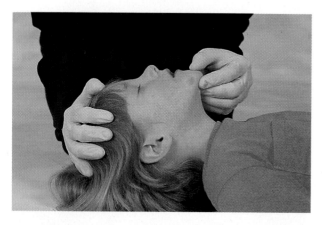

If you suspect a cervical spine injury, you should use the jaw-thrust maneuver without the head tilt to open the child's airway. It should be done the same way as that for an adult.

As soon as the airway is opened, you should assess the patient's breathing. Repeat the look, listen, and feel technique. Place your ear over the patient's mouth and nose and look toward the chest and abdomen. The patient is breathing if you see the chest and abdomen rise and fall, feel air movement from the nose and mouth, and hear air move as the patient exhales.

# SUCTIONING

If a patient has a mouth full of foreign material, whether broken teeth, food, or vomitus, the material must be removed prior to ventilation. If it is not, you will force it into the lungs and possibly cause a complete airway obstruction. *If you hear gurgling, the patient needs suctioning!* Therefore suctioning is your next priority. Make sure that you keep the airway clear so that you can ventilate the patient properly.

## SUCTIONING EQUIPMENT

### Units

Portable and fixed (mounted) suctioning equipment is essential for resuscitation. A portable suctioning unit must provide a vacuum pressure and flow adequate for effective suctioning of the mouth and oropharynx. Hand-operated suctioning units with disposable chambers are reliable, effective, and relatively inexpensive (Figure 8-10). A fixed suctioning unit should generate air flow of more than 30 L per minute and a vacuum of more than 300 mm Hg when the tubing is clamped.

A suctioning unit should be fitted with the following:

- wide bore, thick-walled, nonkinking tubing
- rigid, plastic, pharyngeal suction tips (tonsil tips)

- a nonbreakable collection bottle
- a supply of water for rinsing the tips

You should make sure that the suction yoke, the collection bottle, water for rinsing, and the suction tube are easily accessible at the patient's head.

### Catheters

Plastic pharyngeal suction tips (**tonsil tips**) are best for suctioning the pharynx. Tonsil tips have a large diameter and are somewhat rigid so they do not collapse. Tips with a curved contour allow for easy and rapid placement in the pharynx (Figure 8-11). You should use extreme caution when suctioning a conscious or semiconscious patient. A tonsil tip should only be put in as far as you can visualize. Suctioning may induce vomiting in these patients. A rigid catheter should be used when suctioning infants and children. However, you must not touch the back of the airway. This may activate the gag reflex, cause vomiting, and increase the possibility that contents from the stomach will get into the lungs.

Soft plastic (nonrigid) catheters are used for liquid secretions in the back of the mouth or for suctioning the nose or where you cannot use a rigid catheter (Figure 8-12). For example, if the patient has clenched teeth, you may not be able to insert a rigid catheter. The patient may break off teeth trying to bite it. A flexible catheter may be worked in without injury. Before you insert any catheter, make sure to measure for the proper size. A catheter should not be inserted past the base of the tongue, as this may result in gagging and vomiting.

### TECHNIQUES OF SUCTIONING

You should inspect your suctioning equipment regularly to make sure it is in proper working condition. You should also clean and decontaminate equipment after each use. As you are inspecting your equipment,

### FIGURE 8-10

A manual suctioning unit

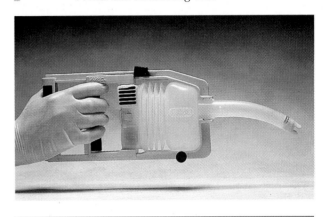

### FIGURE 8-11

A tonsil-tip catheter

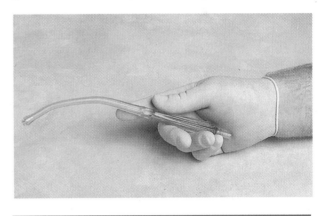

### FIGURE 8-12

A soft plastic suction catheter

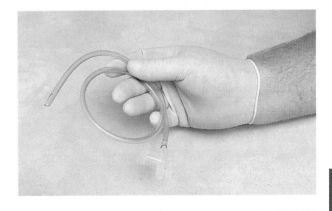

switch on the suction and then clamp the tubing. Make sure that the unit generates a vacuum of more than 300 mm Hg. Also make sure that a battery-charged unit has charged batteries.

You should operate a suctioning unit in the following way:

1. Check the unit for proper assembly of all its parts, as described above.
2. Turn on the suctioning unit.
3. Attach a catheter to the tubing. Use a pharyngeal suction tip (tonsil tip) when suctioning the mouth of an infant or child. Use a bulb suction or soft catheter set at low to medium setting when suctioning the nose.
4. Open the patient's mouth using the jaw-thrust maneuver.
5. Insert the suction tip, without suction if possible, with its convex side along the roof of the mouth until you reach the pharynx. Insert the tip only to the base of the tongue (Figure 8-13).

**FIGURE 8-13**

Suctioning the oropharynx with a tonsil-tip catheter

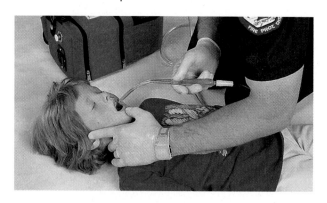

6. After the tip is in place, release the clamp on the tube and suction as you withdraw the suction tip from the pharynx and mouth. Move the suction tip from side to side.

7. Never suction for more than 15 seconds at one time. Suctioning removes oxygen from the airway very effectively. With infants and children, suction for no more than 5 seconds.
8. Rinse the catheter and tubing with water to prevent clogging of the tube with dried vomitus or other secretions.
9. Suctioning may be repeated only after the patient has been ventilated and re-oxygenated.

At times, a patient may have secretions or vomitus that cannot be suctioned quickly and easily. In these instances, you should remove the catheter from the patient's mouth, log roll the patient to the side, and then clear the mouth carefully with your gloved finger. A patient may also produce frothy secretions as quickly as you can suction them from the airway. In these instances, you should suction the patient for 15 seconds, provide artificial ventilation for 2 minutes, then suction again for 15 seconds. In this situation, hyperventilate the patient before and after suctioning and then inform medical control of your situation and ask for guidance.

## ARTIFICIAL VENTILATION

In the prehospital care setting, patients with fewer than 12 breaths per minute or more than 24 breaths per minute are not breathing adequately. Certainly a patient who is not breathing needs artificial ventilation and supplemental oxygen. However, it is important to note that fast, shallow breathing can be as dangerous as a very slow breathing rate. Fast, shallow breathing moves mostly dead space air—air in the larger airways only. This type of breathing does not allow for adequate exchange of air and carbon dioxide in the alveoli. Therefore, patients with fast, shallow breathing need airway care as do patients who are breathing slowly or not at all.

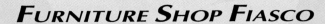

## FURNITURE SHOP FIASCO

It's almost time to get off shift when a call comes in for a woman "acting strange" at Fred's Furniture Fix-it Shop. You arrive a few minutes later to find a 39-year-old woman sitting outside Fred's on the front steps. The other employee at the shop tells you that Fred has been sick for the last 2 weeks and that his sister has been trying to help out. He also says that she had just started stripping some chairs when she started to act strange. She's oriented only to person and place and has respirations of 36/min. Her skin is cool, clammy, and slightly cyanotic. She has audible wheezes in all fields. The patient states that she started feeling sick and was having trouble breathing immediately after spilling a bucket of paint stripper down the front of her coveralls. She states that she isn't ill otherwise and she does not take any medication on a regular basis. She does take ibuprofen every now and then if her back is bothering her.

### For Discussion

1. Why should the patient's contaminated clothing be removed before she is loaded into the ambulance?
2. Why is airway management in the prehospital setting so difficult?

In your BLS class, you learned that you do not need any special equipment to provide simple artificial ventilation. Artificial ventilation by mouth-to-mask delivers exhaled gas from you to the patient. This gas contains 16% oxygen, more than enough to maintain the patient's life. There are several ways you can provide artificial ventilation to a patient who is not breathing. Some methods require equipment, some do not. In order of preference, the four methods for providing artificial ventilation by an EMT-B are as follows:

1. Mouth-to-mask ventilation
2. Two-person bag-valve-mask (BVM)
3. Oxygen-powered manually triggered breathing device
4. One-person bag-valve-mask (BVM)

Once you determine a patient is not breathing or needs assisted ventilations, you should begin artificial ventilation immediately. Continue artificial ventilation, along with your efforts to support the circulation and correct cardiac problems, as you were directed in your BLS training.

## MOUTH-TO-MOUTH VENTILATION

As you learned in BLS training, mouth-to-mouth ventilations are now done routinely with a **barrier device**, such as a mask. Barrier devices feature a plastic barrier placed on the patient's face and a one-way valve to prevent back flow of secretions and gases (Figure 8-14). These devices provide good infection control. Providing mouth-to-mouth ventilations without such a device is appropriate only in extreme conditions. Mouth-to-mouth ventilations are best done with a one-way valve mask to prevent possible disease transmission.

You should perform mouth-to-mouth ventilation with a simple barrier device in an adult in the following way:

1. Open the airway with the head-tilt/chin-lift maneuver, as described earlier.

2. Press on the forehead to maintain the backward tilt of the head. Pinch the patient's nostrils together with your thumb and index finger.

3. Depress the lower lip with the thumb of the hand lifting the chin. This will help keep the mouth open during mouth-to-mouth ventilation.

4. Open the patient's mouth widely and place the barrier device over the patient's mouth.

5. Take a deep breath, make a tight seal with your mouth around the patient's mouth. Breath slowly into the patient's mouth for 1½ to 2 seconds. This slow, gentle method of ventilating keeps from forcing air into the stomach (Figure 8-15).

6. Remove your mouth and allow the patient to exhale passively. Turn your head slightly to watch for movement of the patient's chest.

If you use the jaw-thrust maneuver to open the airway, you must move to the patient's side. Keep the patient's mouth open with both thumbs, and seal the nose by placing your cheek against the patient's nostrils (Figure 8-16).

## MOUTH-TO-MASK VENTILATION

A mask with an oxygen inlet provides oxygen during mouth-to-mouth ventilation

### FIGURE 8-15

Mouth-to-mouth ventilation with a barrier device

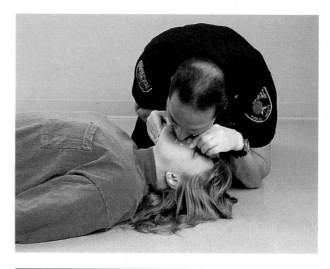

### FIGURE 8-14

A barrier device

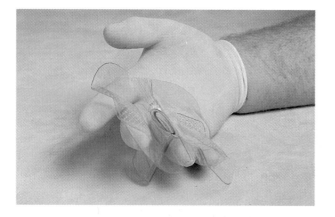

## FIGURE 8-16

Mouth-to-mouth ventilation using the jaw-thrust maneuver

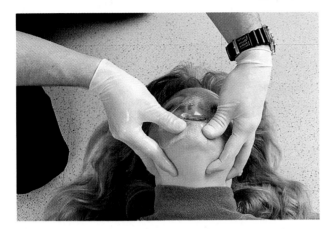
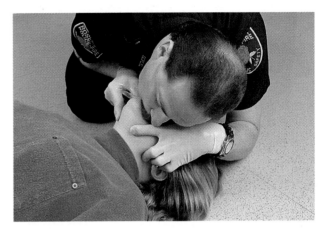

(Figure 8-17). The mask supplies supplemental oxygen as you ventilate the patient with air from your own lungs. You provide the artificial ventilation, but significant oxygen enrichment with inspired air also occurs. This mouth-to-mask system frees both your hands to help keep the airway open. It also helps you to provide a better seal between the mask and the face.

The mask is shaped like a triangle, with the apex (top) placed across the bridge of the nose. The base of the mask is placed in the groove between the lower lip and the chin. In the center of the mask is a chimney with a 15 mL connector.

You should perform mouth-to-mask ventilation in an adult in the following way:

1. Kneel at the patient's head. Open the airway using the head-tilt maneuver, or the jaw-thrust maneuver if indicated.

2. Connect the one-way valve to the face mask.

3. Place the mask on the patient's face. Make sure the apex is over the bridge of the nose and the base is in the groove between the lower lip and the chin.

## FIGURE 8-17

Pocket mask

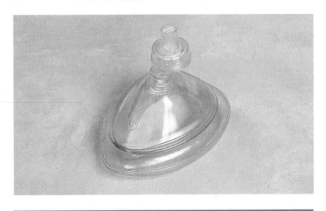

4. Grasp the patient's lower jaw with your first three fingers on each hand. Place your thumbs on the dome of the mask. Make an airtight seal by applying firm pressure between the thumbs and the fingers (Figure 8-18a).

5. Maintain an upward and forward pull on the lower jaw with your fingers to keep the airway open.

6. Take a deep breath and exhale through the open port of the one-way valve.

Breathe slowly into the patient's mouth for 1½ to 2 seconds (Figure 8-18b).

7. Remove your mouth and watch the patient's chest fall during passive exhalation (Figure 8-18c).

You know that you are providing adequate ventilations if you see the patient's chest rise and fall. Feel for resistance of the patient's lungs as they expand. You should also hear and feel air escape as the patient exhales. Make sure that you are providing the correct number of breaths per minute for the patient's age (Table 8-1).

The oxygen concentration given with the mask can be increased by adding gas through the oxygen inlet valve. Any oxygen delivered to the patient is diluted with your exhaled breath. You should give high-flow oxygen at 15 L/min. This, when combined with your exhaled breath, will give the patient 55% oxygen.

The mask also works well for patients breathing on their own who need supplemen-

## FIGURE 8-18

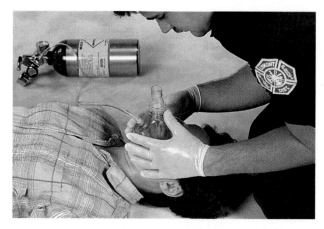

**A**    Apply the mask over the patient's mouth

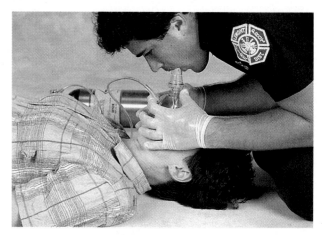

**B**    Inhale deeply and breathe into the chimney of the mask

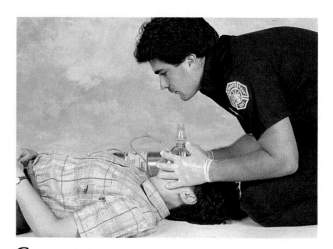

**C**    Watch for chest movement

| **TABLE 8-1** | **NORMAL RESPIRATION RATE CHANGES** |
|---|---|
| **Adults** | 12 to 20 breaths per minute |
| **Children** | 15 to 30 breaths per minute |
| **Infants** | 25 to 50 breaths per minute |

To obtain the breathing rate in a patient, count the number of breaths in a 30-second period and multiply by two. Avoid letting the patient know that you are counting to prevent influencing the rate.

tal oxygen, but do not need full ventilatory assistance. The mask has an elastic strap for patients who can breathe on their own.

## THE BAG-VALVE-MASK DEVICE

Both mouth-to-mouth and mouth-to-mask ventilations can provide large volumes of inspired air—up to 4 L per breath. With mouth-to-mouth ventilation, the concentration of oxygen delivered to the patient is 16%. With mouth-to-mask ventilation connected to high-flow oxygen, the concentration of oxygen, at best, is only 55%.

At the same oxygen flow rate (10 to 15 L/min) as the mask alone, a **bag-valve-mask (BVM) device** with an oxygen reservoir can deliver more than 90% oxygen (Figure 8-19). However, the device can deliver only as much gas as you can squeeze out of the bag by hand. Therefore, you should practice on ventilation mannequins several times before using a bag-valve-mask device on a real patient. Most bag-valve-mask devices on the market today include modifications or accessories that permit the delivery of oxygen concentrations approaching 100%. Without these modifications, it is difficult to achieve oxygen concentrations above 50%.

Therefore, a bag-valve-mask device should be used when you need to deliver oxygen concentrations of greater than 50% to a patient. The device is also used for patients with severe respiratory failure. You will typically use an oropharyngeal or nasopharyngeal airway with the bag-valve-mask device. These airway adjuncts are explained in chapter 9, Airway Adjuncts and Oxygen Equipment. Patients in severe respiratory distress have an inadequate minute volume. The minute volume is the volume of air cycled through the alveoli in 1 minute.

### Bag-Valve-Mask Components

All bag-valve-mask devices should have the following components:

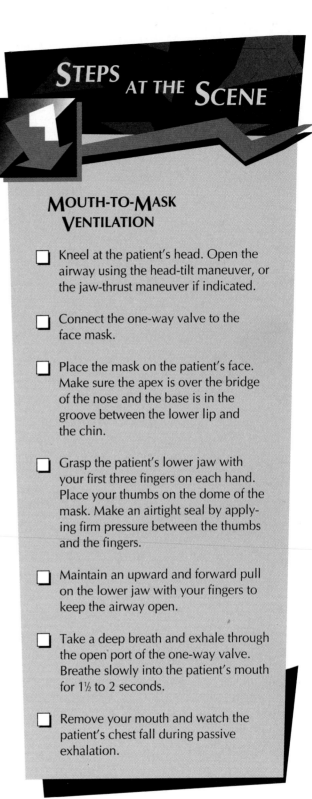

## STEPS AT THE SCENE

### MOUTH-TO-MASK VENTILATION

☐ Kneel at the patient's head. Open the airway using the head-tilt maneuver, or the jaw-thrust maneuver if indicated.

☐ Connect the one-way valve to the face mask.

☐ Place the mask on the patient's face. Make sure the apex is over the bridge of the nose and the base is in the groove between the lower lip and the chin.

☐ Grasp the patient's lower jaw with your first three fingers on each hand. Place your thumbs on the dome of the mask. Make an airtight seal by applying firm pressure between the thumbs and the fingers.

☐ Maintain an upward and forward pull on the lower jaw with your fingers to keep the airway open.

☐ Take a deep breath and exhale through the open port of the one-way valve. Breathe slowly into the patient's mouth for 1½ to 2 seconds.

☐ Remove your mouth and watch the patient's chest fall during passive exhalation.

- a self-refilling bag that is either disposable or easily cleaned and sterilized

- no pop-off valve

## FIGURE 8-19

A bag-valve-mask (BVM) device

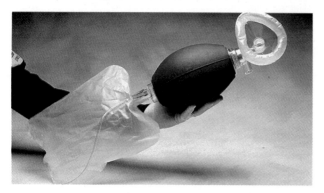

## FIGURE 8-20

Different sizes of BVM devices

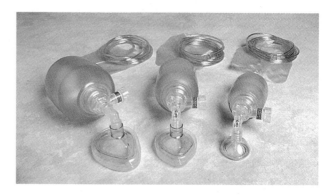

- a true valve for nonrebreathing
- a transparent self-inflating, deflatable reservoir bag or tube to allow for high concentrations of oxygen
- a one-way, no-jam valve that incorporates the following: the exhalation port; oxygen inflow at a maximum of 15 L/min; a standard 15/22 connection between the face mask and the bag; and an attachment for the transparent reservoir bag or tube
- a transparent face mask (Masks are available in adult size, child's size for the smaller face, or one of three infant sizes, including a "preemie" size.) (Figure 8-20)
- ability to perform under extreme heat or cold

The total amount of gas in the reservoir bag of an adult bag-valve-mask device is usually 1,200 to 1,600 mL. The pediatric bag contains 500 to 700 mL, and the infant bag holds 150 to 240 mL. A volume of 10 to 15 mL/kg should be delivered over 2 seconds.

### Bag-Valve-Mask Technique

Whenever possible, both you and your partner should provide bag-valve-mask ventilation. It is very difficult for one EMT-B to maintain a proper seal between the mask and face using just one hand and getting adequate air into the patient with the other hand. With two EMT-Bs, the first can secure the mask to the face with two hands while the second squeezes the bag.

You should perform ventilations with a bag-valve-mask device in an adult in the following way:

1. Kneel above the patient's head. If possible, your partner should be at the side of the head in order to bag the patient while you hold a seal between the mask and the patient's face with two hands. (This assumes that you have enough personnel to do everything else that needs to be done.) Two-person BVM is more effective than one-person BVM, if it is feasible.

2. Maintain the patient's neck in extension, unless there is a possible cervical spine injury. With a possible cervical spine injury, you should immobilize the patient's head and neck. Your partner can hold the head manually. If you are alone, use your knees to immobilize the head.

3. Insert an oropharyngeal or nasopharyngeal airway to maintain an open airway.

4. Select the proper mask size.

5. Place the mask on the patient's face. Make sure the apex is over the bridge of the nose and the base is in the groove

## FIGURE 8-21

Two-person BVM ventilation

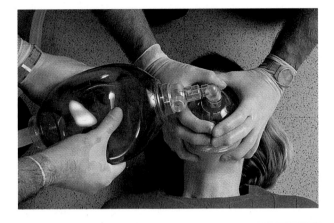

## FIGURE 8-22

The use of a C-clamp to hold mask in place

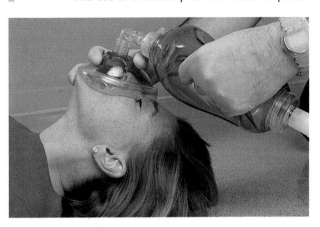

between the lower lip and the chin. If the mask has a large round cuff around the ventilation port, center the port over the patient's mouth. Inflate the collar before use to obtain a better fit and seal to the face.

6. Bring the lower jaw up to the mask with your ring and little fingers. This will help maintain an open airway. If you suspect a possible spinal injury, make sure your partner immobilizes the cervical spine as you move the lower jaw.

7. Hold the mask in position by placing the thumbs over the top part of the mask and the index and middle fingers over the bottom half. Make sure you do not grab the fleshy part of the neck as you may compress structures and create an airway obstruction.

8. Connect the bag to the mask, if you have not already done so.

9. Hold the mask in place while your partner squeezes the bag with two hands until the patient's chest rises. Continue squeezing the bag once every 5 seconds for adults and once every 3 seconds for infants and children (Figure 8-21).

10. If you are alone, hold your index finger over the lower part of the mask and secure the upper part of the mask with your thumb. This is known as the "C-clamp" and will maintain the seal. Make sure the neck is maintained in extension. Squeeze the bag in a rhythmic manner once every 5 seconds with your other hand. Continue squeezing the bag once every 5 seconds for adults and once every 3 seconds for infants and children (Figure 8-22).

When using the device to assist respirations, you should deflate the bag simultaneously with the patient's inspiratory effort and ultimately try to achieve a more normal rate and depth of respiration.

When using the device with external chest compression, you should squeeze the bag during pauses in compression. Ventilate once after every fifth compression, or twice after every fifteenth compression. You should allow at least 1½ to 2 seconds for each ventilation.

As you are assisting ventilations with a bag-valve-mask device, you should evaluate how well the patient is breathing. If the patient's chest does not rise and fall, you may need to reposition the head or use an airway adjunct. If the patient's stomach seems to be rising and falling, you should reposition the head. In a patient with possible spinal injury, you should reposition the jaw rather than the head. If too much air is escaping from under the mask, then you should reposition the mask for a better mask seal. If after correcting the technique, the patient's chest still does not rise and fall, you should try another airway device, such as mouth-to-mask ventilation or an oxygen-powered manually triggered breathing device. Make sure you recheck the airway for any obstruction.

## FLOW-RESTRICTED, OXYGEN-POWERED VENTILATION DEVICES

A third method of providing artificial ventilation is with flow-restricted, oxygen-powered ventilation devices. These devices are widely available, but should not be used on infants and children. You should also follow local protocols carefully when you use these devices.

### Components

Flow-restricted, oxygen-powered ventilation devices should have the following components:

- a peak flow rate of 100% oxygen at up to 40 to 50 L/min

- an inspiratory pressure safety release valve that opens at approximately 60 cm of water and vents any remaining volume to the atmosphere or stops the flow of oxygen

- an audible alarm that sounds whenever the relief valve pressure is exceeded

- the ability to operate satisfactorily under normal and varying environmental conditions

- a trigger (or lever) positioned so both of your hands can remain on the mask to

provide an airtight seal while supporting and tilting the patient's head and keeping the jaw elevated (Figure 8-23)

Proper training is vital if you are to learn how to use these devices correctly. You must make sure there is an airtight fit between the patient's face and mask, as with bag-valve-mask devices. Practice and strict adherence to proper technique will minimize this problem. You must also be alert for gastric distention as a result of such a high flow rate. As stated earlier, follow local medical protocols carefully when you use these devices.

### Technique

You should perform ventilations with a flow-restricted, oxygen-powered ventilation device as follows:

1. Open the patient's airway and suction as needed. Insert an oropharyngeal or nasopharyngeal airway.

2. As with the bag-valve-mask technique, place your thumbs over the top half of

## FIGURE 8-23

A flow-restricted, oxygen-powered device

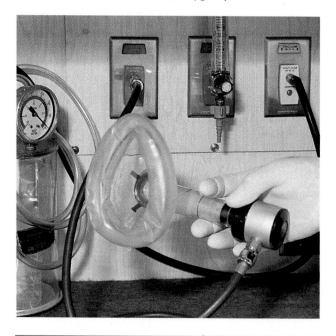

the mask and your index and middle fingers over the bottom half.

3. Place the apex of the mask over the bridge of the nose and then lower the mask over the mouth and upper chin.

4. As with the bag-valve-mask technique, bring the lower jaw up to the mask with your ring and little fingers. This will help maintain an open airway. If the patient has a possible spinal injury, make sure your partner immobilizes the cervical spine.

5. Trigger the device's demand valve until the patient's chest rises (Figure 8-24).

6. Repeat every 5 seconds, as with the bag-valve-mask technique.

7. If the chest does not rise, the patient is not being ventilated. At this point, you need to consider several possible problems:

   a. if the abdomen rises, reposition the patient's head

   b. if air is leaking from under the mask, reposition your fingers and the mask to get a better seal

   c. if, after you try a and b, the chest still does not rise, consider maneuvers for complete airway obstruction. You may also consider different ways of assisting ventilation, such as mouth to mask.

8. If necessary, you may use this device with other airway adjuncts, such as the EOA, EGTA, Combitube, Pharyngotracheal Lumen Airway or endotracheal tube. These airway adjuncts are discussed in chapter 10, Advanced Airway Management.

Remember that the amount of pressure necessary to ventilate a patient adequately will vary according to the size of the patient, the patient's lung volume, and the condition of the lungs. A patient with chronic obstructive pulmonary disease (COPD) will need greater pressure to receive a given volume than would be necessary for a patient with normal lungs.

## PEDIATRIC CONSIDERATIONS

### BLS Technique

Children who are struggling to breathe (partial airway obstruction), but maintaining an airway, will stay in a position that helps them breathe. You should allow them to stay in that position as long as their breathing does not deteriorate. You should closely monitor these patients. For infants, the preferred method of providing artificial ventilation is mouth-to-nose-and-mouth ventilation. You must cover both the mouth and the nose with your mouth and make a seal. If a child is large enough so that a tight seal cannot be made over both mouth and nose, mouth-to-mouth ventilation is performed as in the adult.

Once you make an airtight seal, give two gentle breaths for 1 to 1½ seconds each. These initial breaths help you assess for airway obstruction as you expand the lungs. If air enters freely with these breaths and the chest rises, you can assume that the airway

## FIGURE 8-24

The use of the trigger demand valve on a flow-restricted, oxygen-powered device

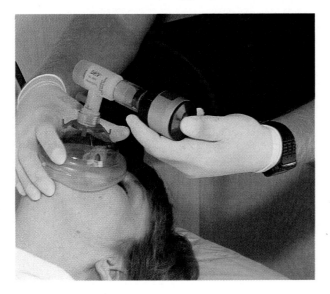

is clear. You should then check the pulse. If air does not enter freely, you should check for an obstruction. Reposition the patient using the chin-lift or jaw-thrust maneuvers to open the airway, and if air still does not enter freely, you should suspect an obstruction. You must then clear the airway.

As you learned in your BLS training, you will have to provide one breath every 3 seconds or 20 times per minute for infants and children alike. These rates will require appropriate pauses in external chest compression, if it is being given. The lungs of a child, especially an infant, are much smaller than those of an adult. Therefore, the volume of air needed for effective ventilation will be less than that in an adult. In fact, the volume should be limited to the amount needed to cause the chest to rise. However, a child has smaller air passages, which provide a greater resistance to air flow. Therefore, the ventilatory pressure needed to inflate the lungs will probably be greater than you expect. You are using the right amount of pressure if the chest rises and falls.

### Bag-Valve-Mask Technique

You should carry a bag-valve-mask device specially designed for neonatal (newborn) resuscitation if you expect to deliver a baby. More than 12% of births in the prehospital setting will require some sort of resuscitation. These self-inflating bags and reservoirs have an intake valve at one end to allow rapid reinflation and blow-by oxygen. Make sure that the bag will deliver oxygen passively through the mask. You should ventilate with only as much pressure as it takes to make the patient's chest rise. Avoid excessive bag pressure by watching the chest rise and fall.

The American Heart Association recommends that bags used for pediatric resuscitation should not have pop-off valves. If the device has a pop-off valve, it should be bypassed. Bypass is necessary because the pressures needed to adequately ventilate an infant during CPR may exceed the pop-off pressure limits. The fit of the face mask is also important. Masks with cushioned rims are most effective.

## SPECIAL CONSIDERATIONS

### STOMAS

Bag-valve-mask ventilation must also be used for patients who have had a laryngectomy (surgical removal of the larynx). These patients have a permanent tracheal **stoma** (an opening in the neck that connects the trachea directly to the skin). It may be seen as an opening at the center, at the front and the base of the neck. In many of these patients, there will be other openings in the neck, according to the type of operation done. Any opening other than the midline tracheal stoma should be ignored. The midline opening is the only one that can be used to put air into the patient's lungs. In general, other neck openings will lie to one side or the other, but not in the midline (Figure 8-25).

### FIGURE 8-25

A tracheal stoma

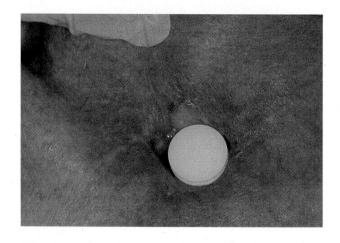

Neither the head-tilt/chin-lift nor the jaw-thrust maneuver is required for ventilating a patient with a stoma. If the patient has a tube in the stoma, you should ventilate through the tube (Figure 8-26). Seal the patient's mouth and nose with one hand to prevent a leak of air up the trachea when you ventilate through a tracheal tube or stoma. Release the seal of the patient's mouth and nose for exhalation. This allows the air to exhale through the upper airway.

## FOREIGN BODY OBSTRUCTION

### Causes

In your BLS training, you learned the techniques used to open an airway that is blocked by a foreign object. Appendix A provides a review of those techniques. This section will only briefly describe how to identify types of obstruction and the proper ways to clear the airway.

Foreign object airway obstruction can occur due to one or a combination of the following:

- relaxation of the tongue and throat tissues in an unconscious patient
- vomited stomach contents
- blood clots, bone fragments, or damaged tissue after an injury
- foreign objects, such as dentures, food, and small toys

Sudden airway obstruction by a foreign object in an adult usually occurs during a meal. In a child, it occurs while eating, playing with small toys, or crawling about the house. An otherwise healthy child who has sudden difficulty breathing has probably aspirated a foreign object. *The earlier you recognize airway obstruction the better.* You must learn to recognize the difference between airway obstruction caused by a foreign object and that resulting from a medical condition. Airway obstruction in a child is usually caused by a foreign object or an infection, resulting in swelling and narrowing of the airway. With infection, attempts at clearing the airway will not be helpful and can be dangerous. These attempts will result in delaying transport.

One sure sign of an obstruction is a sudden inability to speak or cough during or immediately after eating. The person may grasp his or her throat, begin to turn blue, and have extreme difficulty breathing. There is little or no air movement. At first, the person will remain conscious and be able to signal to you what is wrong. Make sure you ask, "are you choking?" If the patient nods "yes," then you know to act. If you do not clear the airway quickly, the oxygen in the lungs will be used up. Unconsciousness and death will follow.

When you find a patient unconscious, you will not know the cause at first. The unconsciousness may have been caused by an airway obstruction, a heart problem, or any number of other problems. Any patient you find unconscious must be managed as if he

## FIGURE 8-26

Ventilate through the tube in a tracheal stoma

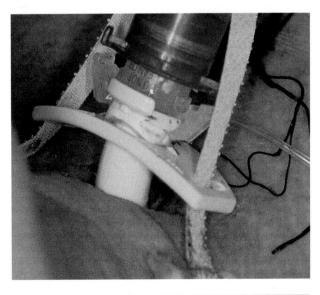

or she is in cardiac arrest. You must first open the airway and then provide artificial ventilation as you would for CPR. If, after opening the airway, you feel resistance after blowing into the patient's lungs, or pressure builds up in your mouth, you should consider the possibility of airway obstruction.

### Removal Techniques

You should use the following manual techniques for relieving complete airway obstruction: 1) the Heimlich maneuver (abdominal thrusts), and 2) finger sweeps and manual removal of the object. The Heimlich maneuver is the most effective method of dislodging and forcing an object out of the airway. Residual air, which is always present in the lungs, is compressed upward and used to expel the object. These techniques are reviewed in detail in appendix A, BLS Review.

You should perform the head-tilt/chin-lift maneuver to open an obstruction caused by tongue and throat muscles relaxing back into the airway. Loose dentures and large pieces of vomited food, mucus, or blood clots in the mouth should be swept forward and out of the mouth with your gloved index finger. Once it becomes available, suctioning should be used to maintain a clear airway. On occasion, a large foreign object will be aspirated and block the upper airway. In these instances, you should perform three cycles of the Heimlich maneuver. If you are not successful in dislodging the object, transport the patient, continuing your efforts to clear the airway en route.

Occasionally, a patient will be able to exchange air in the lungs, but will still have some degree of respiratory distress. This condition is called a **partial airway obstruction.** Breathing is noisy, and the patient may be coughing. With good air exchange, the patient can cough forcefully, although there may be wheezing between coughs. As long as the patient can breathe, cough, or talk, you should not interfere with the patient's attempts to expel the foreign object. Abdominal thrusts are not usually effective for dislodging a partial obstruction. Manual removal is dangerous because the object could be forced farther down the airway, causing a complete obstruction. You must take great care to prevent a partial airway obstruction from becoming a complete airway obstruction.

With a partial airway obstruction, the head-tilt/chin-lift or jaw-thrust maneuvers should be performed to support the airway in its most efficient position. You should also give 100% supplemental oxygen and then provide transport. Of course, if air movement stops completely, you should immediately perform the Heimlich maneuver. The emergency department personnel should be notified of the problem and the expected time of arrival.

## GASTRIC DISTENTION

Artificial ventilation often fills the stomach with air. This condition is called **gastric distention.** Gastric distention most commonly occurs in children, but it also happens in adults. It is most likely to occur when you blow too forcefully or too often in artificial ventilation, or when the airway is obstructed. This is why you are instructed to give slow, gentle breaths during artificial ventilation. Slight gastric distention is not of concern. However, severe inflation of the stomach is dangerous because it causes vomiting during CPR. Gastric distention can also reduce the lung volume by elevating the diaphragm.

You should attempt to relieve gastric distention as soon as you recognize the condition—before the abdomen is so tense that ventilation is ineffective. To relieve gastric distention in children and adults, first log roll the patient onto his or her side. The patient's entire body should be turned, preferably to the left side. Then, use the flat of your hand to apply moderate pressure on the abdomen between the umbilicus and the rib cage (Figure 8-27). To relieve gastric distention in an infant, turn the infant's entire body to the left side, with the head down, and apply firm manual pressure to the abdomen. Expect the patient to vomit a mixture of air, gastric juice, and food. Aspiration of the gastric contents into the lungs must be prevented during this maneuver, and a suction device should be used promptly to remove any vomitus.

## FIGURE 8-27

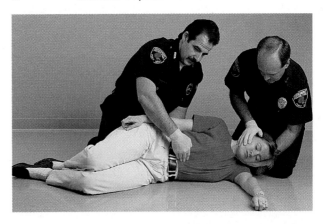

Relieving gastric distention using abdominal pressure

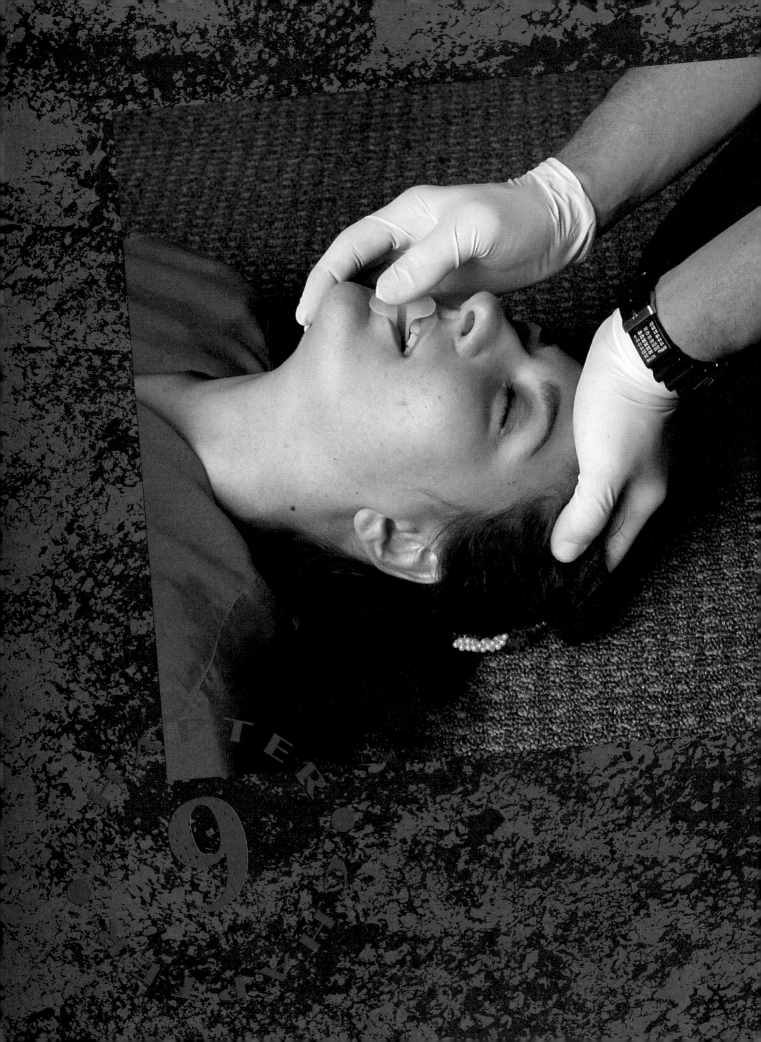

# CHAPTER 9

# Airway Adjuncts and Oxygen Equipment

After you have read this chapter, you should be able to:

- Describe how to measure and insert both an oropharyngeal airway and a nasopharyngeal airway.
- Define the components of an oxygen delivery system.
- Identify a nonrebreathing mask and state the oxygen flow requirements needed for its use.
- Describe the indications for using a nasal cannula versus a nonrebreathing mask.
- Identify a nasal cannula and state the oxygen flow requirements needed for its use.

## Overview

BLS measures for patients who are not breathing or are having difficulty breathing do not require any mechanical equipment. However, you will often use artificial airways, commonly called airway adjuncts, to care for these patients. The primary function of airway adjuncts is to prevent blockage of the upper airway by the tongue.

The proper ways to clear and maintain the airway have been described throughout this section. Simple maneuvers such as the head-tilt/chin-lift will usually open the airway. At times, you will need to insert airway adjuncts and deliver oxygen. Therefore, it is important that you learn how to use all artificial airway equipment. Improper use of this equipment could have serious, even fatal, results for your patient.

The first section of the chapter describes the proper use of oropharyngeal and nasopharyngeal airways. The last sections describe when to use supplemental oxygen and how to store and maintain oxygen equipment.

# **K**ey Terms

**American Standard System** A safety system for large oxygen cylinders to prevent the accidental attachment of a regulator to a wrong cylinder.

**Hypoxia** Dangerous condition in which the body's tissues and cells do not have enough oxygen.

**Nasal cannula** Oxygen delivery device in which oxygen flows through two small, tube-like prongs that fit into the patient's nostrils.

**Nasopharyngeal airway** Airway adjunct inserted into the nostril of a conscious patient who is not able to maintain a natural airway.

**Nonrebreathing mask** A mask and reservoir bag system that is the preferred way to give oxygen in the prehospital setting. With a good mask to mouth seal, it can provide up to 95% inspired oxygen.

**Oropharyngeal airway** Airway adjunct inserted into the mouth to keep the tongue from blocking the upper airway and to make suctioning the airway easier.

# Airway Adjuncts

## Oropharyngeal Airways

An **oropharyngeal (oral) airway** has two principal purposes. The first is to keep the tongue from blocking the upper airway. The second is to make suctioning the airway, if necessary, easier. An oropharyngeal airway should be inserted promptly in unconscious patients who have no gag reflex, but are breathing on their own. An oropharyngeal airway is often used in conjunction with BVM ventilation. Patients with a gag reflex will not tolerate this type of airway. If you insert this airway in a patient with a gag reflex, the patient may vomit or the vocal cords may spasm. An oropharyngeal airway is also a safe, effective way to maintain the airway of the patient with a possible spinal injury. Constant use of the head-tilt or other maneuvers for these patients is less efficient.

It is important to understand when and how this device is used. If the airway is not the proper size or is inserted incorrectly, it could actually push the tongue back into the pharynx. In this case, instead of maintaining the airway, it could actually block the airway.

The oropharyngeal airway has an opening down the center or along either side. The opening permits the free flow of air and allows easy access for suctioning (Figure 9-1). Before you can insert the airway, you must be sure you have selected the proper size. Select the proper size by measuring from the earlobe to the corner of the mouth on the side of the face (Figure 9-2). When inserted properly, the airway will rest in the mouth with the curvature of the airway following the contour of the tongue. The flange should rest against the lips; the other end opens into the pharynx.

### Inserting the Oropharyngeal Airway

You should insert an oropharyngeal airway in an adult in the following way:

1. Select the proper sized airway, as described above. Moisten the airway with a small amount of water to make insertion easier.

2. Open the patient's mouth with one hand.

**FIGURE 9-1**

An oropharyngeal airway

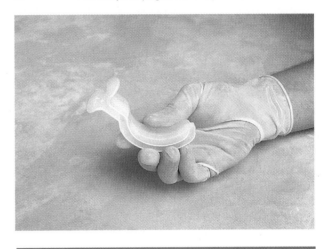

**FIGURE 9-2**

Proper sizing of an oropharyngeal airway

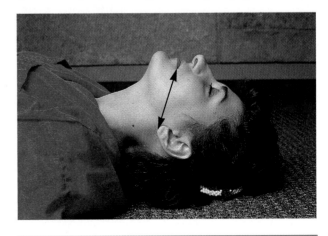

# FIGURE 9-3

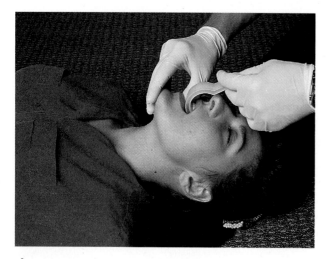

**A**    Inserting an oropharyngeal airway

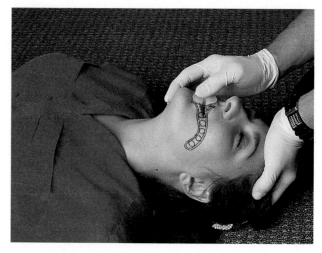

**B**    Proper position of a flange after insertion

3. Hold the airway upside down with your other hand. Insert it into the patient's mouth with the tip facing the roof of the patient's mouth (Figure 9-3a).

4. Rotate the airway 180° until the flange comes to rest on the patient's lips and/or teeth. In this position, the airway will hold the tongue forward (Figure 9-3b).

You should insert an oropharyngeal airway in an infant or child in the following way:

1. Select the proper sized airway, as described above. Moisten the airway with a small amount of water to make insertion easier.

2. Open the patient's mouth with one hand using the jaw-thrust maneuver.

3. Depress the tongue with two or three stacked tongue blades, pressing it forward and away from the roof of the mouth.

4. Slide the airway into place, either right side up or sideways with a 90° rotation.

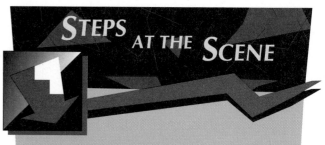

## STEPS AT THE SCENE

### INSERTING THE OROPHARYNGEAL AIRWAY—ADULT

☐ Select the proper sized airway, as described above. Moisten the airway with a small amount of water to make insertion easier.

☐ Open the patient's mouth with one hand.

☐ Hold the airway upside down with your other hand. Insert it into the patient's mouth with the tip facing the roof of the patient's mouth.

☐ Rotate the airway 180° until the flange comes to rest on the patient's lips and/or teeth. In this position, the airway will hold the tongue forward.

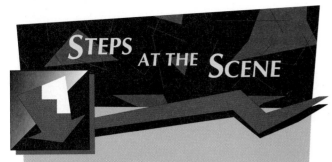
## INSERTING AN OROPHARYNGEAL AIRWAY—CHILD

- ☐ Select the proper sized airway, as described above. Moisten the airway with a small amount of water to make insertion easier.

- ☐ Open the patient's mouth with one hand using the jaw-thrust maneuver.

- ☐ Depress the tongue with two or three stacked tongue blades, pressing it forward and away from the roof of the mouth.

- ☐ Slide the airway into place, either right side up or sideways with a 90° rotation. Lifting the mandible away from the upper jaw will also make inserting the airway much easier.

Lifting the mandible away from the upper jaw will also make inserting the airway much easier.

Take care to avoid injuring the hard palate as you insert the airway. Rough insertion can cause bleeding. This may aggravate airway problems and may even cause vomiting.

## NASOPHARYNGEAL AIRWAYS

A **nasopharyngeal (nasal or trumpet) airway** is usually used for a conscious patient who is not able to maintain an airway

## FIGURE 9-4

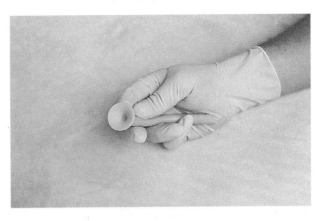

A nasopharyngeal airway

(Figure 9-4). A patient with an altered level of consciousness or a patient experiencing a seizure may also benefit from this airway. If a patient has had severe trauma to the head or face, you should consult medical control before inserting a nasopharyngeal airway. Extreme care must be used with these trauma patients. The airway may be pushed through the hole caused by a basilar skull fracture and may accidentally penetrate through the cranium and into the brain.

This airway is usually well tolerated and is not as likely as the oropharyngeal airway to cause vomiting. It must be well coated with a water-soluble lubricant before it is inserted. Be aware that slight bleeding may occur even when the airway is inserted properly. However, you should never force the airway into place.

One disadvantage to this airway is that it usually does not allow for adequate suctioning. The diameter of the airway is not large enough for a standard suction tip or large suction catheter. You may also need to perform a head-tilt/chin-lift or some other maneuver in conjunction with use of this airway.

Before you can insert the airway, be sure you have selected the proper size. Select the proper size by measuring from the tip of

## FIGURE 9-5

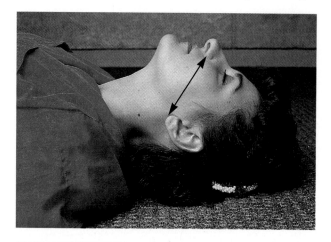

Proper sizing of a nasopharyngeal airway

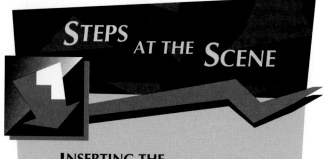
**INSERTING THE NASOPHARYNGEAL AIRWAY—CHILD OR ADULT**

☐ Select the proper sized airway, as described above. Make sure you coat the tip with a water-soluble lubricant.

☐ Gently stretch the nostrils open with your thumb.

☐ Select the nostril large enough for the airway to fit easily.

☐ Gently insert the airway, without force, through the nostril until the flange rests against the skin. Do not force the airway if you feel any resistance or obstruction. Instead, remove the airway and insert it into the other nostril.

the nose to the earlobe (Figure 9-5). In almost everyone, one nostril is larger than the other. The airway should be placed in one nostril with the curvature following the curve of the floor of the nose. The flange, or trumpet-like flare, rests against the nostril. The other end of the airway opens into the posterior pharynx.

### Inserting the Nasopharyngeal Airway

You should insert a nasopharyngeal airway in a child or an adult in the following way:

1. Select the proper sized airway, as described above. Make sure you coat the tip with a water-soluble lubricant.

2. Gently stretch the nostrils open with your thumb (Figure 9-6a).

3. Select the nostril large enough for the airway to fit easily.

4. Gently insert the airway, without force, through the nostril until the flange rests against the skin (Figure 9-6b). Do not force the airway if you feel any resistance or obstruction. Instead, remove the airway and insert it into the other nostril.

## SUPPLEMENTAL OXYGEN

### WHEN TO GIVE SUPPLEMENTAL OXYGEN

You should always give supplemental oxygen to the following patients:

- those who are not breathing on their own

- those who are not breathing well enough to supply adequate oxygen to the lungs

FIGURE 9-6

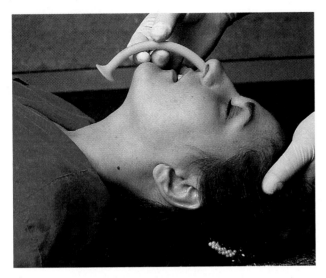

**A**  Inserting a nasopharyngeal airway

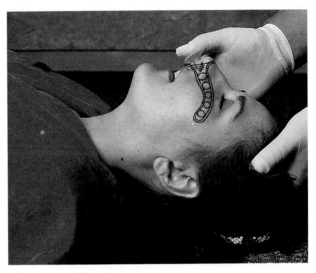

**B**  Proper position of a flange after insertion

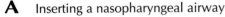

Some tissues and organs, such as the heart, the central nervous system, lungs, kidneys, and liver, need a constant supply of oxygen to function normally. Oxygen should never be withheld from any patient who may benefit from it, even if you must assist ventilations.

If the tissues and cells do not have enough oxygen for a period of time, **hypoxia** will develop. Hypoxia is a very dangerous condition and may result in death. Without supplemental oxygen, a patient's recovery from hypoxia will be slow and often incomplete. Therefore, during resuscitation the principles of oxygen administration are identical for adult, child, and newborn. *All patients should be given oxygen in any arrest situation.*

You should not give low concentrations of oxygen to patients in any arrest situation. These patients are dying and need as much oxygen as possible. High-concentration oxygen given for a short time will not damage the lungs in adults or children. Problems with oxygen toxicity develop only after several days of more than 50% in-spired oxygen delivered at higher than normal pressures. Therefore, you should not withhold oxygen in the prehospital setting.

It is important for you to know when and how to give supplemental oxygen. You must also understand how oxygen is stored and the various hazards associated with its use.

## SUPPLEMENTAL OXYGEN EQUIPMENT

### Oxygen Cylinders

The oxygen you will give to patients is usually supplied as a compressed gas in green seamless steel or aluminum cylinders. However, the bottle may be silver or chrome with a green area around the valve stem on top. Newer bottles are often made of lightweight aluminum or spun-steel, while older bottles are much heavier. Positively verify that the cylinder is labeled for medical oxygen. You should look for letters and numbers stamped into the metal on the collar of the cylinder (Figure 9-7). Of particular importance is the month and

## SHIFTING SANDS

The city that employs you as an EMT started a road construction project to add new sewers on Main Street. You know it's a much needed project, but also know your responses for the next 6 months will be more difficult. Main Street is the primary route for emergency traffic through town. You and your partner are discussing the pros and cons of the project when you're dispatched to 7th and Main for a trapped construction worker. On arrival, you find a 22-year-old man who is trapped chest deep in a trench where a sandy soil wall collapsed. He was buried up to the nipple line before he could get out. Co-workers have shored up the walls around him to protect against further collapse. The patient is conscious and alert, but has pain in the chest and both legs. He also has difficulty breathing.

### For Discussion

1. Why is it important to have a basic understanding of and practice with all the airway adjuncts covered in the text?

2. Would a BVM device or an oxygen-powered manually triggered breathing device be more appropriate for this patient? Explain why.

## FIGURE 9-7

Size D oxygen cylinder with collar etchings

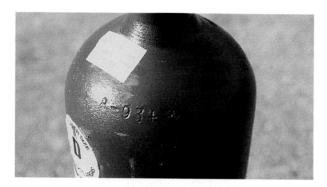

year stamp, indicating when the bottle was last tested. If there is a star stamped next to the date, the bottle is certified as safe for 10 years. If the cylinder does not have a star, it should be retested within 5 years of the stamped date.

Oxygen cylinders are available in several sizes. The two sizes you will most often use are the D (or super D) and M cylinders (Figure 9-8). The D (or super D) cylinder can be carried from your unit to the patient. The M tank remains on board your unit as a main supply tank. Other sizes you will see are A, E, H, and K (Figure 9-9).

## FIGURE 9-8

Size D and M oxygen cylinders

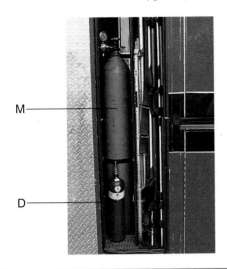

## FIGURE 9-9

Different sizes of oxygen cylinders

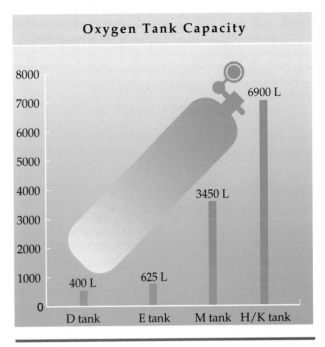

Oxygen Tank Capacity

400 L — D tank
625 L — E tank
3450 L — M tank
6900 L — H/K tank

**Safety considerations** You must always handle and connect oxygen cylinders with great care. Compressed gas cylinders must be handled carefully, because their contents are under pressure. Cylinders are fitted with specific pressure regulators to make sure that patients receive the right amount and type of gas. Make sure that the correct pressure regulator is firmly attached before you transport the cylinders. A loose regulator or a puncture or hole in the tank can cause the cylinder to become a deadly missile. Do not handle a cylinder by the neck assembly alone.

**Pin-indexing system** The compressed gas industry has established a pin-indexing system for portable cylinders that prevents an oxygen regulator from being connected to a carbon dioxide cylinder, and vice versa. Verifying that the pinholes exactly match the corresponding pins on the regulator is an important safety check when preparing to administer oxygen.

The pin-indexing system includes a series of pins on a yoke that must be matched with the holes on the valve stem of the gas cylinder. The arrangement of the

pins and holes varies for different gases according to accepted national standards. Each cylinder of a specific gas has a given pattern and a given number of pins. Other gases supplied in portable cylinders, such as acetylene, carbon dioxide, and nitrogen, use regulators and flowmeters that are very similar to those used with oxygen. Thus, when you must use two or more different gases, these safety measures will not allow you to attach a cylinder of nitrous oxide to an oxygen regulator. The oxygen regulator will not fit.

The outlet valves on D size or smaller cylinders are designed to accept yoke-type pressure-reducing gauges (Figure 9-10). The yoke-type gauge contains the pin-indexing system. The safety system for large cylinders is known as the **American Standard System.** Cylinders larger than D size are equipped with threaded gas outlet valves. The inside and outside thread sizes of these outlets vary depending on the gas in the cylinder. The cylinder will not accept

**FIGURE 9-10**

Yoke connector

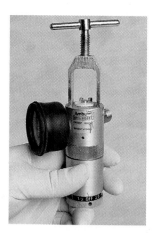

a regulator valve unless it is properly threaded to fit that regulator. The purpose of these safety devices is to prevent the accidental attachment of a regulator to a wrong cylinder.

### Pressure Regulators

The pressure of gas in a full oxygen cylinder is 2,100 psi. This is far too much pressure to be safe or useful for your purposes. Pressure regulators reduce the pressure to a more useful range, usually 40 to 70 psi. Most pressure regulators in use today reduce the pressure in a single stage, although multi-stage regulators do exist. A two-stage regulator will first reduce the pressure to 700 psi and then to 40 to 70 psi. After the pressure is reduced to a workable level, the final attachment for delivering the gas to the patient is usually through one of the following ways:

- a quick-connect female fitting that will accept a quick-connect male plug from a pressure hose or ventilator or resuscitator

- a flowmeter that will permit the regulated release of gas measured in liters per minute

### Flowmeters

Flowmeters are usually permanently attached to pressure regulators on emergency medical equipment. The two types of flowmeters commonly in use are pressure-compensated flowmeters and Bourdon-gauge flowmeters.

A pressure-compensated flowmeter incorporates a float ball within a tapered calibrated tube. The float rises or falls according to the gas flow within the tube. The flow of gas is controlled by a needle valve located downstream from the float ball. This type of flowmeter is affected by gravity and must always be maintained in an upright position for an accurate flow reading (Figure 9-11).

The Bourdon-gauge flowmeter is commonly used because it is not affected by gravity and can be used in any position. It is actually a pressure gauge calibrated to record flow rate (Figure 9-12). The major disadvantage of this flowmeter is that it does not compensate for back pressure. Therefore, it will usually record a higher flow rate when there is any obstruction to gas flow downstream.

## OPERATING PROCEDURES

When placing an oxygen cylinder into service, begin by inspecting the cylinder and its markings. If the cylinder was commercially filled, it will have a plastic seal around the valve stem covering the opening in the stem. Remove the seal and inspect the opening to make sure that it is free of dirt and other debris. The valve stem should not be sealed or covered with adhesive tape or any petroleum-based substances. These can contaminate the oxygen and can contribute to spontaneous combustion when mixed with the pressurized oxygen.

To help make sure that dirt particles and other possible contaminants do not enter the oxygen flow, "crack" the cylinder by

## FIGURE 9-11

A pressure-compensated flowmeter

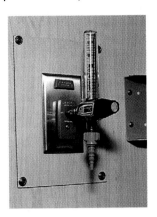

## FIGURE 9-12

A Bourdon-gauge flowmeter

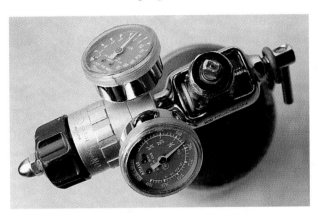

## SMOKIN' IN THE BOYS ROOM

Moments after Firecom gets a call about a bathroom fire at the local high school, EMS is also requested to respond. The attack crew off the pumper quickly extinguishes the fire that apparently started in a large wastepaper basket filled with paper towels. A few minutes later, two patients are brought out of the bathroom stalls where they apparently sought refuge after the fire started. The first patient is alert and walking. He has a headache, is coughing, and has difficulty breathing. The second patient was carried out by a fire fighter who tells you that he found the patient on the floor. This 17-year-old patient responds when you pinch his arm, but only by moaning. His pupils are dilated, but slightly reactive. His skin is slightly gray, and is warm and moist. He has a blood pressure of 138/74 mm Hg, a regular pulse of 130/min, and respirations of 22/min.

### For Discussion

1. Why is patient assessment considered the most important skill of an EMT?

2. What are the advantages and disadvantages to using only one approach to patient assessment?

quickly opening and then reclosing the valve. Open the tank by attaching a tank key to the valve and rotating the valve counterclockwise (Figure 9-13). Close the tank by rotating the valve clockwise. You should be able to easily hear the rush of oxygen coming from the tank.

After clearing the opening, attach the regulator/flowmeter to the valve stem. On one side of the valve stem, you will find three holes. The larger one, on top, is a true opening through which the oxygen flows. The two smaller holes below it do not extend to the inside of the tank. They provide stability to the regulator. These two holes are very precisely located in positions unique to oxygen cylinders (Figure 9-14).

Above the pins on the inside of the collar is the actual port through which oxygen flows from the cylinder to the regulator. A metal or plastic O-ring is placed around the oxygen port to maximize the airtight seal between the collar of the regulator and the valve stem.

Place the regulator collar over the cylinder valve, with the oxygen port and pin-indexing pins on the side of the valve stem with the three holes. Open the screw bolt just enough to allow the collar to freely fit over the valve stem. Move the regulator so

that the oxygen port and the pins fit into the correct holes on the valve stem (Figure 9-15). The screw bolt on the opposite side should be aligned with the dimpled depression. As you hold the regulator securely against the valve stem, tighten the screw bolt until the regulator is firmly attached to the cylinder. When sufficiently tight, there should not appear to be any open spaces between the sides of the valve stem and the interior walls of the collar.

With the regulator firmly attached, open the cylinder and read the pressure level on the regulator gauge. Most portable cylinders have a maximum pressure of 2,100 psi. Most EMS services consider a cylinder with less than 500 psi to be too low to keep in service. Learn your department's policies in this regard.

The flowmeter will have either a second gauge or a selector dial that indicates the oxygen flow rate. Several popular types of devices are widely used. Attach the selected oxygen device to the flowmeter by connecting the universal oxygen connective tubing to the "Christmas-tree" nipple on the flowmeter (Figure 9-16). Most oxygen delivery devices such as nasal cannula come with this tubing permanently attached. Some oxygen masks do not come equipped with

## FIGURE 9-13

Opening or "cracking" the oxygen cylinder

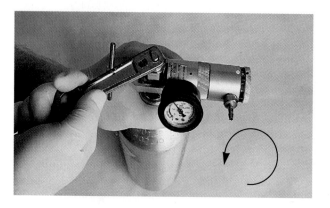

## FIGURE 9-14

A valve stem with pin-index holes

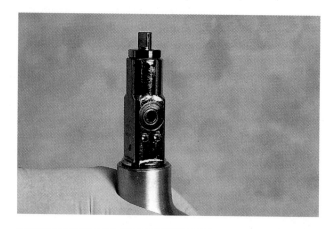

tubing. BVM devices do not include tubing. Therefore, it must be added when oxygen is being supplied to the BVM device.

Next, open the flowmeter to the desired flow rate. How to do this will vary depending on the device. *Remember that you must be completely familiar with the equipment before attempting to use it on a patient!* Once the oxygen is flowing at the desired rate, apply the oxygen device to the patient and make any necessary adjustments. Monitor the patient's reaction to the oxygen and to the oxygen device, and periodically recheck the regulator gauge to make sure there is sufficient oxygen in the cylinder.

When oxygen therapy is complete, or when the patient has been transferred to the hospital and has been switched to the hospital's oxygen system, disconnect the tubing from the flowmeter nipple and turn off the cylinder valve. In a few seconds, the sound of oxygen flowing from the nipple will cease. This indicates that all the pressurized oxygen has been removed from the flowmeter. Then turn off the flowmeter. The gauge on the regulator should read zero with the tank valve closed. This confirms that there is no pressure left above the valve

stem. *As long as there is a pressure reading on the regulator gauge it is not safe to remove the regulator from the valve stem!*

## HAZARDS OF SUPPLEMENTAL OXYGEN

Oxygen does not burn or explode; however, it does support combustion. The more oxygen there is around, the faster the combustion progresses. A small spark can become a flame in an oxygen-rich atmosphere. For example, a glowing cigarette can burst into flames. Therefore, any possible source of fire must be kept away from the area while oxygen is in use. Any area where oxygen is being given to a patient should be adequately ventilated. This is especially true in industrial settings where hazardous materials may be present and where sparks are easily generated.

## EQUIPMENT FOR OXYGEN DELIVERY

In general, the oxygen delivery equipment used in the field should be limited to nasal

### FIGURE 9-15

Proper position of the regulator on a valve stem with pins in view

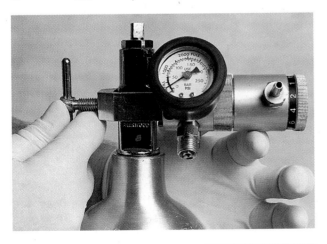

### FIGURE 9-16

Attaching the flowmeter to the Christmas tree nipple

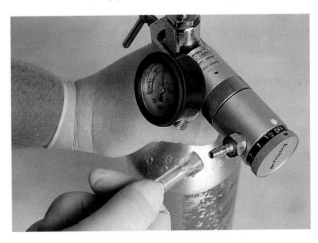

cannulas and nonrebreathing masks. However, you may encounter other devices during transports between medical facilities.

### Nonrebreathing Mask

The **nonrebreathing mask** is the preferred way of giving oxygen in the prehospital setting. With a good mask to mouth seal, it is capable of providing up to 95% inspired oxygen.

The nonrebreathing mask is a mask and reservoir bag system. The mask is similar to a simple face mask. However, with this system, oxygen fills a reservoir bag that is attached to the mask by a one-way valve. The system is called a nonrebreathing mask because the exhaled gas escapes through flapper valve ports at the cheek areas of the mask (Figure 9-17). The valve also prevents the patient from "rebreathing" exhaled gases as the gas in the reservoir bag flows into the mask during inhalation.

If you remove the flapper valves on the mask, the system becomes a partial rebreathing mask and reservoir bag (Figure 9-18). The valves may be removed to provide for proper fit or when necessary to handle large exhalation volumes. Oxygen concentrations of more than 60% inspired air can be delivered with a partial rebreathing mask.

In both of these systems, you must be sure that the reservoir bag is full before the mask is placed on the patient. The flow rate should be adjusted so that when the patient inhales, the bag does not fully collapse. This is about ⅔ of the bag volume or 15 L per minute. Make sure you use a smaller reservoir bag with infants and children, as the volume inhaled each time will be less.

### Nasal Cannula

With a **nasal cannula,** oxygen flows through two small, tube-like prongs that fit into the patient's nostrils (Figure 9-19). A nasal cannula can provide 35% to 50% inspired oxygen if the flowmeter is set at 6 to 7 L per minute. The nasal cannula delivers dry oxygen directly into the nostrils. Therefore, when you anticipate a long transport time, you should consult medical control about humidification. Humidifying the oxygen will prevent discomfort and possible damage to the mucous membranes in the nose.

**FIGURE 9-17**

A nonrebreathing mask

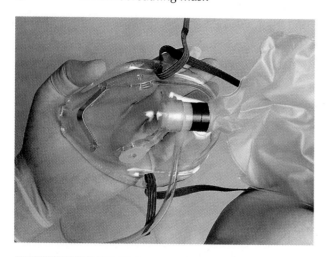

**FIGURE 9-18**

Conversion of a nonrebreathing mask to a partial rebreathing mask

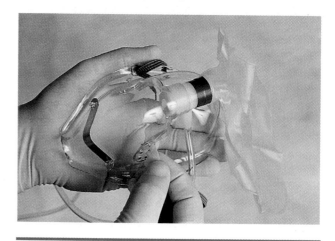

A nasal cannula is rarely the best method of delivering oxygen in the prehospital care setting. For example, a patient who breathes through the mouth or who has a nasal obstruction will get little or no benefit from a nasal cannula. A patient who is breathing on his or her own, but whose condition is not stable, should be given oxygen through a nonrebreathing mask. A nasal cannula is best used for more stable patients as either a preventive measure or mild treatment, according to your local protocols. For example, a patient who had chest pain an hour ago, but now has none, would benefit from a nasal cannula.

FIGURE 9-19

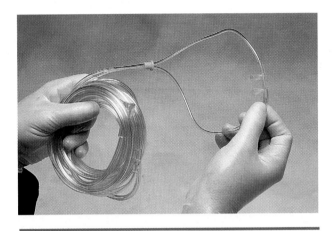

A nasal cannula

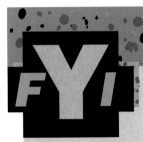

## Replacing Oxygen Cylinders

Part of your routine as an EMT-B will include switching to a fresh oxygen cylinder before the one in use is completely emptied—normally at 200 psi. This level is the safe residual level. You can calculate any cylinder's remaining "useful life" if you know its current pressure reading and flow as well as its factor.

### Cylinder Factors

| Type | Factor |
|------|--------|
| D | 0.16 |
| E | 0.28 |
| G | 2.41 |
| H | 3.14 |
| K | 3.14 |
| M | 1.56 |

One formula for calculating a cylinder's remaining life is as follows:

$$\frac{(\text{Gauge pressure} - \text{Safe residual}) \times \text{Factor}}{\text{Flow rate}}$$

For example, you have an M cylinder (factor = 1.56) with a gauge registering a pressure of 1,200 psi. Like most cylinders, the safe residual is 200 psi. And the flowmeter is set for 5 L/min.

To determine the cylinder's remaining life, you first subtract the safe residual from the cylinder's gauge pressure:

$$1,200 - 200 = 1,000$$

Next, you multiply that number by the cylinder's factor:

$$1,000 \times 1.56 = 1,560$$

Finally, you divide that result by the cylinder's flow rate:

$$1,560 \div 5 = 312$$

Thus this cylinder has 312 minutes (or 5 hours and 12 minutes) of useful life left.

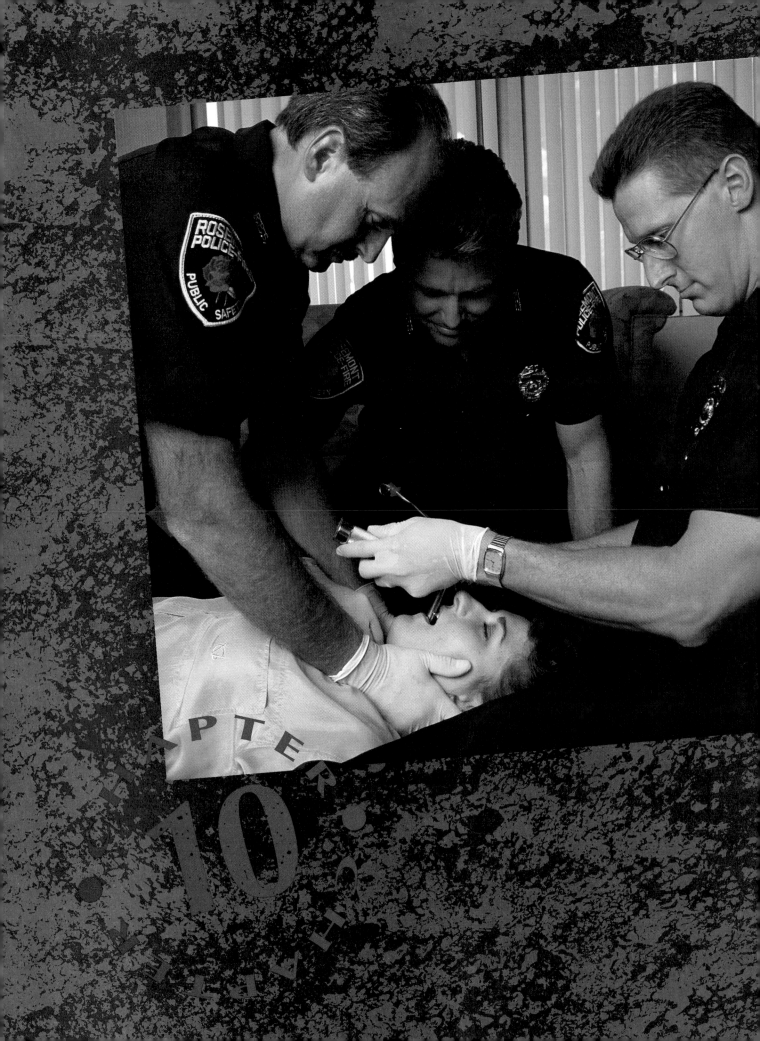

# Advanced Airway Management

## Objectives

After you have read this chapter, you should be able to:

- Describe the proper use of airway adjuncts.
- Review the use of oxygen therapy in airway management.
- Describe the indications for advanced airway management.
- Describe the indications, contraindications, and technique for inserting a nasogastric tube.
- Describe how to perform the Sellick maneuver.
- List the equipment needed for orotracheal intubation.
- Describe the proper use of both curved and straight blades for orotracheal intubation.
- State the reasons for and proper use of the stylet in orotracheal intubation.
- Describe how to select the proper-sized endotracheal tube for an adult.
- State the formula, along with alternative ways, for sizing an endotracheal tube for infants and children.
- List complications associated with advanced airway management.
- Explain the process of orotracheal intubation in adults and children.
- Explain how to confirm placement of an endotracheal tube in infants, children, and adults.
- Explain the consequences of and need to recognize unintentional esophageal intubation.
- Explain how to secure an endotracheal tube in infants, children, and adults.

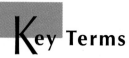

# Overview

At times it may be necessary for you to insert a tube into the patient's nose or throat to keep the airway open. This is called endotracheal intubation or simply, intubation. Intubation prevents aspiration, and it provides an open channel for you to give the patient oxygen. Four types of devices are used in advanced airway management: the endotracheal tube, the esophageal obturator airway (and the esophageal gastric tube airway), the esophageal tracheal combitube, and the pharyngeotracheal lumen airway. The endotracheal tube is discussed in detail in this chapter. The other devices are covered in an FYI feature at the end of this chapter.

Once you have learned how to insert these artificial airways, you will be able to protect the patient's airway and provide effective ventilation in any situation. However, you must have consent of your medical director, and you must follow local protocols.

This chapter begins with a brief review of airway adjuncts and a discussion of nasogastric tubes. Orotracheal intubation is discussed next, including detailed discussions of indications, pediatric considerations, proper equipment, and proper procedure for endotracheal intubation. An explanation of the importance of confirming tube placement follows. The next section describes the most common complications and errors of intubation. To avoid duplication, procedures are described once, with both adult and pediatric considerations discussed. The chapter ends with an FYI feature that covers the proper use of other advanced airway adjuncts.

# Key Terms

**Endotracheal intubation** A method of intubation in which an endotracheal tube (ETT) is placed through a patient's mouth or nose and directly through the larynx between the vocal cords into the trachea to open and maintain an airway.

**End tidal carbon dioxide detector** Plastic disposable indicator that signals, by color change, that the ETT is in the proper place.

**Laryngoscope** An instrument used to give a direct view of the patient's vocal cords during endotracheal intubation.

**Nasotracheal intubation** The placement of a tube through the nose into the trachea to improve ventilation.

**Orotracheal intubation** The placement of a tube through the mouth into the trachea to improve ventilation.

**Sellick maneuver** Technique in which pressure is applied on the cricoid cartilage to prevent aspiration. Involves pressing posteriorly on the cricoid cartilage to compress and shut off the esophagus behind it.

**Stylet** Plastic-coated wire that gives added rigidity and shape to the ETT.

**Vallecula** Space between the base of the tongue and the epiglottis.

# BASIC AIRWAY ADJUNCTS

The primary function of an artificial airway is to prevent obstruction of the upper airway by the tongue and allow passage of air and oxygen to the lungs.

The airway of an unconscious patient who is breathing spontaneously can be maintained with greater ease if an oropharyngeal airway is in place rather than with the constant use of the head-tilt or other maneuvers. The oropharyngeal airway should be used promptly for an unconscious patient who tolerates the airway and is breathing spontaneously. In the patient who is suspected of having a spinal injury, the oropharyngeal airway is a safe and effective means of keeping the airway open.

A conscious patient who is not able to maintain a natural airway may benefit from the use of a nasopharyngeal airway. A semiconscious or seizing patient may also benefit from this type of airway. This adjunct is usually well tolerated and is not as likely as the oropharyngeal airway to stimulate vomiting. A disadvantage is that it is usually not large enough in diameter, however, to allow passage of a standard suction tip or large suction catheter. Also, airway positioning techniques to ensure an open airway may still need to be applied with this type of airway. Length sizing is accomplished by measuring from the tip of the nose to the earlobe. Chapter 9 provides a detailed discussion of both oropharyngeal and nasopharyngeal airways.

Artificial ventilation can cause gastric distention, especially if high ventilatory pressures are used. Massive distention can interfere with artificial ventilation. Distention elevates the diaphragm, decreases lung volume, and increases the possibility for vomiting. You can minimize gastric distention by using slow, 1- to 1½-second breaths, with just enough pressure to make the chest rise. Attempt to relieve gastric distention by inserting a nasogastric tube when you recognize the condition and before the abdomen is so tense that ventilation is ineffective. The danger of aspiration into the lungs is great in this situation. Thus, you should have a suctioning unit available at all times.

## ADVANCED AIRWAY ADJUNCTS

A nasogastric or orogastric tube serves four principal purposes, as follows:

1. It relieves gastric distention.
2. It clears the stomach of poisons.
3. It clears the stomach of blood.
4. It provides a clear channel to give feedings or medications.

You will use a gastric tube primarily to decompress the stomach of a patient with gastric distention. This problem is most common in children. If you are unable to effectively ventilate a child, or the child is unconscious, you should attempt to insert a gastric tube. It is best to insert an orogastric tube, if possible, because it is safer and easier to insert. If the patient has head, spinal, or major facial trauma, you must insert the tube carefully, according to local protocol. The gastric tube should not make the child's condition worse. A nasogastric tube can cause nasal trauma with bleeding. Inserting a gastric tube can activate the gag reflex and cause vomiting and aspiration, or it can be passed into the trachea. If the patient has a basilar skull fracture, a gastric tube can be passed into the brain. However, this is more of a problem with nasogastric tubes.

### EQUIPMENT

You will need the following equipment for gastric intubation (Figure 10-1):

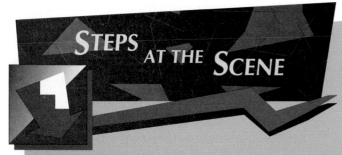

## STEPS AT THE SCENE

### INSERTING A NASOGASTRIC TUBE

☐ Prepare and assemble the proper equipment.

☐ Measure the tube from the tip of the nose, around the ear, to the epigastric area below the xiphoid process. (If you are using an orogastric tube, measure from the teeth to the angle of the jaw and down to the epigastric area.) Mark the tube with a piece of tape.

☐ Lubricate the distal tube with the proper lubricant.

☐ Place the patient in the proper position. If you do not suspect a spinal injury, place the patient supine, with the head turned to the side.

☐ Pass the tube along the nasal floor (or, for an orogastric tube, over the tongue to the back of the throat) until you reach the tape marker.

☐ Confirm tube placement by aspirating stomach contents with the syringe or injecting 20 mL of air and listening for gurgling over the stomach with the stethoscope.

☐ Aspirate air and stomach contents with the syringe to decompress the stomach. Irrigate the tube with 10 to 20 mL of water if it becomes plugged with material.

☐ Secure the tube in place with tape.

## FIGURE 10-1

Equipment for gastric intubation

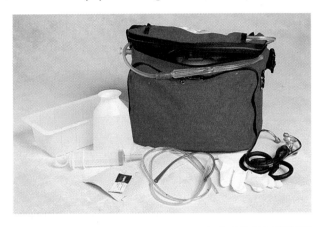

- proper-sized tube:
  - newborn/infant, 8 French
  - toddler/preschool, 10 French
  - school-age child, 12 French
  - adolescent, 14–16 French
- catheter-tipped 20-mL syringe
- water-soluble lubricant
- emesis container

- tape
- stethoscope
- suctioning unit

## SELLICK MANEUVER

Unresponsive patients who have no cough and gag reflexes are at risk for vomiting and aspiration. Without proper drainage, vomitus can travel up through the esophagus and then be aspirated into the lungs. Once in the lungs, vomitus can damage tissues and block the lower airway passages. This can easily happen in patients receiving artificial ventilations and CPR.

A procedure originally developed for intubating patients during surgery can be helpful to you. Applying pressure on the cricoid cartilage, commonly called the **Sellick maneuver,** can help to prevent aspiration (Figure 10-2a). This maneuver involves pressing posteriorly on the patient's cricoid cartilage to compress and shut off the esophagus behind it (Figure 10-2b).

## FIGURE 10-2

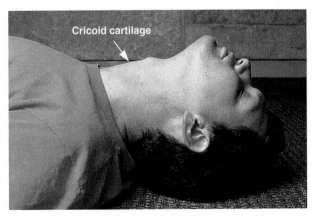

**A**   Identify the cricoid cartilage

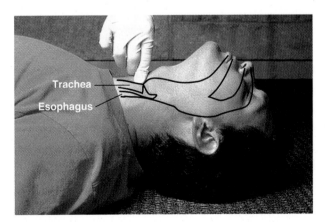

**B**   Apply pressure with your thumb and index finger to the cartilage

## ANATOMY REVIEW

The cricoid cartilage, located just below the thyroid cartilage (Adam's apple), is a ring-shaped structure that completely encircles the larynx at the top of the trachea. While this ring is not as strong or rigid as bone, it is strong enough to keep the trachea open. The depression between the thyroid cartilage and the cricoid cartilage is called the cricothyroid membrane. In certain cases, ALS providers will insert an emergency airway in the cricothyroid membrane.

The esophagus is much softer than the trachea and does not have rings of cartilage to hold it open. The esophagus is normally closed. It opens only as we eat or drink to allow fluids or pieces of food to travel along to the stomach. You can squeeze the esophagus shut by applying pressure on the cricoid cartilage. This may prevent solids and fluids from leaving the esophagus and eventually being aspirated into the larynx and the trachea.

## TECHNIQUE

Cricoid pressure is applied with the thumb and the index finger. When two-person CPR is being performed, a third EMT-B usually locates the cartilage and applies the pressure (Figure 10-3). The thumb and index finger should be placed just to each side of the midline of the cricoid cartilage. While you should apply firm pressure, you must also be sure you do not press too hard. Too much pressure could collapse the larynx. You should maintain pressure until the patient begins breathing on his or her own, is intubated, or begins coughing and gagging.

The cricoid cartilage can be difficult to locate in infants, children, and small adults. You must be certain you have located the cricoid cartilage before you apply pressure.

## FIGURE 10-3

The use of the Sellick maneuver during two-person CPR

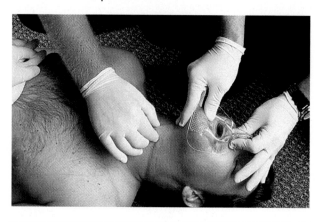

The Sellick maneuver should be performed by a third EMT-B. Therefore, this technique may not be possible if you and your partner are alone.

## OROTRACHEAL INTUBATION

The purpose of advanced airway management is to protect and improve ventilation through orotracheal intubation in patients who are not breathing on their own. **Orotracheal intubation** involves placing an endotracheal tube (ETT) into a patient's airway through the mouth to maintain the airway.

## INDICATIONS

Your initial assessment must focus on airway, breathing, circulation, and disability. This rule applies to every patient—infant, child, or adult. The obviously broken leg or amputated finger may be eye-catching, but the blocked airway must be cleared immediately or the patient will die. As discussed throughout this section of the text, the single most important skill you will perform as an EMT-B is establishing and maintaining a patient's airway. Most conscious patients are able to maintain an adequate airway on their own. As long as the gag reflex is present, most patients can clear their own airways. Thus, in the management of the conscious patient, you may need only to provide oxygen and monitor the patient closely for any changes. Semiconscious patients may require an oropharyngeal or nasopharyngeal airway and suctioning, as described in chapter 8, Airway and Ventilation.

However, patients who are unresponsive and not breathing on their own will fare better with advanced airway techniques. Orotracheal intubation is indicated for patients who cannot protect their own airways due to unconsciousness or cardiac arrest. Other situations in which orotracheal intubation is indicated include patients who need prolonged artificial ventilation. *Be advised that you should not immediately intubate an unresponsive or arrested patient!* First you must try to open the airway with the appropriate BLS maneuver. When BLS maneuvers fail to open the airway, or if the patient is unconscious, you should consider orotracheal intubation based on your local medical protocols.

## PEDIATRIC CONSIDERATIONS

Airway management of children presents some special challenges due to some key differences in anatomy. Children have larger heads in relation to their bodies than do adults. A child's larynx is higher and more anterior than in an adult's airway. The diameter of a child's airway is smaller at all levels. This means that something that would cause only partial airway obstruction in an adult would completely obstruct a child's airway. A child's tongue is also relatively larger for body size. This means that the tongue can easily cause an airway obstruction. An illness or injury that causes the tongue or other parts of the airway to swell affects a child much more seriously than an adult. For example, while epiglottitis occurs in both adults and children, it only rarely causes a serious airway problem in adults. However, it is commonly life threatening in children.

Other anatomic differences are equally important. All the supporting cartilages of the larynx, cricoid, and trachea are less rigid in children than in adults. Thus, even a moderate amount of external pressure will close off a child's airway. The same amount of pressure would not affect adults or would affect them minimally.

It is important for you to remember that a child's airway is much more at risk for obstruction than is the airway of an adult. It is more difficult to establish and maintain a child's airway than that of an adult. It is also much more difficult to bring a child's airway into alignment. This affects your ability to visualize the vocal cords for intubation. The cricoid cartilage below the larynx is the narrowest part of the airway. Pediatric tube sizes are based on the likely size of the airway opening at this level.

## ADVANTAGES

There are many advantages to orotracheal intubation, including the following:

- it completely controls and protects the airway

- it delivers better minute volume without the difficulty of maintaining an adequate mask seal as needed with a BVM device

- it may be left in place for a long time, if necessary

- it prevents gastric distention, which means less regurgitation of stomach contents

- it prevents aspiration of stomach contents because the trachea is sealed off by a balloon
- it allows for direct access to suctioning of the trachea
- it allows for the delivery of high volumes of oxygen at higher than normal pressures
- it allows for administration of certain medications

The insertion of a tube directly into the trachea is called **endotracheal intubation.** The ETT is placed through the patient's mouth or nose, directly through the larynx between the vocal cords, and then into the trachea. Endotracheal intubation, or simply "intubation," is a difficult skill to master and requires more training, but the extra effort provides a more effective airway. As an EMT-B, you will be intubating only those patients who are unconscious, unresponsive, or in cardiac arrest. Endotracheal intubation on patients who are conscious or drifting in and out of consciousness is much more difficult. You should not immediately intubate an unresponsive or arrested patient. First you must try to open the airway with the appropriate BLS maneuver and ventilate.

## COMPLICATIONS

While endotracheal intubation has several advantages, there are a number of possible complications. As mentioned earlier, endotracheal intubation is a difficult skill to master. If intubation takes too long, the resulting delay in oxygenation may lead to brain damage. You should not interrupt CPR for more than 30 seconds as you insert the ETT. Thus, you need a great deal of practice and expert instruction in endotracheal intubation. These are explained in more detail in a later section of this chapter.

1. *Intubating the right mainstem bronchus.* This is the most common error made during intubation. If you push the tube in too far or accidentally slip it in too far, the ETT will pass into the right mainstem bronchus. In this position, it will ventilate the right lung only. Thus, you will hear breath sounds on only one side. The patient may become more short of breath and perhaps even turn blue. The best way to correct this problem is to pull the tube back slightly. Even when placed properly, the ETT will move if it is not secured. Never let go of the ETT until it is taped securely in place. Even then, you must continuously check the tube to make sure it is secure and in the correct place.

2. *Intubating the esophagus.* This will commonly occur when the ETT is inserted without first seeing the vocal cords. Usually, the ETT will be inserted into the esophagus rather than into the trachea. In this position, intubation will not ventilate the lungs. Rather, it will rapidly inflate the patient's stomach. Therefore, you must be very careful about verifying tube placement. As you insert the ETT, carefully watch as it passes through the vocal cords. Next, check breath sounds in four locations and watch for the rise and fall of the chest. If there is any doubt, pull out the ETT, reventilate the patient for 2 to 3 minutes and then try again.

3. *Aggravating a spinal injury.* Whenever there is concern about a spinal injury, you must intubate without moving the patient's neck from the neutral, in-line position. The major problem when intubating a trauma patient is lifting the lower jaw and tongue enough to see the vocal cords while maintaining the neck in a neutral position. This is a two-person procedure.

4. *Taking too long to intubate.* You should never spend more than 30 seconds trying to intubate. This will make the patient more hypoxic. Your partner or another member of the team should actually time the intubation. If you cannot intubate the patient within 30 seconds, then ventilate the patient again with a BVM device at 100% oxygen for 2 to 3 minutes and try again. To better see the vocal cords, you should ask a third EMT-B to perform the Sellick maneuver. If after two tries at intubation the tube cannot be passed, try another airway technique or ask another qualified rescuer to try. If the patient is difficult to intubate, you should not waste time in the field. Provide immediate transport and use another airway adjunct and assist ventilations, as needed.

5. *Vomiting and/or removing the tube.* A patient who is not totally unresponsive may begin to gag or may try to remove the tube. Gagging may cause the patient to vomit and aspirate stomach contents into the lungs. You must be careful to avoid intubation in a patient who still has a gag reflex. You can check for a gag reflex with a tongue blade or the laryngoscope blade. Always be aware that you can make the patient vomit as you check for a gag reflex. You should always have a suctioning unit ready. Trying to insert an ETT through the vocal cords can also cause the cords to spasm. This is called laryngospasm. If this occurs, stop intubating and try to ventilate the patient with positive pressure.

6. *Causing soft tissue trauma.* The laryngoscope and the tip of the ETT can injure the lips, teeth, tongue, gums, and other airway structures. If the laryngoscope blade is used as a lever, the patient's teeth can be broken easily. If the tube is blindly pushed forward without watching the vocal cords, it can lacerate the oropharynx.

Once the ETT is secured in place, you must carefully assess the patient's vital signs, particularly the heart rate. With endotracheal intubation, the heart rate may decrease when the airway has been stimulated. Also make sure you evaluate the patient's lung sounds any time you move the patient. A summary of the advantages and disadvantages of endotracheal intubation is presented in Table 10-1.

**TABLE 10-1**  ADVANTAGES AND DISADVANTAGES OF ENDOTRACHEAL INTUBATION

| Advantages | Disadvantages |
| --- | --- |
| Provides complete protection of airway | Intubating the right mainstem bronchus |
| Can be left in for long periods of time | Intubating the esophagus |
| Delivers better oxygen concentration than BVM device | Aggravating a spinal injury |
| Prevents gastric distention and aspiration | Taking too long to intubate |
| Allows for deep suctioning of the trachea | Vomiting and/or removing the tube |
| Allows for administration of certain medications | Causing soft tissue trauma |

## EQUIPMENT

If you and your partner find that you will be intubating a patient, you must first assemble all the equipment you need (Figure 10-4). Endotracheal intubation requires all your attention. You should not be searching for forgotten or misplaced equipment. As with all patient care situations, follow BSI techniques, as you will be exposed to blood or other body fluids.

### FIGURE 10-4

Equipment for endotracheal intubation

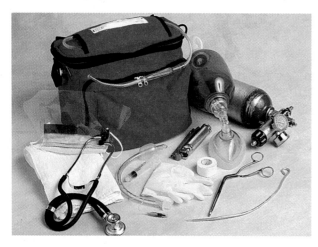

You will need the following equipment for endotracheal intubation:

- proper-sized endotracheal tube
- laryngoscope
- stylet
- 10-mL syringe
- oxygen, with BVM device or oxygen-powered breathing device
- a suctioning unit
- Magill forceps
- towels
- gloves
- stethoscope
- face mask
- eye protection

### FIGURE 10-5

An aligned airway

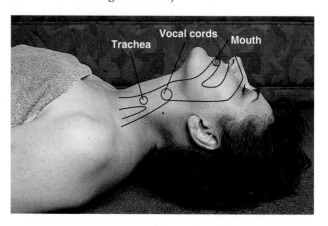

#### Laryngoscope

The **laryngoscope** gives you a direct view of the patient's vocal cords. The purpose of a laryngoscope is to align the airway so that the vocal cords can be seen and the ETT passed through them (Figure 10-5). The handle of the laryngoscope contains two C or D cell batteries and has a locking bar. Be sure you keep spare batteries in your unit. The blade of the laryngoscope is detachable from the handle. Blade sizes range from 0 to 4, all either curved or straight (Figure 10-6). The curved blade is inserted into the vallecula to allow for visualization of the glottic opening and vocal cords. The **vallecula** is the space between the base of the tongue and the epiglottis. A curved blade is preferred for use in older children due to its broader base and flange. These features provide better displacement of the tongue in older children (Figure 10-7a). A straight blade

**FIGURE 10-6**

A laryngoscope with curved and straight blades

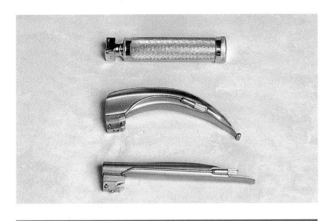

You must check your equipment daily to be certain that it is properly assembled and working, especially before you try to intubate a patient. There is a notch on the blade that locks onto the locking bar of the handle. Adequate lighting is essential for intubation. For this purpose, there is a light bulb near the tip of the blade. You can activate the light by lifting the blade away from the handle until it locks at a right angle (Figure 10-8). The light should be bright white. However, it will not come on if the blade is not attached properly, if the bulb is burned out or loose, or if the batteries in the handle are dead. Always carry extra batteries for the handle and extra light bulbs.

actually lifts the epiglottis to allow for visualization of the vocal cords. A straight blade is preferred for use in infants, as it provides greater displacement of the tongue and better visualization in general. Simply put, the straight blade is inserted past the epiglottis and the curved blade goes just in front of the epiglottis (Figure 10-7b).

**Endotracheal Tubes**

**Selecting tube size** Endotracheal tubes come in many sizes—from 2.5 to 9 mm inside diameter. The outside of the tube is marked in centimeters. You must carry a complete selection of tube sizes. The usual length of an adult tube is 33 cm. It is generally 15 cm to

**FIGURE 10-7**

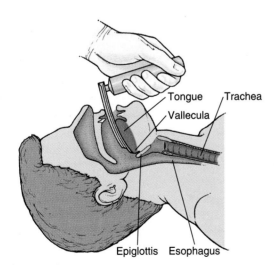

Tongue   Trachea
Vallecula

Epiglottis   Esophagus

**A**   The insertion of a curved blade in front of the epiglottis

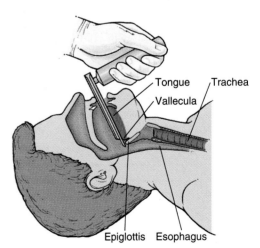

Tongue   Trachea
Vallecula

Epiglottis   Esophagus

**B**   The insertion of a straight blade past the epiglottis

## FIGURE 10-8

Turning on the laryngoscope light

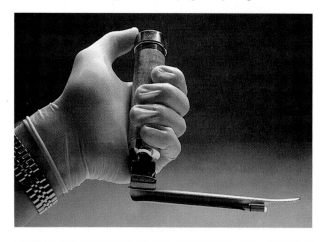

## FIGURE 10-9

Tape for sizing ET tubes in children

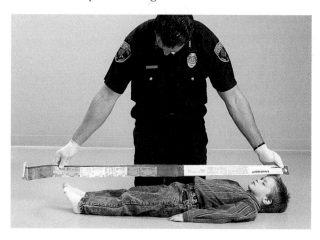

the vocal cords, 20 to 21 cm to the sternal notch, and 25 cm to the carina. You must also remember to carry a water-soluble lubricant for use on the tube and the stylet. Check with your medical director regarding local protocol on lubricating the stylet. The proper size for most adult males ranges from 7.5 to 8.5 mm; for most adult females it ranges from 6.5 to 8.0 mm. Thus, for adults, the best sized tube for emergencies is 7.5 mm.

For children, it is best to have a chart or tape device to help you with sizing the ETT (Figure 10-9). Generally, for newborns and small infants, the proper tube size ranges from 3.0 to 3.5 mm and for infants up to 1 year, 4.0 mm. You may also follow a formula for sizing tubes in children. You can calculate tube size in children by adding 16 + the child's age, and then dividing by 4. Another method is to select a tube that roughly equals the size of the diameter of the patient's little finger across the nailbed (Figure 10-10). No matter what size you decide to use, you should also have one tube larger and one tube smaller available should you need it.

**Other tube components**    The parts of an endotracheal tube include a standard

## FIGURE 10-10

Selecting the proper-sized ET tube using a child's finger

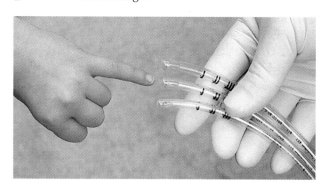

15-mm adapter. This adapter is attached to either the BVM or oxygen-powered breathing device, whichever is used. You must make sure that the adapter is securely pushed into the tube so that it does not pull off when you ventilate the patient. The tube has a pilot balloon at the top to indicate how well the balloon cuff at the end is inflated. The cuff at the end holds about 10 mL of air. The small hole at the distal end of the tube across from the bevel end is called a Murphy eye. The Murphy eye helps prevent tube obstruction (Figure 10-11).

You will use uncuffed tubes in children younger than 8 years old. The circular nar-

## FIGURE 10-11

Adult (top) and pediatric (bottom) ET tubes

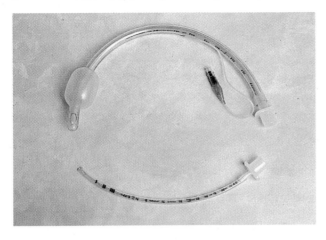

## FIGURE 10-12

Stylets for adults (bottom) and children (top)

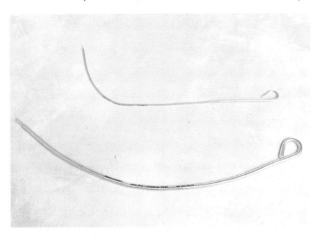

## FIGURE 10-13

Testing the balloon for air leaks

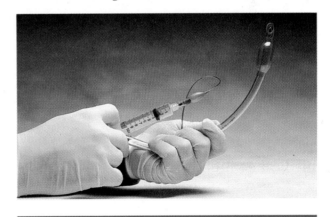

rowing of a child's trachea at the level of the cricoid cartilage serves as a functional cuff. However, for children older than 8 years, you will use cuffed tubes, just as you would for adults. Watch the tube pass through vocal cords in a child to make sure that the tip of the ETT is in the proper position.

### Stylet

A plastic-coated wire stylet may be inserted into the ETT in both adults and children (Figure 10-12). The **stylet** gives added rigidity and shape to the tube. You should bend the tip of the stylet to form a gentle curve in adults. The stylet should be bent in the shape of a hockey stick in infants and children. This difference in shape is because the airway in infants and children is more angular and less aligned than that in an adult. You should also apply a little water-soluble lubricant to the end of the stylet for all patients. This makes removing the stylet much easier once the tube is in place. The stylet must not be inserted past the Murphy eye, as it could puncture or lacerate delicate airway tissues. A good rule of thumb is to keep the stylet ¼" from the cuff in adults and 1" from the end of the tube in infants and children.

### Syringe

After you select the proper tube, use a 10-mL syringe to inflate the balloon to test for air leaks (Figure 10-13). This step is done only for cuffed tubes. Thus, you will not perform this step with the uncuffed tubes used on infants and small children. After you have tested the balloon, completely deflate the balloon. However, the syringe should be left attached to the tube and filled with another 10 mL of air. The second time you inflate the balloon, the ETT should be inserted into the patient's airway.

## Other Equipment

You must also have either tape or a commercial securing device available, along with any other equipment necessary for airway and ventilation assistance. This includes oxygen, a suctioning unit, a BVM device, Magill forceps, and towels if the patient's head and/or shoulders need to be raised. The BVM will help you ventilate the patient before you first try to intubate. It can also be used to ventilate the intubated patient after detaching the mask. With difficult intubations, you can use the Magill forceps to direct the tip of the ETT toward and through the vocal cords. If you are inserting the ETT, you should guide the tube with the Magill forceps under direct visualization of the laryngoscope. Your partner will then push in the tube when instructed (Figure 10-14).

## ENDOTRACHEAL INTUBATION

You may only intubate if allowed by off-line medical control or confirmed with on-line medical control, based on your local medical protocols. Once you and medical control have made the decision to intubate, you must act quickly and carefully. Intubation should be done as quickly and efficiently as possible. No more than 30 seconds should be needed to place the ETT in the proper position. Your first step is to open the airway with a BLS maneuver and clear the airway of any foreign material. Be sure to follow BSI techniques. Intubation is a three-person task, as follows:

- EMT-B #1 prepares the patient and intubates
- EMT-B #2 continues CPR
- EMT-B #3 provides 100% oxygen with a BVM device once every 4 to 6 seconds

## FIGURE 10-14

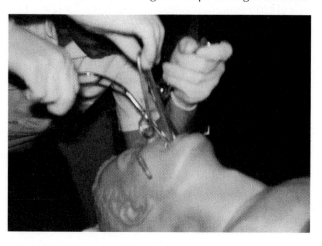

The use of Magill forceps during intubation

Each breath given to the patient should last 1½ to 2 seconds. During the initial phase after a cardiac arrest, you should give 12 to 15 breaths/min and later 10 to 12 breaths/min. However, this rate will vary depending on the age of the patient. The patient must get oxygen continuously! You should hyperventilate the patient for at least 1 minute before attempting intubation. Just prior to intubation, the patient must be well oxygenated. Remember also that defibrillation is the top priority. Intubation is only done after defibrillation and 1 minute of CPR, if necessary.

You must then quickly assemble and test your equipment: gloves, mask, eye protection, proper-sized ETT, laryngoscope, lubricating gel, syringe, stylet, suctioning unit, Magill forceps, suction tubes, and tonsil sucker. Lubricate the tube and the stylet. Make sure you have towels available to help with positioning the head, if needed.

## POSITIONING THE PATIENT

Once the equipment is ready, the patient's head and neck should be positioned properly. Use the following procedure for nontrauma patients. To simplify intubation,

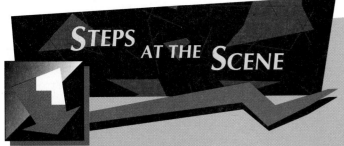

## INSERTING THE ENDOTRACHEAL TUBE

- ☐ Open the airway and hyperventilate the patient. Follow BSI techniques.

- ☐ Assemble the proper equipment.

- ☐ Check your equipment, including the light, balloon cuff, syringe, and suctioning unit. Also lubricate the tube and stylet.

- ☐ Position the patient's head and neck (nontrauma and trauma positions).

- ☐ Clear dentures, vomitus, or blood from the mouth. Use Magill forceps for objects.

- ☐ Open the airway.

- ☐ Gently position the laryngoscope.

- ☐ Move the lower jaw and tongue to expose the vocal cords. A straight blade goes past the epiglottis. A curved blade goes in front of the epiglottis. Use the Sellick maneuver, if needed, to bring the cords into view.

- ☐ Slip the tube and the stylet through the vocal cords.

- ☐ Remove the laryngoscope, turn off the light, and hold the tube.

- ☐ Remove the stylet while holding the tube.

- ☐ Inflate the cuff with 5 to 10 mL of air and ventilate the patient.

- ☐ Check breath sounds to confirm placement. Look for chest to rise.

- ☐ Insert the oral airway.

- ☐ Secure the tube.

- ☐ Continually monitor the tube and patient.

- ☐ Suction as required, but never for more than 10 seconds.

---

align the mouth, the pharynx, and the trachea in a straight line. First, flex the neck on the chest to align the pharynx and trachea (Figure 10-15a). Then extend the head on the neck, lining up the mouth and pharynx (Figure 10-15b). It may be useful to place a towel under the patient's occiput or shoulders for better flexion of the neck and better visualization of the vocal cords.

Once you have aligned the airway, clear the mouth of any loose or obstructing materials. Remove dentures or partial plates. Use suctioning to remove vomitus, blood clots, or other material in the upper airway.

Use Magill forceps to grasp objects obstructing the airway.

A patient in cardiac arrest that is not due to trauma should be positioned as described above. However, a patient who is unconscious because of injury presents a more difficult situation. You must take care to prevent further injury to a patient who may have a spinal injury. With these patients, controlling the airway with the modified jaw-thrust maneuver, an oropharyngeal airway, and BVM device is usually adequate. However, if you must intubate, the patient's head must be held in a neutral, in-line

## FIGURE 10-15

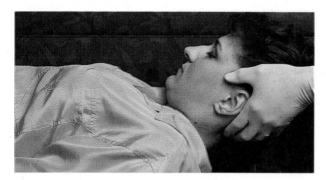

**A** Flex the neck to prepare for insertion of the ET tube

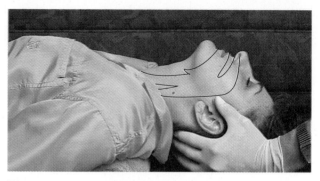

**B** Extend the head on the neck to align the pharynx with the trachea

position during intubation. You or your partner should kneel, straddling the patient, to maintain the head in a neutral position. The major difficulty is lifting the lower jaw and tongue sufficiently to visualize the cords while maintaining vertebral alignment in a neutral position. Practically speaking, the EMT-B who will insert the ETT will likely need to lie on his or her stomach or sit straddling the patient's head, leaning back. One of these positions is necessary to adequately visualize the vocal cords (Figure 10-16).

## INSERTING THE LARYNGOSCOPE

A laryngoscope is used to view the vocal cords as the ETT passes through them. In some instances, medical control will direct you to insert the ETT using the sounds of labored respirations as a guide, or place it by feel through the vocal cords. For injured patients, medical control may recommend the blind orotracheal technique of feeling the epiglottis and then passing the ETT through the vocal cords by feel. This technique is called digital intubation. The laryngoscope is used to make sure the ETT is in the proper position. Direct visualization of

## FIGURE 10-16

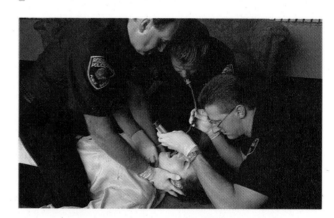

**A** Visualize the vocal cords by lying on your stomach

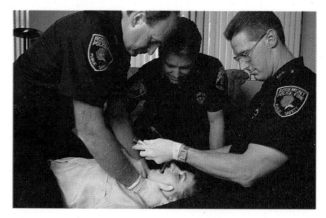

**B** Visualize the vocal cords by sitting at the patient's head and leaning back

the vocal cords also minimizes damage to the larynx and trachea.

Once the airway is aligned and any foreign matter removed, you are ready to gently insert the laryngoscope. Remember that very little force is necessary during intubation. Grasp the laryngoscope handle in your left hand. Open the patient's mouth with the gloved fingers of your right hand. Place your right thumb on the lower teeth and hook your index finger behind the thumb under the jaw. Exert force just behind the lower front teeth (Figure 10-17). Place the blade in the right side of the patient's mouth. Next, move it to the center, gently pushing the tongue to the left.

The final position of the blade will vary, depending on the shape of the blade, as

## FIGURE 10-18

Proper use of a laryngoscope

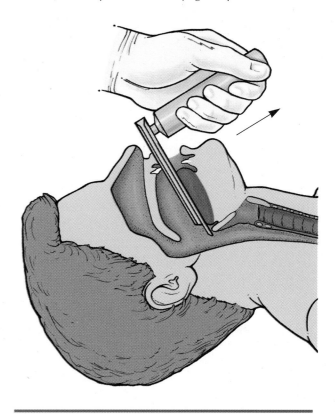

## FIGURE 10-17

Lift the mandible as you insert the laryngoscope

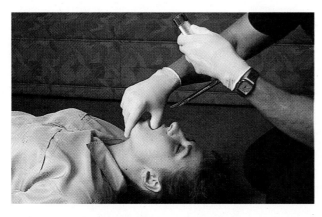

shown earlier in this chapter. A curved blade is advanced along the base of the tongue until its tip rests at the vallecula. The vallecula is the space between the base of the tongue and the epiglottis. A straight blade is advanced slightly farther, catching and pulling the epiglottis itself anteriorly. The laryngoscope must then be lifted away from the posterior pharynx enough so you can see the vocal cords. The lifting force is directed straight up, parallel to the long axis of the laryngoscope handle. This force should feel as if you are picking the patient's head up with his or her jaw. The direction of force is not back toward you at the head of the patient. *Never use the blade as a lever against the upper teeth!* By doing so, you will not see the vocal cords and you could break the patient's teeth (Figure 10-18).

### Performing the Sellick Maneuver

You can improve visualization of the vocal cords by having a third EMT-B, if available, perform the Sellick maneuver. Remember that with this maneuver, you apply light pressure over the cricoid cartilage to close off the esophagus. This also protects the patient from aspiration of the stomach contents. Pressure should be maintained until the ETT cuff is inflated. Do not lose sight of the vocal cords at any time.

## INSERTING THE ETT

With the patient's vocal cords now in direct view, hold the ETT in your right hand. Advance the tube from the right side of the patient's mouth. You must keep the vocal cords and the tip of the tube in sight at all times. Do not advance the ETT down the center of the laryngoscope blade, because you will not be able to see its tip. You must be able to see the tip of the ETT as it passes through the vocal cords. Also, watch the

uninflated balloon as it passes through the vocal cords. Then advance the ETT 1" beyond the upper edge of the balloon (Figure 10-19). At this point, the tip of the ETT should be halfway between the carina and the vocal cords. Make sure you note the cm markings on the ETT at the upper teeth or gum line and then record its position. Once the tube has been inserted through the vocal cords into the trachea, gently remove the laryngoscope and stylet.

You should next inflate the soft balloon cuff near the end of the tube with 5 to 10 mL of air. This will seal the trachea and anchor the tube, so that air can be blown directly into the lungs. The syringe must then be detached or the air in the balloon will empty back into it. After you inflate the balloon,

## FIGURE 10-19

Adult airway with an ET tube in place

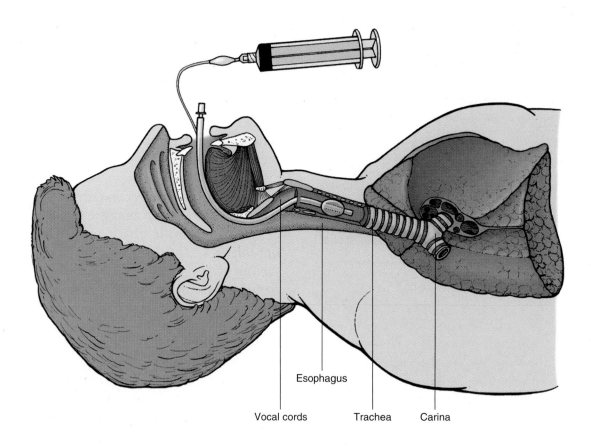

Esophagus

Vocal cords          Trachea          Carina

continue to hold the tube in place until it is secured with tape or with a device approved by your medical director. However, do not secure the tube at this time. You or your partner (whoever is not holding the ETT in place) should first begin ventilating the patient with a BVM device once every 3 to 5 seconds. Each breath lasts 1½ to 2 seconds. During the initial phase after a cardiac arrest, you should give 12 to 15 breaths/min and later 10 to 12 breaths/min.

## CONFIRMING PLACEMENT

Your next step is to confirm that the ETT is in the proper position. Listen with a stethoscope over both lungs and the stomach as you ventilate the patient through the tube (Figure 10-20). You should be able to hear breath sounds over both right and left lung fields and in the axillae. Also listen at the sternal notch in children. You should *not* be able to hear breath sounds in the stomach. You should also see both sides of the chest rise and fall with each ventilation. This is especially important in children, as breath sounds in children may be misleading. You may hear them even if the tube is

in the esophagus. At this point, you should also reassess the patient's vital signs. Check the heart rate and skin color, especially in children. Remember to reassess breath sounds each time you move the patient. If you see and hear each of the above, you should next secure the ETT in place.

Even with the balloon inflated, the ETT can move into the trachea. Therefore, you must secure the ETT in the proper position. Never let go of the tube until it has been secured in place with tape. Use adhesive tape or a 30" length of umbilical tape. Wrap the tape around the tube and then around the patient's head to maintain its proper position. Remember to note the distance that the tube has been inserted. Commercial devices, such as a plastic bite block with Velcro fasteners, are also available, but they must be approved by your medical director.

Proper placement of the ETT may also be confirmed by obtaining a pulse oximetry reading and by using an end tidal carbon dioxide detector. A pulse oximetry reading of an oxygen saturation greater than 90% is helpful (Figure 10-21). However, this is only a small piece of the puzzle in confirming proper tube placement. You must also see the tube go through the vocal cords, or

### FIGURE 10-20

Confirm proper placement of the ET tube

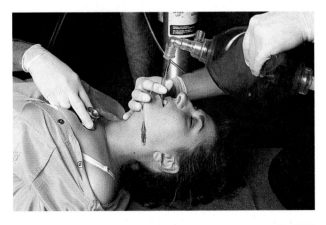

### FIGURE 10-21

Obtain a pulse oximetry reading

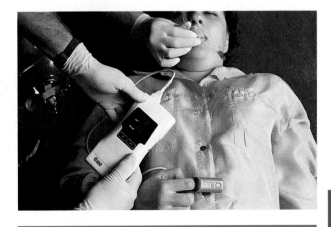

hear good bilateral breath sounds and see the patient's chest rise and fall. Another helpful adjunct is the **end tidal carbon dioxide detector.** This adjunct is a plastic disposable indicator that signals, by color change, that the ETT is in the proper place (Figure 10-22). The color may vary with inhalation and exhalation as the levels of carbon dioxide rise and fall in the airway. The device is placed over the end of the ETT where the gases can pass through it. The chemically treated paper in the device changes from purple to yellow in the presence of carbon dioxide. If the ETT is properly placed in the trachea, and if carbon dioxide is being produced, then the device will indicate proper placement. Patients in full cardiac arrest may not be producing carbon dioxide. Thus, the color indicator may not change, even though the ETT is in the proper place. In general, this device has become a standard of care in confirming proper tube placement. Consult your medical director for more information.

Once you have secured the ETT and confirmed its placement, place an oropharyngeal airway or a bite block between the

### FIGURE 10-22

End tidal carbon dioxide detector

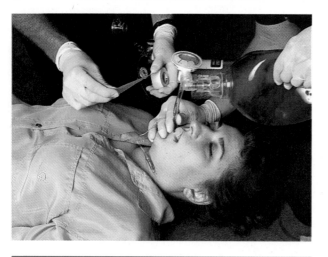

### FIGURE 10-23

Insert bite block to protect the secured ET tube

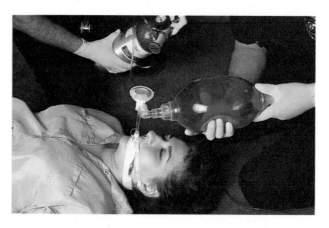

patient's teeth. This will prevent the patient from biting on the tube (Figure 10-23).

### Intubating the Bronchus

The most common error made during endotracheal intubation is to advance the tube too far. The ETT then ends up in the right mainstem bronchus where it will ventilate only the right lung. This is why it is essential that you hear good breath sounds on both sides of the chest to confirm placement. If you hear breath sounds on the right side only, you should deflate the cuff and pull the ETT back about 1". Reinflate the cuff and then listen again for bilateral breath sounds.

### Intubating the Esophagus

The other common error occurs when the ETT is inserted without adequate visualization of the vocal cords. In this situation, the ETT usually ends up in the esophagus. If you hear breath sounds in the stomach and not the lungs, you have intubated the esophagus. Intubating the esophagus means that oxygen will be blown into the stomach, not the lungs. If not corrected, the patient will die. Thus, it is essential that you see the vocal cords and watch the tip of the tube as it passes between them. Be warned that although this maneuver may help to bring the vocal cords into view, it also may cause the patient to gag and vomit. As long as you maintain firm pressure on the cricoid cartilage, the esophagus will be blocked, preventing vomiting. Therefore, once you apply pressure to the cricoid cartilage, you must maintain it until the ETT is properly placed and the balloon is inflated. If the ETT is in the esophagus, it should be removed. You should then hyperventilate the patient for 2 to 3 minutes before a second attempt is made.

### Extubating

While it is rare, sometimes the patient will regain a gag reflex or regain consciousness and not be able to tolerate the ETT. You should not remove the ETT unless it has moved to the esophagus or the patient will no longer permit the tube to remain in place. Before extubating the patient in these circumstances, you should make sure that the suctioning unit is nearby and turned on. If you must remove the ETT, first consult medical control. The recommended procedure is to deflate the cuff and withdraw the ETT as the patient inhales. Provide immediate suctioning if the patient vomits, assess the airway, and then give supplemental oxygen.

### Mechanical Failure

It is easy to dislodge the ETT when moving the patient. You should recheck tube placement after moving the patient to the stretcher, or after moving from one stretcher to another.

You may notice a large air leak when ventilating the patient. In an adult, this means that the balloon cuff does not have enough air in it or that the balloon has broken. If this occurs, you must get more air into the cuff (check the pilot balloon), or you must replace the tube. In a child, either the uncuffed tube is too small or the child is large enough (usually over 8 years old) to need a cuffed tube.

In children, if the ventilations are still inadequate, check that the pop off valve has been deactivated. In all patients, make sure that the BVM system does not have a leak in it or that the ventilator is delivering the proper tidal volume at the proper rate.

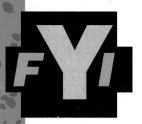

# Atlas of
# Other Advanced Airway Adjuncts

## ESOPHAGEAL OBTURATOR AIRWAY AND THE ESOPHAGEAL GASTRIC TUBE AIRWAY

Advanced airway management is also possible with an esophageal obturator airway (EOA) or its more modern form, the esophageal gastric tube airway (EGTA). The EOA has been used since 1973 to help with airway management in CPR. A properly placed ETT provides the most effective possible delivery of oxygen to the lungs. However, some studies have shown that the EOA may be just as effective when used for a short time and in combination with a flow-restricted oxygen-powered ventilation device. Less practice and skill are required to insert the EOA, because you do not have to use a laryngoscope to visualize the vocal cords during intubation.

The EOA is a plastic, semirigid tube that is 34 cm long and 13 mm in diameter (Figure 10-24). The lower end is smooth, rounded, and closed. The esophageal tube of the EGTA differs from that of the EOA. The tube of the EGTA has a valve designed to permit a tube to be passed through it and into the stomach (Figure 10-25). This allows for decompression and suctioning of the stomach. The upper one third of both tubes is designed to function as an airway. Each tube has 16 holes in its wall at the junction of the middle and upper thirds. When properly placed, these holes will lie at the level of the pharynx and provide free passage of oxygen to the lungs. The lower two thirds of the EOA or the EGTA should lie in the esophagus. The balloon surrounding the end of the tube is normally inflated to block the esophagus.

**FIGURE 10-24**

An esophageal obturator airway (EOA)

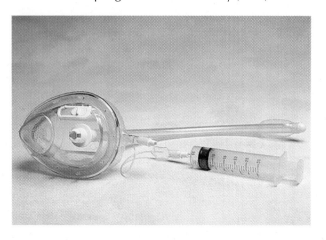

**FIGURE 10-25**

An esophageal gastric tube airway (EGTA)

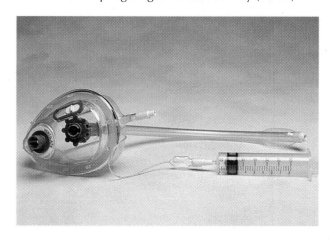

## FIGURE 10-26

The airflow in a properly placed EOA

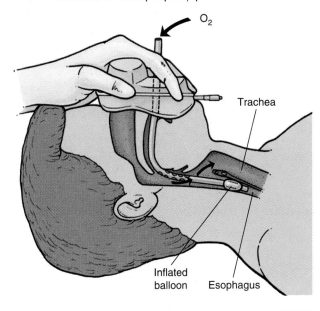

This prevents regurgitation of stomach contents into the airway.

The face mask on an EOA or EGTA is designed to fit snugly over the patient's nose and mouth. The mask must provide a tight seal. Oxygen-rich air given through the 15-mm opening in the tube first passes to the face mask. The oxygen then passes through the upper portion of the airway and into the lungs through the side holes in the esophageal tube. Oxygen moves this way because the esophagus is blocked by the inflated balloon and the obturator (Figure 10-26). The oxygen inlet port on the EGTA is in the face mask, not the esophageal tube. This provides for a greater volume flow of oxygen to the lungs than with the EOA.

### Contraindications

You should not insert an EOA/EGTA in any of the four following situations:

1. *On patients who are awake.* The EOA/EGTA will cause vomiting and aspiration.

The EOA/EGTA should be used only in deeply unconscious patients, usually after an endotracheal intubation has failed.

2. *On small children.* The EOA/EGTA should not be used for children under 16 years of age. The EOA/EGTA is made in only one size. Thus, it is too large for children and does not work effectively.

3. *On patients with known esophageal disease.* The EOA/EGTA may cause serious problems for a patient with esophageal cancer or esophageal varices. If a patient has swallowed a caustic agent, such as lye, the EOA/EGTA may perforate the injured esophagus.

4. *On patients with significant upper airway bleeding.* Blood from the nose or mouth will pass directly into the lungs once the esophageal cuff is inflated. If blood, mucus, or saliva collects in the upper airway once an EOA/EGTA is in place, it must be cleared by suctioning under the mask.

### Complications

INTUBATING THE TRACHEA    The most common complication in using the EOA/EGTA is placement in the trachea rather than the esophagus. Once the EOA/EGTA has been inserted, you must listen carefully for breath sounds over all lung fields. You can confirm improper position if breath sounds are absent on one (usually the right) or both sides of the chest. In this instance, you must remove and replace the tube promptly. Tracheal intubation is more likely to occur if the head is extended on the neck. The head should be flexed or held in a neutral in-line position when you insert the EOA/EGTA. Excessive curvature to the EOA/EGTA will also increase the likelihood of entering the trachea. This can happen if the EOA/EGTA is stored in too small a plastic bag. As a result, it stays bent for some time prior to use. It can also become kinked. The EOA/EGTA should always be stored in its original packaging to prevent this problem.

**RUPTURE OF THE ESOPHAGUS**    Rupture or tearing of the esophagus can also result from the use of the EOA/EGTA. Thus, you should never insert the EOA/EGTA roughly or with excessive force. Although the cuff will hold up to 35 mL of air, 20 to 30 mL is usually sufficient to block the esophagus. This smaller volume of air is less likely to injure the esophagus. In addition, the EOA/EGTA should not be stored in a cold ambulance or kept in a cold environment, as it will become stiff and be more likely to injure the esophagus when inserted.

**INADEQUATE VENTILATION**    A third complication is inadequate ventilation, despite proper placement of the airway. This usually happens due to persistent leakage of air around the face mask. A firm seal between the mask and the face must be maintained at all times. There is an inflatable, balloon-like seal around the edge of the mask to provide a leak-proof contact with the contours of the face. This balloon should contain just enough air to allow the finger, when pressed against it, to make contact with the edge of the underlying plastic mask. Another cause of inadequate ventilation is the delivery of an inadequate volume of air to the airway via a BVM device. You should always use a flow-restricted oxygen-powered ventilation device.

## INSERTING THE **EOA/EGTA**

1. Assemble and check the proper equipment. Also lubricate the esophageal tube.
2. Snap tube into lock at mask-tube connection.

3. Position the head and neck (nontrauma and trauma positions).
4. Open and clear the airway.
5. Hyperventilate the patient with 100% oxygen.
6. Gently guide the esophageal tube into place.
7. Inflate the obturator balloon cuff.
8. Insert an oropharyngeal airway.
9. Seal the mask to the patient's face.
10. Ventilate the patient.
11. Check the chest for breath sounds.
12. Use flow-restricted oxygen-powered ventilation device.
13. Maintain effective mask-face seal.

## *EOA/EGTA* INTUBATION

Once you have confirmed with medical control your decision to intubate, you must act quickly and carefully. Remember that you should follow BSI techniques any time you may be exposed to blood or other body fluids. Your first step is to quickly assemble the proper equipment, including the following:

- EGTA or EOA
- 30-mL syringe
- water-soluble lubricant
- suctioning unit
- oral airway
- flow-restricted oxygen-powered ventilation device
- gloves
- eye protection
- mask

Always check to make sure the EOA/EGTA is working properly before you try to insert it. Inflate the face mask with 20 to 30 mL of air. Then fill the 30-mL syringe with air and attach it to the valve supplying the obturator's cuff. Inflate the cuff with 20 mL of air and check for leaks. Then deflate the cuff, but leave the syringe attached. Next, attach the mask to the tube. It is designed to lock into proper position with a definite snap. Lubricate the lower two thirds of the tube with a water-soluble gel. Before you insert the EOA/EGTA, you must hyperventilate the patient for 2 to 3 minutes with a BVM device with 100% oxygen.

### Positioning the Patient

The tube is designed to be inserted with the patient's head slightly flexed or in a neutral position. Thus, you should gently position the head this way if the patient does not have a possible spinal injury. Flexing the head onto the trunk will decrease the risk of inserting the tube into the larynx and trachea. This flexed position brings the opening of the esophagus into a more exposed position. However, with an unconscious trauma patient, you must maintain the head in an in-line neutral position while your partner opens the airway and inserts the EGTA or EOA.

### Inserting the EOA/EGTA

Open the patient's airway and then grasp the tongue and the lower jaw between your gloved thumb and index finger. Lift the tongue and the lower jaw with your left hand (Figure 10-27). Grasp the EOA/EGTA with the mask attached with your right hand. Insert it along the tongue and against the posterior wall of the pharynx in the midline (Figure 10-28a). ***Do not use great force to insert the airway!*** Only light to moderate pressure is needed. The EOA/EGTA is inserted until the mask makes good contact with the face, and the bite block lies at the level of the incisor teeth (Figure 10-28b).

### Confirming Placement

Using both hands, hold the face mask firmly against the patient's face and check the EOA/EGTA for proper placement. Give mouth-to-mask or BVM ventilation. Your partner will listen for breath sounds over both lung fields. You will hear breath sounds over both lung fields if the EOA/EGTA is in the esophagus. However, you will not hear breath sounds if it has been placed in the trachea. If it has been placed in the right mainstem bronchus, you will hear breath sounds on the left side only. If you are not certain about its position, remove the EOA/EGTA. You should then ventilate the patient before you try to insert the EOA/EGTA again. If you hear good breath sounds over both lung fields, inflate the cuff with 20 to 30 mL of air and remove the syringe to keep the cuff inflated (Figure 10-29).

With the tube in the proper position, you must hold the mask firmly against the patient's face. Remain at the patient's head. Hold the mask to the patient's face with your thumb and index finger. Use the other three fingers to hold the lower jaw against

---

**FIGURE 10-27**

Lift the tongue and lower jaw to insert the EOA

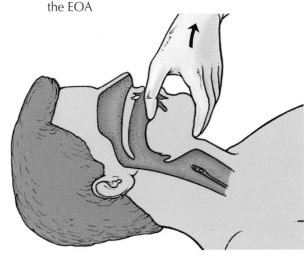

---

**FIGURE 10-28**

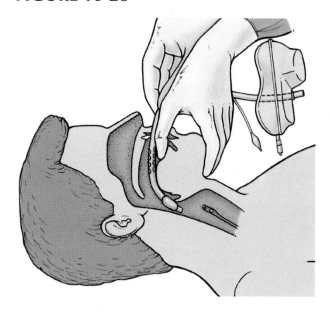

**A**   Insert the EOA along the tongue

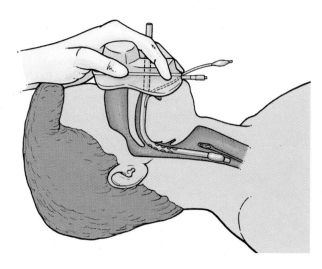

**B**   Apply the face mask over the patient's mouth

the mask. If there is no concern about neck injury, you can extend the head to further open the airway. Then attach the opening in the face mask to a flow-restricted oxygen-powered ventilation device. This device provides the necessary volume and pressure of oxygen for effective ventilation with an EOA/EGTA. These levels cannot be achieved with a BVM device.

## REMOVAL OF THE *EOA/EGTA*

Remember that the EOA/EGTA should be used for short-term airway management only. It should be removed when the unconscious patient awakens and is able to protect the airway or when an ETT has been inserted. Once the cuff is deflated and the airway removed, there is a very high risk of vomiting. Therefore, you should log roll a conscious patient onto his or her side and have a suctioning unit available prior to removal, unless an ETT has been inserted. Once the patient is ready, the EOA/EGTA

is easily removed by fully deflating the balloon and sliding it out.

If long-term airway management is required in the hospital, the EOA/EGTA should be replaced by an endotracheal tube. In this situation, the EOA/EGTA must be left in place until the ETT is securely and properly placed (Table 10-2).

**FIGURE 10-29**

Inflate the EOA balloon

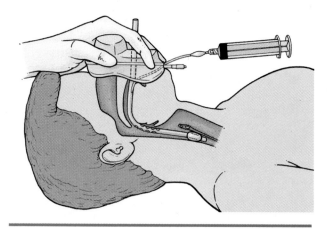

## TABLE 10-2    EOA/EGTA AIRWAY

| Advantages | Disadvantages |
|---|---|
| Rapid, blind insertion | Requires good mask seal |
| Can be placed with minimal neck movement | Requires frequent practice |
| Can be used in all types of arrests | Blood and vomitus may be forced into lungs |
| Prevents gastric distention | Patients do *not* tolerate it |
| Prevents gastric regurgitation | Laceration of esophagus |
| Permits easy ETT placement over it | |

## PHARYNGEOTRACHEAL AIRWAYS

Pharyngeotracheal airways have been designed to provide lung ventilation when placed either in the trachea or the esophagus. Several devices are available, including the Esophageal Tracheal Combitube (ETC) and the Pharyngeotracheal Lumen Airway (PtL). These devices are designed to be inserted blindly into the oropharynx and esophagus, but you must be trained and authorized to use them.

### Esophageal Tracheal Combitube

The ETC consists of a double lumen tube and two balloon cuffs. One is a clear cuff at the tip (distal cuff) and the other is a larger, flesh-colored cuff near the midway point (Figure 10-30). The blue lumen (No. 1) is the primary ventilation port when the tube is inserted in the esophagus. The clear lumen (No. 2) is the ventilation port if the tube is placed in the trachea. The large flesh-colored cuff seals off the oropharynx and nasopharynx. The distal cuff seals off the esophagus or the trachea. A blue pilot balloon and a white pilot balloon correspond to the flesh-colored and distal cuffs. Two syringes are also included in the kit.

### FIGURE 10-30

Components of the Combitube

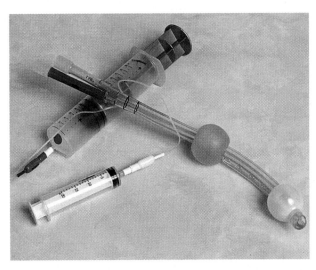

The ETC is a single-use item and must be discarded after use. It should not be cleaned and reused. The ETC is similar to the EOA/EGTA, but it is designed to function like an ETT. For example, when blindly inserted, if the tube happens to go into the trachea (Figure 10-31), it acts like an ETT. If the tube goes into the esophagus, it acts like

**FIGURE 10-31**

The ETC inserted into the trachea functions as an ET tube

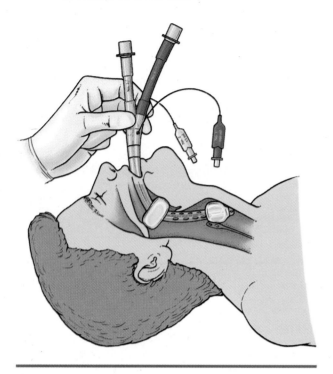

**FIGURE 10-32**

The ETC inserted into the esophagus functions as an EOA/EGTA

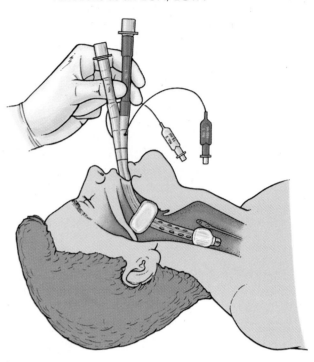

an EOA/EGTA (Figure 10-32). However, if the ETC functions like an EOA/EGTA, you need not maintain a constant face mask seal. The ETC forms an inflated cuff seal in the oropharynx, and the trachea may be ventilated via a tube rather than a mask. This ease of ventilation is an advantage of the ETC over the EOA/EGTA.

### Contraindications

You should not attempt to insert an ETC in a conscious or semiconscious patient with a gag reflex. It should not be used in children under the age of 16 years or in adults under 5' tall. Check with your medical director for local protocol regarding patient age. Of course, like the EOA/EGTA, it should not be used in patients who are known to have ingested a caustic substance, or those who have known esophageal disease.

## INSERTING THE ETC

1. Assemble and check the proper equipment. Also lubricate the ETC.

2. Position the head and neck (nontrauma and trauma positions).

3. Open and clear the airway.

4. Hyperventilate the patient with 100% oxygen.

5. Lift the lower jaw and tongue away from the posterior pharynx.

6. Gently guide the ETC along the base of the tongue and into the airway.

7. Inflate the blue pilot balloon (flesh-colored cuff) with the blue-tipped 100-mL syringe.

8. Inflate the white pilot balloon with 15 mL of air from the smaller predrawn syringe.

9. Ventilate (bag-to-tube or with an oxygen-powered ventilation device) the patient through the blue (No. 1) tube.

10. Check the patient's chest for breath sounds.

11. If the ETC is not in the esophagus, ventilate the patient through the clear (No. 2) tube. (In this case, the ETC will function as an ETT).

12. Listen for breath sounds.

13. Ventilate the patient with a flow-restricted oxygen-powered ventilation device.

**ETC INTUBATION**    Once you have confirmed with medical control your decision to intubate, or if it is permitted by off-line protocol, you must act quickly and carefully. Remember that you should follow BSI techniques any time you may be exposed to blood or other body fluids. Your first step is to quickly assemble the proper equipment, including the following:

- ETC kit with syringes
- water-soluble lubricant
- suctioning unit
- flow-restricted oxygen-powered ventilation device
- gloves
- eye protection

Always check to make sure the ETC is working properly before you try to insert it. Begin the procedure by preparing and checking the materials while the patient is being hyperventilated with 100% oxygen. Lubricate the tube with a water-soluble lubricant.

**Positioning the Patient**    Once the equipment is assembled and checked, open the patient's mouth and clear it of any foreign objects, including vomitus, dentures, and blood clots. Remove the oropharyngeal airway, if one has been inserted. Open the airway by hyperextending the patient's head and neck. Perform this airway maneuver only if the patient does not have a possible spinal injury. However, with an unconscious trauma patient, you must maintain the neck in a neutral, in-line position during intubation.

**Inserting the ETC**    Insert your thumb deep into the patient's mouth, grasping the tongue and lower jaw between your thumb and index finger. Lift the tongue and lower jaw directly away from the posterior pharynx. Hold the ETC so that it curves in the same direction as the natural curvature of the pharynx. Insert the tip into the mouth and advance it carefully along the tongue. Do not force the ETC. If resistance is met, pull back and redirect the ETC. When the ETC is at the proper depth, the teeth or alveolar ridge will be between the heavy black lines.

Next, inflate the blue pilot balloon (and flesh-colored cuff) with the predrawn 100-mL blue-tipped syringe. Once that cuff is inflated and the pilot balloon is tense, immediately inflate the white pilot balloon (and the distal cuff) with the smaller predrawn 15-mL syringe. The ETC may move forward a little bit, but this is normal. Ventilate the blue lumen with a BVM device or an oxygen-powered ventilation device.

**Confirming Placement**    Observe the chest and listen for lung sounds. If the chest rises and falls, and you hear breath sounds, the ETC is in the esophagus. Thus, you are ventilating the patient as with an EOA/EGTA. When this is the case, continue to ventilate through the blue (No. 1) tube. If the chest does not rise, and you do not hear breath sounds, the ETC is in the trachea. In this case, put the BVM device or the oxygen-powered ventilation device on the shorter clear tube and ventilate the patient through it. Again, listen for breath sounds in all lung fields and in both axillae. Also listen over the stomach to verify the proper position and that effective ventilation is occurring.

Once you are certain that the patient is being properly ventilated, connect the ETC to a flow-restricted oxygen-powered ventilation device. Continuously monitor the patient. Occasionally, the balloon cuffs leak. You must watch for leaks by carefully squeezing the pilot balloon. Use the syringes to keep the balloon cuffs properly inflated. Balloon cuffs may be torn by jagged, broken teeth, dentures, and bones. Thus, you must use special care with this device, especially in the event of facial trauma.

### Removing the ETC

Removal of the ETC airway is fairly simple. If you are ventilating a deeply unconscious patient via the blue (No. 1) tube, then you should intubate with an ETT around the ETC. Or, you should remove the tube if the patient will no longer tolerate it. Remember, the patient will vomit when the ETC is removed from the esophagus. You must have a suctioning unit readily available. Make sure to turn the patient on his or her side to keep the airway clear of vomitus. When you are ready, simply deflate the balloon cuffs and gently remove the tube.

### Pharyngeotracheal Lumen Airway

The PtL consists of two tubes, two balloon cuffs, a bite block, and a neck retaining strap (Figure 10-33). The long, clear (No. 3) tube contains a stylet and a low-pressure balloon cuff near its tip. The No. 3 tube remains plugged by the stylet if it is placed in the esophagus. The stylet is removed if the tube ends up in the trachea. In either case, the balloon cuff prevents gastric contents from entering the lungs when the cuff is inflated. The No. 3 tube passes through the larger diameter green (No. 2) tube. The No. 2 tube has a large balloon cuff designed to seal the oropharynx. This allows ventilation gas to pass through it into the trachea (should the

**FIGURE 10-33**

Components of the PtL

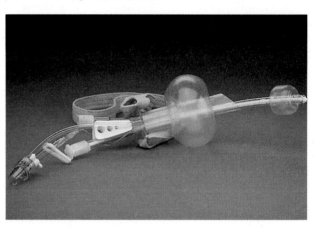

No. 3 tube be placed in the esophagus), but also prevents blood and debris from entering the airway from above. The balloon cuff in the No. 2 tube functions as the mask seal. The No. 1 tube is connected to these balloon cuffs to assist with inflation of these important airway seals.

Like the ETC, this device is designed to be inserted blindly into the oropharynx and esophagus, but you must be trained and authorized to use it. The PtL is similar to the EGTA, but it is designed to function like an ETT. If the tube happens to go into the trachea when blindly inserted (Figure 10-34), it acts like an ETT. If the long tube goes into the esophagus (Figure 10-35), it functions like an EGTA. However, with the PtL, you need not maintain a constant face mask seal. The PtL forms an inflated cuff seal in the oropharynx, and the trachea may be ventilated via a tube rather than a mask.

### Contraindications

The PtL is contraindicated in conscious or semiconscious patients with a gag reflex. It should not be used in children under the age of 14 years or adults under 5' tall. Like

## FIGURE 10-34

The PtL inserted into the trachea functions as an ET tube

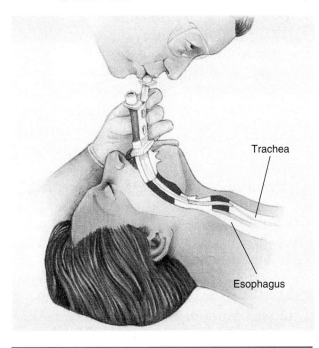

Trachea

Esophagus

## FIGURE 10-35

The PtL inserted into the esophagus functions as an EOA/EGTA

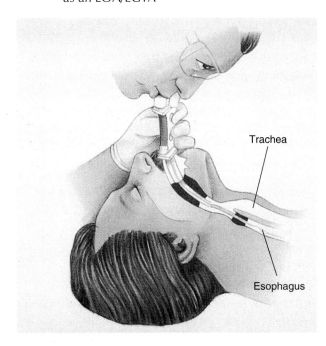

Trachea

Esophagus

the EOA/EGTA, the PtL should not be used in patients who have ingested a caustic substance or who have a known esophageal disease.

## INSERTING THE PtL

1. Assemble and check the proper equipment. Also lubricate the tube on the PtL.

2. Position the head and neck in extension (neutral in-line position for trauma patients).

3. Open and clear the airway.

4. Hyperventilate the patient with 100% oxygen.

5. Lift the lower jaw and tongue away from the posterior pharynx.

6. Gently guide the PtL along the base of the tongue and into the airway until the teeth are against the teeth strap.

7. Inflate balloon cuffs with the No. 1 tube. Be sure to close the white cap.

8. Ventilate (mouth-to-tube) the patient through the short, green No. 2 tube.

9. Check the patient's chest for breath sounds.

10. If the No. 3 tube is not in the trachea, ventilate the patient using the No. 2 tube.

11. If the No. 3 tube is in the trachea, remove the stylet and ventilate the patient using the No. 3 tube.

12. Check the patient's chest for breath sounds.

13. Ventilate the patient with a flow-restricted oxygen-powered ventilation device.

14. If ventilating via the No. 2 tube, consider using an ETT with the No. 3 tube sealing the esophagus during the procedure.

**PtL INTUBATION**    Once you have confirmed with medical control your decision to intubate, or if it is permitted by off-line protocol, you must act quickly and carefully. Remember that you should follow BSI techniques any time you may be exposed to blood or other body fluids. Your first step is to quickly assemble the proper equipment, including the following:

- PtL
- water-soluble lubricant
- suctioning unit
- flow-restricted oxygen-powered ventilation device
- gloves
- eye protection

Begin by preparing and checking the materials listed above while the patient is being hyperventilated with 100% oxygen. Lubricate the long clear No. 3 tube with a water-soluble lubricant.

**Positioning the Patient**    First, open the patient's mouth to clear any foreign objects, including vomitus, dentures, and blood clots. Remove the oropharyngeal airway, if one has been inserted. If the patient does not have a spinal injury, open the airway by hyperextending the patient's head and neck. However, with a trauma patient, either you or your partner must maintain the neck in a neutral in-line position during intubation.

**Inserting the PtL**    Insert your thumb deep into the patient's mouth, grasping the tongue and lower jaw between your thumb and index finger and lift them directly away from the posterior pharynx. Hold the PtL so that it curves in the same direction as the natural curvature of the pharynx. Insert the tip into the mouth and advance it carefully along the tongue until the teeth strap touches the patient's teeth. Do not force the PtL. If resis-

tance is met, pull back and redirect the PtL. When the PtL is at the proper depth, place the neck strap over the patient's head and tighten it with the Velcro closures on both sides.

Next, attempt ventilation via the green No. 2 tube. If you do not hear breath sounds, use the No. 3 tube as you would an ETT. Immediately inflate both cuffs at once using the No. 1 tube. Blow into the inflation valve using a steady, gentle, sustained breath. Then, close the white cap. Once the cuffs are inflated and the little pilot balloon is tense, immediately blow forcefully into the short, green No. 2 tube.

**Confirming Placement**    Observe and listen to the chest. If the chest rises and you hear breath sounds, the long, clear No. 3 tube is in the esophagus, working as an EOA. When this is the case, continue to ventilate through the green No. 2 tube. If the chest does not rise, and you do not hear breath sounds, the long, clear No. 3 tube is likely in the trachea. In this case, remove the stylet from the long, clear No. 3 tube and ventilate the patient through that tube. Listen to the lungs on both sides of the chest anteriorly and in both axillae. Also listen over the stomach to verify the tube position and that the patient is receiving adequate ventilation. Once you are certain, connect the PtL to a flow-restricted oxygen-powered ventilation device. Continuously monitor the patient.

Occasionally, the balloon cuffs leak. Thus, you must watch to make sure the equipment is working properly. Use inlet tube No. 1 to keep the balloon cuffs properly inflated. Balloon cuffs are easily torn by jagged, broken teeth, dentures, and bones. Therefore, you must use special care if the patient has facial trauma.

**REMOVAL OF THE PtL**    Removal of the PtL airway is simple. If you are ventilating the patient via the short, green No. 2 tube (with the long, clear No. 3 tube being used as an esophageal obturator), you have two choices. You may choose to perform endotracheal intubation over the No. 3 tube if the patient is in a deep coma. Or, you should remove the tube if the patient will no longer tolerate it.

Remember, the patient will vomit when the No. 3 tube is removed from the esophagus. Keep a suctioning unit nearby. Also remember to turn the patient to the side to help keep the airway clear of vomitus. Simply deflate the balloon cuffs and gently remove the tube (Table 10-3).

**TABLE 10-3**            **PtL AND ETC Airways**

| Advantages | Disadvantages |
|---|---|
| Difficult to place improperly | Loses effectiveness (cuff malfunction) |
| No mask seal necessary | Requires deeply comatose patient |
| Requires minimal skill and practice to maintain | Requires constant balloon observation |
| Easily used in spinal injury patients | Cannot be used on patients under 5' tall |
| May be inserted blindly | Requires great care in listening for |
| Protects the airway from upper airway secretions |   breath sounds |
| Stays in place well (ETC) | Large balloon is easily broken and tends to |
| Sturdy balloon (ETC) |   push the PtL out of the mouth when inflated |

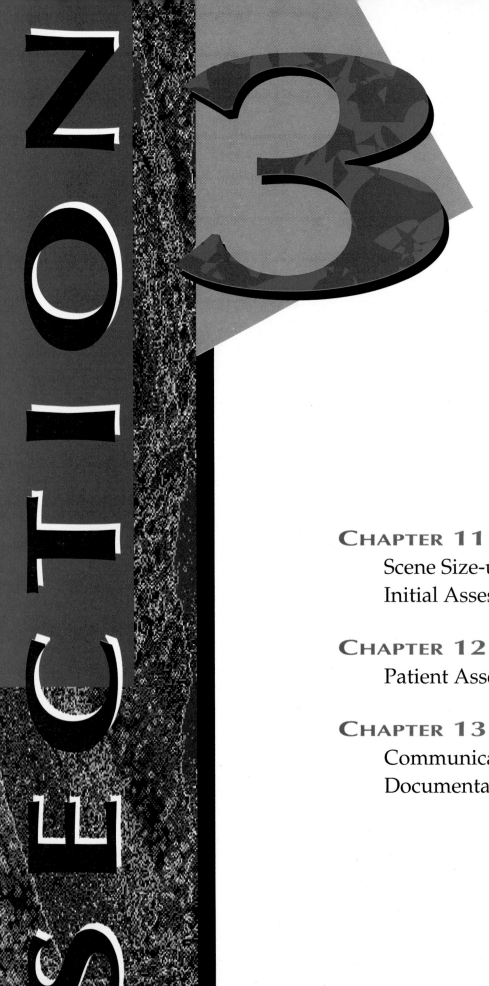

# SECTION 3

# Patient Assessment

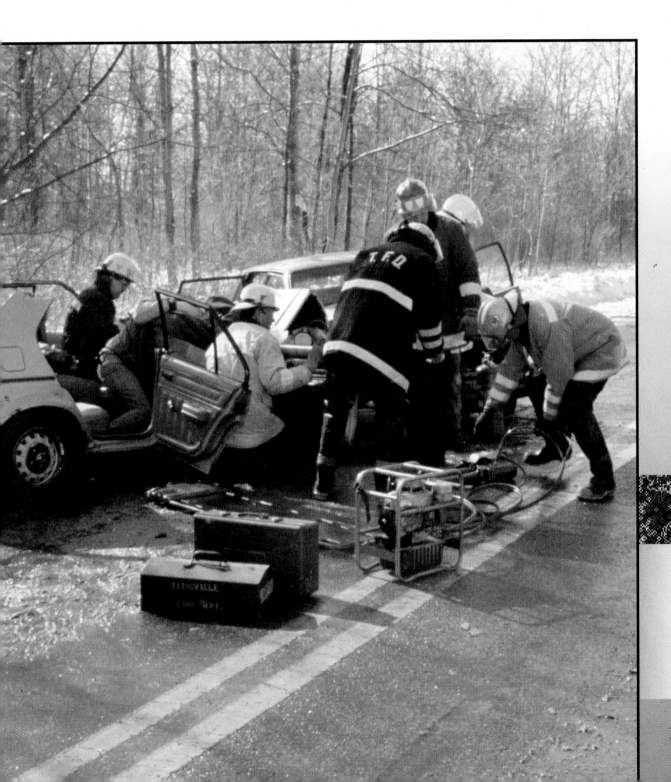

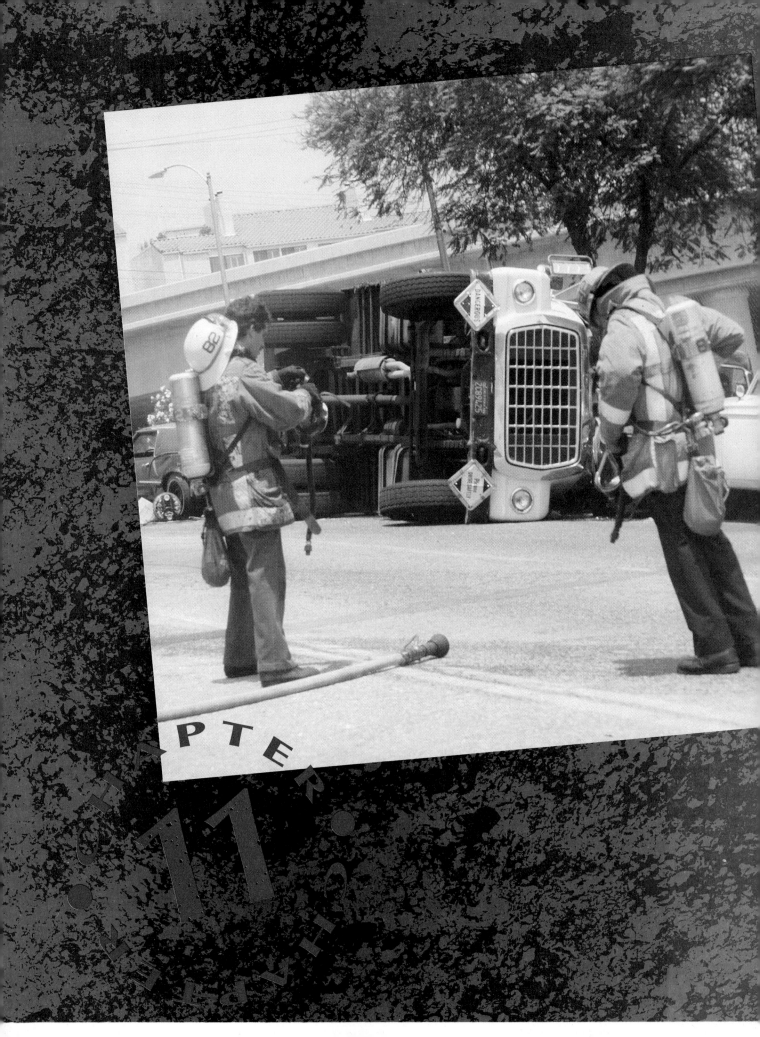

# Scene Size-up and Initial Assessment

## Objectives

After you have read this chapter, you should be able to:

- Recognize and describe hazards and potential hazards at the scene.
- Determine if a scene is safe to enter.
- Discuss common mechanisms of injury and illness.
- Discuss why it is important to identify the number of patients and the need for additional resources at the scene.
- Explain the importance of obtaining a general impression of the patient.
- Discuss the methods of assessing level of consciousness in adults and children.
- Discuss the methods of assessing airway and breathing in adults and children.
- Describe proper emergency care for adults and children who are breathing adequately and for those not breathing adequately.
- Differentiate between adequate and inadequate ventilations.
- Discuss the methods of assessing ventilations in adults and children.
- Describe proper respiratory care for adults and children.
- Describe the methods of obtaining a pulse in adults and children.
- Discuss the need for assessing a patient who has external bleeding.
- Describe normal and abnormal findings when assessing the skin.
- Describe normal and abnormal findings when assessing capillary refill in children.
- Explain the reason for prioritizing a patient for care and transport.

- Define the term "chief complaint."
- Describe management of the cervical spine in a trauma patient.

# Overview

As an EMT-B, your first, most important step in caring for patients is to identify and treat life-threatening injuries and illnesses. To do this, you must first evaluate the scene to make sure it is safe for you and your partner to enter. You must look at the "big picture" because the scene may present many dangers to both you and the patient. Second, you should carefully assess the patient for other problems that may require emergency treatment or transportation to a hospital. These two important steps will be emphasized repeatedly during your training for a single reason. If you do not know how to thoroughly assess your patients, they may be permanently injured, or they may die. Often, your care means the difference between life and death. Simple things forgotten in the field, especially a careful examination of the scene, may result in serious problems for both you and your patient. Therefore, your approach to the scene and patient assessment must be a systematic one.

You must use a consistent, methodical approach to assessment to avoid missing important problems. One important task is gathering as much information about the scene as possible. You must also be willing and able to adjust to different situations. As an EMT-B, you will find yourself in many different settings caring for many different types of patients. A patient thrown from a speeding car has different needs than a patient who is complaining of chest pain. Therefore, the patient's situation will sometimes affect how much time you spend on any one step. The patient's situation will also dictate what protective equipment you will need. Remember that you must always complete a full survey of the scene and every step of the patient assessment in the proper sequence.

Assessment of both the scene and the patient is an ongoing process. From the minute you begin the initial (or first) assessment, until you turn over care of the patient at the hospital, you will be engaged in patient assessment.

This chapter describes the steps and the reasons for scene size-up and the initial assessment. These are your first steps at any scene. The chapter begins by explaining the importance of checking the scene and obtaining a general impression of the patient. The ABCD of initial assessment is discussed, as are the ways in which you evaluate each element.

# Key Terms

**AVPU scale**   Method of assessing the patient's level of consciousness.

**Barrier device**   A protective item, such as a valved pocket mask, that limits your exposure to the patient's body fluids.

**Body substance isolation (BSI)**   An infection control concept and practice that assumes all body fluids as being potentially infectious.

**Capillary refill**   The ability of the circulatory system to restore blood to the capillaries after you squeeze the fingertip.

**Chief complaint**   The patient's response to a general question such as "What's wrong?" or "What happened?"

**General impression**   Overall initial impression formed to determine the priority for patient care.

Based on the patient's surroundings, the mechanism of injury, or the patient's chief complaint.

**Look, Listen, and Feel technique**   Way of assessing the airway of an unconscious patient.

**Recovery position**   Position used to help maintain a clear airway in a patient with a decreased level of consciousness who has not had traumatic injuries and is breathing on his or her own.

**Scene size-up**   A quick assessment of the scene and the surroundings that provides you and your partner as much information as possible about the safety of the scene before you begin patient assessment.

**Triage**   The process of establishing treatment and transportation priorities according to severity of injury and medical need.

# YOUR FIRST STEPS AT THE SCENE

Before you arrive at the scene, think about what might have happened to cause the problem or injury. Preparing for the scene once you are dispatched is important. Think about the types of danger you may be faced with upon arrival. Once you arrive at the scene, quickly perform a scene size-up before you step out of your unit. This also includes looking at weather conditions. A **scene size-up** is a quick assessment of the scene and the surroundings (Figure 11-1). This will provide you and your partner as much information as possible about the safety of the scene before you begin patient assessment. Your first step at any scene is to make sure that you and your partner are safe. *Never become a victim yourself.*

Before you step out of the unit, look for the following possible dangers:

- on-coming traffic
- wet or icy patches on the ground
- leaking gasoline or diesel fuel
- downed electrical lines
- hostile bystanders

## FIGURE 11-1

Size up the scene upon arrival

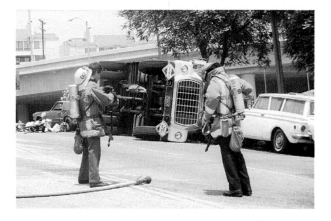

- fire
- possible hazardous materials

Park your unit in a place that will offer you and your partner the greatest safety. In most instances, law enforcement will be at the scene before you arrive. You should talk with them before entering the scene. Make sure to follow instructions if the scene is a

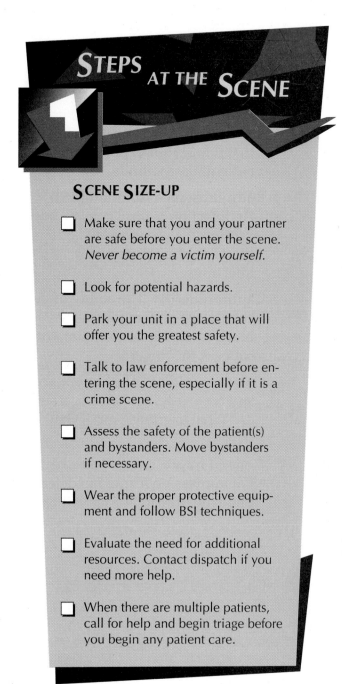

## STEPS AT THE SCENE

### SCENE SIZE-UP

☐ Make sure that you and your partner are safe before you enter the scene. *Never become a victim yourself.*

☐ Look for potential hazards.

☐ Park your unit in a place that will offer you the greatest safety.

☐ Talk to law enforcement before entering the scene, especially if it is a crime scene.

☐ Assess the safety of the patient(s) and bystanders. Move bystanders if necessary.

☐ Wear the proper protective equipment and follow BSI techniques.

☐ Evaluate the need for additional resources. Contact dispatch if you need more help.

☐ When there are multiple patients, call for help and begin triage before you begin any patient care.

crime scene. Also be sure to have law enforcement accompany you if the patient is a suspect in the crime. Consider your unit a "safe haven." You are no help to the patient if you enter the scene without first protecting yourself and your partner. Your next concern is the safety of the patient(s) and bystanders. This is not an easy task. Bystanders can become a problem when they try to help. Protect yourself and bystanders alike by moving them to a safe area or assigning them a specific task that you can monitor.

## THE NEED FOR PROTECTIVE EQUIPMENT

Your next step is to make sure you are wearing the proper protective equipment. Wearing protective equipment will reduce your risk of exposure to a communicable disease. The best way to reduce your risk of exposure is to follow **body substance isolation (BSI)** techniques. The concept of BSI assumes that all fluids present a possible risk. Once you are ready to step out of the unit, you and your partner must have the proper protective equipment ready. Vinyl or latex gloves are always indicated. Eye protection, masks, and gowns may also be indicated, if there is a lot of blood or other body fluids in the patient area (Figure 11-2). Eye protection is needed when there may be the risk that blood or other body fluids will splatter. You should put on a mask and gown, if needed, right before you enter the area immediately around the patient. If the scene involves hazardous materials or fire, wear the appropriate gear for the situation.

## THE NEED FOR ADDITIONAL RESOURCES

Occasionally, you and your partner will not be able to safely enter a scene. This is due to the need for extrication, possible

## FIGURE 11-2

Protective equipment for BSI

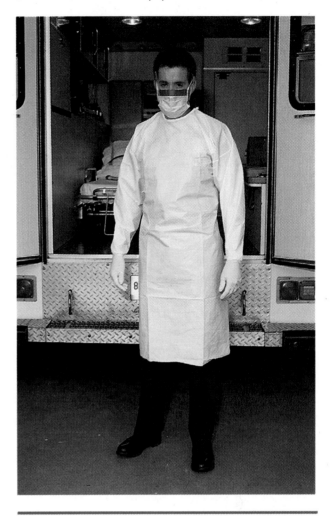

hazardous conditions, or the presence of more patients than you can handle alone. These situations seem very difficult when you want to provide medical care to sick or injured patients. However, the safety of you and your partner is most important. If you need more help, do not hesitate to ask for it. Be as specific as possible about the type of help you need. Remember, though, it takes time for additional resources, such as an extrication team, law enforcement, or another EMS unit, to arrive at the scene.

As you evaluate the need for additional resources, ask yourself the following questions:

- How many patients need medical care?
- What is the nature of the patient's illness or the mechanism of injury?
- Who contacted EMS?
- Is the scene a possible crime scene in which evidence may need to be preserved?
- Are hazardous materials, such as chemicals, leaking fuel, etc. involved?

### Triage

With multiple patients, you should call for assistance and begin triage before you begin any patient care. **Triage** is a process of establishing treatment and transportation priorities according to severity of injury and medical need. One EMT-B, usually the most experienced, should be assigned to perform triage. The process will help you to provide care more effectively and efficiently in a multiple-patient situation. If there is a large number of patients or if the patient needs are greater than the available resources, put your local mass-casualty plan into action.

You should always call for additional resources before you begin caring for patients. It is never wrong to call for backup, even if the extra units are sent back. Remember, you are less likely to ask for help after you begin patient care because at that point you are part of the scene. For more information about triage, see chapter 28, Scene Techniques.

## THE INITIAL ASSESSMENT

Next, try to find out as much as you can about the patient's condition. As you approach the patient, determine the mechanism of injury or the nature of the patient's illness. With this information, you can begin forming a general impression of the patient and the patient's condition. A **general impression** is formed to determine the priority for patient care. You will form this impression by looking at the patient's surroundings and the mechanism of injury or the patient's chief complaint. It includes information about the patient's age, sex, and race, if necessary. The following questions offer a systematic way in which you can base your first decisions about patient care:

- Was the patient in an accident? If so, what was the mechanism of injury?
- Does the patient have a life-threatening problem? If so, you must provide immediate care and then transport to the hospital.
- Does the patient have a medical problem? If so, what are the patient's complaints?

Remember to use all your senses at all times—before, during, and after the assessment. As you approach, check to see if the patient is moving or still, awake or unconscious, cut or bleeding. Listen to what the patient and bystanders have to say. You may be able to smell chemical hazards, smoke, or the odor of alcohol on the patient's breath. You can feel for pulses, pain, and deformities when you reach the patient. At this time, you should identify yourself as an EMT and that you are there to help. If the patient is alert, begin a conversation. With a responsive patient, try to learn as much as possible about what is wrong before you begin. You should continue to ask questions and talk to a responsive patient during the next phase of assessment.

Usually the patient's response to a general question such as, "What's wrong?" or "What happened?" is called the chief complaint. The **chief complaint** is usually the symptom that is bothering the patient the most. Despite what you have already seen, do not jump to any conclusions about what is troubling the patient. Now is the time to listen. It is important to understand the patient's problems in the patient's own words.

## STEPS AT THE SCENE

### INITIAL ASSESSMENT

☐ Determine the mechanism of injury so that you can form a general impression of the patient.

☐ Listen to what the patient and/or bystanders have to say.

☐ Ask the patient, "Are you okay?" to assess if the airway is open.

☐ Open the airway, if necessary, using the chin-lift or jaw-thrust maneuvers.

☐ Assess breathing. Give high-flow oxygen or assist ventilations if necessary.

☐ Assess circulation by taking the radial pulse in adults or carotid pulse in children.

☐ Begin CPR or apply AED, if necessary, depending on your situation.

☐ Control any external bleeding.

☐ Assess skin color, temperature, and condition.

☐ Assess capillary refill in infants and children.

The first steps in caring for any patient focus on finding and treating the most life-threatening illnesses and injuries. You should assess and stabilize the following systems in this order of importance:

A = Airway
B = Breathing
C = Circulation
D = Disability

In all cases, the patient's airway, breathing, circulation, and disability (ABCD) will govern the extent of your assessment and treatment at the scene. *Always give priority to emergency care of the ABCD to ensure life- and limb-saving treatment.*

## ASSESSING LEVEL OF CONSCIOUSNESS

The "A" of ABCD is "Airway." Assessment of the patient's airway begins by evaluating the patient's level of consciousness. Once you are at the scene, you should first make sure it is safe to begin patient care. Then, you should approach the patient, identify yourself as an EMT, and explain that you are there to help. The way the patient responds will tell you about the airway. A conscious patient is likely breathing, but you must always watch for airway problems to develop. Therefore, you should always have a pocket mask or some other airway adjunct available in case airway problems develop.

The patient's level of consciousness (or disability) is assessed by how well the patient responds to the question, "Are you okay?" The patient's level of consciousness or "mental status" can be described using one of the following four terms of the **AVPU scale:**

- *Alert.* The patient's eyes open spontaneously, and the patient can answer questions clearly. The patient knows and can correctly tell you the date, the location, and his or her own name. If the patient knows these facts, the patient is said to be "alert and oriented times three."

- *Responsive to verbal stimulus.* The patient's eyes do not open spontaneously. The patient may not be oriented to time, place, and person but does respond in some meaningful way when spoken to.

- *Responsive to pain.* The patient does not respond to your questions, but moves or cries out in response to a painful stimulus. This response is tested by gently, but firmly, pinching the patient's skin. An appropriate response is withdrawal from the pinch. If the patient has a paralyzed arm or leg, you should not use painful stimuli. Use of extremely painful stimuli is never appropriate.

- *Unresponsive.* The patient does not respond to painful stimuli, such as the pinch test described above.

Occasionally, a patient will attempt to fake unconsciousness. If you suspect this, hold the patient's hand above his or her face and then allow the hand to rapidly drop. If the patient is unconscious, the hand will hit the face.

## ASSESSING THE AIRWAY

As you move through the steps of assessment, you must always watch the patient's airway for signs of trouble. A patient who regains consciousness after a head injury, or a patient who has taken a drug overdose may develop airway problems.

## RESPONSIVE PATIENTS

The easiest way to assess whether a patient is responsive is to ask a basic question, as described above. A responsive patient will be able to talk. Ask the patient if he or she knows the time, date, and place. Have the patient cough. If the patient can do all of these things with ease, the airway is open. However, you must always watch for airway problems to develop.

## UNRESPONSIVE PATIENTS

Airway obstruction in an unconscious patient is most commonly due to relaxation of the muscles of the tongue. The airway is obstructed by the tongue, which tends to fall back into the throat to create the block. Dentures, blood clots, vomitus, mucus, food, or other foreign objects may also create a block. You can check an unconscious patient's airway using the **Look, Listen, and Feel technique.** Place your head slightly above the patient's face. Look at the patient's chest for smooth, even movement. Listen and feel for air moving in and out of the nose and/or mouth (Figure 11-3). If the patient does not appear to be breathing or has an inadequate airway, start airway management immediately. The following two steps can be done in nearly one motion:

1. Place your face squarely in front of the patient's face while grasping the patient's wrist nearest to your hand.

2. Ask the patient "Are you okay?" while you take the pulse. Watch the patient's response carefully and then continue your assessment.

### Basic Airway Maneuvers

Once you have determined that the patient is not breathing, your first step in airway management is to open the airway. The way in which you open the airway depends on the patient's condition. For an unresponsive patient with no spinal injury, you should use the head-tilt/chin-lift maneuver (Figure 11-4). The five basic steps of the head-tilt/chin-lift maneuver are as follows:

1. Extend the neck with firm pressure applied to the forehead.

2. Move the patient's head back as far as possible and leave your hand in place.

3. Place the tips of the fingers of your other hand under the bony part of the chin.

4. Lift the chin forward, bringing the entire lower jaw with it.

5. Make sure the chin is lifted enough to bring the teeth together, but the mouth should not close.

For an unresponsive patient with a possible spinal injury, you should use the modified jaw-thrust maneuver (Figure 11-5). This maneuver should be used when you believe that the patient has had a cervical spine injury. Only a deeply unconscious patient will tolerate this technique, as it is very unpleasant. The four basic steps of the jaw-thrust technique are as follows:

1. Place the fingers of both your hands behind the angles of the patient's lower jaw.

2. Forcefully move the jaw forward.

3. Tilt the head back without significantly extending the patient's cervical spine.

## FIGURE 11-4

The head-tilt/chin-lift maneuver

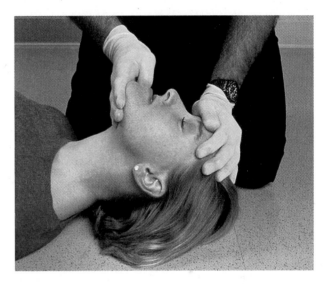

## FIGURE 11-3

The Look, Listen, and Feel technique

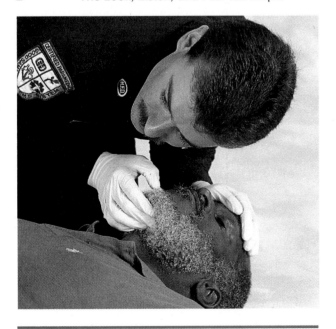

## FIGURE 11-5

The modified jaw-thrust maneuver

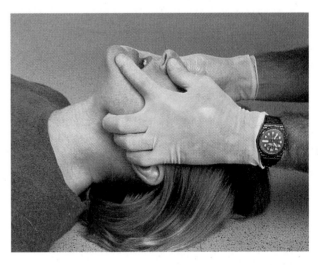

4. Pull the patient's lower lip down using your thumb so that the patient can breathe through both the nose and mouth.

After you have completed one of these two techniques, check the patient's airway again using the Look, Listen, and Feel technique. If the patient is not breathing, you should begin rescue breathing.

# ASSESSING BREATHING

As you assess the patient's breathing, look at how much work it takes for the patient to breathe. An adult's breathing rate will vary widely, from 12 to 20 breaths/min. Normal respirations are not usually shallow or deep. So as you assess the patient, ask yourself the following questions:

1. Are the respirations shallow or deep?

2. Does the patient appear to be choking?

3. Is the patient cyanotic (blue)?

If the patient seems to have trouble breathing, you should immediately start airway management.

You should give high-concentration (15 L/min) oxygen to any patient if you think airway problems may develop. You should give high-concentration oxygen via a nonrebreathing mask. *Never withhold oxygen from any patient at the scene!*

## RESPONSIVE PATIENTS

A responsive patient may need oxygen, even though he or she appears to be breathing normally. You should assist ventilations with a BVM device for all responsive patients who have respirations of greater than 24/min or less than 8/min. Medical patients with no suspected cervical spine in-

jury should remain in a comfortable position. However, any patient with a possible cervical spine injury should be fully immobilized.

## UNRESPONSIVE PATIENTS

An unresponsive patient who is breathing and has no history of traumatic injury should be placed in the recovery position. The **recovery position** is used to help maintain a clear airway in a patient who has not had traumatic injuries and is breathing on his or her own. In this position, the patient is rolled onto his or her right or left side. The rolling motion occurs so that the head, shoulders, and body move at the same time without twisting. The patient's hands are then placed under the cheek (Figure 11-6). This position is used to help the patient continue to breathe independently. It also allows for excretions, such as vomitus, to spontaneously drain from the mouth. The recovery position is also used after a patient has been resuscitated following CPR. A patient in the recovery position should be given high-concentration oxygen via a nonrebreathing mask.

An unresponsive patient who is not breathing, but is believed to have neck or

## FIGURE 11-6

The recovery position

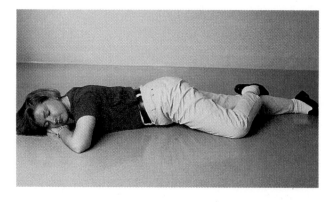

## TOO CLOSE FOR COMFORT

A young woman steps off the curb in the parking lot at a shopping mall without looking. A car driven by an elderly man speeds by in pursuit of a parking place that just opened up. The car is so close that it knocks the woman's purse and shopping bags from her hand, but miraculously misses her. She's visibly shaken, and her two friends are not able to calm her, prompting a call to EMS. On arrival, you find a 16-year-old girl who is alert and oriented. She is breathing at a rate of approximately 40 times a minute, and you also observe nasal flaring. She has a regular pulse of 128/min, and pale, moist skin. Her pupils are dilated, but reactive to light.

### For Discussion

1. For a patient with a fast heartbeat (tachycardia), why is it important to treat the underlying cause?

2. Compare and contrast hyperventilation with at least three other conditions it could be mistaken for.

---

back injuries, must be handled with extreme care. You must roll the patient's head, neck, and back as a single unit onto a flat surface or backboard. Once the patient is properly positioned, and the airway is opened, you should begin rescue breathing. Any type of rescue breathing will deliver exhaled gas containing 16% oxygen from the rescuer. This level is more than adequate to maintain the patient's life.

You do not need any special equipment for rescue breathing. You will, however, want to use a barrier device to limit your exposure to any saliva and/or blood at the patient's mouth. A **barrier device** is a protective item, such as a valved pocket mask, that limits your exposure to the patient's body fluids. The three most commonly used devices for giving oxygen are mouth-to-mask devices, bag-valve-mask devices, and oxygen-powered mechanical devices. Of these three devices, the valved pocket mask provides the easiest and most efficient delivery of oxygen. The bag-valve-mask device and the oxygen-powered mechanical device (demand valve) require more training and are more difficult to use.

The four basic steps of mouth-to-mask rescue breathing for an unresponsive patient with suspected neck and back injuries are as follows:

1. Open the patient's airway using the jaw-thrust maneuver, as described above.

2. Place the mask over the patient's mouth, or mouth and nose, depending on the device.

3. Give two slow breaths, each lasting 1½ to 2 seconds.

4. Check for a pulse.

## ASSESSING CIRCULATION

### ASSESSING THE PULSE

A patient's pulse rate will give you a rough idea of the strength of the heart's contractions. Pulse is one of the vital signs you should monitor continuously in most patient situations, including while en route to the hospital (Table 11-1). You measure the pulse by palpating (feeling) an artery at a pulse point. A pulse point is an area where an artery lies close to the surface of the skin.

#### Adults

For an alert, responsive patient, your hands taking the radial pulse can be a very reassuring gesture. The most common place to palpate for the pulse in a responsive patient is at the wrist, along the radial artery. You will usually feel the radial pulse if the blood pressure is 80 mm Hg or higher.

If you cannot feel a pulse at either wrist, you should try to find it in the neck at the carotid artery. You should always palpate the carotid pulse in an unresponsive patient. The carotid pulse is easier to feel than the radial pulse, especially if the patient has a low blood pressure. The carotid pulse is most easily felt by first finding the patient's Adam's apple at the front of the neck. You should then slide your index and

middle fingers along one side of the neck until you feel the pulse. The carotid pulse can be felt along a groove between the larynx (voice box) and one of the neck muscles. You will usually feel a carotid pulse if the blood pressure is at least 60 mm Hg.

| TABLE 11-1 | AVERAGE PULSE RATE RANGES |
|---|---|
| Adults | 60 to 100 beats per minute |
| Children | 80 to 100 beats per minute |
| Toddlers | 100 to 120 beats per minute |
| Newborns | 120 to 140 beats per minute |

To obtain a pulse rate from most patients, count the number of beats over a 30-second period and multiply by two.

#### Infants and Children

You can feel the pulse of a child at the carotid artery, similar to an adult. However, palpating this pulse in an infant may present a problem. Because an infant's neck is often very short and fat, you may have a hard time finding the carotid pulse. In infants younger than 1 year then, you should feel the brachial artery to assess the pulse.

You must assess the pulse to determine if rescue breathing has been effective in an unresponsive patient. If the patient has a pulse but is still not breathing, continue rescue breathing at a rate of 12 to 20 breaths/min for an adult, or 20 to 25 breaths/min for a child, until the patient begins breathing again.

## Apical Pulse

If you still cannot feel a pulse, you can confirm the absence of heart activity by listening over the left side of the chest using your ear or a stethoscope (Figure 11-7). Your next step in caring for the patient depends on the following three conditions:

1. *The patient has a medical problem.* If the patient is older than 12 years of age and has a medical problem, you should immediately start CPR and prepare the patient for automated external defibrillation (AED). Attach the AED to the patient as soon as possible and turn on the power. Activate the AED analyzer and follow the directions, as described in chapter 16, Cardiac Emergencies.

2. *The patient is a child.* If the patient is younger than 12 years of age and has a medical problem, you should immediately start CPR. Defibrillation is not commonly performed on children who are younger than 12 or who weigh less than 90 lb.

3. *The patient has traumatic injuries.* If the patient has had a traumatic injury, you should immediately start CPR.

## FIGURE 11-7

Listening to the heart over the left side of the chest

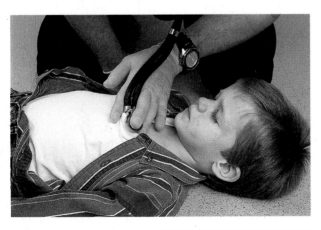

## ASSESSING FOR EXTERNAL BLEEDING

The next step in the initial assessment is to control any external bleeding. In some instances, blood loss can be very rapid and can result in shock and even death. Therefore, this step demands your immediate attention, as soon as the patient's airway is cleared and breathing is stabilized. Controlling external bleeding is often very simple. In almost all instances, your first step is to apply direct pressure with your gloved hand and a sterile bandage at the bleeding site. This pressure stops the flow of blood and helps the blood to coagulate (clot naturally). Remember that you must wear gloves whenever you may be exposed to blood or other body fluids.

You can control active external bleeding using one of six methods. The three most practical and most often used methods are as follows: 1) direct pressure and elevation; 2) splinting; and 3) air pressure splinting. Of these, direct pressure is the most effective way to control bleeding. Three less common ways of controlling bleeding include: 4) arterial pressure points; 5) pneumatic air pressure devices; and 6) tourniquets. Each of these six methods is described in detail in chapter 22, Bleeding and Shock.

## ASSESSING THE SKIN

You should also assess circulation by examining the patient's skin color, temperature, and condition. As you evaluate the skin, you should continue to look for bleeding.

### Skin Color

Skin color depends on the amount of blood circulating in the vessels of the skin. That is one reason you look at skin color to assess circulation. Skin color also depends

# THE BROWN BOTTLE BLUES

It's 6 am on a cold Sunday morning, and you are dispatched to a local trailer park for a "man not feeling well." On arrival, you enter the trailer and immediately notice the obvious signs of a recent party. There are empty wine and beer bottles scattered throughout the trailer along with a half-dozen pizza boxes. You find a 46-year-old man lying on the couch. As you approach, you note that he appears very pale and sweaty. He tells you that he hosted a bachelor party for a friend last night that lasted until 4 am. He states that he has vomited three times since the party wrapped up. A quick assessment shows that he has a blood pressure of 96/64 mm Hg, a pulse of 118/min, and respirations of 26/min.

## For Discussion

1. What is the importance of taking two or more sets of vital signs on serious or critical patients?

2. Discuss the relationship between a patient's vital signs and his or her initial signs and symptoms.

---

on the kind and amount of pigment in the skin. Deeply pigmented skin may hide color changes that result from illness or injury. Therefore, in all patients, you should look for changes in color at the fingernail beds, the sclera (whites of the eyes), conjunctivae (lining of the eyelids), and the mucous membranes of the mouth. Normal skin color is pink. Skin colors that should alert you to possible medical problems include cyanosis (blue), flushed (red), pale (white), and jaundice (yellow).

Assessment of the patient's skin color can help you to make some immediate decisions about treatment. Oxygen may be needed, you may need to control severe bleeding, or you may need to start CPR. For example, a patient with cyanosis lacks adequate oxygen in the blood. Such a patient should be given high-concentration oxygen. A patient with jaundiced skin (or sclera or mucous membranes) is very sick. The presence of jaundice should alert you to use appropriate infectious disease precautions. Pale or white skin, sometimes described as ashen skin, means that the patient has inadequate circulation. In these cases, there is literally not enough blood circulating in the skin.

Another way to assess circulation is to check capillary refill, especially in infants and children. **Capillary refill** is the ability of the circulatory system to restore blood to the capillaries after you squeeze the fingertip. Checking capillary refill is very simple. First, you gently squeeze the patient's fingernail bed. The area under the fingernail will turn white once you squeeze it.

Next, you should let go of the patient's finger and then watch for the finger to turn pink. Normally, the area under the fingernail bed will turn pink within 2 seconds. If the area remains white, or becomes blue, then you know that circulation is inadequate. This assessment does not work well if the patient has been exposed to a cold environment.

### Skin Temperature and Condition

The skin is actually an organ, not just soft tissue. Like all other organs, the skin has many functions. It maintains the water content of the body. It acts as insulation and protection from infection. It also regulates body temperature. Normal body temperature is 98.6°F (37°C). Changes in skin temperature result from illness or injury.

Assess the skin temperature by touching the patient's skin with your wrist or the back of your hand. Does it feel warm, hot, cool, or cold? Finally, determine whether the patient's skin is dry or moist and wet.

# IDENTIFYING PRIORITY PATIENTS

Once you have completed your initial assessment, you have to make some decisions about patient care. First, you must care for life-threatening injuries and/or illnesses. Next, you must identify "priority" patients, or those who need immediate care and transport. Patients with one of the following conditions should be considered priority patients and given care and/or transport first:

- poor general impression
- unresponsiveness, with no gag or cough reflexes
- responsive, but unable to follow commands
- difficulty breathing
- shock (hypoperfusion)
- complicated childbirth
- uncontrolled bleeding
- severe pain in any area of the body
- severe chest pain, especially when the systolic blood pressure is less than 100 mm Hg

Once you have identified priority patients, you can turn to the focused history and detailed physical exam, as described in the next chapter.

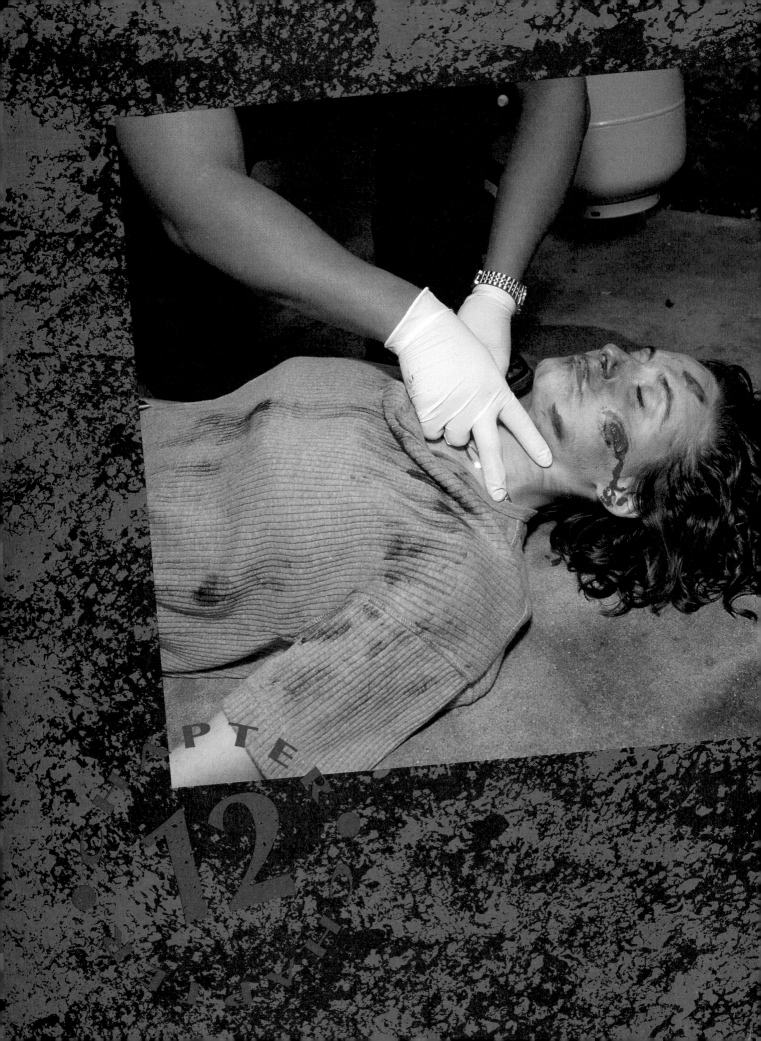

# CHAPTER 12

# Patient Assessment

## Objectives

After you have read this chapter, you should be able to:

- Describe the unique needs for assessing a patient with a chief complaint with no known prior history.
- Explain the differences in performing a focused history/exam for responsive patients with no known prior history and those with a known prior history.
- Describe the unique needs for assessing a patient who is unresponsive or has an altered level of consciousness.
- Explain the differences in the assessment of a patient who is unresponsive or has an altered level of consciousness and other medical patients requiring assessment.
- Discuss the reasons for reconsideration concerning the mechanism of injury.
- Explain the importance of performing a rapid trauma assessment, a focused history/exam, the detailed physical exam, and on-going assessment.
- List the steps of the rapid trauma assessment and discuss what should be evaluated during each step.
- Explain when the steps in the rapid assessment may be altered in order to provide patient care.
- List the steps of and any additional care that should be provided during the detailed physical exam.
- Explain how the detailed physical exam differs for trauma patients and medical patients.
- List the components of the extended vital signs and why an accurate set of vital signs is important.
- Explain why the steps of the initial assessment are repeated as part of the on-going assessment.

**249**

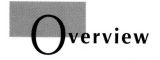

# Overview

This chapter reviews the steps of patient assessment. Assessment and treatment of all patients should be carried out in a systematic way. However, the chapter presents the different approaches necessary for assessing medical patients and trauma patients, and conscious and unconscious patients. Thus, the order in which the steps are presented for each type of patient is significant.

The first section discusses the proper way to approach caring for trauma patients. The second section focuses on the history and physical exam of medical patients. The steps of the rapid trauma assessment and the detailed physical exam are also described. You will immediately see that many of the steps are the same for both types of patients. However, the entire sequence for each type of patient is presented for completeness.

# Key Terms

**Auscultate**  Listening to sounds within the body. This is usually done with a stethoscope.

**Breath sounds**  An indication of air movement in the lungs. Breath sounds are heard by listening to the lungs with a stethoscope.

**Chief complaint**  The patient's response to a general question such as "What's wrong?" or "What happened?"

**Crepitus**  A crackling sound often heard when two ends of a broken bone rub together. Also air bubbles under the skin, giving the skin a crinkly feeling.

**Distention**  The act or state of being swollen or stretched.

**Golden Hour**  The period of time during which treatment of a patient in shock or with traumatic injuries is most critical. This period of time is generally thought to be the first 60 minutes after injury.

**Guarding**  Tensing of the abdomen during palpation.

**Inspect**  Assessing the body by looking.

**Mechanism of injury**  The way in which traumatic injuries occur. With a traumatic injury, the body has been exposed to some force or energy that has resulted in permanent damage or even death.

**OPQRST** The six "pain questions." Onset, Provoke, Quality, Radiation, Severity, Time.

**Palpate** Examination by touch.

**Paradoxical motion** Chest movement that is in the opposite direction of the normal rise and fall of breathing. Paradoxical motion is occurring if part of the chest wall expands outward as the patient exhales and inward as the patient inhales.

**Rapid trauma assessment** A quick area by area examination of a trauma patient to identify life-threatening injuries.

**Rapport** A trusting relationship that you build with your patient.

**Sign** A condition displayed by the patient that you observe, such as bleeding or a contusion.

**Symptom** A condition that the patient tells you about, such as "I feel dizzy."

# THE SETTING OF ALL PATIENT ASSESSMENT

As an EMT-B, you will find yourself in many different settings caring for many different types of patients. A patient thrown from a speeding car has different needs than a patient who is complaining of chest pain. An infant or child will oftentimes need special care that you would not give to an adult. Therefore, the patient's situation often affects how much time you spend on any one step. You will find yourself assessing and reassessing the patient, perhaps several times from the time you arrive at the scene until the patient is delivered to the emergency department. You will also need to be in constant contact with medical control should the patient's condition change. However, every time you provide patient care, you must begin with a consistent, methodical approach to assessment. With a consistent approach to assessment, you are less likely to miss important problems. Therefore, you must always complete every step of the patient assessment in the proper sequence.

The first steps in caring for any patient, the initial and rapid assessments, focus on finding and treating the most life-threatening emergencies. You should always assess and stabilize the following systems in this order of importance:

A = Airway
B = Breathing
C = Circulation
D = Disability

*Always give priority to emergency care of the ABCD to ensure life- and limb-saving treatment.* In all cases, the patient's airway, breathing, circulation, and disability (ABCD) will govern the extent of your assessment and treatment at the scene. When dealing with trauma patients, you may need to remove some of the patient's clothing to complete your assessment. This step is sometimes called Expose, or "E."

Therefore, you may see or hear about ABCDE. This is merely the ABCD with "Expose" added.

Once you have completed the initial and rapid assessments, you may begin a head-to-toe assessment or the detailed physical exam. A patient who has a life-threatening illness or injury must be stabilized and transported immediately. With these patients, you may not have the time to perform a detailed physical exam at the scene. In fact, the detailed physical exam is often done en route to the hospital. Only after a patient has been stabilized and transport has been arranged, or you are en route, can you begin this more detailed assessment. Your detailed physical exam of a patient who has a medical problem will focus on a particular problem. Your detailed assessment of a trauma patient may focus on a specific part of the body or multiple body systems. Detailed physical exams are most likely to occur en route to the emergency department.

## THE TRAUMA PATIENT

Some trauma patients have life-threatening injuries that cannot be treated in the field. These patients must arrive at the hospital for definitive care within 60 minutes from the time of injury. You will often hear this period of time called the **Golden Hour.** The Golden Hour is the time during which treatment of shock or traumatic injuries is most critical (Figure 12-1). After the first 60 minutes have passed, the body has increasing difficulty in keeping the vital signs going.

Therefore, with trauma patients, your goal is to use as little of the Golden Hour as possible. Generally, you should stay at the scene only long enough to manage treatable life- and/or limb-threatening injuries. Your

## FIGURE 12-1

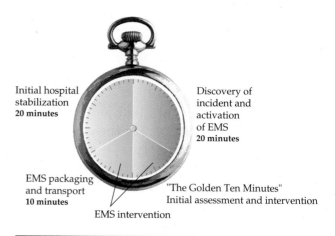

The Golden Hour

Initial hospital stabilization
20 minutes

Discovery of incident and activation of EMS
20 minutes

EMS packaging and transport
10 minutes

"The Golden Ten Minutes"
Initial assessment and intervention

EMS intervention

care focuses on stabilizing injuries so that the patient's condition does not become worse before you reach the hospital. You should begin with the patient's ABCD, as described in the following:

- provide ventilation, if necessary (Airway)
- give oxygen (Breathing)
- control bleeding (Circulation)
- continue cervical spinal immobilization
- continue to assess level of consciousness (Disability)
- rapidly package the patient on a long spine board
- provide rapid transport to the emergency department
- consider air medical transport or transfer to ALS, if long transport time

This section of the chapter focuses on the history and physical exam of the trauma patient. The section begins with a discussion of mechanism of injury and is followed by an area-by-area description of the rapid trauma assessment.

## MECHANISM OF INJURY

As an EMT-B, you will be called to accidents or situations in which patients have had life-threatening traumatic injuries. To properly care for these patients, you must understand how traumatic injuries occur, or the **mechanism of injury.** With a traumatic injury, the body has been exposed to some force or energy that has resulted in a temporary injury, permanent damage, or even death. You will commonly hear the terms blunt trauma and penetrating trauma. With blunt trauma, the force of the injury occurs over a large area, and the skin is not broken. However, the tissues and organs below the area are damaged. With penetrating trauma, the force of the injury occurs in a small point of contact between the skin and the object. The object pierces the skin and creates an open wound. The type of injury that occurs depends on the amount of force or energy, whether the skin is broken, and the part of the body affected. For example, soft tissues, such as the skin and cartilage, stretch and break with relatively little force, as with a punch in the nose. A gentle punch will cause a temporary deformity, such as swelling. A harder punch, however, may actually cause permanent damage.

As you might expect, some parts of the body are more easily injured than others. The brain and the spinal cord are very fragile and easy to injure. They are protected from injury by the skull, the vertebrae, and several layers of soft tissues. The eyes are also easily injured. Even small forces on the eye may result in serious injury. The bones and certain organs are hardier and can absorb small forces without resulting injury.

You should be prepared to see many types of traumatic injuries. Some will be the result of car accidents. Some will be the result of violence. Some will be the result of work-related accidents, such as construction or farm accidents. The area in which you work will determine how often you see certain kinds of traumatic injuries. Be prepared, however, to see everything.

While it is impossible to predict exact injuries, understanding how traumatic injuries occur will better prepare you for providing proper patient care. For example, the driver in a head-on collision who goes up and over the steering wheel is likely to injure the face, head, and spine. The driver's chest and abdomen will strike the steering wheel injuring the lungs, heart, and chest (Figure 12-2). With this mechanism of injury, serious chest or abdominal injuries may result. The more serious injury is usually the chest or abdominal injury, but

### FIGURE 12-2

Mechanism of injury

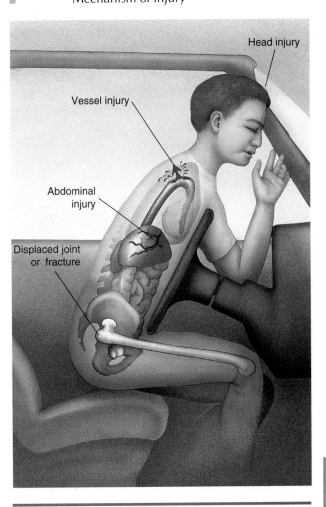

Head injury

Vessel injury

Abdominal injury

Displaced joint or fracture

# THE MECHANISM MATTERS

It's about 3 am on a rainy Sunday morning when you and your partner are dispatched to a motor vehicle crash on Old Mountain Highway. On arrival, a state trooper has secured the scene, and tells you that there are two patients still in the pickup. A third patient was ejected from the truck and is lying approximately 60' from the vehicle. The trooper tells you the truck hit a tree, careened off the road, and in his opinion, rolled over at least three times. Your partner goes to check out the patient who was ejected, while you go to the truck. He returns and tells you that the patient is in full cardiac arrest. The driver of the vehicle was not wearing a seat belt, and he too is in cardiac arrest. The passenger was wearing a seat belt and responds to your voice. This patient also complains of pain in the right shoulder, chest, and hip.

## For Discussion

1. Why does a patient in cardiac arrest due to blunt trauma mechanism of injury have such a poor chance for survival?

2. When you are dispatched on a call, what can the evaluation of the time of occurrence tell you?

---

because the face is bleeding, you may spend all your time trying to control this bleeding.

Patients with significant mechanisms of injury can have life-threatening problems. Significant mechanisms of injury include the following:

- ejection from a vehicle
- severe damage to the vehicle, resulting in death of other passenger
- falls from higher than 20 feet
- rollover in a vehicle
- high-speed vehicle collision
- pedestrian-vehicle collision
- motorcycle crash
- blunt head injury
- penetration injuries of the head, chest, or abdomen
- hidden injuries, such as seat belt or air bag injuries

Significant mechanisms of injury in infants and children include the above, along with the following:

- falls from higher than 10 feet
- bicycle collision
- medium-speed vehicle collision

## HIDDEN INJURIES

It is important to learn if a patient involved in an automobile accident was wearing a seat belt, or if an air bag was deployed. There is no doubt that these safety devices save lives. However, they can also result in injuries that you should know about. When preparing a patient for transport from the scene of an automobile accident, you should always look to see or ask if seat belts and/or an air bag was involved. If a patient is unconscious after any type of accident, you should make sure the patient's cervical spine is immobilized. You should also monitor the patient for signs of shock and breathing difficulties.

### Seat Belts

Seat belts have prevented many thousands of injuries and have saved many thousands of lives. Patients who otherwise would have been thrown out of a smashed car owe their lives to the use of seat belts. If the force of a crash is significant enough, patients can have bruises under the seatbelts and possible internal injuries (Figure 12-3). However, these injuries are less severe than if they had not been wearing seat belts. Seat belts worn improperly across the abdomen rather than across the pelvic bones increase the potential for internal injuries.

Lap seat belts must be worn so that they lie below the iliac crests, snugly up against the hip joints. If the seat belt is worn too high, sudden slowing or an abrupt stop might result in abdominal injuries (Figure 12-4). Occasionally, injuries of the lumbar spine can occur, even if the patient is wearing the seat belts properly.

## FIGURE 12-3

Bruising due to a seat belt injury

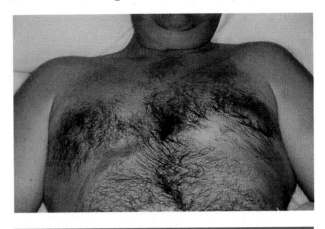

## FIGURE 12-4

The improper (A, B) and proper (C) use of seat belts

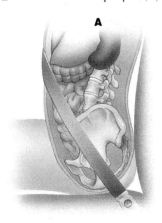
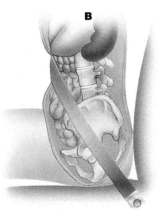
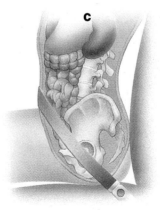

Lap belts and shoulder belts are now commonly combined into a single unit. Some cars have separate lap and shoulder belts. Used alone, shoulder belts can cause injuries of the chest, ribs, and liver.

### Air Bags

Air bags represent a great advance in automotive safety. Before air bags were commonplace, patients in head-on crashes would have significant facial injuries and bleeding—clear, visible signs that they had been injured. With air bags, patients will occasionally have facial burns from the explosive chemical that causes the air bag to expand. However, with air bags and seat belts, patients may or may not have visible injuries. While patients involved in serious crashes may look fine, they may have internal injuries.

You should always look under a deployed air bag to see if the steering wheel is bent or deformed in any way. If an air bag has deployed, you should first remove the patient from the car. Then lift the air bag and check the steering wheel (Figure 12-5). If the wheel is bent or deformed in any way,

## FIGURE 12-5

Lifting a deployed air bag to check the steering wheel

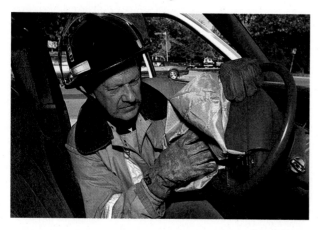

you should suspect possible internal injuries, as the patient has hit the steering wheel. Internal injuries may be possible even if the steering wheel is not bent or deformed. The general health of the patient, the patient's age, and other factors can also increase the possibility for internal injuries.

Therefore, you should tell hospital personnel if seat belts were worn and if so, correctly (if you can tell), and if the air bag deployed. The fact that the air bag deployed indicates a potential severe mechanism of injury.

## THE RAPID TRAUMA ASSESSMENT

After you are certain that the scene is safe, you should turn your full attention to completing a **rapid trauma assessment**. The rapid trauma assessment consists of two major parts: 1) a rapid, initial assessment of ABCD, and 2) a quick area-by-area examination to identify life-threatening injuries. It is important that you stay focused on performing the assessment. Do not become distracted by graphic injuries that may not be life threatening. If the airway needs assistance, the breathing is difficult, the patient appears to be in shock or is unconscious, you should strongly consider completing the assessment en route to the hospital.

The rapid trauma assessment is "systematic" in two ways. First, the steps should be done in the same order every time you assess any patient. Second, the order in which you complete the assessment is body area by body area. Thus, the systematic way in which you do a rapid assessment is both practical and efficient.

When caring for any trauma patient, you must always keep the cervical spine immobilized "in line," even as you begin assess-

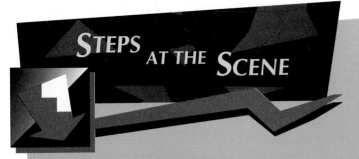

## STEPS AT THE SCENE

### RAPID TRAUMA ASSESSMENT

☐ Perform a rapid, initial assessment of ABCD. Keep the cervical spine immobilized in line.

☐ Inspect and palpate each area of the body. Look and feel for deformities, bruises, abrasions, punctures/penetrations, burns, tenderness, lacerations, or swelling.

☐ Assess the head, neck, and cervical spine. Apply a cervical collar at this time.

☐ Assess and feel the chest area. Listen for breath sounds.

☐ Assess the abdomen for injuries, bruising, bleeding, pain, tenderness, and guarding.

☐ Assess the pelvis for signs of obvious injuries, bleeding, or swelling.

☐ Assess the extremities. Feel for pulses, assess for strength, sensation, and motor function.

☐ Examine the back and cervical spine before securing the patient onto a backboard.

☐ Take the patient's baseline vital signs and complete the SAMPLE history.

☐ Reassess the vital signs every 15 minutes in a stable patient, every 5 minutes for a patient who is not stable.

ing the airway. Ask questions and talk to a responsive patient during the rapid trauma assessment. This will help you to continue to monitor the patient's level of consciousness. As you inspect and palpate each area of the body, look and feel for the following examples of injury or signs of injury:

- deformities
- contusions (bruises)
- abrasions
- punctures/penetrations
- burns
- tenderness
- lacerations
- swelling

## AREA-BY-AREA EXAMINATION

### Head, Neck, and Cervical Spine

Recognizing a possible spinal injury is one of your major responsibilities as an EMT-B. You should assume a spinal injury with any patient who: 1) has traumatic injuries; 2) is under the influence of drugs and/or alcohol; 3) is unconscious; and/or 4) cannot move. First, quickly look at the head, neck, and cervical spine. Gently feel the head and cervical spine for deformity or tenderness (Figure 12-6). Ask a responsive patient if he or she feels any pain or tenderness. With a trauma patient, you should apply a cervical spine immobilization device at this time.

## FIGURE 12-6

Palpate the head and neck for deformity

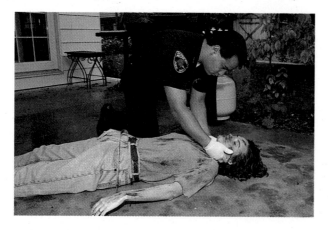

Next, check the jugular (neck) veins for distention (swelling). If the jugular veins are swollen, you should gently press them with two widely spread fingers to see if they refill from below (Figure 12-7). Report and record your findings immediately, especially if the area of injury is under a cervical collar. Do not move on to the next step until you are sure the airway is clear and that the cervical collar is in place. Be sure to check for subcutaneous air, abnormal masses, and a midline trachea.

### Chest

Next, look at and feel over the chest area for injury or signs of injury (Figure 12-8). Look for bruising, sternal tenderness, or splinting of the chest wall. Also look for **paradoxical motion.** Paradoxical motion is chest movement in the opposite direction of the normal rise and fall of breathing. Paradoxical motion is occurring if part of the chest wall expands outward as the patient inhales and inward as the patient exhales. If the patient has broken ribs, sometimes as you feel the chest, you may feel bone grating on bone. This is called bony **crepitus.** Other times you will feel air bubbles under the skin, which feel crinkly. This is called air crepitus or subcutaneous emphysema (air). This is caused by a pneumothorax (rupture of the lung) or an injury to the airway passages. You should report these findings to hospital personnel, because they indicate severe underlying injuries. You may need to provide rapid transport.

Certain traumatic injuries make breathing difficult. These injuries result in decreased or absent breath sounds on one or both sides of the chest. So, before you continue the rapid trauma assessment, you should listen for breath sounds.

## FIGURE 12-7

Press on distended jugular veins

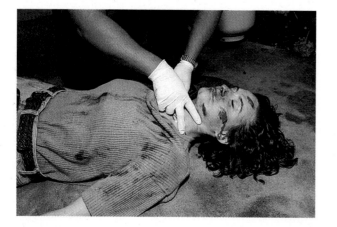

## FIGURE 12-8

Palpate the chest for injuries

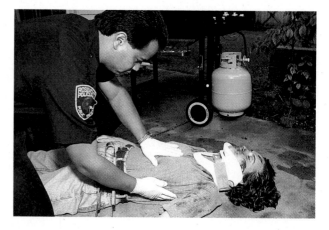

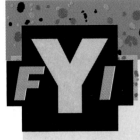

# What is Trauma?

**Trauma,** or injury, occurs when the body is forced to suddenly absorb energy (such as heat, electricity or motion). Energy cannot be created or destroyed—only transformed. One common mechanism is when the body rapidly absorbs **kinetic energy,** the energy of a moving object (such as a car).

The body can absorb a limited amount of energy without sustaining permanent damage. Soft tissues (such as skin) can stretch or deform, while firmer tissues (such as bone or the liver) can resist or absorb small forces. However, damage will worsen until all kinetic energy is spent. Soft tissues will eventually tear; firmer tissues will break apart. The brain, spinal cord and eye are especially vulnerable, even from small forces. High-energy injuries (resulting from car wrecks, certain gunshots and falls) may damage several structures; a victim can be permanently, sometimes fatally, damaged.

A moving object's kinetic energy is calculated as follows:

Kinetic energy = $M/2 \times V^2$

[M = mass (weight) and
V = velocity]

Note that kinetic energy *quadruples* when an object's <u>speed</u> doubles but *doubles* when its <u>weight</u> doubles. Thus the speed, rather than the size, of a car involved in a collision is important.

This fact is especially significant with firearms. As bullet speed rises, damage increases greatly. Fast bullets cause significantly more damage than slow ones, requiring different surgical treatment. Therefore, it is essential to report the firearm used to the hospital.

Significant injury can also occur when a moving body strikes a stationary object, or when parts of the body come to a stop more rapidly than do others. Sudden **deceleration** (decreased speed) occurs at impact.

When the head strikes the dashboard in a car wreck, the skull quickly stops moving. However, the brain continues to move forward until it strikes the skull's inner surface. This "second impact" often causes brain injury. Deceleration injury of the internal organs may be fatal, although outward signs, such as laceration or bruising, may not be great.

The critical determinant of an injury's severity is the amount of kinetic energy absorbed. It is imperative to identify high-energy injuries quickly. They often produce such severe damage the patient can only be saved by rapid transportation to a trauma center.

With certain mechanisms of injury, particularly a car accident, specific injuries frequently occur together. For example, in a front-end collision, the front-seat passenger might strike his knee against the dashboard, resulting in a patellar fracture or knee dislocation. In addition, the femur or pelvis might fracture and/or the hip might dislocate. In a head-on collision, the driver could injure his lungs, heart, great vessels or abdominal organs in addition to his face, head and spine.

**Breath sounds** are an indication of air movement in the lungs. To listen for breath sounds, you need a stethoscope. Make sure that you place the ear pieces facing forward in the ears. Note that breath sounds are usually reported in one of the following ways:

- present and equal
- absent
- decreased at the apices of the lungs, at the midclavicular line bilaterally
- or at the bases of the lungs, at the midaxillary line bilaterally (Figure 12-9)

## FIGURE 12-9

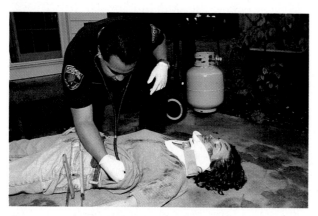

**A**   Auscultate for breath sounds

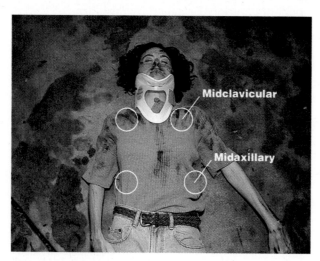

**B**   Points of auscultation

Make sure that the patient is breathing adequately, or is being assisted with breathing, if necessary. Also be sure to assess circulation before you move on to the abdomen.

### Abdomen

Look over the abdomen for any obvious injuries, bruising, and bleeding. Feel over the abdominal area (Figure 12-10). If the patient is awake and alert, ask about pain and tenderness. Do not palpate obvious injuries. Use the terms hard, soft, tender, or distended (swollen) to report your findings. Ask the patient to cough. If the patient grimaces and the pain gets worse, he or she may have what is called rebound tenderness. Some patients may tense the abdomen as you feel it. This is called **guarding.**

### Pelvis

First, look for any signs of obvious injuries, bleeding, or swelling. If the patient reports no pain, gently press on the pelvic bones (Figure 12-11). If you feel them moving or if the patient reports any pain or tenderness, it may indicate a severe injury in this region.

## FIGURE 12-10

Palpate the abdomen

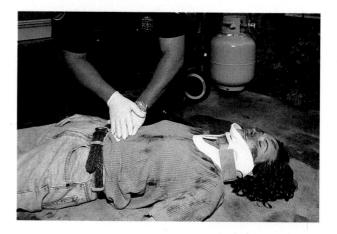

## FIGURE 12-11

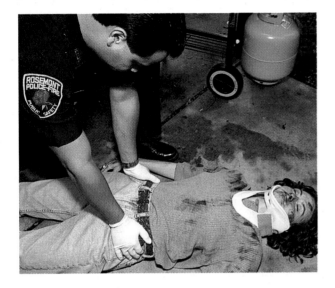

Gently compress the pelvis

### Extremities

Look for lacerations, bruises, swelling, obvious injuries, and bleeding. Next, feel along each extremity for deformities. Ask the patient about any tenderness and pain (Figure 12-12). During this part of the assessment, ask the patient if he or she can feel what you are doing.

## FIGURE 12-12

Palpate the lower extremities

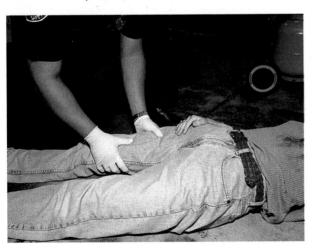

Next, feel for pulses on the top of each foot (dorsalis pedis), at the medial side of each ankle (posterior tibial), and at each wrist (radial) (Figure 12-13). Assess the strength of the extremity by asking the patient to press his or her foot or hand against your hand (Figure 12-14). Compare the strength of each extremity. Note the presence of sensation (feeling) and motor function (movement). If the patient has any type of injury, make sure that you properly immobilize that extremity. Report and record any absence of pulse, any loss of motor-

## FIGURE 12-13

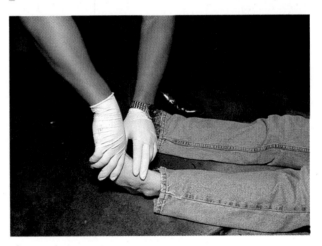

**A**   Palpate the dorsalis pedis pulses

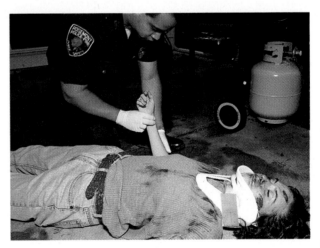

**B**   Palpate the radial pulse

**FIGURE 12-14**

Check strength in the feet

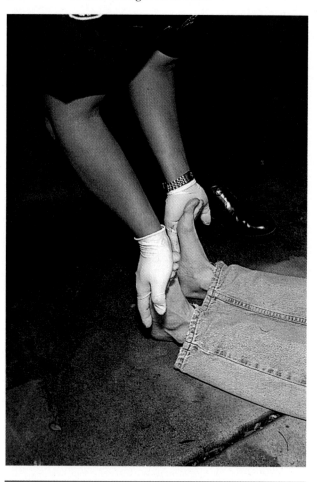

function, and any loss of sensation. Assess the above both before and after you immobilize the extremity.

### Back

The back should be thoroughly examined before you secure the patient onto a backboard. This part of the rapid trauma assessment is especially important if the patient is unconscious. An unconscious patient cannot tell you about any injuries.

Look for any signs of obvious injury, including bruising or deformity. If you suspect a spinal injury, make sure that the patient's spine is stabilized in line at all times during your assessment. This is best done by log rolling the patient. Next, carefully palpate the cervical spine for tenderness or deformity. Also, feel along the length of the spine and ribs for possible injury (Figure 12-15).

## BASELINE VITAL SIGNS AND SAMPLE HISTORY

The purpose of the rapid trauma assessment is to identify any injuries and life-threatening problems. You should now take

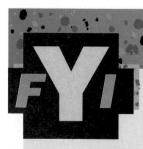

# How Trauma Affects the Vital Signs

The vital signs are affected by trauma in the following ways:
- weak, rapid pulse and low blood pressure suggest significant bleeding

- shallow, rapid breathing often occurs with serious injuries to the head, neck, and chest
- extremes in body temperature suggest exposure and/or possible infection

**FIGURE 12-15**

Palpate the spine

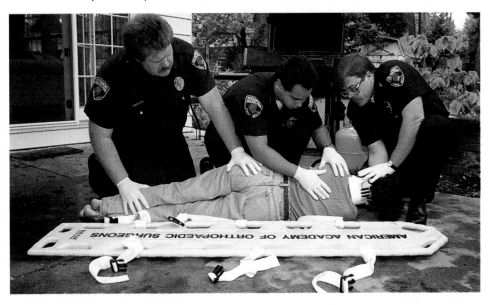

the patient's baseline vital signs and complete the SAMPLE (**S**igns/symptoms, **A**llergies, **M**edications, **P**ertinent past history, **L**ast oral intake, **E**vents leading to injury/illness) history, as described in chapter 5. If the patient is critically injured, you may need to quickly speak with bystanders or law enforcement officials about the mechanism of injury. However, you must not delay transport in order to obtain the SAMPLE history.

Next, assess the patient's respirations, pulse, skin temperature and condition, pupils, and blood pressure. If the patient's condition is stabilized, you should reassess the vital signs every 15 minutes until you reach the emergency department. If the patient's condition has not been stabilized, you should reassess the vital signs every 5 minutes. A trauma patient must be reassessed often because the vital signs may begin to deteriorate at any time.

A patient's vital signs may not deteriorate right away. Even when seriously injured, the body can compensate for blood loss or moderate respiratory insufficiency

for a short time. However, with severe trauma, the body eventually loses its ability to keep the vital signs going. The vital functions then deteriorate rapidly. This is why it is important to record and recheck the vital signs often. Also note any changes in the patient's pulse, motor function, and sensation.

## CARING FOR OTHER TRAUMA PATIENTS

For trauma patients who do not have life-threatening injuries, your approach to assessment and treatment should be a bit different. As with all patients, you should first assess ABCD. The next step is to obtain a SAMPLE history, baseline vital signs, and complete a focused assessment based on the patient's major injuries. Reassess the vital signs every 15 minutes. As long as the vital signs and the ABCD remain stable, you can proceed to the detailed physical exam.

# RIDE 'EM COWBOY!

It is a hot August night and your team is on standby for a rodeo that is in town. The grandstand is packed for the final event of the evening—the bull riding competition. The first rider comes out of the chute. The bull executes a series of quick jumps and turns that cuts the ride short, as the cowboy is launched into the air. He hits the ground and struggles to get to his feet, but the bull hooks him with his horns and flips the cowboy back into the air. He lands on his side on top of a fence, and falls over onto the ground. You find the 26-year-old cowboy alert and oriented, complaining of chest pain over the ribs on his left side. He is also having difficulty catching his breath. The patient has a blood pressure of 146/76 mm Hg, a pulse of 108/min, and respirations of 24/min. His skin is flushed and moist, and his pupils are equal and reactive to light. He has no other complaints or obvious injuries.

## For Discussion

1. Why is it important to evaluate the patient's signs and symptoms in light of the physical surroundings?

2. What is the value of comparing the patient's initial signs and symptoms with those a few minutes later, and then again at transport?

## THE MEDICAL PATIENT

For patients with medical problems, you must complete a thorough assessment and begin stabilizing treatment at the scene. This does not mean that you should delay transport or treatment of these patients. For example, patients with chest pain must be taken to the hospital quickly so that immediate treatment may be given to minimize heart damage. The care you give to patients who are in shock or are unconscious is different from care for patients who are talking and have stable vital signs. Patients in shock must be assessed quickly and their ABCD stabilized as much as possible. Patients with medical problems can deteriorate quickly en route to the hospital.

Patients with medical problems also present other challenges. First, you may arrive at the scene at the beginning, in the middle, or at the end stages of a particular problem. That is why your approach should differ from that of a trauma situation. Listen carefully to the patient's complaints. These complaints may give you an important clue to what body system needs your attention.

Second, you should immediately inform medical control about a patient with medical problems who has no known medical history. You should not help give any medication to such a patient unless medical control directs you to do so.

Caring for a very sick patient can be bewildering unless you approach it in a systematic fashion, focusing on ABCD as your priority. Before you can tailor your assessment to the specific needs of the medical patient, you must understand the basics of patient assessment. The basics include assessing the patient's signs and symptoms, the chief complaint, and the patient's history. Of course, the way in which you actually carry out these steps will depend on whether the patient is alert and responsive or unconscious.

## THE PATIENT HISTORY

### Signs and Symptoms

The words signs and symptoms are often used incorrectly, even by experienced medical personnel. You will hear these words often; therefore, it is important that you understand what they mean. You will also be responsible for reporting a patient's signs and symptoms. All signs and symptoms must be noted and reported to medical control or higher level emergency care personnel when you transport the patient.

A **symptom** is something that the patient experiences and tells you, such as "My arm hurts," "I feel dizzy," "I can't breathe," or "I feel like I'm going to die." A symptom is considered subjective information (Figure 12-16a). A **sign** is something that you see in the patient, such as deformity or bleeding in an injured arm. A blood pressure reading, the pulse rate, and rate of breathing are also signs (Figure 12-16b). Wheezing in a patient who is struggling to breathe is also considered a sign. Because you actually see, hear, or feel signs, they are considered to be more reliable than symptoms. Signs are considered an objective finding.

### The Chief Complaint

Usually the patient's response to a general question such as, "What's wrong?" or "What happened?" is called the **chief complaint.** The chief complaint is usually the symptom that is bothering the patient the most. Despite what you have already seen, do not jump to any conclusions about what is troubling the patient. Now is the time to listen. It is important to understand the patient's problems in the patient's own words.

## FIGURE 12-16

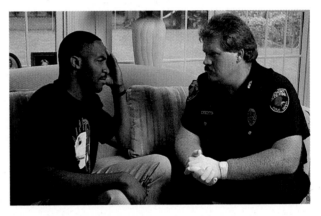

**A**   Taking a patient history (symptoms)

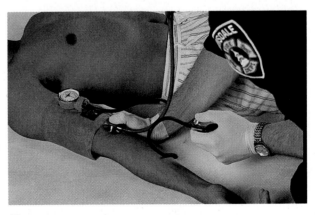

**B**   Checking the blood pressure (signs)

You should record the chief complaint in a few of the patient's own words, along with how long the patient has had the symptoms: "I fell and hurt my arm 2 hours ago," or "I have had chest pain since last night." If the patient is not able to tell you what is wrong, you should ask a family member or bystander. The relationship of this person to the patient should be written on the ambulance form. For example, "Wife: He passed out and stopped breathing 5 minutes ago."

One of the most common chief complaints is pain. Pain can, and will, be described in many different ways. It is important to ask the patient about the nature and the extent of the pain. You can remember the six "pain questions" by the letters **OPQRST:**

**O** *Onset.* When did the pain first start?

**P** *Provoke.* What causes the pain? What makes the pain worse? What makes the pain better?

**Q** *Quality.* What does the pain feel like? Sharp? Dull? Burning? Stabbing? Crushing? Throbbing?

**R** *Radiation.* Does the pain travel from one area to another? For example, does the patient's chest pain seem to go up into his or her jaw?

**S** *Severity.* Does the patient think the pain is mild, moderate, or severe? It is often useful to ask the patient to rate the pain on a scale of 1 to 10. One is almost no pain and 10 is the worst pain ever. This type of rating scale helps to better quantify changes in pain, should they occur.

**T** *Time.* Is the pain constant or intermittent? Has the pain occurred before? When did it start? Does it change (get better, then worse)?

## THE RAPID ASSESSMENT

After you have obtained basic information, as described above, your next step is to perform a rapid assessment, focusing on ABCD. The rapid trauma assessment and the rapid assessment of a medical patient are done for the same reasons. The rapid assessment of a medical patient helps you to identify possible injuries or medical conditions that need attention, such as airway problems or assisted ventilations. It also helps you determine if the patient feels pain and has sensation. The rapid assessment is systematic in two ways. First, the steps should be done in the same order every time you assess any patient. Second, the order in which you complete the assessment is area by area. Thus, the systematic way in which you do a rapid assessment of a medical patient is both practical and efficient.

## THE DETAILED PHYSICAL EXAM

The purpose of the detailed physical exam is to gather more information about the patient. Up to now, you have completed the initial and rapid assessments, and you have obtained the SAMPLE history. At this time, you should spend more time assessing each area of the body. What this means is that you must **inspect** (look), **palpate** (feel), and **auscultate** (listen to) each area of the body, starting at the head and ending at the feet.

Remember that the patient is likely to be frightened and concerned about what is happening. As a result, the patient may not understand or may misinterpret your gestures, body movements, and attitude. *Remember that an essential part of providing high-quality patient care is caring, professional communication.* As you begin the detailed

# THE HEART OF THE MATTER

Your quiet Wednesday evening is interrupted as the radio crackles to life. You are dispatched to a private residence for a possible heart attack. On arrival, you find a 39-year-old man sitting in a large recliner in his living room. He is alert and oriented and tells you that the pain came on suddenly about 2 hours ago. He states that he had a similar episode about a year ago, but that he has no other significant medical history. The patient points to the center of his chest and describes the pain as "tight and squeezing." The patient has a blood pressure of 160/92 mm Hg, a pulse of 112/min, and respirations of 16/min.

## For Discussion

1. Why is recording the time of onset an important part of the cardiac history?

2. When questioning a possible cardiac patient about medication, why is it also important to ask about over-the-counter (OTC) medications as well as illicit drug use?

physical exam, you should explain the answers to the following questions:

1. What is happening now?

2. What will happen next?

3. Why is this happening?

Effective communication is important throughout the assessment process, starting with the initial assessment. As you begin the detailed physical exam, remember that the patient needs reassurance. Often, it takes only a kind word, a caring look, and thoughtful touch to establish **rapport** with the patient. Establishing rapport is building a trusting relationship with your patient. This will make the job of caring for the patient much easier for both you and the patient.

## AREA-BY-AREA EXAMINATION

In the earlier phases of assessment, you identified and provided care for life-threatening conditions. You also obtained the SAMPLE history. In this next phase of assessment, you are carefully looking and feeling for the following signs of injury:

- deformities
- contusions (bruises)
- abrasions
- penetrations
- lacerations
- tenderness
- burns
- swelling

*Remember that patients who seem to be medical patients can have injuries and trauma patients can have medical problems!*

Any change in the level of consciousness is the most important assessment you can make after identifying life-threatening conditions. During the first phases of assessment, you are constantly evaluating the patient's level of consciousness. You should also look for changes in level of consciousness during the detailed physical exam. Your on-going assessments should include an evaluation of level of consciousness every 10 minutes. Any changes should be reported to medical control and recorded in the patient's record.

### Head, Neck, and Cervical Spine

This step begins the same as with the rapid assessment. First, make sure the nose and mouth are clear. If a foreign object appears to be in the mouth, you should carefully remove it with your gloved fingers. *Never insert an unprotected finger into the patient's mouth.* A gloved hand can be placed in the mouth if a bite block is used, or another hand is holding the jaw. Make sure that the cervical spine remains immobilized as you clear the object from the mouth. Once a foreign object has been removed, you should make sure that air flows freely through the nose and mouth. You should then give the patient high-concentration oxygen via a nonrebreathing mask at 15 L/min. If the patient is still not breathing well, use one of the techniques for giving oxygen, as described in chapter 9. In all cases, you should give high-concentration oxygen, no matter what device is used for delivery.

After you have checked the airway, carefully look at the face, scalp, ears, eyes, nose, and mouth for any swelling, deformity, or lacerations (Figure 12-17). Examine the eyes and eyelids, checking for redness and for contact lenses. Use a penlight to check for unequal pupils, look for any fluid drainage or blood, particularly around the ears and nose (Figures 12-18, 12-19). Also check for foreign objects and/or blood in the anterior chamber of the eye. If the patient has had a head injury, you may find discoloration or bruising around the eyes (Raccoon eyes) or behind the ears (Battle's sign).

Next, palpate gently, but firmly, around the face, scalp, eyes, ears, and nose for tenderness or instability. Tenderness or abnormal movement of bones often signal a serious injury. Look and feel inside the mouth next. Loose or broken teeth or a foreign object may block the airway. You should also look for lacerations, swelling, bleeding, and any discoloration in the mouth and the tongue. Smell the patient's breath. Unusual odors, such as a strong alcohol odor or fruity breath odor, should be reported and recorded (Figure 12-20).

Recognizing a possible spinal injury is one of your major responsibilities as an EMT-B. First, quickly look at the head, neck, and cervical spine for any obvious injuries or swelling. Gently feel the cervical spine for deformity or tenderness (Figure 12-21). You should assume a spinal injury with any patient who 1) has traumatic injuries, 2) has an altered level of conscious, and/or 3) cannot move. With a patient who has a possible spinal injury, you should apply a cervical spine immobilization device at this time. It is vital to maintain and record in the patient record that you have immobilized the cervical spine. Ask a responsive patient if he or she feels any pain or tenderness.

Next, check the jugular veins for distention. Also check the neck for crepitance. If the neck veins are swollen, you should gently press them with two widely spread fingers to see if they refill from below (Figure 12-22). The trachea should always appear to be in the middle of the neck at the suprasternal notch (Figure 12-23). Report and record your findings immediately,

## FIGURE 12-17
Examine the scalp

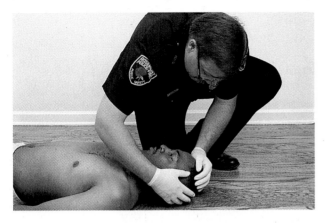

## FIGURE 12-20
Examine the nose and mouth

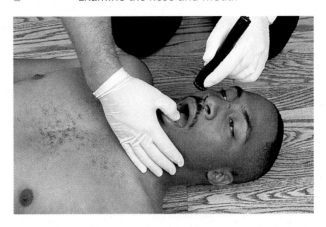

## FIGURE 12-18
Examine the eyes and eyelids

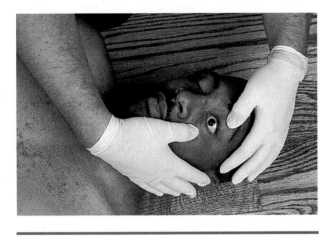

## FIGURE 12-21
Palpate the cervical spine

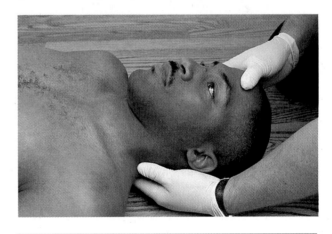

## FIGURE 12-19
Examine the ears for drainage

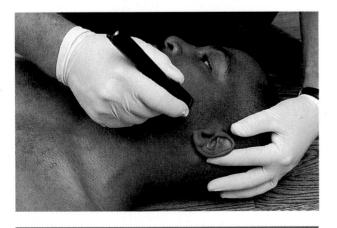

## FIGURE 12-22
Check distended neck veins

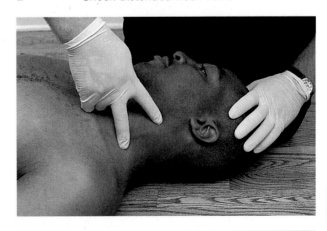

especially if the area of injury is under a cervical collar. Do not move on to the next area until you are sure the airway is clear and that the cervical collar is in place.

## FIGURE 12-23

Palpate the trachea

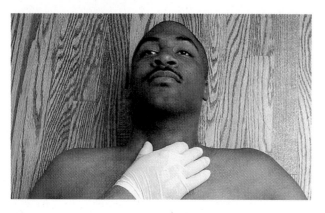

exhales. Also check for crepitance, which is a sensation of bones grating or a crackling feeling when you touch the chest wall (Figure 12-24).

## FIGURE 12-24

Palpate the chest wall

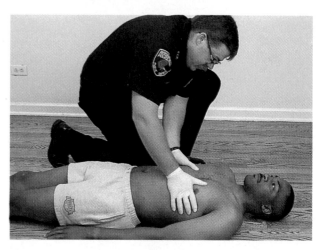

### Chest

Throughout the initial and rapid assessments, you should carefully monitor the patient's breathing. During the detailed physical exam, you should continue to monitor the patient's breathing as you look at the chest for any obvious injuries.

You should next turn your attention to how the chest itself looks. Look carefully for any signs of obvious injury. Gently press on the ribs to determine if there is any tenderness. Do not press on bruises or breaks in the skin. Look for the normal rise and fall of the chest with breathing. Does the chest wall move in the opposite direction from which you would normally expect? Movement in the opposite direction from the normal rise and fall of breathing is called paradoxical motion. Paradoxical motion is occurring if part of the chest wall expands outward as the patient inhales and inward as the patient

Certain injuries and medical conditions make breathing difficult for the patient. These injuries and illnesses may result in decreased or absent breath sounds on one or both sides of the chest. Therefore, your last step in assessing the chest is to listen for breath sounds. Breath sounds are an indication of air movement within the lungs. To listen for breath sounds, you need a stethoscope. Make sure that you place the ear pieces facing forward in your ears.

First, place the end of the stethoscope on the chest at the top of each lung. Listen to both lungs at the top, just below the clavicles. Next, listen at the nipple level at the midaxillary line and finally at both bases near the rib margins (Figure 12-25). You should record if the breath sounds are present or absent and if they are the same on both sides. Listen for wheezing or gurgling sounds. You should also listen for breath sounds from the back. In trauma patients,

## FIGURE 12-25

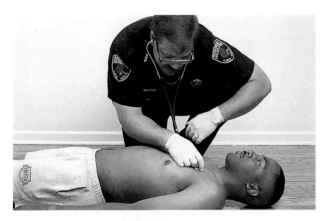

**A**   Auscultate breath sounds

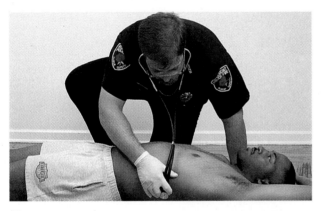

**B**   Auscultate breath sounds at the bases of the lungs

you can easily do this as you log roll the patient to inspect the back.

### Abdomen

The next area of assessment is the abdomen. Look first for any signs of obvious injury, including swelling and bruising. All injuries, including contusions, lacerations, and penetrating objects, should be noted.

Next begin gently feeling the abdomen. Ask the patient if there is any pain or tenderness as you press over the abdomen (Figure 12-26). Report to medical control if there is significant pain or tenderness. This may signal a serious problem. As you report your

findings, you should describe the abdomen as soft (which is normal) or hard (rigid). You should also report any stretching or swelling (**distention**) or guarding.

## FIGURE 12-26

Palpate the abdomen

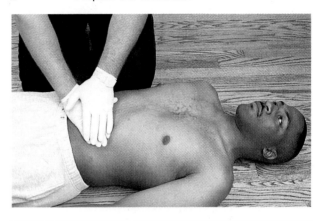

### Pelvis

The large bone that surrounds the lower abdomen is called the pelvis. It is composed of several bones that are tightly bound together. During this part of the assessment, check for tenderness and any signs of injury. If the patient does not complain of pain, or if the patient is unresponsive, gently flex and compress the entire ring of the pelvis to determine if there is any tenderness or instability (Figures 12-27 and 12-28).

### Extremities

Begin your assessment of the extremities at the thigh and work down to the foot. Look for lacerations, bruises, swelling, obvious deformities, and bleeding (Figure 12-29). Next, feel along the calves and shins for tenderness and pain. During this part of the assessment, ask the patient if he or she can feel what you are doing.

## FIGURE 12-27

Compress the pelvis from the sides

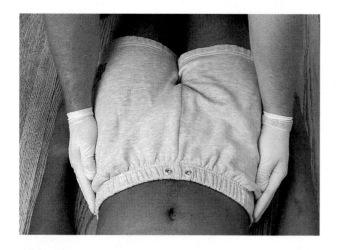

## FIGURE 12-29

Examine the lower extremities

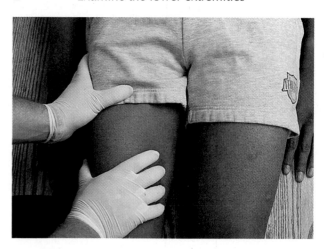

## FIGURE 12-28

Compress the pelvis from the front

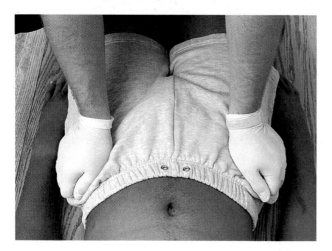

## FIGURE 12-30

Test the strength of the lower extremities

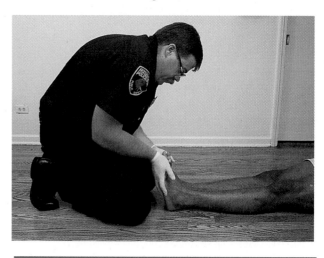

Next, feel for pulses on the top of each foot (dorsalis pedis) and at the medial side of each ankle (posterior tibial). Assess the strength of each foot by having the patient press the foot against your hand. Compare the strength of each foot. Note the presence of sensation and movement (Figure 12-30). If the patient has a leg injury, make sure that the leg is properly immobilized. Report

and record any absence of pulse, any loss of motor function, and any loss of sensation.

You should next examine the arms. Look for lacerations, bruises, swelling, obvious deformities, and bleeding. Next, feel along the upper and lower parts of the arm for tenderness and pain (Figure 12-31). During this part of the assessment, ask the patient if he or she can feel what you are

## FIGURE 12-31

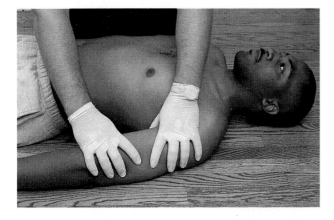

Palpate the upper extremities

## FIGURE 12-32

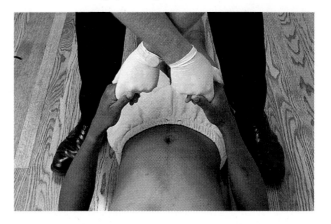

Test grip strength

doing. If the patient has not been able to feel your light touch during other parts of the assessment, gently pinch along the arms to test for pain.

Next, check the radial pulses at the wrist in each arm. Test the patient's sensation of light touch by gently stroking the top of the index finger. Test the patient's ability to move each hand. Ask the patient to open and close the fist to test neurologic function. This is also a way to test how well the patient can follow commands. Finally, ask the patient to grasp both your hands in a test of grip strength. Compare the patient's grip strength (Figure 12-32). If the patient has an injury, make sure that the arm is properly immobilized. Report and record any absence of pulse, any loss of motor function, and any loss of sensation.

### Back

The last area that you should examine is the posterior side of the body, particularly the back. The back should be thoroughly examined before you secure the patient onto a backboard. This part of the detailed physical exam is especially important if the patient is unconscious or unable to communicate.

Look for any signs of obvious injury, including bruising or deformity. If you suspect a spinal injury, make sure that the patient's spine is stabilized "in line" at all times during your assessment. This is best done by log rolling the patient (Figure 12-33). At this time, you may also listen for breath sounds from the back. Next, carefully palpate the cervical spine for tenderness or deformity. Also, feel along the length of the spine for possible injury.

## FIGURE 12-33

Log roll the patient to inspect for spinal injury

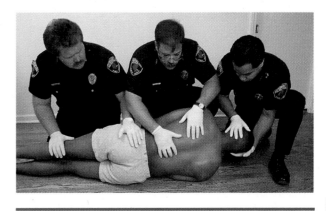

## STAIR SCARE

In preparation for moving out of her duplex, a young lady is mopping her kitchen floor. She slips in the soapy water, tumbles down eight stairs, and ends up on the basement floor. A neighbor, who was helping her clean, hears the commotion and calls 9-1-1. On arrival, you find a 29-year-old woman in obvious pain still lying on the basement floor. At first she simply says that she is scared and that everything hurts. She also thinks that she may have lost consciousness, but she isn't sure. She has multiple abrasions, a number of which are slightly oozing blood. The patient is alert and oriented to person, place, and time. She has good circulation, motor, and sensory functions in all extremities, and her skin is pink, warm, but slightly moist. Other than the abrasions, there are no other obvious signs of trauma. Her pupils are slightly dilated, but reactive. The patient has a blood pressure of 130/68 mm Hg, a pulse of 106/min, and respirations of 22/min. The patient states that she has no allergies, but takes Ventolin for asthma.

### For Discussion

1. What makes assessment of the airway the most essential part of the on-going assessment?

2. Why is it important to repeat the initial assessment as part of the on-going assessment?

## REASSESSMENT OF VITAL SIGNS

Once you have completed the detailed physical exam, you should keep a mental list of problem areas. Your care will then be directed to stabilizing these areas and constantly watching the ABCD. At this point, you should also reassess the patient's vital signs. Look for and record any changes in the patient record. Hospital personnel will be especially interested in changes in vital signs and level of consciousness during transport.

# ON-GOING ASSESSMENT

Blood pressure, pulse, respirations, and neurologic status are essential components of patient on-going assessment. These vital signs must be monitored at 5- to 15-minute intervals en route to a receiving facility.

If the patient at any time has a change in mental status or vital signs, the initial assessment should be repeated. It is critical to document all components of patient re-assessment for hospital personnel. Care is not complete until the assessment is carefully recorded.

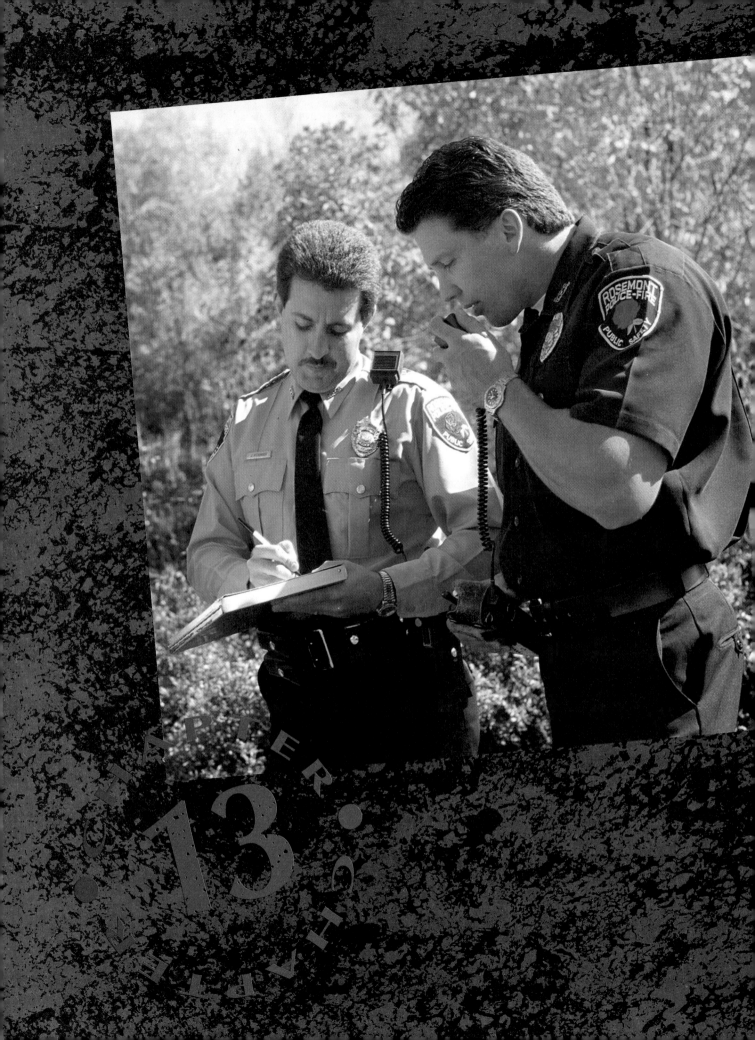

# CHAPTER 13

# Communications and Documentation

## Objectives

After you have read this chapter, you should be able to:

- List the correct radio use procedures in the following phases of a typical call:
  — en route and at the scene
  — en route and at the medical facility
  — in service
  — en route and at the station.
- List the proper ways of beginning and ending a call.
- State the proper order for reporting patient information.
- Explain the importance of effective communication of patient information in the oral report.
- Identify the essential components of the oral report.
- Describe the attributes for increasing effectiveness and efficiency of oral communications.
- State legal aspects to consider in oral communication.
- Discuss the communication skills that should be used to interact with the patient, as well as family, bystanders, individuals from other agencies, and hospital personnel.
- Explain the components of the written report and list the information that should be included on the written report.
- Identify the various sections of the written report.
- Describe what information is required in each section of the prehospital care report and how it should be entered.
- Define the special considerations concerning patient refusal.

- Describe the legal implications associated with the written report.
- Discuss all state and/or local record and reporting requirements.

# 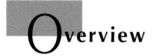verview

Radio and telephone communications link you and your team with other members of your EMS system. This link helps the entire team to work together more effectively. You must know what your communications system can and cannot do, and you must be able to use your system efficiently and effectively. You must be able to send precise, accurate reports about the scene, the patient's condition, and the treatment you provide.

This chapter describes the skills that you need to be an effective communicator. The chapter identifies the kinds of equipment used, along with standard radio operating procedures and standard radio protocols. It also describes the role of the Federal Communications Commission (FCC) in EMS. A discussion of the principles of effective interpersonal communication, particularly with patients and family members, is also included.

The chapter also discusses the written report. We all know that paperwork is not the exciting, "save-a-life" part of your job. Nevertheless, it is a vital part of providing emergency medical care. Adequate reporting and accurate records ensure the continuity of patient care. Complete patient records also guarantee proper transfer of responsibility, comply with the requirements of health departments and law enforcement agencies, and fulfill your administrative needs. Reporting and record keeping duties are essential, but they must never come before patient care. As you become more experienced, you will learn to obtain most of the necessary information by simply watching, listening, and questioning the patient as you provide care.

# Key Terms

**Base station**   Any radio hardware containing a transmitter and receiver that is located in a fixed place.

**Cellular telephone**   A low-power portable radio that communicates through an interconnected series of repeater stations called "cells."

**Channel**   An assigned frequency or frequencies used to carry voice and/or data communications.

**Dedicated line**   A special telephone line used for specific point-to-point communications. Also known as a "hot line."

**Duplex**   The ability to transmit and receive simultaneously.

**Federal Communications Commission (FCC)**   Federal agency with jurisdiction over interstate and international telephone and telegraph services and satellite communications—all of which may involve EMS activity.

**Hot line**   Same as a dedicated line.

**MED channels**   VHF and UHF channels designated by the FCC exclusively for EMS use.

**Paging**   Involves the use of a radio signal and a voice or digital message that is transmitted to pagers ("beepers") or desktop monitor radios.

**Rapport**   A trusting relationship that you build with your patient.

**Repeater**   A special base station radio that receives messages and signals on one frequency and then automatically retransmits them on a second frequency.

**Scanner**   A radio receiver that searches or "scans" across several frequencies until the message is completed. The process is then repeated.

**Simplex**   Single-frequency radio; transmissions can occur in either direction but not simultaneously in both; when one party transmits the other can only receive, and when one party is transmitting it is unable to receive.

**Standing orders**   Written documents, signed by the EMS system's medical director, that outline specific directions, permissions, and sometimes prohibitions regarding patient care. Also called protocols.

**Telemetry**   A process in which electronic signals are converted into coded, audible signals. These signals can then be transmitted by radio or telephone to a receiver at the hospital with a decoder.

**UHF**   Ultra High Frequency. Radio frequencies between 300 and 3,000 MHz.

**VHF**   Very High Frequency. Radio frequencies between 30 and 300 MHz. The VHF spectrum is further divided into "high" and "low" bands.

# COMMUNICATIONS SYSTEMS

## SYSTEM COMPONENTS

As an EMT-B, you must be familiar with two-way radio communications and have working knowledge of the mobile and hand-held portable radios used in your unit. You must also know when to use them and what to say when you are transmitting.

### Base Station Radios

The dispatcher usually communicates with field units by transmitting through a fixed radio base station controlled from the dispatch center. A **base station** is any radio hardware containing a transmitter and receiver located in a fixed place. The base station may be used in a single place by an operator speaking into a microphone connected directly to the equipment. It also works remotely through telephone lines or by radio from a communications center.

A "two-way" radio consists of two units—a transmitter and a receiver. Some base stations may have more than one transmitter and/or more than one receiver. They may also be equipped with one multi-channel transmitter and several single channel receivers. Regardless of the number of transmitters and receivers, they are commonly called base radios or stations. Base stations usually have more power (often 100 watts or more) and higher, more efficient antenna systems than mobile or portable radios. This increased broadcasting range allows the base station operator to communicate with field units and other stations at much greater distances.

The base radio must be physically close to its antenna. Therefore, the actual base station cabinet and hardware are commonly found on the roof of a tall building or at the bottom of an antenna tower (Figure 13-1).

The base station operator may be miles away in a dispatch center or hospital communicating with the base station radio by dedicated lines or special radio links. A **dedicated line,** or **hot line,** is always open or under the control of the individuals at each end. This type of line is immediately "on" as soon as you lift the receiver and cannot be accessed by outside users.

### FIGURE 13-1

A typical base station

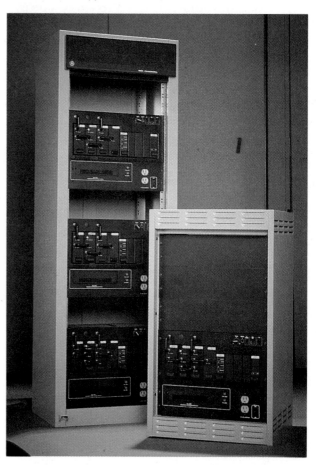

### Mobile and Portable Radios

In the ambulance, you will use both mobile and portable radios to communicate with the dispatcher or with medical control. An ambulance will often have more than

**FIGURE 13-2**

Mobile radio

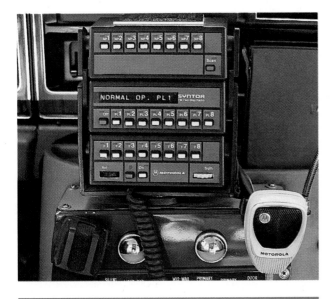

one mobile radio, each on a different frequency (Figure 13-2). One radio may be used to communicate with the dispatcher or other public safety agencies. A second radio is often used for communicating patient information to medical control.

A mobile radio is installed in a vehicle and usually operates at lower power than a base station. Most **VHF** (Very High Frequency) mobile radios operate at 100 watts of power. **UHF** (Ultra High Frequency) mobile radios usually have only 40 watts of power. Cellular telephones operate on 3 watts of power or less. Mobile antennas are much closer to the ground than base station antennas, so communications from the unit are typically limited to 10 to 15 miles over average terrain.

Portable radios are hand-carried or hand-held devices that operate at 1 to 5 watts of power. Since the entire radio can be held in your hand, when in use the antenna is often no higher than the EMT using the radio. The transmission range of a portable radio is more limited than that of mobile or base station radios. Portable radios are essential in helping to coordinate EMS activities at the scene of a multiple-casualty incident. They are also helpful when you are away from the ambulance and need to communicate with dispatch, another unit, or medical control (Figure 13-3).

### Repeater-Based Systems

A **repeater** is a special base station radio that receives messages and signals on one frequency and then automatically retransmits them on a second frequency. Because a repeater is a base station, it is able to receive low power signals, such as those from a portable radio, from a long distance away. The signal is then rebroadcast with all the power of the base station. EMS systems that use repeaters usually have outstanding system-wide communications and are able to get the best signal from portable radios.

### Digital Equipment

Although most people think of voice communications when they think of two-way radios, digital signals are also a part of EMS communications. Some EMS systems

**FIGURE 13-3**

Portable radio

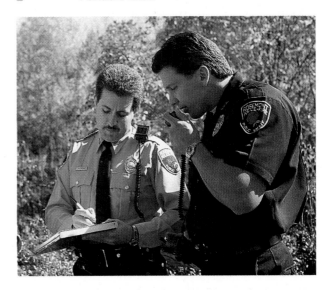

use telemetry to send an ECG from the unit to the hospital. With **telemetry,** electronic signals are converted into coded, audible signals. These signals can then be transmitted by radio or telephone to a receiver at the hospital with a decoder. The decoder converts the signals back into electronic impulses that can be displayed on a screen or printed. Another example of telemetry is a fax message.

Digital signals are also used in some kinds of paging and tone alerting systems because they transmit faster than spoken words and allow more choices and flexibility.

### Cellular Telephones

**Cellular telephones** are becoming more common in EMS communications systems. These telephones are simply low-power portable radios that communicate through a series of interconnected repeater stations called "cells" (hence the name "cellular"). Cells are linked by a sophisticated computer system and connected to the telephone network (Figure 13-4). Cellular telephones are also popular with other public safety agencies, particularly as more cell sites are constructed in rural areas.

Unlike typical two-way mobile communications, which are free access, a cellular system charges fees for its use. Your system can buy portable or mobile radios on the local EMS frequency and use them at no cost. However, buying a cellular telephone is only half of the process of being able to use it. A cellular telephone cannot simply access the telephone network. The user must be assigned a specially coded number that the cellular system's computers will recognize. It is that access and the amount of time a user spends on the telephone for which the cellular system charges. However, once you are connected to the network, you can call any other telephone in the world and can send voice, data, and telemetry signals.

Many cellular systems make equipment and air time available to EMS services at

**FIGURE 13-4**

Map of cell sites for cellular phone

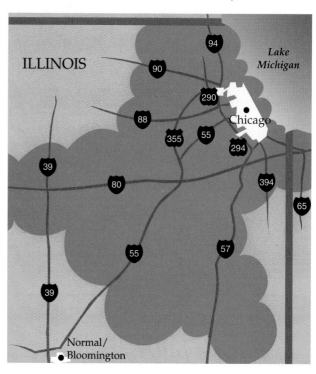

little or no cost as a public service. The public is often able to call 9-1-1 or other emergency numbers on a cellular telephone free of charge. Cellular systems can become overloaded and jammed in mass casualty and disaster situations.

As with all repeater-based systems, a cellular telephone is useless if the equipment fails, loses power, or is damaged by severe weather or other circumstances. Like all voice radio communications systems, cellular telephones can be easily overheard on scanners. Although cellular telephones are more private than most other forms of radio communications, they can still be overheard. Therefore, you must always speak in a professional manner every time you use the EMS communications system.

### Other Communications Equipment

Ambulances and other field units are usually equipped with an external public address system. This system may be a part of the siren or the mobile radio. The intercom between the cab and the patient compartment may also be a part of the mobile radio. These components do not involve radio wave transmission, but you must understand how they work and practice *before* you really need them.

EMS systems may use a variety of two-way radio hardware. Some systems operate VHF equipment in the **simplex** (push-to-talk, release-to-listen) mode. In this mode, radio transmissions can occur in either direction but not simultaneously in both. When one party transmits, the other can only receive. Other systems conduct **duplex** (simultaneous talk-listen) communications on UHF frequencies and also use cellular telephones. In the full duplex mode, radios can transmit and receive communications simultaneously on one channel. This is sometimes called "a pair of frequencies." A number of VHF and UHF channels are re-

served exclusively for EMS use, commonly called **MED channels.** However, hundreds of other commercial, local government, and fire service frequencies are also used for EMS communications.

Some EMS systems rely on dedicated lines (hot lines) as control links for their remotely located base stations and antennas. Other systems are more simply configured and require no off-site control links. No matter what type of equipment is used, all EMS communications systems have some basic limitations. Therefore, you must know what your equipment can and cannot do.

The ability for you to communicate effectively with other units or medical control depends on how well the weaker radio can "talk back." Base and repeater station radios often have much greater power and higher antennas than mobile or portable units. This increased power affects your communications in two ways. First, signals are generally heard and understood from a much greater

## RADIO REPORT

You are transporting a man who states he is "feeling depressed" to the Allswell Memorial Hospital. He tells you that he has been feeling this way for about the last 3 weeks. You've completed your initial assessment and the detailed physical exam. You have also obtained two complete sets of vital signs.

### For Discussion

1. List at least three legal aspects to consider with regard to the prehospital radio report.

2. Effective communication with family members involves some affective attitudes and behaviors. List at least three and briefly explain why they are important.

YOU ARE THE EMT

distance than the signal produced from a mobile unit. Second, signals are received clearly from a much greater distance than with a mobile or portable unit. *Remember when you are at the scene, you may be able to clearly hear the dispatcher or hospital on your radio, but you may not be heard or understood when you transmit.*

Even small changes in your location can significantly affect the quality of your transmission. Also remember that the location of the antenna is critically important for clear transmission. Commercial aircraft flying at 37,000 feet can transmit and receive signals over hundreds of miles, yet their radios have only a few watts of power. Their "power" comes from their 37,000 foot high antenna!

At times you may be able to communicate with a base station radio, but you will not be able to hear or transmit to another mobile unit that is also communicating with that base. Repeater base stations eliminate such problems. They allow two mobile or portable units that cannot reach each other directly to communicate through the repeater—using its greater power and antenna.

The success of communications is dependent on the efficiency of your equipment. A damaged antenna or microphone often prevents high-quality communications. Check the condition and status of your equipment at the start of each shift, and then correct or report any problems.

## RADIO COMMUNICATIONS

### RADIO FREQUENCIES

All radio operations in the United States, including those used in EMS systems, are regulated by the **Federal Communications Commission (FCC)**. The FCC has jurisdiction over interstate and international tele-

phone and telegraph services and satellite communications—all of which may involve EMS activity.

The FCC has five main EMS-related responsibilities, as follows:

1. *Allocating specific radio frequencies for use by EMS providers.* Modern EMS communications began in 1974. At that time, the FCC assigned 10 MED channels in the 460-470 MHz (UHF) band to be used by EMS providers. These UHF channels were added to the several VHF frequencies that were already available for EMS systems. However, these VHF frequencies had to be shared with other "special emergency" uses, including school buses and veterinarians. In 1993, the FCC created an EMS only block of frequencies in the 220-MHz portion of the radio spectrum.

2. *Licensing base stations and assigning appropriate radio call signs for those stations.* An FCC license is usually issued for 5 years, after which time it must be renewed. Each FCC license is granted only for a specific operating group. Often, the longitude and latitude (location) of the antenna and the address of the base station determine the call signs.

3. *Establishing licensing standards and operating specifications for radio equipment used by EMS providers.* Before it can be licensed, each piece of radio equipment must be submitted by its manufacturer to the FCC for type-acceptance, based on established operating specifications and regulations.

4. *Establishing limitations for transmitter power output.* The FCC regulates broadcasting power to reduce radio interference between neighboring communications systems.

5. *Monitoring radio operations.* This includes making spot field checks to help ensure compliance with FCC rules and regulations.

The FCC's rules and regulations fill many volumes and are written in technical and legal language. Only a very small section (part 90, subpart C) deals with EMS communications issues. You are not responsible for reading these detailed and often confusing documents. For appropriate guidance on technical issues, contact your EMS system supervisor. In fact, many EMS systems look to radio and telephone communications experts for advice on technical issues.

## RESPONSE TO THE SCENE

EMS communications systems may operate on several different frequencies and may use different frequency bands. Some EMS systems may even use different radios for different purposes. However, all EMS systems depend on the skill of the dispatcher. The dispatcher, not the EMT-B, receives the first call to 9-1-1. You are part of the team that responds to calls once the dispatcher notifies your unit of an emergency.

### Alert and Dispatch

The dispatcher has several important responsibilities during the alert and dispatch phase of EMS communications. The dispatcher must do all of the following:

- properly screen and assign priority to each call

- select and alert the appropriate EMS response unit(s)

- dispatch and direct EMS response unit(s) to the correct location

- coordinate EMS response unit(s) with other public safety services until the incident is over (Figure 13-5)

- provide emergency medical instructions to the telephone caller so that essential care (e.g. CPR) may begin before the EMTs arrive

When the first call to 9-1-1 comes in, the dispatcher must try to judge its relative importance to begin the appropriate EMS response. First, the dispatcher must find out the exact location of the patient and the nature and severity of the problem. Next, some description of the scene, such as the number of patients or special environmental hazards, is needed. Then, if possible, the dispatcher should ask for the caller's telephone number, the patient's age and name, and other information, as directed by local protocol.

From this information, the dispatcher will assign the appropriate EMS response unit(s) based on the following:

- the dispatcher's perception of the nature and severity of the problem

- the response time to the scene

- the level of training (First Responder, BLS, ALS) of available EMS response unit(s)

- the need for additional EMS units, the fire department, a HazMat team, air medical support, or law enforcement

The dispatcher's next step is to alert the appropriate EMS response unit(s). Alerting these units may be done in a variety of ways. The dispatch radio system may be used to contact those units already in service

## FIGURE 13-5

An EMS dispatcher

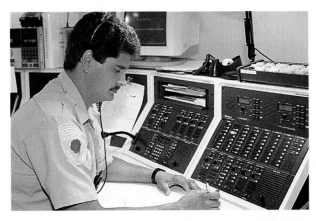

# NO BINGO THIS TIME

Your team is dispatched to a local bingo hall where you find a 58-year-old man complaining of shortness of breath. He can answer your questions, but appears to be confused. The patient tells you he's had a cough for the last couple of weeks and really hasn't felt very good. He has pink, warm, and slightly moist skin, except around the mouth and lips, which appear cyanotic (blue). The patient also states that he has been taking antibiotics for the last couple of days and he uses an inhaler for his asthma. You find also that he smokes two to three packs of cigarettes a day. He has a blood pressure of 160/86 mm Hg, a pulse of 104/min, and respirations of 24/min.

## For Discussion

1. Describe the relationship between the prehospital assessment and the radio report.

2. Why is effective communication between the provider and the patient so crucial to the evolution of the call?

---

and monitoring the channel. Dedicated (hot) lines between the control center and the EMS station may be used.

The dispatcher may also page EMS personnel. Pagers are commonly used by both volunteer and full-time EMS personnel. **Paging** involves the use of a coded tone or digital radio signal and a voice or display message that is transmitted to pagers (beepers) or desktop monitor radios. Paging signals may be sent to alert only certain personnel, or as blanket signals to activate all the pagers in the EMS service. Pagers and monitor radios are convenient because they are usually silent until their specific paging code is received. Alerted personnel contact the dispatcher to confirm the message and receive details of their assignments.

Once EMS personnel have been alerted, they must be properly dispatched and sent to the incident. Every EMS system should use a standard dispatching procedure. The dispatcher should give the responding unit(s) the following information:

- the nature and severity of the injury, illness, or incident
- the exact location of the incident
- the number of patients
- responses by other public safety agencies
- special directions or advisories, such as adverse road or traffic conditions, or severe weather reports
- time at which the unit(s) are dispatched

Your unit must confirm to the dispatcher that you have received the information and that you are en route to the scene. Local protocol will dictate whether it is the job of the dispatcher or your unit to notify other public safety agencies that you are responding to an emergency. In some areas, the emergency department is notified whenever an ambulance responds to an emergency.

You should report any problems during your run to the dispatcher. You should also inform the dispatcher that you have arrived at the scene. The arrival report to the dispatcher should include any obvious details you see during size up. For example, "Dispatch, Medic One is on scene at Main Street with a two-vehicle collision" would be appropriate.

All radio communications during dispatch, as well as other phases of operations, must be brief and easily understood. Although speaking in plain English is best, many areas find that 10 codes are shorter and simpler for routine communications. The development and use of such codes requires strict discipline. When used improperly or not understood, codes create rather than clear up confusion.

## COMMUNICATING WITH MEDICAL DIRECTION AND HOSPITALS

### MEDICAL CONTROL

Every EMS system needs input and involvement from physicians. A team of physicians will provide medical direction (medical control) for your EMS system. The EMS director, medical control officers, and other providers must develop standard medical treatment and radio communications protocols for use by the physicians and EMS in your area. Protocols help decrease confusion and misunderstanding between hospital personnel and EMS regarding patient reports and orders. They also help reduce scene time. Medical control must be readily available on the radio at the hospital or on a mobile or portable unit when you call.

In most areas, medical direction comes from the receiving hospital (Figure 13-6). However, many variations have developed across the country. For example, some EMS units receive medical direction from one hospital, even though they are taking the patient to another hospital. In other areas, they receive medical direction from the receiving hospital only. Medical direction may come from a free-standing center or even from an individual physician.

### FIGURE 13-6

Hospital-based medical direction

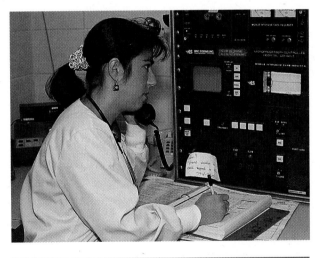

Regardless of your system's design, your link to medical control is vital. You will need directions on how best to care for your patient. How often you need to call medical control varies. It often depends on your system's protocols and how much care you can provide before you must call for guidance.

## Calling Medical Control

You can use the radio in your unit or a portable radio to call medical control. A cellular telephone can also be used. Regardless of the type of radio, you should use a channel that is relatively free of other radio traffic and interference. There are a number of ways to control access on ambulance-to-hospital channels. In some EMS systems, the dispatcher monitors and assigns appropriate, clear medical control channels. Other EMS systems rely on special communications operations, such as CMEDs (Centralized Medical Emergency Dispatch) or resource coordination centers, to monitor and allocate the medical control channels.

Due to the large number of EMS calls to medical control, your radio report must be well organized, precise, and contain only important information. In addition, because you need specific directions on patient care, the information you provide to medical control must be accurate. *Remember that the physician on the other end bases his or her instructions on the information you provide.*

*You should never use codes when communicating with medical control.* You should use proper medical terminology when giving your report. Never assume that medical control will know what a "10-50" or a "Signal 70" means. Medical control handles many different EMS systems and will not know your unit's special codes or signals.

Once you receive an order from medical control, you must repeat the order back word for word and then receive confirmation. No matter if the physician gives an order for medication, a specific treatment, or denies a request for a particular treatment, you must repeat the order back word for word. This "echo" exchange helps to eliminate confusion and the possibility for poor patient care. *Orders that are unclear or seem inappropriate or incorrect should be questioned.* Do not blindly follow an order that does not make sense to you. The physician may have misunderstood or missed part of your report. Therefore, he or she may not be able to respond appropriately to the patient's needs.

## Giving the Patient Report

The patient report should follow a standard format established by your EMS system. The patient report commonly includes the following seven elements:

1. Your unit identification and level of service. For example, "Brimfield Medic 71-BLS."

2. The receiving hospital and your estimated time of arrival. For example, "Robinson Memorial Hospital—ETA 10 minutes."

3. The patient's age and sex. For example, "A 33-year-old female." (Note: The patient's name should not be given over the radio because it may be overheard. This is an invasion of the patient's privacy.)

4. The patient's chief complaint or your perception of the problem and its severity. For example, "The patient complains of pain in the right lower leg."

5. A brief history of the patient's illness or injury. For example, "The patient takes insulin and is allergic to penicillin." Other important information about the patient, such as a history of heart problems, recent surgery, or pregnancy should also be included.

6. A brief report of physical findings. This report should include vital signs, level of consciousness, the patient's general appearance, and degree of pain. For example, "The patient is alert and responsive and has warm skin. The blood pressure is 132 over 84, the pulse is 72, and ventilations are 14."

7. A brief summary of the care given and any patient response. For example, "We

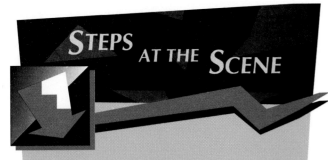

## GIVING THE ON-SCENE ORAL REPORT

☐ Report your unit identification and level of service.

☐ Identify the receiving hospital and your estimated time of arrival.

☐ Give the patient's age and sex. Do not give the patient's name over the radio.

☐ Report the patient's chief complaint or your perception of the problem and its severity.

☐ Give a brief history of the patient's illness or injury. Include all relevant information about the patient's condition.

☐ Give a brief report of physical findings, including vital signs, level of consciousness, general appearance, and degree of pain.

☐ Provide a brief summary of the care given and any patient response.

have immobilized the injured leg in a padded cardboard splint. The patient is now on a backboard. The patient still has motor, sensory, and circulatory function distal to the injured area. He also reports a decrease in pain since the splint was applied."

Be sure you report all patient information in a professional manner. People with scanners are listening. You could be successfully sued for slander if you describe a patient in a way that injures his or her reputation.

## STANDARD PROCEDURES AND PROTOCOLS

Use your radio communications system effectively from the time you acknowledge a call until you complete your run. Standard radio operating procedures are designed to reduce the number of misunderstood messages, to keep transmissions brief, and to develop effective radio discipline. Standard radio communications protocols help both EMT-Bs and dispatchers to communicate properly. Protocols should include the following:

- a preferred format for transmitting messages
- definitions of key words and phrases
- procedures for troubleshooting common radio communications problems

The "call up" from one unit to another begins by identifying the called unit first, followed by the unit calling. For example, "Dispatch, this is Medic One." This exchange alerts the dispatcher to listen for both the identity of the unit calling and the message.

### Guidelines for Effective Radio Communication

1. Monitor the channel before transmitting to avoid interfering with other radio traffic.

2. Plan your message before pushing the transmit switch. This will keep your transmissions brief and precise. You should use a standard format for your transmissions.

3. Press the "push-to-talk" (PTT) button on the radio, then wait for 1 second before

starting your message. By waiting, you can be sure that the transmitter will "power up." Your message has a better chance of being heard clearly if the transmitter is working at full power.

4. Hold the microphone 2" to 3" from your mouth. Speak clearly, but never shout, into the microphone. Speak at a moderate, understandable rate, preferably in a clear, even voice (Figure 13-7).

5. Identify the person or unit you are calling first, then identify your unit as the sender. You will rarely work alone, so say "we" instead of "I" when describing yourself.

6. Acknowledge a transmission as soon as you can by saying "go ahead" or whatever is commonly used in your area. You should say, "over," when you are finished. If you cannot take a long message, simply say "stand by."

7. Use plain English. Avoid meaningless phrases ("Be advised"), slang, or complex codes. Avoid words that are difficult to hear, such as "yes" and "no." Use "affirmative" and "negative."

8. Keep your message brief. If your message takes more than 30 seconds to send, pause after 30 seconds and say, "break." The other party can then ask for clarification, if needed. Also someone else with emergency traffic can break through, if needed.

9. Avoid showing negative emotions, such as anger or irritation, when transmitting. Courtesy is assumed, making it unnecessary to say "please" or "thank you," which wastes air time.

10. When transmitting a number with two or more digits, say the entire number first and then each digit separately. For example, say, "Sixty-seven," followed by "six-seven."

11. Do not use profanity on the radio. This is a violation of FCC rules and can result

## FIGURE 13-7

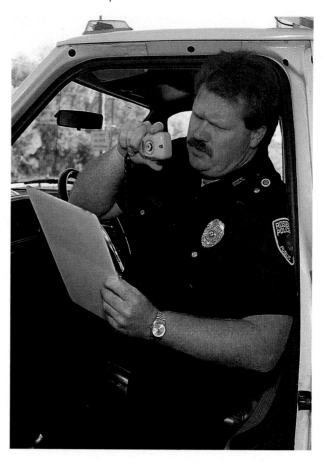

Proper position for holding a radio microphone

in substantial fines and even loss of your radio license.

12. Use EMS frequencies for EMS communications. Do not use these frequencies for any other type of communications.

13. Reduce background noise as much as possible. Move away from wind, noisy motors, or tools. Close the window if you are in a moving ambulance.

## REPORTING REQUIREMENTS

Proper use of the EMS communications system will help you do your job more effectively. From acknowledgment of the call until you are cleared from the medical emergency, you will use radio communications. You must report in to dispatch at least six times during your run, as follows:

1. To acknowledge the dispatch information and to confirm that you are responding to the scene

2. To announce your arrival at the scene

3. To announce that you are leaving the scene and are en route to the receiving hospital (At this point you must state the number of patients transported, your ETA to the hospital, and run status.)

4. To announce your arrival at the hospital or other facility

5. To announce that you are clear of the incident or hospital and available for another assignment

6. To announce your arrival back at quarters or other off the air location

While en route to and from the scene, you should report to the dispatcher special hazards or road conditions that might affect other responding units. Report any unusual delays, such as road blocks or elevated bridges. Once you are at the scene, you may request additional EMS or other public safety assistance, and then help coordinate the response.

During transport, you must periodically reassess the patient's vital signs, overall condition, and response to care provided. You should immediately report any significant changes in the patient's condition, especially if the patient seems worse. Medical control can then give new orders and prepare to receive the patient.

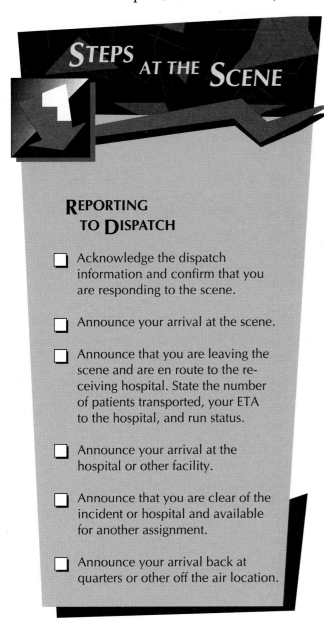

## STEPS AT THE SCENE

### REPORTING TO DISPATCH

☐ Acknowledge the dispatch information and confirm that you are responding to the scene.

☐ Announce your arrival at the scene.

☐ Announce that you are leaving the scene and are en route to the receiving hospital. State the number of patients transported, your ETA to the hospital, and run status.

☐ Announce your arrival at the hospital or other facility.

☐ Announce that you are clear of the incident or hospital and available for another assignment.

☐ Announce your arrival back at quarters or other off the air location.

## MAINTENANCE OF RADIO EQUIPMENT

Like all other EMS equipment, radio equipment must be serviced by properly trained and equipped personnel. Remember that the radio is your lifeline to medical control, and it must perform under emergency conditions. Radio equipment that is operating properly should be serviced at least once a year. Any equipment that is not working properly should be immediately removed from service and sent for repair.

Sometimes radio equipment will stop working during a run. In the worst case scenario, it will stop just as you are trying to consult with medical control about treatment orders. Your EMS system must have several backup plans and options. The goal of a backup plan is to make sure that you can maintain contact with medical control when the usual procedures do not work. There are quite a few options.

The simplest backup plan relies on written standing orders. **Standing orders,** often called protocols, are written documents signed by the EMS system's medical director. These orders outline specific directions, permissions, and sometimes prohibitions regarding patient care (Figure 13-8). When properly followed, standing orders or formal protocols have the same authority and legal status as orders given over the radio. They exist to one extent or another in every EMS system and can be applied to all levels of EMT providers.

## FIGURE 13-8

Standing orders (protocols)

INFECTION CONTROL (cont)                                          VI   4

RECOMMENDED PERSONAL PROTECTION EQUIPMENT FOR WORKER
PROTECTION AGAINST TRANSMISSION OF INFECTION IN PEHOSPITAL SETTING

SKILLS AND/OR PROCEDURES

| TASK/ACTIVITY | GLOVES | GOWN | MASK | GOGGLES |
|---|---|---|---|---|
| Bleeding Control Spurting Blood | YES | YES | YES | YES |
| Bleeding Control Minimal Bleeding | YES | NO | NO | NO |
| Childbirth | YES | YES | YES | YES |
| Blood Drawing | YES | NO | NO | NO |
| Starting IV | YES | NO | NO | NO |
| Intubation ET/EOA | YES | NO | YES | YES |
| Suctioning Oral/Nasal | YES | NO | YES | YES |
| Manual Clearing of Airway | YES | NO | YES | YES |
| Handling & Cleaning Soiled Equipment | YES | YES | NO | NO |
| Giving an Injection | YES | NO | NO | NO |
| Measuring Rectal Temp. | YES | NO | NO | NO |

CONTAGIOUS DISEASES

| DISEASE | GLOVES | GOWN | MASK | GOGGLES |
|---|---|---|---|---|
| Tuberculosis | NO | NO | YES | NO |
| Chicken Pox | YES | YES | YES | NO |
| Meningitis | NO | NO | YES | NO |
| Whooping Cough | NO | NO | YES | NO |

RMH EMS   4/94

# THE ORAL REPORT

Your reporting responsibilities do not end when you arrive at the hospital. In fact, they have just begun. The transfer of care officially occurs during your oral report at the hospital, not as a result of your radio report en route. Once you arrive at the hospital, a hospital staff member will take responsibility of the patient from you. Depending on the hospital and the condition of the patient, the person who takes over the care of the patient varies. However, you can only transfer the care of your patient to someone with at least your level of training.

Once a hospital staff member is ready to take responsibility for the patient, you must provide that person with a formal oral report of the patient's condition (Figure 13-9). Giving a report is a long-standing and well-documented part of transferring the patient's care from one provider to another. Your oral report is usually given at the same time that a hospital staff member is doing something for the patient. For example, a nurse or physician may be looking at the patient, beginning assessment, or helping you to move the patient from the stretcher to an examination table. Therefore, you must report important information in a complete, precise way.

The oral report should include the following six elements:

1. *The patient's name (if you know it) and the mechanism of injury or chief complaint.* For example, "This is Mr. Campbell. His wife told us that he has been acting confused all day."

2. *A summary of the information that you gave in your radio report.* For example, "He has a history of high blood pressure and had a stroke 4 years ago. He has little permanent damage from the stroke. His wife states that he is usually alert and oriented."

## FIGURE 13-9

Giving an oral report at the hospital

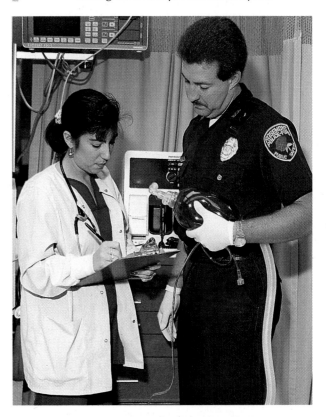

3. *Any important history that was not given already.* For example, "His wife told us that he takes his medicine regularly. On the way in, she told us that Mr. Campbell's medicine was just changed 2 days ago."

4. *Patient response to treatment given en route.* It is especially important to report any changes in the patient or the treatment provided since your radio report. For example, "We started oxygen by face mask at 10 L/min. His LOC improved and he started to fight the mask. We were able to get him to hold the mask next to his mouth and nose for the rest of the trip."

5. *The vital signs assessed during transport and after the radio report.* For example, "His vitals during transport were blood pressure 184 over 110, pulse 96, ventilations 22. They are generally unchanged since we reported earlier."

6. *Any other information you may have gathered that was not important enough to report sooner.* Information gathered during transport, any patient medications you have brought with you, and any other details about the patient provided by family members or friends may be included. For example, "Mrs. Jones' husband rode in with us. Her daughter is coming from home and should be here soon."

## THE WRITTEN REPORT

Along with your radio report and oral report, you must also complete a formal written report about the patient before you leave the hospital. You may be able to do the written report en route, if the trip is long enough and the patient needs minimal care. Usually you will finish the written report after you have transferred the care of the patient to a hospital staff member (Figure 13-10). Be sure to leave the report at the hospital before you leave.

### MINIMUM DATA SET

The information you collect during a call becomes part of the data set. The minimum data set includes both patient information and administrative information.

The patient information included in the minimum data set should be as follows:

- chief complaint
- level of consciousness (AVPU) or mental status
- systolic blood pressure for patients older than 3 years
- capillary refill for patients younger than 6 years
- skin color and temperature
- pulse
- respiratory rate and effort

The administrative information included in the minimum data set should be as follows:

- time that the incident was reported
- time that the EMS unit was notified
- time that the EMS unit arrived at the scene
- time that the EMS unit left the scene
- time that the EMS unit arrived at the receiving facility
- time that patient care was transferred

You will begin gathering the patient information as soon as you reach the patient. Continue collecting information as you provide care, until you arrive at the hospital.

### PREHOSPITAL CARE REPORT

Prehospital care reports help to ensure efficient continuity of patient care. This report describes the nature of the patient's injuries or illness at the scene and the initial treatment you provide. While this report may not be read immediately at the hospital, it may very well be referred to later for important information.

The prehospital care report has the following six functions:

1. continuity of care
2. legal documentation
3. education
4. administrative
5. research
6. evaluation and continuous quality improvement

A good prehospital care report documents the care that was provided and the patient's condition on arrival at the scene. It also documents any changes in the patient's condition upon arrival at the hospital. The information in the report also serves to prove

# FIGURE 13-10

A written report

that you have provided proper documentation. In some instances, it also shows that you have properly handled unusual or uncommon situations. Both objective and subjective information are included in this report. *It is critical that you document everything in the clearest manner possible.* If a patient brings legal action against you, you and your prehospital care report will have to go to court.

These reports also provide valuable administrative information. For example, the report provides information for patient billing. It can also be used to evaluate response times, equipment usage, and other areas of administrative responsibility.

Data may be obtained from the prehospital care forms to analyze causes, severity, and types of illness or injury requiring emergency medical care. These reports may also be used in an on-going program for evaluation of the quality of patient care. All records are reviewed periodically by your system. The purpose of this review is to make sure that trauma triage and/or other prehospital care criteria have been met.

There are many requirements on a prehospital care report. Often, these requirements vary from jurisdiction to jurisdiction, mainly because so many agencies obtain information from them. There is no universally accepted form. However, all forms should include at least the following information:

- patient's name, sex, date of birth, and address
- nature of call
- mechanism of injury
- location of patient when first seen (specific details noted, especially if incident is a car accident or criminal activity is suspected)
- rescue and treatment given prior to your arrival
- signs and symptoms found during your patient assessment

- care and treatment given at site and during transport
- baseline vital signs
- SAMPLE history
- changes in vital signs and condition
- date of call
- time of call
- the location of the call
- time of dispatch
- time of arrival at scene
- time of leaving the scene
- time of arrival at hospital
- patient's insurance information
- names and/or certification numbers of EMT-Bs responding to call
- the base hospital involved in the run
- type of run to scene, emergency/routine

## TYPES OF FORMS

You will most likely use one of two types of forms. The first type is the traditional written form with check boxes and a narrative section. The second type is a computerized version in which you fill in information using an electronic clipboard or similar device (Figure 13-11). If your service uses written forms, be sure to fill in the boxes completely and avoid making stray marks on the sheet. Make sure you are familiar with the specific procedures for collecting, recording, and reporting the information in your area.

If you must complete a narrative section, be sure to describe what you see and what you do. Be sure to include significant negative findings and important observations about the scene. Do not record your conclusions about the incident. For example, you may write, "The patient's breath smelled of alcohol." This is a clear description that does not make any judgments about the patient's condition. However, a report that says, "The patient was drunk,"makes a conclusion about the patient's condition. Also avoid radio codes and use only standard abbreviations. When information is of a sensitive nature, note the source of the information. Be sure to spell words correctly, especially medical terms. If you do not know how to spell a particular word, find out how to spell it, or use another word. Also be sure to record the time with all assessment findings.

Remember that the report form itself and all the information on it are considered confidential documents. Be sure to be familiar with state and local laws concerning confidentiality. All prehospital forms must be handled with care and stored in an appropriate manner once you complete them. After you have completed a report, distribute the copies to the appropriate locations, according to state and local protocol. In most instances, a copy of the report will remain at the hospital and will become a part of the patient's record.

## REPORTING ERRORS

Everyone makes mistakes. If you leave something out of a report, or record information incorrectly, do not try to cover it up. Rather, write down what did or did not happen, and the steps that were taken to correct the situation. Falsifying information on the prehospital report may result in suspension or revocation of your certification/license. More importantly, falsifying information results in poor patient care, because other health care providers have a false impression of assessment findings or the treatment given. Document only those vital signs that were actually taken. If you did not give the patient oxygen, do not chart that the patient was given oxygen.

## FIGURE 13-11

An electronic report

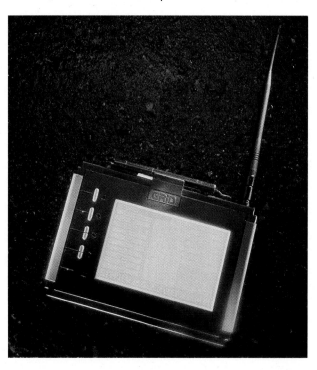

If you discover errors as you are writing your report, draw a single horizontal line through the error, initial it, and write the correct information next to it (Figure 13-12).

## FIGURE 13-12

Correcting an error on a written report

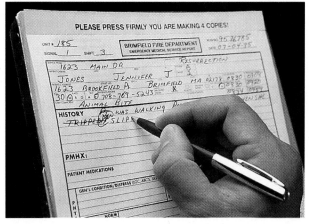

cross with one line only
& put initials next to it
& date it

Do not try to erase or cover the error with correction fluid. This may be interpreted as an attempt to cover up a mistake.

If errors are discovered after you submit your report, draw a single line through the error, preferably in a different color ink, initial, and date it. Make sure to add a note with the correct information. If you left out information accidentally, add a note with the correct information, the date, and your initials.

When you do not have enough time to complete your report before the next call, you will need to fill it out later.

## DOCUMENTING RIGHT OF REFUSAL

Competent adult patients have the right to refuse treatment. If you are faced with this situation, you must inform medical control immediately. Before you leave the scene, try to persuade the patient to go to the hospital and consult medical direction as directed by local protocol. Also make sure that the patient is able to make a rational, informed decision and is not under the influence of alcohol or other drugs or illness/injury effects. Explain to the patient why it is important to be examined by a physician at the hospital. Also explain what may happen if the patient is not examined by a physician. If the patient still refuses, suggest other means for the patient to obtain proper care. Explain that you are willing to return. If the patient still refuses, document any assessment findings and emergency medical care given, then have the patient sign a refusal form. You must also have a family member, police officer, or bystander sign the form as a witness. If the patient refuses to sign the refusal form, have a family member, police officer, or bystander sign the form verifying that the patient refused to sign.

Be sure to complete the prehospital report, including the patient assessment findings. Also include the care you wished to provide for the patient. You must also in-clude a statement explaining that you informed the patient about the possible consequences of failure to accept care, including potential death, and alternative methods of obtaining care you suggested.

## SPECIAL REPORTING SITUATIONS

In some instances, you may be required to file special reports with appropriate authorities. These may include incidents involving gunshot wounds, dog bites, certain infectious diseases, suspected physical, sexual, or substance abuse. Learn your local requirements for reporting these incidents. Failure to report them may have legal consequences. It is important that the report is accurate, objective, and submitted in a timely manner. Also remember to keep a copy for your own records.

Another special reporting situation is a multiple-casualty incident (MCI). The local MCI plan should have some means of recording important medical information temporarily (triage tag that can be used later to complete the form). The standard for completing the form in an MCI is not the same as for a typical call. Your local plan should have specific guidelines.

# INTERPERSONAL COMMUNICATIONS

## COMMUNICATIONS SKILLS

As an EMT-B, you must master many communications skills, including radio operations, verbal communications, and written reports. Your skill in communicating with the patient and the rest of the team has a great impact on the quality of patient care. You must be able to find out what the patient needs and then tell others on the team. *Remember you are the vital link between the patient and medical control.* As an EMT-B, you must learn the following communications skills:

- good judgment and common sense at all times

- the ability to concentrate, listen, and follow instructions and protocols

- the ability to speak so that others can understand you

- familiarity and ability to use all the communications tools available in the EMS system

These tools include the radio, telephone, vehicle lights, siren and PA system, hand signals, and written messages and reports.

Remember that someone who is sick or injured is scared and may not understand what you are doing and saying. Therefore, your gestures, body movements, and attitude toward the patient are critically important in gaining a patient's trust. These Ten Golden Rules will help you to calm and reassure your patients.

### Ten Golden Rules of Patient Interaction

1. *Make and keep eye contact with your patient at all times.* Give the patient your undivided attention. This will let the patient know that he or she is your top priority. Look the patient straight in the eye to establish rapport. Establishing **rapport** is building a trusting relationship with your patient. This will make the job of caring for the patient much easier for both you and the patient.

2. *Tell the patient the truth.* Even if you have to say something very unpleasant, telling the truth is better than lying. Lying will destroy the patient's trust in you and decreases your own confidence. You may not always tell the patient everything, but if the patient or a family member asks a specific question you should answer truthfully. A direct question deserves a direct answer. If you do not know the answer to the patient's question, say so. For example, a patient may ask, "Am I having a heart attack?" "I don't know" is an adequate answer.

3. *Use language that the patient can understand.* Do not talk up or talk down to the patient in any way. Avoid technical medical terms that the patient may not understand. Instead, ask the patient if he or she has a history of "heart problems." This will usually result in more accurate information than if you ask about "previous episodes of myocardial infarction" or a "history of cardiomyopathy."

4. *Be careful of what you say about the patient to others.* A patient may hear only part of what is said. As a result, the patient may seriously misinterpret (and remember for a long time) what was said. Therefore, assume that the patient can hear every word you say, even if you are speaking to others and even if the patient appears to be unconscious or unresponsive.

5. *Be aware of your body language.* Nonverbal communication is extremely important in dealing with patients. In stressful situations, patients may misinterpret your gestures and movements. Be particularly careful not to appear threatening. Instead, position yourself at a level lower than the patient, when practical. Remember that you should always, always conduct yourself in a calm, professional manner.

6. *Always speak slowly, clearly, and distinctly.*

7. *Use the patient's proper name when you know it.* Ask the patient what he or she wishes to be called. Do not use terms

## FIGURE 13-13

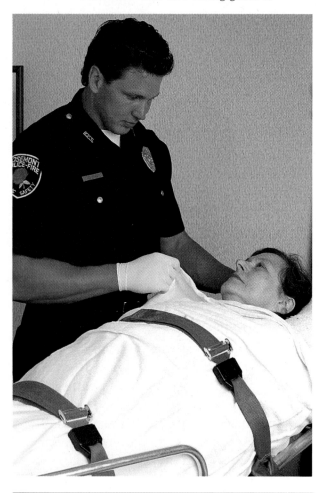

Use kind words and caring gestures

such as "Pops," "Lady," "Kid," or "Dear." Avoid using a patient's first name, except if the patient is a child or if the patient asks you to use his or her first name. Rather, use what is called a courtesy title, such as Mr. Peters, Mrs. Garoni, Ms. Butler.

8. *If the patient is hearing impaired, speak clearly and face the person so that he or she can read your lips.* Do not shout at a person who is hearing impaired. Shouting will not make it any easier for the patient to understand you. Instead, it may frighten the patient and make it even more difficult to understand you. Never

assume that an elderly patient is hearing impaired or otherwise unable to understand you. Also, never use baby talk with elderly patients.

9. *Allow time for the patient to answer or respond to your questions.* Do not rush a patient unless there is immediate danger. Sick and injured people may not be thinking clearly and may need time to answer even simple questions.

10. *Act and speak in a calm, confident manner while caring for the patient.* Make sure you attend to the patient's pains and needs. Try to make the patient physically comfortable and relaxed (Figure 13-13). Find out if the patient is more comfortable sitting or lying down. Is the patient cold or hot? Does the patient want a friend or relative nearby?

Patients literally place their lives in your hands. They deserve to know that you can provide medical care and that you are also concerned about their well-being.

## COMMUNICATING WITH ELDERLY PATIENTS

By the year 2000, about 13% of the U.S. population will be considered geriatric, or over 65 years old. A person's actual age may not be the most important factor in making him or her "elderly." More important to determine is a person's functional age. The functional age relates more to the person's ability to function in daily activities, the person's mental state and activity pattern.

Most elderly people think clearly, can give you a clear medical history, and can answer your questions. **Do NOT assume that an elderly patient is senile or confused.** Remember, though, that communicating with some elderly patients is extremely difficult. Some may be hostile, unkempt, irritable, and/or confused. You need great patience and compassion when you are called upon to

## THEY AREN'T JUST WORDS

You are dispatched for a routine transfer to take a patient from General Hospital back to the Golden Years extended-care facility. Your patient is an 82-year-old woman who was admitted 2 days ago for a possible obstructed bowel. The 1/2-mile trip to Golden Years takes a couple of minutes. You pour a cup of coffee while your partner fills out the prehospital care report. As she writes in the vital signs, she comments, "Those will work." When you question her, she admits that she regularly makes up vitals on patients returning home from the hospital. "After all," she says, "they are going home from the hospital. They are supposed to be better. Besides taking their vital signs is a waste of time."

### For Discussion

1. Why would a set of vital signs and a brief assessment be indicated for a patient returning from the hospital?

2. Describe some of the problems that might result if false or fabricated vital signs are recorded on a prehospital care report?

care for such a patient. Think of the patient as someone's grandmother or grandfather, or even yourself when you reach that age.

Approach an elderly patient slowly and calmly. Allow plenty of time for the patient to respond to your questions. Watch for signs of confusion, anxiety, or impaired hearing or vision. The patient should feel confident that you are in charge and that everything possible is being done for him or her.

Elderly patients often do not feel much pain. An elderly person who has fainted or has difficulty breathing may report no pain. Even minor changes in breathing or mental state may signal major problems.

Remember to attend to an elderly patient's family members and friends. Seeing his or her loved one taken away in an ambulance can be a particularly frightening experience. Take a few minutes to explain to an elderly patient's spouse or family what is being done and why such action is being taken.

### COMMUNICATING WITH CHILDREN

Everyone who is thrust into an emergency situation becomes frightened to some degree.

However, fear is probably most severe and most obvious in children. Children may be frightened by your uniform, the ambulance, and by the number of people who have suddenly gathered around. Even a child who says little may be very much aware of all that is going on.

Familiar objects and faces will help to reduce this fright. Let a child keep a favorite toy, doll, or security blanket to give the child some sense of security and a lot of comfort. Having a family member or friend nearby is also helpful. However, you will have to make sure this person will not upset the child. Sometimes adult family members are not helpful because they become too upset by what has happened. An overly anxious parent or relative can only make things worse. Be careful about selecting the proper adult for this role.

Children can easily see through lies or deceptions, so you must always be honest with them. Make sure you explain to the child over and over again what and why certain things are happening. If treatment is going to hurt, such as applying a splint, tell the child ahead of time. Also tell the child that it will not hurt for long and that it will help "make it better."

***Respect a child's modesty.*** Both little girls and little boys are embarrassed if they have to undress or be undressed in front of strangers. When a wound or site of injury has to be exposed, try to do so out of sight of strangers. Again, it is extremely important to tell the child what you are doing and why you are doing it.

You should speak to a child in a professional, yet friendly, way. A child should feel reassured that you are there to help in every way possible. Maintain eye contact with a child, as you would with an adult, to let the child know that you are helping and that you can be trusted. It is helpful to position yourself to their level so that you do not appear to tower above them.

## COMMUNICATING WITH HEARING-IMPAIRED PATIENTS

Patients who are hearing impaired or deaf are rarely ashamed or embarrassed by their disability. Often it is the people around a deaf or hearing-impaired person who have the problem coping. Remember that you must be able to communicate with hearing-impaired patients so that you can provide necessary or even lifesaving care.

First, you should always assume that hearing-impaired patients have normal intelligence. These patients can usually understand what is going on around them, provided that you can successfully communicate with them. Second, most patients who are hearing impaired can read lips to some extent. Therefore, you should place yourself in a position so that the patient can see your lips. Third, many hearing-impaired patients have hearing aids that may have been lost in an accident or fall. Hearing aids may also be forgotten if the patient is confused or ill. Look around or ask the patient or the family about a hearing aid.

Remember the following five steps to help you efficiently communicate with patients who are hearing impaired:

1. *Make sure you have paper and a pen.* This way you can write down questions and the patient can write down answers, if necessary. Make sure you print so that your handwriting is not a communications barrier.

2. *If the patient can read lips, you should speak slowly, clearly, and distinctly.* Do not cover your mouth or mumble.

3. *Never shout!*

4. *Make sure you listen carefully, ask short questions, and give short answers.* Remember that although many hearing-impaired patients can speak distinctly, some cannot.

5. *Learn some simple phrases used in sign language.* For example, knowing the signs for "sick," "hurt," and "help" may be useful if you cannot communicate in any other way.

## COMMUNICATING WITH VISUALLY IMPAIRED PATIENTS

Like hearing-impaired patients, visually impaired and blind patients have usually accepted and learned to deal with their disability. Of course, not all visually impaired patients are completely blind. Many can perceive light and dark, or can see shadows or movement. Ask the patient whether he or she can see at all. Also remember that as with other patients who have disabilities, you should expect that visually impaired patients have normal intelligence.

As you begin caring for a visually impaired patient, explain everything you are doing in detail as you are doing it. Make sure that you stay in physical contact with the patient as you begin your care. Hold your hand lightly on the patient's shoulder or arm. Try to avoid sudden movements. If the patient can walk to the ambulance, place his or her hand on your arm, taking care not to rush. Transport any mobility aids, such as a cane, with the patient to the hospital.

A visually impaired person may have a guide dog. Guide dogs are easily identified by their special harnesses. They are trained not to leave their masters and not to respond to strangers. A visually impaired patient who is conscious can tell you about the dog and give instructions for its care. If circumstances permit, bring the guide dog to the hospital with the patient. If the dog has to be left behind, you should arrange for its care.

## COMMUNICATING WITH NON-ENGLISH-SPEAKING PATIENTS

As part of the focused physical exam, you must obtain a medical history from the patient. You cannot skip this step simply because the patient does not speak English. Most patients who do not speak English fluently will still know certain important words or phrases.

Your first step is to find out how much English the patient can speak. Use short, simple questions and simple words whenever possible. Avoid difficult medical terms. You can help patients to better understand if you point to specific parts of the body as you ask questions.

In many areas, particularly large urban centers, major segments of the population do not speak English. Your job will be much easier if you learn some common words and phrases in their language, especially common medical terms. Pocket cards are available that show the pronunciation of these terms. If the patient does not speak any English, find a family member or friend to act as an interpreter.

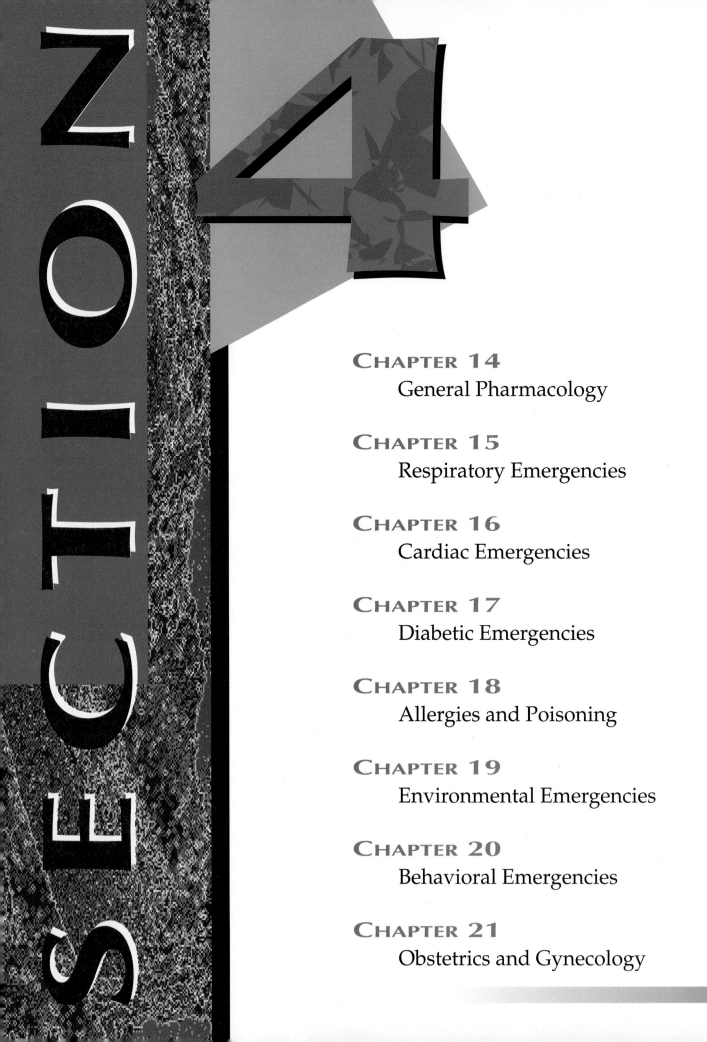

# SECTION 4

# Medical Emergencies

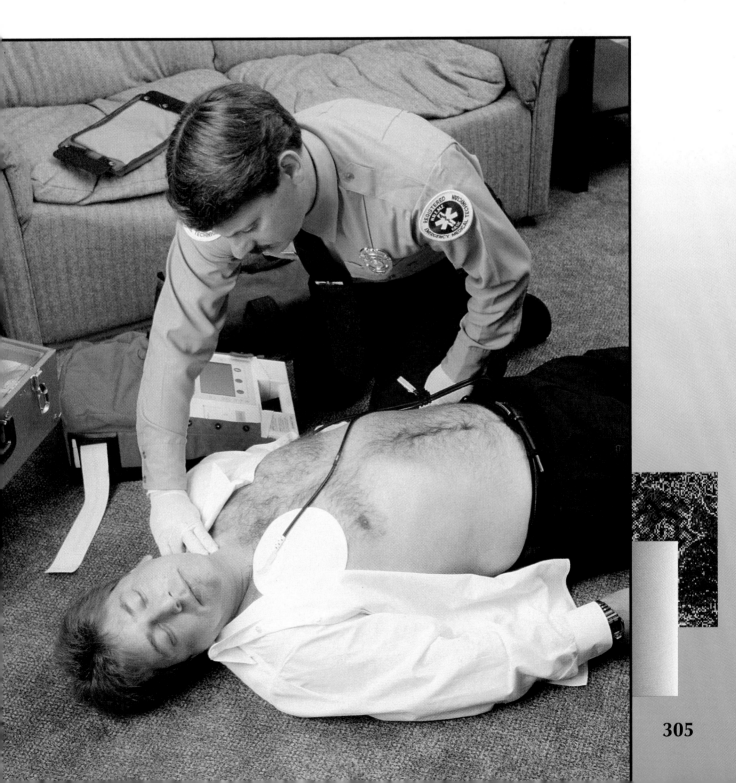

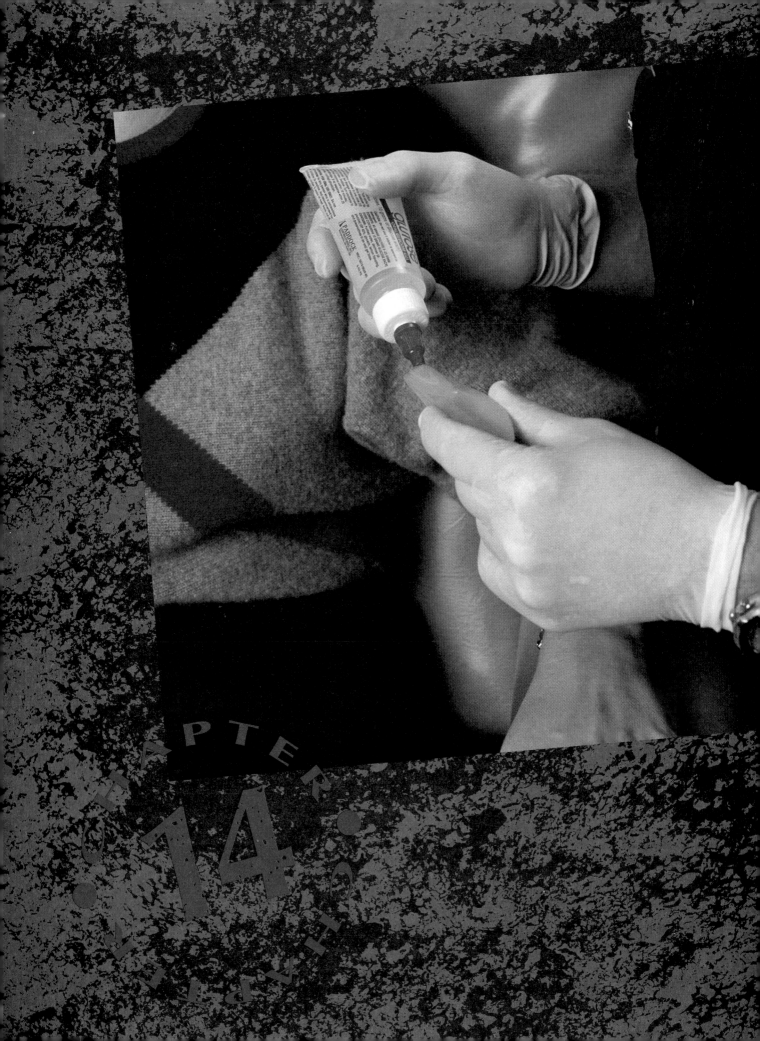

# CHAPTER 14

# General Pharmacology

## Objectives

After you have read this chapter, you should be able to:

- Identify which medications will be carried on the unit.
- List the medications carried on the unit and those you may help administer by generic name.
- Identify the medications that you may help the patient administer.
- Discuss the forms in which medications may be found.

## Overview

Pharmacology is the study of drugs and medications. While you will administer only a limited number of medications, it is useful to have a general understanding of medications. A patient's history may include medications. In some cases, you will be able to assess the situation more easily because you know something about the medications involved. You must also report the patient's medication history to hospital personnel.

Understanding how certain medications work will help you use them more effectively. Plus, you will understand why you are authorized to administer those medications.

This chapter begins with a general discussion of where medications work and how that affects the way they are manufactured and given. You will then learn more detail about the medications you can carry on the unit and those you may help the patient administer.

# Key Terms

**Absorption**   The process by which medications travel through body tissues until they reach the bloodstream.

**Actions**   The effects that a drug is expected to have on the patient's body.

**Contraindications**   Situations in which a drug should not be given because it would either harm the patient or have no positive effect on the patient's condition.

**Dose**   The amount of the drug that is given.

**Generic name**   The name of a drug as listed in *United States Pharmacopoeia;* also generally the simple chemical name.

**Indications**   The most common uses of a drug in treating a specific illness.

**Intramuscular (IM)**   The injection of medication into muscle tissue.

**Intravenous (IV)**   The injection of medication into the blood through the wall of a vein.

**Metered-dose inhaler**   A miniature spray can designed to deliver medica-

tions inhaled into the lungs. Each use delivers the same dose.

**Side effects**   Any actions of a drug other than the desired effect.

**Solution**   A liquid containing dissolved medication, which generally passes through a filter and does not settle. Solutions do not need to be shaken.

**Subcutaneous (SC)**   The injection of a medication into the tissue between the skin and the muscle.

**Sublingual (SL)**   Medications placed under the tongue that are absorbed through the mucous membranes.

**Suspension**   A liquid containing particles of medication, which will generally settle when left standing. Suspensions need to be shaken.

**Trade name**   The brand name a manufacturer gives a drug.

**Transdermal**   Medication absorbed through the skin (topically). With transdermal patches, the medication is in direct contact with the skin until it is absorbed into the blood.

# HOW MEDICATIONS WORK

Like any tool, medications perform certain jobs. Some medications work in specific areas of the body. Given the proper dose, most medications use the body's circulatory system to reach the right job site. A **dose** is the amount of the drug that is given. **Actions** are the effects that a drug is expected to have on the patient's body. For example, nitroglycerin relaxes the walls of the blood vessels, dilating the coronary arteries. This is important during a common cardiac emergency called angina. Angina is characterized by squeezing or crushing pain in the chest. The actions of nitroglycerin increase blood flow, and ultimately the supply of oxygen, to the heart muscle. This relieves the pain that occurs with angina. Because nitroglycerin has this effect, its use is **indicated** for chest pain associated with angina.

Administering medications is certainly helpful in many situations. However, there are times when you should not give a patient medication, even if the medication is indicated for the patient's condition. These situations are called contraindications. **Contraindications** are situations in which a drug should not be given because it would either harm the patient or have no positive effect on the patient's condition. For example, giving activated charcoal is indicated in instances where a patient has swallowed a poison. Generally, activated charcoal premixed with water is given to prevent a poison from being absorbed by the body. However, giving activated charcoal would be contraindicated if the patient is unconscious and could not swallow. Activated charcoal may cause vomiting, especially if the patient already has nausea. In this case, the vomiting is a side effect of the activated charcoal. **Side effects** are any actions of a drug other than the desired effect.

# ROUTES OF ADMINISTRATION

**Absorption** is the process by which medications travel through body tissues until they reach the bloodstream. Sometimes a medication must enter the blood immediately, so it is injected directly into a vein. This is called an **intravenous (IV)** injection. Medications that enter the blood via any other route of administration are absorbed.

Many medications are quickly absorbed when injected into a muscle. This is called an **intramuscular (IM)** injection, because muscles have a lot of blood vessels. However, some medications irritate or damage tissues when they are injected into a muscle. Some are absorbed well if they are injected into the tissue between the patient's muscle and skin. This is called a **subcutaneous (SC)** injection. Because the blood flow is not as great here as in a muscle, absorption will generally be slower and the effect more prolonged. However, if a medication does not irritate or damage the tissue, an SC injection is a useful way to administer medications that cannot be taken by mouth.

Most medications enter the bloodstream through the digestive system. The majority of these are given by mouth (PO). However, many medications can also be absorbed from the rectum, so some are given per rectum (PR). Most medications given by mouth are absorbed in the small intestine. This generally means it will take at least 1 hour before absorption begins.

Some medications cannot survive the stomach's acid or passing through the liver when taken by mouth. One alternative is to place the medication where it can be absorbed through the skin (topically) or mucous membranes. Several medications are marketed in **transdermal** patches. With these patches, the medication is in direct contact with the skin until it is absorbed into the blood. Medications absorbed through the mucous membranes are commonly placed under the tongue. This **sublingual (SL)** route not only protects medications from the digestive system but also gets them into the bloodstream quickly.

A final route of administration is inhalation. Some medications are inhaled into the lungs to get them into the blood. Others are inhaled because they work in the lungs. Sometimes inhalation is preferred because it produces an effect quickly; other times, because it minimizes the effects in other body tissues.

## MEDICATION NAMES

A medication may have many different names, which may be a bit confusing for you at first. Medications are often known by their well-known trade name, such as Valium or Tylenol. A **trade name** is the brand name a manufacturer gives the drug. We are used to trade names in every aspect of our daily lives. For example, we know Jell-O gelatin, Band-Aid adhesive bandages,

and Life Savers candy. Thus, you may hear many different trade names for the same drug. You may also hear about drugs that are OTC. This means over-the-counter drugs that do not require a physician's prescription.

Drugs also have generic names. A drug's **generic name** is the name listed in the *United States Pharmacopoeia*, a governmental publication that lists all the drugs in the United States. The generic name of a drug is commonly its simple chemical name. Sometimes a drug is referred to by its generic name more often than one of its many trade names. For example, you may hear "charcoal" more often than the many trade names for activated charcoal, such as Actidose. Tables 14-1 and 14-2 provide a listing of the generic and common trade names for medications you will likely administer as an EMT-B. Of course, the list is not comprehensive, especially if you can administer other medications as your local protocol allows.

## TABLE 14-1    MEDICATIONS CARRIED ON THE UNIT

| Generic name | Trade name(s) | Dosage form(s) | Condition(s) |
|---|---|---|---|
| Activated charcoal | SuperChar, InstaChar, Actidose, LiquiChar | Suspension | Poisoning/overdose |
| Oral glucose | Glutose, Insta-glucose | Oral gel | Diabetic emergencies |
| Oxygen | — | Compressed gas | Variety of conditions |

**TABLE 14-2**      MEDICATIONS YOU MAY HELP ADMINISTER

| Generic name | Trade name(s) | Dosage form(s) | Condition(s) |
|---|---|---|---|
| Epinephrine | Adrenalin | IM, SC | Allergic reactions |
| Albuterol | Proventil, Ventolin | Inhaler | Asthma |
| Metaproterenol | Alupent, Metaprel | Inhaler | Asthma |
| Isoetharine | Bronkosol, Bronkometer | Inhaler | Asthma |
| Nitroglycerin | Nitrobid, Nitrony, Nitrostat | SL tablet or spray | Cardiac emergencies |

# DOSAGE FORMS OF MEDICATION

## TABLETS AND CAPSULES

Most medications given by mouth to adult patients are in tablet or capsule form. Capsules are gelatin shells filled with powdered or liquid medication. If the capsule contains liquid, the shell is sealed and generally soft. Most capsules that contain powder can be pulled apart, allowing the medication to spill out (Figure 14-1). Tablets often mix medications with other materials, which are compressed under high pressure. Some tablets are designed to dissolve very quickly in small amounts of liquid so they can be given sublingually.

It is important for you to remember that medications taken by mouth need time to be absorbed. Thus, it generally does not make sense to ask a patient to swallow a medication in an emergency. Also remember that, if a patient is likely to need surgery, his or her stomach should be empty.

## FIGURE 14-1

Tablets and capsules

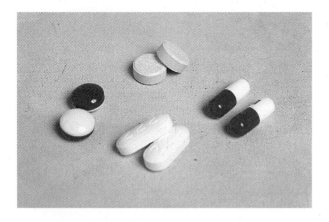

## FIGURE 14-2

A metered-dose inhaler

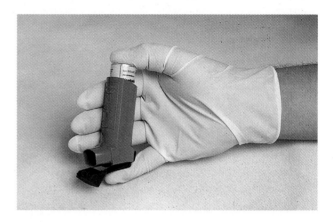

## SOLUTIONS AND SUSPENSIONS

When one or more substances are mixed into a liquid and cannot be separated by filtering or by letting the mixture stand, it is called a **solution.** Solutions can be given by almost any route. When given by mouth, solutions may be absorbed from the stomach quickly because the drug is already dissolved. Many solutions can be given in an IV, IM, or SC injection. If they are irritating to the stomach, solutions might also be given rectally or topically, sprayed sublingually or into the airway, where the solution is inhaled.

Many substances do not dissolve well in liquids. Some can be ground into fine particles and then evenly distributed throughout a liquid when shaken or stirred. This type of mixture is called a **suspension.** Suspensions separate if they stand or are filtered so it is important for you to shake or swirl a suspension before it is administered. If you don't, the patient might not get the right amount of medication in the measured liquid. Activated charcoal is commonly given as a suspension or a slurry.

Suspensions are commonly administered by mouth. However, they are sometimes given rectally and are occasionally used to treat skin problems. Suspensions cannot be given IV. Injectable suspensions are intended only for IM or SC use.

## INHALERS AND TOPICAL MEDICATIONS

If liquids (or solids) are broken into small enough droplets (or particles), they can be inhaled. **Metered-dose inhalers** are miniature spray cans that have two tasks: 1) to spray droplets that travel into the lungs when inhaled through the mouth, and 2) to spray the same amount of medication each time (Figure 14-2).

Most creams and ointments are intended to work directly on the skin. However, others are absorbed into the bloodstream from the skin, especially if the medication is covered. Adhesive patches, which are attached to the skin, allow controlled absorption of a drug.

## MEDICATION MYSTERY

Your unit is returning to quarters when dispatch requests that you respond to the No Tell Motel for a "sick man." On arrival, you stop at the front desk and are directed down a dark, dingy hall to room #9. Inside you find a messy 49-year-old man lying on a bed in a dried puddle of vomit. He says he is sick and wants to go to the hospital, but first he wants you to find his medications. He has slurred speech and his breath odor suggests that he's been drinking. However, when you ask him about drinking today, he denies it. A search of his room turns up a large pill bottle with no label. He asks you to open it and get out a yellow pill and a small white pill and give them to him.

### For Discussion

1. Why is it essential to have a fundamental knowledge of any drug before you give it to a patient?

2. What is the importance of checking expiration dates on a drug before you give it to a patient?

## MEDICATIONS CARRIED ON THE UNIT

As an EMT-B, you will carry three medications on the unit so you can give them in life-threatening emergencies. Your local protocols may authorize you to carry and administer other medications as well.

### OXYGEN

If a patient is not breathing, or is having trouble getting air into the lungs, you should give supplemental oxygen. In general, you will give oxygen via nasal cannula and nonrebreathing mask. However, you may encounter other devices, such as a simple face mask or a Venturi mask during transports between medical facilities. The nonrebreathing mask is the preferred way of giving oxygen in the prehospital setting. With a good mask to mouth seal, it is capable of providing up to 95% inspired oxygen. With a nasal cannula, oxygen flows through two small, tube-like prongs that fit into the patient's nostrils. A nasal cannula can provide 35% to 50% inspired oxygen if the flowmeter is set at 6 to 7 L per minute. Specific instructions for giving oxygen are presented in chapter 9, Airway Adjuncts and Oxygen Equipment.

Also remember that there are hazards associated with giving oxygen. Oxygen does not burn—it allows other things to burn. Thus, it is easier for an object to burn when there is extra oxygen in the air around it. For this reason, make sure there are no open flames, lit cigarettes, or sparks in the area where you are administering oxygen. Otherwise, your patient's clothing and blankets, which could be saturated with oxygen, might burst into flame if exposed to these triggers.

## ACTIVATED CHARCOAL

Of the poisoning emergencies you will encounter, many will involve overdoses of drugs taken by mouth. Fortunately, many drugs bind (stick to the surface) to activated charcoal, preventing the drug from being absorbed by the body. Activated charcoal is ground into a very fine powder to provide the greatest possible surface area. You will likely carry a container with a premixed suspension of activated charcoal powder and water.

When drugs "adsorb" (stick to the surface), it is not a permanent attachment. If activated charcoal remains in the digestive system through a normal 1-day digestive process, the drug may break free and be absorbed into the bloodstream. That is why activated charcoal is given as a suspension. It is usually suspended as a concentrated solution that acts as a laxative. Thus, it causes the entire suspension to move through the digestive system quickly.

Activated charcoal is given in suspension, by mouth, for many poisonings or drug overdoses. While sorbitol sweetens the suspension, the charcoal's black color makes the fluid look unappealing (Figure 14-3). For

**FIGURE 14-3**

Activated charcoal

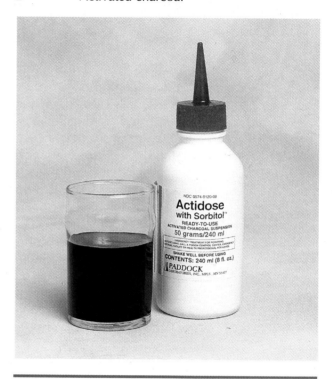

this reason, you should use a covered container and have the patient drink the fluid through a straw so he or she can't see it. Specific instructions for giving activated charcoal are presented in chapter 18, Allergies and Poisoning.

## ORAL GLUCOSE

Glucose is a sugar that our cells use as fuel. While some cells can use other sugars, brain cells must have glucose. Patients whose blood glucose (blood sugar) level gets too low can lose consciousness, convulse, and die.

Hypoglycemia is the medical term for an excessively low blood glucose level. One cause of this condition may be an insulin reaction. This occurs when a patient who takes insulin to control blood glucose levels injects too much, given the combination of food and exercise in subsequent hours.

Oral glucose can counter the effects of hypoglycemia. The advantage of glucose over other sugars is that it is a "simple" sugar. Common table sugar, or sucrose, on the other hand, is a double sugar and must be split before it can be absorbed. Glucose, however, is ready for the body to use and is more rapidly absorbed.

Hospital personnel can give glucose through an IV line. In the prehospital setting, you will give glucose by mouth (Figure 14-4). There are glucose gels, which are basically thick solutions. The gels were developed to be spread on the mucous membranes between the cheek and the gum. However, this absorption is not reliable so it is better to have a conscious hypoglycemic patient, who is able to swallow, take the glucose by mouth. Specific instructions for giving oral glucose are presented in chapter 17, Diabetic Emergencies.

## MEDICATIONS YOU MAY HELP ADMINISTER

### EPINEPHRINE

Epinephrine is the principal hormone for the body's fight or flight response. Because it is secreted by the adrenal glands, it is also known as adrenaline. Epinephrine has many effects on different body tissues and is used as a medicine in several forms.

#### Administering by Metered-Dose Inhaler

Another condition that excessively constricts the airways is asthma. Asthma, which can be a life-threatening condition, is also known as "reactive airway disease." Inhaling epinephrine can help relieve this condition. Thus, some patients use epinephrine inhalers, such as Primatene Mist, Bronitin Mist, Bronkaid Mist, and Medihaler-Epi.

**FIGURE 14-4**

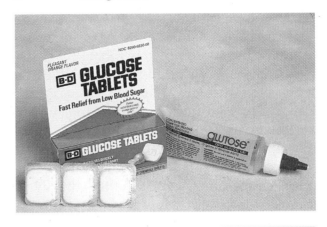

Oral glucose

Remember, though, epinephrine tends to increase heart rate. Thus, most people suffering from asthma have prescriptions for chemical cousins of epinephrine. Designed to produce fewer side effects, the most widely used substitutes are metaproterenol (Alupent or Metaprel) and albuterol (Proventil or Ventolin). These and others—terbutaline (Brethaire), bitolterol (Tornalate) and isoproterenol (Isuprel or Medihaler-Iso)—specifically relieve asthma symptoms. Other medications help prevent asthma. These include anti-inflammatory steroids like beclomethasone (Vanceril or Beclovent), flunisolide (Aerobid), and triamcinolone (Azmacort). All of these medications are available in metered-dose inhalers.

Patients with asthma can generally inhale, but they have difficulty exhaling. Wheezing is a common sign. As you can imagine, patients with asthma experience a great deal of distress. On top of this, using the inhaler requires a great deal of coordination. The patient must aim properly and spray just as he or she starts to inhale. If the patient uses the adapter, which fits over the inhaler like a sleeve, most of the medication often ends up on the roof of the mouth. For this reason, many patients are prescribed "spacer" devices (Figure 14-5). The inhaler fits into an opening on one end of the spacer's chamber. There is a mouthpiece on the other end. With this device, the patient can spray the prescribed dose into the chamber and then breathe in and out of the chamber until the mist is completely inhaled.

If the patient does not have this device, you can improvise a spacer by using the cardboard tube from a roll of paper towels or toilet paper. Have the patient open his or her lips inside one end of the tube. Place the adapter on the inhaler and hold the mouthpiece at the other end of the tube. Activate the spray by pressing the can into the adapter; try to spray just as the patient starts to inhale. Wait about 3 minutes before repeating this sequence.

### Administering by Injection

Patients who know they have allergic reactions to insect stings will often have prescribed epinephrine for SC or IM injections. They use this medication after they are stung. In such cases, epinephrine serves as a specific antidote to the histamine released by the allergic reaction. Histamine lowers blood pressure by relaxing the small blood vessels and allowing them to leak. Epinephrine counters this effect by constricting or tightening the vessels. The reverse is true of the lung's airways. Histamine constricts them, while epinephrine dilates or enlarges these passages.

You may be trained to administer SC and IM injections of epinephrine, depending on local protocol. Remember that an SC injection puts the epinephrine into the tissue between the skin and the muscle. Therefore, it is usually helpful to pinch the skin lightly to lift it away from the muscle (Figure 14-6). A syringe intended for SC use has a short, thin needle, typically between ½" and ⅝" long. The syringe for IM use has a longer, thicker needle, typically between 1" and 1½" long so it can reach the muscle.

For either type of injection, you should draw the syringe's plunger back slightly after inserting the needle and before injecting the medication. Check to see if any blood seeps into the syringe. If it does, you have accidentally placed the needle into a small blood vessel. You should withdraw the needle and start again. Epinephrine causes a burning sensation where it is

### FIGURE 14-5

A metered-dose inhaler with a spacer device

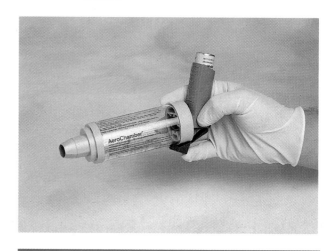

### FIGURE 14-6

Preparing the skin for an SC injection

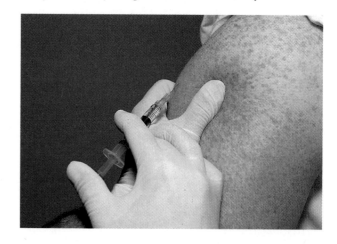

injected. You can also expect the patient's heart rate to increase after the injection.

## NITROGLYCERIN

Many patients, particularly the elderly, use nitroglycerin. If you think this sounds like an explosive, you're right. This is the same substance as TNT (trinitrotoluene). However, the medical forms of nitroglycerin are stabilized so they are not explosive (Figure 14-7).

Nitroglycerin is most commonly used to treat a condition called "angina." If you use a muscle so much that it runs out of oxygen, it develops a painful, burning sensation. As a result, you will probably rest that muscle until the pain goes away. When your heart muscle develops a similar pain, it cannot stop to rest. The resulting pain or discomfort is angina.

Angina most commonly occurs after many years of a narrowing of the arteries due to fatty buildup. Occasionally it occurs when these same blood vessels spasm. Nitroglycerin relieves arterial spasms. It can also help the more common angina by relaxing veins throughout the body. If less blood returns to the heart from the veins, the heart will not have to work as hard each time it beats. Thus, if the patient's legs are below the level of the heart, the relaxed veins leave more blood in the legs, reducing the heart's work load. On the other hand, if the patient is standing when the nitroglycerin starts to work, there may not be enough blood for the heart to pump up to the brain. The patient may faint. For this reason, it is best for patients who take nitroglycerin to be seated.

During a heart attack, the blood flow to a section of heart muscle is blocked when a clot forms in a narrowed artery. If the blockage is not cleared in time, a section of heart muscle will die. In some cases, nitroglycerin

## FIGURE 14-7

Nitroglycerin preparations

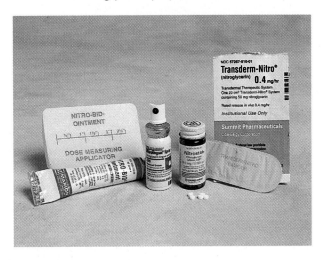

can help open a blocked vessel. When a patient who has previously experienced relief from chest pain by taking nitroglycerin no longer gets relief, he or she may be having a heart attack. Therefore, how much nitroglycerin the patient has needed in the past and how much he or she has taken during the current emergency are important facts. Remember to report this information to medical control.

### Administering by Tablet

Nitroglycerin is used sublingually to relieve chest pain. Most patients place a tiny tablet under the tongue, where it dissolves. These tablets should create a slight tingling or burning sensation. If the nitroglycerin has lost its usual "bite," it may have lost potency through aging or improper storage.

Sublingual nitroglycerin tablets should be stored in their original glass container with the cap screwed on tightly. The "cotton" in the container is made of rayon. If real cotton or other medications are placed in the container, they can absorb nitroglycerin from

## FAST FOOD FRENZY

Even though it's a weeknight, it's almost 8 pm before things slow down enough for dispatch to give you the OK to try to catch a quick bite to eat. No sooner do you pull into a local burger joint and park the rig when a young woman rushes out to the ambulance. She frantically tells you that her 3-year-old son has just eaten a partially cooked hamburger, and she's concerned about E. coli. She demands that you "give him some medicine right away to fix him." You assess the boy, and he appears to be completely healthy. The patient says that he doesn't feel sick, and that he wants to go to the playland next to the restaurant. He is alert and oriented and does not appear to be in any distress.

### For Discussion

1. Why is medication given in the prehospital setting? What are some of the risks? Some of the benefits?

2. What is the purpose of reassessing the patient after the administration of medication?

---

the tablets, reducing their potency. If you notice any signs of improper storage, include that information in the patient's medical history.

### Administering by Metered-Dose Spray

A few patients who use nitroglycerin to relieve chest pain use a metered-dose spray, which deposits nitroglycerin on or under the tongue. Each spray is equal to one tablet.

Whether using tablets or a spray, wait 5 minutes before repeating a dose—unless the patient has learned otherwise. And remember, the best effects are obtained if the patient is seated.

## REASSESSMENT STRATEGIES

It is crucial that you document every dose of medication administered or taken by the patient in your presence. For those medications that you would expect to produce a response during the time the patient is under your care, you need to reassess the patient and record vital signs.

For example, because blood delivers oxygen to tissues, it is likely that giving oxygen will ease a patient's breathing and possibly reduce a rapid heart rate. However, injecting epinephrine and some of the inhalers that contain epinephrine or similar drugs make it easier for the patient to breathe. These drugs may also increase heart rate. In some patients, nitroglycerin may increase heart rate. Reporting these side effects can be important to the physician who treats the patient. Since patients with low blood glucose levels normally have elevated heart rates, giving glucose could be expected to lower the heart rate to a normal range.

In addition to reassessing vital signs, you should also record a verbal description of the patient's status, such as a description of breathing, level of consciousness, or level of comfort.

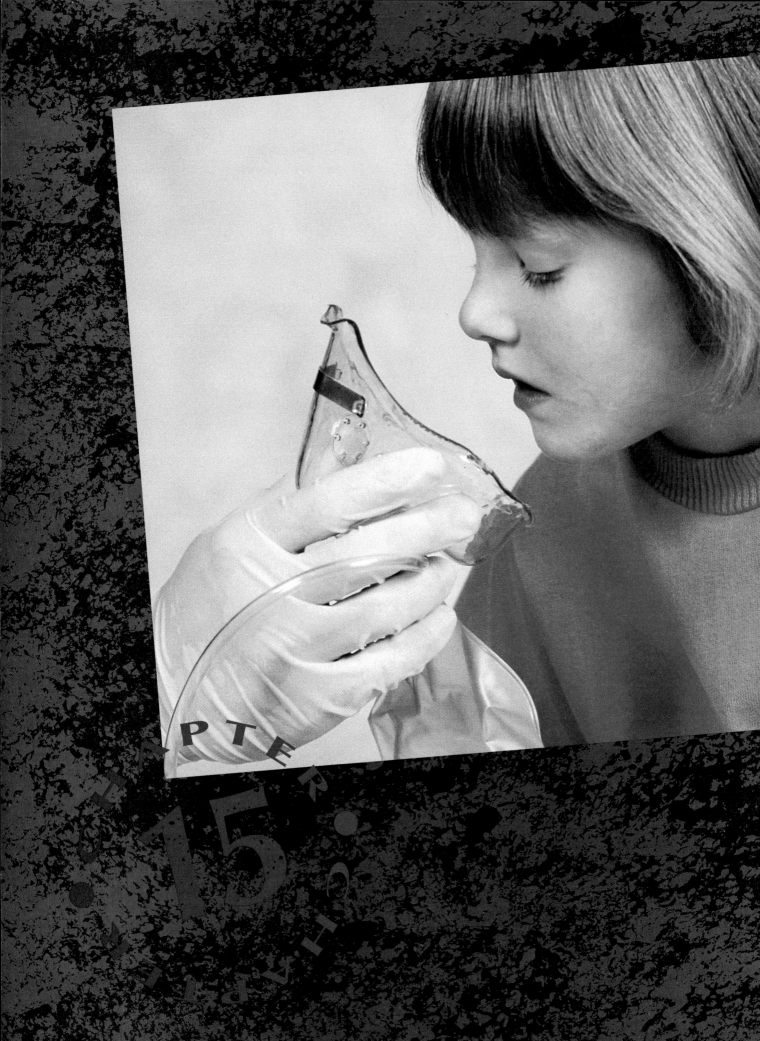

# Respiratory Emergencies

After you have read this chapter, you should be able to:

- List the structures and functions of the respiratory system.
- List the signs and symptoms of a patient with breathing problems.
- Describe the emergency medical care of a patient with breathing problems.
- Explain why medical direction is needed to assist with emergency medical care of a patient with breathing problems.
- Describe the emergency medical care of a patient with breathing distress.
- Establish the relationship between airway management and a patient with breathing problems.
- List the signs of adequate air exchange.
- State the generic name, dosage forms, dose amount, methods of administration, actions, indications, and contraindications of prescribed inhalation medications.
- Describe the differences in care of respiratory distress between pediatric and adult patients.
- Explain the difference between upper airway obstruction and lower airway disease in infants and children.

## Overview

Breathing difficulty is a common reason for calling an ambulance. The reasons for respiratory emergencies are many and complex. Shortness of breath may result from a variety of medical conditions or trauma. This chapter focuses on the medical, nontraumatic causes of shortness of breath.

Shortness of breath is a symptom. It may be accompanied by distinct signs of respiratory distress. It is often difficult to sort out why a patient is having trouble breathing. For example, many patients with heart conditions also have chronic lung disease. In fact, it may not be easy to determine what is causing their breathing problems, even when they get to the hospital.

The chapter begins with a brief review of the anatomy and physiology of the pulmonary system. The role of the lungs in exchanging oxygen and carbon dioxide is reviewed. Also discussed are the many disorders that prevent or obstruct that exchange. The next section presents the signs and symptoms of a patient with breathing difficulty. The third section provides the detailed procedures for the proper treatment of shortness of breath, including assisting with a metered-dose inhaler. A section of pediatric considerations is presented last, but children are discussed throughout, as needed.

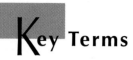

# Key Terms

**Asthma**  A disease of the lungs in which muscles spasm in the small air passageways and large amounts of mucus are produced, resulting in airway obstruction.

**Beta agonists**  Agents that act like epinephrine by relaxing the smooth muscles in the bronchial tubes, causing them to open up.

**Chronic obstructive pulmonary disease (COPD)**  A slow process of dilation and disruption of the airways and alveoli, caused by chronic bronchial obstruction.

**Dyspnea**  Shortness of breath or difficulty breathing.

**Respiration**  The process in which oxygen enters the blood as we inhale and carbon dioxide and waste products are removed as we exhale.

**Sympathomimetic drugs**  Agents that mimic the hormone epinephrine (adrenaline).

## ANATOMY REVIEW

As discussed earlier in this text, the respiratory system consists of all the structures of the body that contribute to the breathing process. Important anatomic features include the upper and lower airways, the lungs, and the diaphragm. Air enters the trachea and moves to the lungs, where oxygen and carbon dioxide are exchanged. The major function of the lungs is respiration. **Respiration** is the process in which oxygen enters the blood as we inhale and carbon dioxide and waste products are removed as we exhale.

For adequate exchange between oxygen and carbon dioxide to occur, the airways and the lungs must be clear. That is why airway management is such a critical part of patient care. Oxygen must be able to reach the alveoli in the lungs. There must be no obstruction to and from the alveoli. Oxygen and carbon dioxide must also pass freely between the alveoli and the pulmonary capillaries (Figure 15-1). Respiratory problems sometimes develop if this passage is blocked or somehow inadequate.

With certain medical conditions, the lungs are damaged or unable to function normally, resulting in one or more of the following:

- muscle spasm, or mucus obstructs the airways
- air fills the pleural space and the lungs cannot expand
- oxygen and carbon dioxide do not exchange due to damaged alveoli
- fluid or infection actually separate the pulmonary vessels from the alveoli
- blood clots obstruct blood flow to the lungs

## FIGURE 15-1

An enlarged view of an alveolus

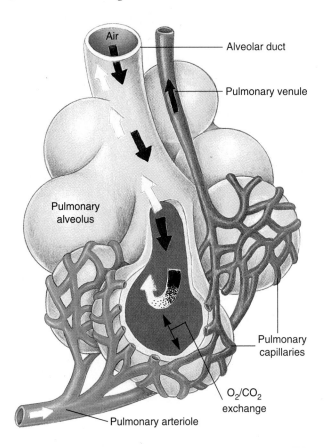

All these conditions prevent the proper exchange of oxygen and carbon dioxide. Abnormalities of the pulmonary blood vessels may also interfere with blood flow, and ultimately, the exchange of oxygen and carbon dioxide.

## NORMAL BREATHING PATTERNS

Remember that normal breathing should appear easy, not labored. As with a bellows used to move air to start a fire, breathing should be a smooth flow of air moving in and out of the lungs. Normal breathing has the following characteristics:

## YOUNG LOVE

It's already been a busy Friday—with four calls since 6 pm. Once again, dispatch calls to check on your availability. Your unit clears the hospital and is dispatched to a high school dance for a girl having "difficulty breathing." On arrival, you are directed to a hallway at the end of the gym where you find a 17-year-old girl who is sitting hunched forward, breathing at a rate of 40/min. Her friends tell you that she just had a fight with her boyfriend, and that he has since left with another girl. The patient is alert and oriented, but is obviously very anxious. She has warm, moist skin, and her pupils are equal and reactive to light. Her lungs are slightly wheezy in all fields. While your partner is taking her vital signs, the patient states that she takes Ventolin for asthma, and that she also takes birth control pills. She smokes about a pack of cigarettes a day. She has a blood pressure of 148/74 mm Hg, a regular pulse of 138/min, and respirations of 40/min.

### For Discussion

1. Discuss the similarities and differences between respiration and gas exchange.

2. Describe the actions of a beta-agonist bronchodilator.

---

- a normal rate and depth
- a regular pattern of inhalation and exhalation
- good audible breath sounds on both sides of the chest
- regular rise and fall movement on both sides of the chest
- movement of the abdomen

An adult who is awake, alert, and talking to you has no *immediate* airway or breathing problems. An adult who is not breathing well will have labored breathing. Labored breathing requires effort. The person may be breathing either much slower (less than 8) or much faster (more than 24) than normal. An adult who is breathing normally will have respirations of 12 to 20 breaths per minute (Table 15-1). Other signs that a person is not breathing normally include the following:

- muscle retractions above the clavicles, between the ribs, and below the rib cage, especially in children

- pale or cyanotic skin
- cool, damp (clammy) skin
- shallow or irregular respirations

## PEDIATRIC CONSIDERATIONS

Normal breathing patterns in infants and children are essentially the same as those in adults. However, infants and children breathe faster than adults. An infant who is breathing normally will have respirations of 25 to 50 breaths per minute. A child will have respirations of 15 to 30 breaths per minute (Table 15-1). Like adults, infants and children who are breathing normally will have smooth, regular respirations, equal breath sounds, and the regular rise and fall movement on both sides of the chest.

Exhalation becomes active when infants and children have trouble breathing. Normally, inhalation alone is the active, muscular part of breathing, as described earlier. However, with labored breathing, both inhalation and exhalation are hard work. With labored breathing, exhalation is not passive. Instead, air is forced out of the lungs during exhalation, and the child may begin to wheeze. This type of labored breathing is also described as use of the accessory muscles of breathing. Other signs that an infant or child is not breathing normally include the following:

- muscle retractions, in which the muscles of the chest and neck are working extra hard in breathing
- nasal flaring in children, in which the nostrils flare out as the child breathes
- see-saw respirations in infants, in which the chest and abdominal muscles alternately contract to look like a see-saw

## RECOGNIZING RESPIRATORY EMERGENCIES

### SIGNS AND SYMPTOMS

Shortness of breath or difficulty breathing (dyspnea) is the primary symptom of respiratory difficulty. Because a lack of oxygen affects all organs, you will see many other signs and symptoms of breathing problems, including the following:

- restlessness and anxiety
- increased pulse rate
- increased or decreased respirations
- changes in skin color
- breathing through pursed lips
- noisy breathing
- inability to speak
- retractions
- shallow, slow, or irregular breathing
- abdominal breathing
- coughing

**TABLE 15-1** NORMAL RESPIRATION RATE RANGES

| | |
|---|---|
| Adults | 12 to 20 breaths per minute |
| Children | 15 to 30 breaths per minute |
| Infants | 25 to 50 breaths per minute |

To obtain the breathing rate in a patient, count the number of breaths in a 30-second period and multiply by two. Avoid letting the patient know that you are counting to prevent influencing the rate.

## COURTSIDE CRISIS

You are called to the local YMCA for a child who is having difficulty breathing. On arrival, you find an 11-year-old girl sitting at the sidelines of a basketball court with her coach. She is crying, and can only speak in two to three word bursts. The coach is answering most of your questions. The coach tells you that the patient got into a fight with her father at halftime about how poorly she was playing. As a result, the girl started crying. Suddenly, she told the coach that she couldn't catch her breath and was having difficulty breathing. The coach, who just received training in first aid, called EMS to check the girl out. The patient appears flushed, and her skin is warm and slightly moist. She has a blood pressure of 126/70 mm Hg, a pulse of 104/min, and respirations of 38/min.

### For Discussion

1. At what point should you intervene and provide care for a patient having respiratory difficulties?

2. What is the role of medical control when you are caring for a patient with a respiratory emergency?

---

- unusual patient position or appearance

A patient may be restless and anxious because it is so difficult to breathe. Normally, breathing takes no conscious effort. The lack of oxygen to the brain also makes the patient anxious, even though the patient is not aware of this effect on the brain.

## EXAMINING PATIENTS WITH RESPIRATORY EMERGENCIES

As you assess the patient, you should obtain the usual vital signs but also note the pattern and quality of respirations. Carefully assess the following for any signs of respiratory difficulty.

### Pulse and Respirations

Both pulse and respirations increase in an attempt to get more oxygen into the blood and around to the other organs. With some conditions, such as a stroke, the patient may have slow, inadequate respirations and eventually slip into unconsciousness. This can also happen in a patient with a severe episode of asthma or exacerbation of a chronic lung disease when that patient starts to tire out and then proceeds into respiratory failure. **Asthma** is a disease of the lungs in which muscles spasm in the small air passageways and large amounts of mucus are produced, resulting in airway obstruction. Thus, you must always be prepared to assist ventilations and use an airway adjunct, if needed, in patients with respiratory problems.

### Noisy Breathing

A patient in severe respiratory distress will often have trouble telling you what is wrong. These patients often cannot catch their breath enough to speak in complete sentences. Some patients may be wheezing or leaning forward breathing with *pursed lips* because it makes breathing easier for them (Figure 15-2). Listen for a cough. Is it a severe cough or a weak one?

Children with breathing problems may make sounds like crowing, snoring, bark-

ing, or wheezing. These sounds are more likely to be heard in children than in adults. This is because a child's larynx and trachea has a smaller diameter and is less rigid. Another indication of a high airway obstruction is stridor—a howling sound on inspiration. You may also hear gurgling and snoring. These sounds indicate there are secretions in the airway or there is a partial airway obstruction. In this instance, an airway maneuver or suctioning is needed.

### Patient Position

In general, the most severely distressed patients will not lie down. In a sitting position, they are able to get more oxygen into their blood. The patient may also lean forward as he or she breathes. However, these same patients may slump over when they reach the point of respiratory failure. You must always be ready to assist with airway and ventilations.

### Skin

Other findings involve the skin. When oxygen levels are low, the skin often becomes cyanotic, especially around the lips, in the mouth, and in the nail beds of the fingers and toes. If the breathing problems are due to shock, then the patient may be pale, and the skin may feel cool and clammy. In this situation, you should turn your attention to the patient's underlying shock. In some situations, such as septic shock (a severe infection in which bacteria enters into the blood) or an allergic reaction (including its most severe form, anaphylactic shock), the skin may become flushed or much redder in appearance. This is due to the blood vessels in the skin opening wider (vasodilation).

### Patient Appearance

A patient who has chronic obstructive pulmonary disease may appear to have an

## FIGURE 15-2

Patient in respiratory distress

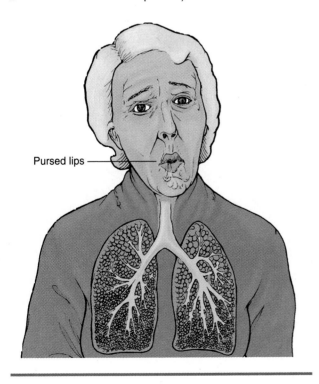

Pursed lips

obvious "barrel chest." **Chronic obstructive pulmonary disease (COPD)** is a slow process of dilation and disruption of the airways and alveoli, caused by chronic bronchial obstruction, usually from smoking. Some patients may appear to be using the accessory muscles of breathing, those in the shoulder girdle and neck. Check to see if the patient has retractions between the ribs due to heavy use of the intercostal muscles. Both of these indicate that the patient is working hard to breathe.

# EMERGENCY MEDICAL CARE

## GENERAL PRINCIPLES

Because the public generally tends to call all lung trouble "asthma," it is important for you to obtain a SAMPLE history. Ask the patient or the family to confirm whether the patient has recurrent episodes of breathing trouble, but can breathe normally at other times. The patient or family should always be asked to describe what "asthma" means to them. Not all wheezing is asthma. Wheezing has many other causes, including some forms of heart failure, foreign body airway obstruction, or inhalation of toxic gases. A history of repeated episodes is critical to identifying patients who truly have asthma.

Once you are at the patient's side, begin your assessment and obtain baseline vital signs and a SAMPLE history. As you are obtaining the history, you should ask the patient the following five questions, which will provide helpful information at the hospital:

1. Have you had an episode like this before? How often? Under what circumstances?

2. Do you have prescribed medication for these episodes? Have you been using your inhaler a lot, or have you recently run out of your medications? Have you ever been on steroids or prednisone? (Also an indicator of previous severe disease.)

3. Do you have a lot of problems with allergies?

In addition, if the episode seems to be severe, it is appropriate to ask the following questions:

4. How long has this episode been going on? Episodes lasting for more than 48 hours increase the possibility that the patient will become tired and possibly go into respiratory arrest.

5. Have you ever had a tube in your windpipe or been on a breathing machine? A patient with one or more previous episodes of respiratory failure is more likely to have another one.

Breathing difficulties that occur as a result of a bee or wasp sting may progress rapidly to full anaphylactic shock. Thus, it is important to find out what caused the attack. Many individuals wear or carry medical identification tags that may provide a clue in the most extreme cases (Figure 15-3).

## FIGURE 15-3

Medical identification tag and bracelet

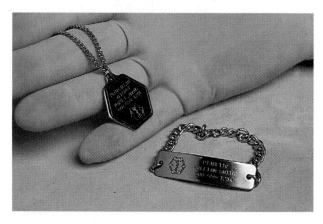

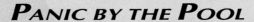
## PANIC BY THE POOL

The afternoon shift has been slow, so you stop by the communications center to visit with dispatch. No sooner do you pour a cup of coffee, when the dispatcher takes a call from a hysterical woman who states "I need an ambulance quick. My baby has drowned!" You are quickly out the door and en route. Traffic is light, so it's only a matter of a couple of minutes before you arrive to find an obviously cyanotic 2-year-old boy lying on the grass by a small backyard pool. The mother is crying and shaking him. Initial assessment reveals that he is unresponsive and is not breathing.

### For Discussion

1. Why is providing psychological support for the mother an essential part of this call?

2. Describe the importance of proficiency with both physical and psychological patient care skills on critical calls.

Your first step in providing patient care is to give oxygen, as you normally would by medical protocol. Allow the patient to sit up, because breathing is much easier in this position. Next, assess the vital signs. The pulse will likely be normal or elevated. The blood pressure may be slightly elevated. This is due to either tension and anxiety or from a medication taken in an attempt to relieve the episode. Respirations will be increased. A patient with asthma often complains of a tight feeling in the chest. However, this feeling resolves as the bronchospasm is relieved. In some situations, the patient's chest pain persists or is a prominent complaint. If the patient is over 35 and has these complaints, you must consider the possibility of heart-related chest pain. Treat the patient for a heart-related condition.

If the patient *has* a verified prescribed beta inhaler, inform medical control (or off-line medical control from your medical director). After consulting with medical control, you can help administer the beta inhaler as directed. If the patient *does not* have a prescribed beta inhaler, proceed with airway and ventilation interventions and provide transport. Be sure to inform the receiving facility about your patient. As in other emergencies, reassure the patient. This will help relieve the tension and anxiety that make these episodes worse.

You must also watch for airway problems to develop. Patients may produce large amounts of mucus that need suctioning. You should then give the patient oxygen. With an unconscious patient, airway maintenance and occasionally CPR, may be needed.

The effort to breathe during an episode of asthma is very tiring. The patient may be exhausted by the time you arrive. He or she may no longer be anxious or even struggling to breathe due to exhaustion. If this is the case, remember that the patient is not recovering. In fact, he or she is actually at a very critical stage and is likely to stop breathing. Aggressive airway management, oxygen administration, an attempt to use the patient's prescribed inhaler, and prompt transport are essential in this situation.

## ASSISTING WITH A PRESCRIBED INHALER

Many people with asthma or known allergies to bee stings or certain foods carry medication to take when an episode occurs. These medications can be obtained and administered with your help. One of the most helpful groups of agents are **sympathomimetic drugs.** These agents mimic the hormone epinephrine (adrenaline), which is secreted by the sympathetic nervous system. They are also called beta agonists because they act like the beta effects of epinephrine. When inhaled, **beta agonists** relax the smooth muscles in the bronchial tubes, which causes them to open up. Thus, breathing becomes easier. Many of these drugs on the market are prescribed as hand-held metered-dose inhalers (Table 15-2).

### Assisting with a Prescribed Inhaler

1. Confirm that the patient is having breathing difficulty, taking care of airway and assisting ventilations if necessary.

2. Confirm that the patient has a prescribed beta agonist inhaler and that it has not expired. (The patient must be conscious to be able to cooperate with the use of the inhaler.)

**TABLE 15-2** METERED-DOSE INHALER BETA AGONISTS

| Trade Name | Generic Name |
| --- | --- |
| Ventolin | albuterol |
| Proventil | albuterol |
| Brethine | terbutaline |
| Bricanyl | terbutaline |
| Alupent | metaproterenol |
| Metaprel | metaproterenol |
| Bronkosol | isoetherine |
| Primatene* | epinephrine |

(*Primatene is OTC. Since the patient may buy it without a prescription, you will not likely assist a patient using it.)

3. Ask the patient if he or she has already taken any doses.

4. Make sure that the inhaler is at room temperature. An inhaler used straight out of the refrigerator may make bronchospasm worse.

5. Shake the inhaler several times to mix the medication and propellant.

6. Remove oxygen from the patient.

7. Tell the patient to exhale deeply.

8. Tell the patient to put the mouthpiece in his or her mouth and make a seal with his or her lips. Some physicians and pharmacists provide a spacer with the inhaler to facilitate good dispersal of the medication into the lungs (Figure 15-4).

### ASSISTING WITH A PRESCRIBED INHALER

☐ Confirm that the patient is having breathing difficulty, taking care of airway and assisting ventilations if necessary.

☐ Confirm that the patient has a prescribed beta agonist inhaler and that it has not expired. (The patient must be conscious to be able to cooperate with the use of the inhaler.)

☐ Ask the patient if he or she has already taken any doses.

☐ Make sure that the inhaler is at room temperature. An inhaler used straight out of the refrigerator may make bronchospasm worse.

☐ Shake the inhaler several times to mix the medication and propellant.

☐ Remove oxygen from the patient.

☐ Tell the patient to exhale deeply.

☐ Tell the patient to put the mouthpiece in his or her mouth and make a seal with his or her lips. Some physicians and pharmacists provide a spacer with the inhaler to facilitate good dispersal of the medication into the lungs.

☐ Tell the patient to depress the inhaler body as he or she inhales. This will squeeze medication into the airstream where it can be sucked into the lungs.

☐ Tell the patient to hold his or her breath as long as he or she can comfortably do so. This will allow the medication to stay in the lungs as long as possible.

☐ Reapply the oxygen.

☐ Allow the patient to breathe a few times. The patient will often take two puffs at one time. Use of a second puff depends on the patient's prescription and what your medical director allows.

## FIGURE 15-4

A metered-dose inhaler with spacer device

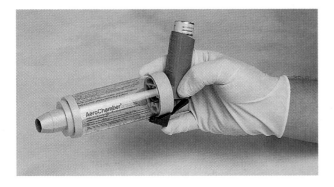

9. Tell the patient to depress the inhaler body as he or she inhales. This will squeeze medication into the airstream where it can be sucked into the lungs.

10. Tell the patient to hold his or her breath as long as he or she can comfortably do so. This will allow the medication to stay in the lungs as long as possible.

11. Reapply the oxygen.

12. Allow the patient to breathe a few times. The patient will often take two puffs at one time. Use of a second puff depends

on the patient's prescription and what your medical director allows.

These drugs are considered very safe. Their side effects are a nuisance more than anything. Beta agonists may increase heart rate and make the patient shaky and nervous. Many times the pulse rate will actually decrease as the airway obstruction is relieved. Remember that a metered-dose inhaler cannot be used if it has not been prescribed for the patient. The prescription was written for that patient. Therefore, you should not use any other inhaler on the patient, including one from a friend or family member. Also remember that you cannot assist with an inhaler if the patient cannot cooperate to use it or if medical control does not permit it.

Once the patient has taken the medication and has had the opportunity to breathe a few times, reassess the patient. Perform another assessment and obtain another set of vital signs. Patients who have severe episodes that progress to anaphylactic shock may become unconscious. These patients need assisted ventilations, oxygen, and prompt transport.

# PEDIATRIC CONSIDERATIONS

Many children have asthma, so metered-dose inhalers are very commonly seen with children. Children will often cough, not wheeze, when they are experiencing bronchospasm, although coughing occurs in adults as well. The indications, considerations, and procedures for using a metered-dose inhaler in children are the same as those outlined for adults. Retractions and use of accessory muscles are more common in children than in adults in respiratory distress. When children are working hard to breathe, they can lose a great deal of moisture from their respiratory tracts. This can lead to dehydration. Children need to be watched carefully for dehydration in this situation.

# Atlas of
# Common Respiratory Emergencies

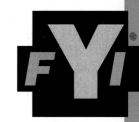

Patients often have breathing problems in association with one of the following medical problems:

- infections of the upper or lower airway
- acute pulmonary edema
- chronic obstructive pulmonary disease (COPD)
- spontaneous pneumothorax
- asthma or allergic reactions
- mechanical obstruction of the airway
- pulmonary embolism
- hyperventilation

## AIRWAY INFECTIONS

Infectious diseases that cause breathing difficulty may affect any or all parts of the airway. With some conditions, patients have only mild discomfort, while in others patients have signs of acute airway obstruction. Generally, all respiratory emergencies involve some type of obstruction. Air flow to the major passages may be blocked, such as with colds, diphtheria, epiglottitis, and croup. The exchange of gases between the alveoli and the capillaries may not be adequate, such as with pneumonia. Shortness of breath is quite common with airway infections, but it is rarely serious. You should give these patients oxygen.

### Common Cold

With the common cold, the mucous membranes in the nose become swollen, and fluid drains from the sinuses and the nose. Breathing difficulties are usually not severe with a cold. Patients often complain of stuffiness or difficulty in breathing. Despite years of research, no sure treatment exists for colds. Fortunately, the common cold rarely causes a severe emergency, unless the patient has underlying heart or lung disease. The congestion and stuffiness of a common cold rarely require emergency care. In fact, people with colds usually treat themselves with over-the-counter medications.

### Diphtheria

Diphtheria, although well controlled in the past decade, is still highly contagious and severe. With diphtheria, a membrane made up of debris, inflammatory cells, and mucus forms in the pharynx. This membrane can rapidly cause a severe airway obstruction.

### Epiglottitis

Epiglottitis is a bacterial infection of the epiglottis. With this infection, the epiglottis can swell two to three times its normal size, especially in children. Complete airway obstruction can develop as a result of this swelling. Therefore, you should not try to suction the airway or insert an airway adjunct. Both could cause complete airway obstruction. Acute epiglottitis can also occur in adults (Figure 15-5). It is often missed because epiglottitis is usually considered a children's disease. Acute epiglottitis in an adult is characterized by a severe sore throat. Airway obstruction may develop quickly. You should provide prompt transport for all patients believed to have epiglottitis.

## FIGURE 15-5

X ray of epiglottitis in an adult

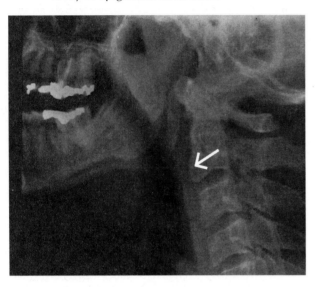

### Croup

Croup is an inflammation and swelling of the lining of the larynx. The larynx is where the airway is normally at its narrowest. A common sign of croup is stridor, a high-pitched, barking, rough sound heard during inhalation. Stridor indicates further narrowing of the air passages, which occasionally may result in airway obstruction.

### Pneumonia

Pneumonia is an acute bacterial or viral infection of the lung. The infection damages and destroys lung tissue. In addition, fluid builds up in the surrounding normal lung tissue and separates the alveoli from the capillaries. As a result, the lung cannot effectively exchange oxygen and carbon dioxide. The patient with pneumonia may breathe faster than normal to compensate for the reduced amount of healthy, working lung tissue. This shortness of breath is not caused by upper airway obstruction. Therefore, inserting an airway adjunct would not help the patient. A patient with pneumonia needs oxygen.

## ACUTE PULMONARY EDEMA

Sometimes the heart muscle is so injured after a heart attack or some other heart disease that it cannot circulate blood properly. With pulmonary edema, the left side of the heart cannot remove blood from the lung as fast as the right side delivers it. Fluid then builds up in the alveoli and also between the alveoli and the capillaries. This buildup of fluid is called pulmonary edema. With this condition, fluid separates the alveoli from the capillaries. This separation interferes with the exchange of carbon dioxide and oxygen (Figure 15-6). The patient usually takes rapid, shallow breaths because with the fluid buildup, there is not enough room in the lung to allow slow, deep breaths. In very severe instances, the patient will have frothy pink sputum at the nose and mouth.

In some instances, patients will have pulmonary edema without accompanying heart disease. Inhaling smoke, toxic chemical fumes, or experiencing a sudden compression injury of the chest can all produce pulmonary edema. In these cases, pulmonary edema occurs from direct damage or irritation to the lung or bronchi. However, the result is the same. Fluid col-

## FIGURE 15-6

Pulmonary edema

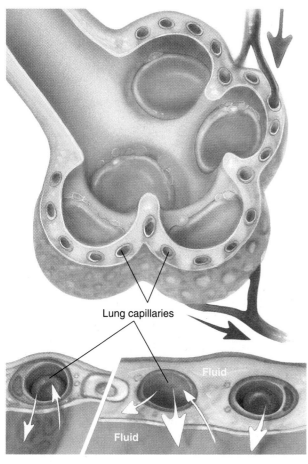

Lung capillaries

Fluid

Fluid

Normal                    Pulmonary edema

lects in alveoli and lung tissue, resulting in breathing difficulty.

When the problem is associated with lung damage rather than heart disease, you should give the patient 100% oxygen. You may also need to suction heavy secretions or mucus from the airway. An airway adjunct is rarely needed, because there is no upper airway obstruction problem. You should then prepare the patient for transport. Place a conscious patient in a position in which it is easiest for him or her to breathe. Usually that is a sitting position. An unconscious patient with acute pulmonary edema may require full ventilatory support, including an airway adjunct, oxygen, and suctioning.

## CHRONIC OBSTRUCTIVE PULMONARY DISEASE

Chronic obstructive pulmonary disease (COPD), or emphysema, is a common problem of the lungs. You are likely to see many older patients with this condition. These patients are usually thin, and their chests often have a barrel-like appearance. This characteristic appearance is due to the fact that air is gradually and continuously trapped within the lung in increasing amounts. With COPD, damage to the airways, the alveoli, and the pulmonary blood vessels occurs slowly, often over a period of several years (Figure 15-7).

Patients may complain of tightness in the chest and constant fatigue. They may or may not appear cyanotic. They may be only semiconscious, or they may even be unconscious due to hypoxia or carbon dioxide narcosis. Carbon dioxide narcosis is elevated levels of $CO_2$ in the blood resulting in changes in mental status. They may also appear to be in respiratory distress. Patients with COPD may use their accessory muscles to breathe, including those in the neck and shoulders. They may also breathe through pursed lips in an attempt to "puff" out air.

COPD may be a result of lung damage from any one of the following:

- cigarette smoking
- repeated infections, such as pneumonia
- inhaling toxic agents, such as industrial gases

## FIGURE 15-7

Damage to alveolus and bronchiole due to COPD

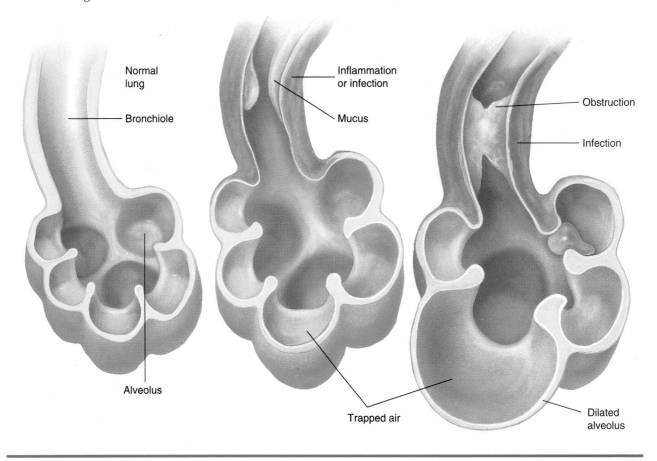

Normal
lung

Bronchiole

Alveolus

Inflammation
or infection

Mucus

Trapped air

Obstruction

Infection

Dilated
alveolus

It is well known that cigarette smoking causes lung cancer. However, its role in COPD is far more significant and less well known. Tobacco smoke irritates the bronchi and can cause chronic bronchitis, an irritation of the trachea and bronchi. Excess mucus is produced constantly and obstructs the small airways and alveoli. When these passages are constantly obstructed, pneumonia often develops. As COPD becomes worse, the level of oxygen in the arteries falls, and the level of carbon dioxide rises.

There is a direct relationship between the number of pack-years and the incidence of COPD. Smoking one pack of cigarettes per day per year equals 1 pack-year.

If a patient has pneumonia along with COPD or any other chronic lung condition, the level of oxygen in the arteries may fall rapidly. In many patients, the level of carbon dioxide is high enough to produce a condition called carbon dioxide narcosis. Patients with COPD do not handle pulmonary infections well. The damage to their airways makes coughing up the mucus or sputum produced by the infection very difficult. Patients often report a recent chest cold and may remember having a recent fever as well as the inability to cough up mucus. Those who can produce sputum will cough up thick, green or yellow sputum. Patients with chronic airway obstruction often have trouble breathing deeply enough to clear their lungs, but rarely report any chest pain. These patients require respiratory support and careful administration of oxygen.

As you obtain the baseline vital signs, pay particular attention to the patient's respirations. They may be rapid or very slow, as in carbon dioxide narcosis. The blood pressure will likely be normal, but the pulse will be rapid and occasionally irregular. When listening to the chest, you will hear abnormal breath sounds, including rales (crackling breath sounds), wheezing (whistling sounds), and rhonchi (rough, gravelly sounds). Breath sounds are often hard to hear in these patients and often are detected only high up on the posterior chest.

You will usually give oxygen, although you must take great care to monitor respirations. Reassess respirations and the patient's overall response to oxygen every 5 minutes until arrival at the hospital.

Monitoring the patient is important, because oxygen may cause a rapid increase in the level of arterial oxygen. This, in turn, can abolish the secondary respiratory oxygen drive while the carbon dioxide level remains high. If a COPD patient depends on a low oxygen level to maintain breathing, this rapid increase in arterial oxygen might abolish the stimulus. The patient could then go into respiratory arrest. However, the patient will still need the oxygen. Thus, you should not withhold oxygen for fear it will depress or even stop the patient's breathing. You should assist breathing if the respiratory rate slows. Slowing respirations in a COPD patient who is receiving oxygen does not mean that the patient no longer needs oxygen. In fact, the patient may need it even more.

## SPONTANEOUS PNEUMOTHORAX

When the surface of the lung is torn or broken in some way, air escapes into the pleural cavity. Normally, the negative pressure in the pleural space keeps the lungs inflated. If air gets into the pleural space, the negative pressure is lost. Then the natural elasticity of the lung tissue causes the lung to collapse. The buildup of air in the pleural space is called a pneumothorax. In most cases, pneumothorax is caused by trauma. However, it may be caused by a medical condition without any injury, or in people who were born with weak areas of the lung. In these instances, the condition is called a spontaneous pneumothorax.

Spontaneous pneumothorax may be the cause of a sudden breathing problem in a patient who has COPD. A patient may be coughing when a weakened portion of lung ruptures. The patient may then have difficulty breathing and pain on one side of the chest that is worse during breathing. Absence of breathing problems and chest pain is also possible. However, the patient will rarely be cyanotic. As you listen to the chest, you will likely note that the breath sounds are absent or decreased on the side with the pneumothorax. However, these altered breath sounds are very difficult to hear in a patient with severe COPD.

You should give these patients supplemental oxygen. If the patient has COPD, medical control may advise you to give oxygen by Venturi mask. You should then prepare the patient for transport. Like most patients with breathing problems, those with spontaneous pneumothorax are usually more comfortable sitting up. Watch for sudden airway problems. Be ready to establish an airway, assist ventilations, and give full CPR, if it becomes necessary.

## ASTHMA OR ALLERGIC REACTIONS

About 6 million Americans have asthma, and between 4,000 and 5,000 people die from it each year. Asthma is an acute spasm of the smaller air passages (bronchioles) that occurs due to excessive mucus production (Figure 15-8). With asthma, when the patient inhales, breathing is normal. The bronchioles open easily during inhalation. However, when the patient exhales, breathing is not normal. Patients with asthma will wheeze as they try to exhale through partially obstructed air passages. This characteristic wheezing occurs only during exhalation. Sometimes the wheezing is so loud that you can hear it without a stethoscope. In some instances, the actual work of exhaling is very tiring, and the patient may become cyanotic.

Asthma usually results from inhaling, ingesting, or injecting an allergen (an agent to which the patient is allergic or sensitive). When exposed to the allergen, the airways react by producing an excessive amount of mucus. This is what is often called an episode or an asthma attack. Between episodes, patients have normal lung function. An allergic reaction to a bee sting or other substance, such as a particular food, may result in an asthma attack. In its most severe form, an allergic reaction can result in anaphylactic shock. A patient in anaphylactic shock may have severe respiratory distress, possibly resulting in coma and even death. Asthma attacks may also occur

## FIGURE 15-8

A normal bronchiole (left). A bronchiole in spasm due to asthma (right)

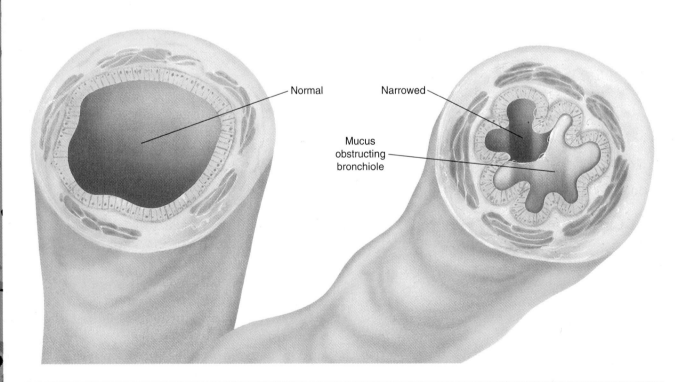

Normal

Narrowed

Mucus obstructing bronchiole

in response to respiratory infections or even severe emotional stress.

Occasionally, a patient has a prolonged asthma attack that is unrelieved by epinephrine. This condition is known as status asthmaticus. This is a true emergency; the patient is frightened, frantically trying to breathe, using all the accessory muscles. In this situation, you should give the patient oxygen and provide rapid transport.

A much milder and much more common allergy problem is hay fever. This is caused by an allergic reaction to pollen. In some areas of the country where pollen is present in the air throughout the year, it is almost a universal illness. Generally, it does not produce major emergencies, but it does cause a number of problems, such as a stuffy or runny nose, and sneezing.

## MECHANICAL OBSTRUCTION OF THE AIRWAY

Mechanical obstruction may occur as a result of improper head position, obstruction by the tongue, aspiration of vomitus, or aspiration of a foreign body. The first thing to do is clear the upper airway. You may open the airway with the head-tilt or chin-lift maneuvers, but first be sure the patient has no head or neck injuries. If these maneuvers do not open the airway, you must check for a foreign body in the upper airway. You should always check for foreign body obstruction in patients who have difficulty breathing during or after eating a meal. You should also check for foreign body obstruction in young children, especially crawling babies, who might have swallowed and choked on a small object, such as a bead or a piece of popcorn. Hot dogs are one of the leading killers of children younger than 5 years, as even small pieces of hot dog create airway obstruction.

Acute upper airway obstruction is usually considered a traumatic cause of breathing problems. Management of airway obstruction is presented in appendix A, BLS Review.

## PULMONARY EMBOLISM

An embolus is anything in the circulatory system that passes from its point of origin and comes to rest at a distant site within the system. Emboli can be blood clots in the arteries or the veins. They can also be foreign bodies, such as a bullet or a bubble of air. Circulation on the other side of the clot or obstruction is cut off or markedly decreased. An embolism is a very serious condition and can cause sudden death.

Pulmonary embolism occurs when a blood clot from a vein breaks off and moves through the veins to the right side of the heart. Almost always, a large, long clot will break off in the large veins of the legs or pelvis. The clot then becomes lodged in the pulmonary artery where it can significantly interrupt arterial blood flow. Pulmonary embolism may occur as a result of the following:

- slow blood flow
- damage to the lining of the vessels
- a tendency for blood to clot unusually fast

Pulmonary embolism is usually seen in patients who are inactive and/or confined to bed, such as during hospitalization. Thus, you will rarely see this condition, although if you are involved in facility-to-facility transfer you may. This condition is of particular concern in the days or weeks after a patient has had a hip fracture or hip surgery. Blood flow to the legs decreases, and the veins often collapse. A person who is wearing a cast, in traction, dehydrated, or who has sustained an injury to the leg can also be at risk. Only rarely do they develop in active, healthy individuals.

Patients usually do not know they have a pulmonary embolism. It depends on how much lung tissue is damaged and how much pain they experience as they breathe. Signs and symptoms include shortness of breath, sharp, stabbing chest pain, coughing up blood, cyanosis, and rapid respirations. Lung damage, along with inflammation of the pleural surfaces, often causes pleuritic (sharp, stabbing) chest pain with each breath. Patients with pulmonary embolism have inadequate exchange of oxygen and carbon dioxide, even though their lungs are working to breathe. With pulmonary embolism, the level of carbon dioxide in the arteries usually rises. The level of oxygen in the arteries may drop enough to cause cyanosis. Complete, sudden blockage of the right side of the heart will result in sudden death.

Usually, it is not necessary to clear the airway, because no obstruction exists. However, you must give the patient oxygen, since much of the lung tissue may not be working properly. You may need to suction mucus or secretions from the airway. You should also expect an unusually rapid and sometimes irregular heartbeat. Acute reflex responses to pulmonary emboli may result in cardiac arrest. When a patient is believed to have a pulmonary embolism, place the patient in a position of comfort, usually sitting, give oxygen, and provide transport.

## HYPERVENTILATION

A patient who is hyperventilating has the feeling that it is impossible to get enough oxygen, even though a larger quantity than usual is being exchanged in the lungs. The patient is often very anxious, perhaps even hysterical. Not all patients are hysterical; some may be quite calm, although they are obviously hyperventilating. Dizziness is common. Patients often experience numbness or tingling in the hands and feet, which may also be described as "being cold." Sticking, stabbing chest pain that becomes worse with each breath may also occur. The patient will often have rapid respirations and pulse, but normal blood pressure. Cyanosis does not develop, which is your key that the patient is hyperventilating.

It is important that you assess the patient carefully and obtain a SAMPLE history. The presence or absence of chest pain, coughing of blood, and a history of heart problems or diabetes should be noted.

Other illnesses may cause a reaction that looks like simple overbreathing. Alterations in the body's acid or alkali balance may produce hyperventilation. This may be seen in the patients with untreated diabetes, severe shock, or after ingestion of certain poisons. Pulmonary embolism may also produce hyperventilation. Many of the symptoms, such as tingling of the fingers and dizziness, are caused by alkalosis secondary to low carbon dioxide in the blood. However, the blood carbon dioxide level will not reach a dangerously low level.

Hyperventilation is common in psychological stress—affecting up to 10% of the population at some time. Symptoms can be self-induced by breathing deeply and rapidly for 3 to 5 minutes. Most people undergoing breathing this way do not know they have been hyperventilating. Signs and symptoms include numbness, tingling in the hands and feet, and a sense of shortness of breath. Respirations are generally more than 40/min. Recent studies indicate that this type of "panic attack" can be associated with major differences in blood flow to specific areas of the brain. A patient may also have a specific organic defect that explains this reaction.

In the absence of any other cause for hyperventilation, you should begin by reassuring the patient in a calm, professional manner. The "old-fashioned" method of dealing with hyperventilation—breathing into a brown paper bag—is dangerous and is not recommended for use. Thus, you should provide prompt transport to the hospital. Although hyperventilation by itself is not a serious condition, patients who hyperventilate should be evaluated by a physician in the hospital.

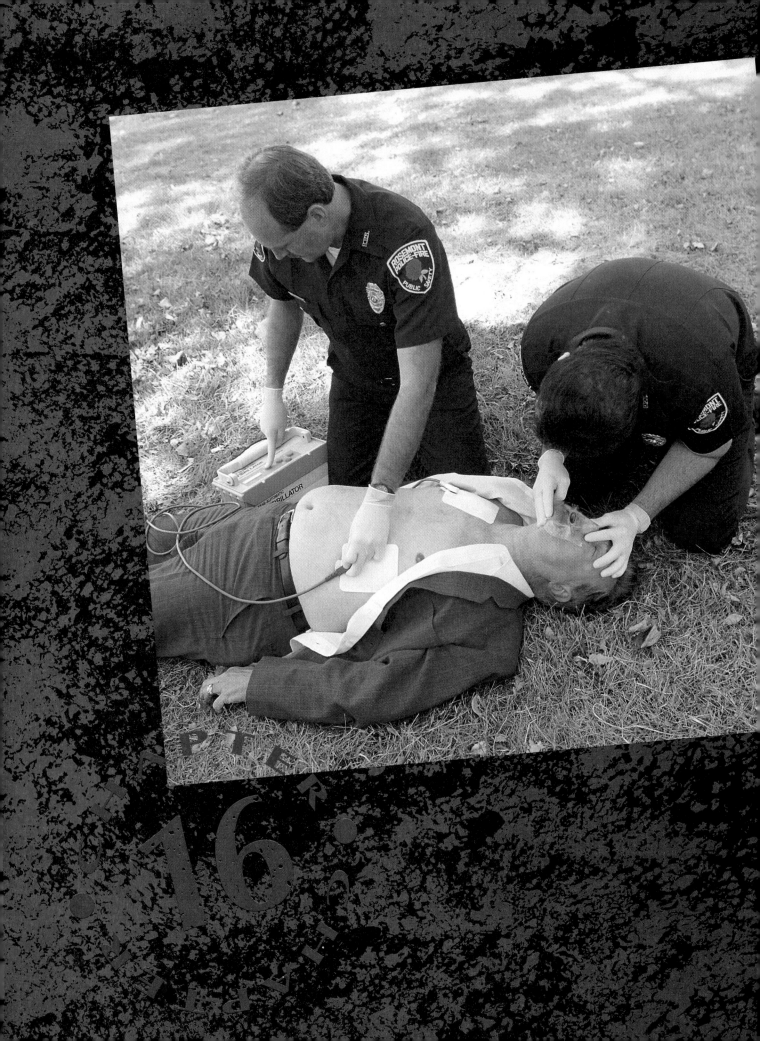

# Cardiac Emergencies

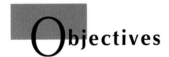

## Objectives

After you have read this chapter, you should be able to:

- Describe emergency medical care for a patient with chest pain and/or discomfort, including the following considerations: positioning, airway management, the role of BLS, care of ventricular fibrillation, and transport issues.
- Describe indications, contraindications, and side effects of nitroglycerin.
- Explain the rationale for and the fundamentals of early defibrillation and discuss the role of the EMT-B in the Chain of Survival.
- Describe the differences between a semiautomated and a fully automated defibrillator.
- Identify various types of AEDs, their standard operating procedures, and the advantages and disadvantages of each type.
- List the indications and contraindications for the use of the AED including the following considerations: age/weight of the patient, the status of the patient's ABCD and vital signs, and when a shock may be given inappropriately.
- Differentiate between single-rescuer and multi-rescuer care with the AED.
- Discuss the role of the American Heart Association in the use of the AED.
- List the steps in the operation of the AED.
- Discuss the special considerations for rhythm monitoring.

- Describe the functional controls of an AED, the process of event documentation, and the care and maintenance of the AED and its battery.
- Explain the importance of frequent practice with the AED, including the need to complete the Automated Defibrillator: Operator's Shift Checklist.
- Explain the importance of prehospital ACLS intervention, including coordinating personnel and transport issues.
- Describe the components and importance of post-resuscitation care.
- Describe the components and importance of case review, quality improvement, and medical direction as it applies to the AED.

# Overview

Heart attacks and other cardiac emergencies affect over 5 million people a year in the United States. Currently, heart disease causes more than 1 million deaths annually. Death rates in recent years have tended to level off rather than increase. However, heart disease remains a leading cause of death. In fact, about one third of the population will die as a result of heart disease. Thus, many of your calls will involve some type of cardiac emergency.

This chapter begins with a brief review of the heart and how it works, and then explains how improper function results in heart disease. The chapter next describes chest pain and discomfort. You must become familiar with the signs and symptoms of cardiac problems, as well as the treatment options. The next section describes the automated external defibrillator (AED) and how you will use this device. Also included in this chapter is a discussion of the use of nitroglycerin for heart problems.

The final section of this chapter is an atlas of common cardiac conditions. It includes descriptions of common conditions and the proper emergency medical care of these problems. Also included is a discussion of patients who have had prior heart surgery and those who have a cardiac pacemaker.

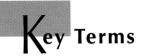

# Key Terms

**Arrhythmia**  An irregular or abnormal heart rhythm. Also called dysrhythmia.

**Asystole**  Complete absence of electrical activity in the heart.

**Bradycardia**  Abnormally slow but regular heart rhythm or pulse.

**Defibrillation**  Delivery of a direct current electric shock (or counter-shock) to the chest over the heart.

**Dilation**  Widening of the blood vessels, such as the coronary arteries.

**Dyspnea**  Shortness of breath or difficulty breathing.

**Ischemia**  Tissue deprived of its blood supply and therefore of its oxygen and nutrients.

**Myocardium**  Heart muscle.

**Nitroglycerin**  Medication used to treat chest pain. Works by dilating the blood vessel walls.

**Premature ventricular contractions (PVCs)**  Abnormal heartbeats that result from uncoordinated electrical impulses in the heart.

**Tachycardia**  Abnormally rapid but regular heart rhythm or pulse.

**Ventricular fibrillation (VF)**  Disorganized, ineffective quivering of the heart.

**Ventricular tachycardia (VT)**  Rapid, regular heart rhythm that results when several PVCs occur together.

## ANATOMY REVIEW

A detailed description of the circulatory system and its components is presented in chapter 4, The Human Body. The discussion presented below reviews critical elements of the circulatory system and how they are affected by cardiac emergencies.

### THE HEART

The heart is a hollow muscular organ about the size of a clenched fist. It is an involuntary muscle made of special tissue called cardiac muscle or **myocardium.** To carry out its pumping function, the heart muscle must have a continuous supply of oxygen and nutrients. The heart can tolerate a serious interruption of its blood supply for only a very few seconds before the signs of heart ischemia develop. Thus, its blood supply is as rich and well distributed as possible.

The coronary arteries supply blood to the heart muscle. They originate at the first part of the aorta, just above the aortic valve. Thus, the heart receives its first blood from the aorta. The right coronary artery supplies the right ventricle and, in most people, part of the left ventricle. The left coronary artery divides into two major branches. Both branches supply the left ventricle (Figure 16-1). The right side of the heart receives oxygen-poor (deoxygenated) blood from the veins of the body. The left side of the heart receives oxygen-rich (oxygenated) blood from the lungs through the pulmonary veins. The left side of the heart is more muscular than the right because it must pump blood into the aorta and then to the arteries.

The heart is always working. When the heart works hard, as when we exercise or experience stress, the heart muscle needs more oxygen and more blood flow. A normal, healthy heart gets the additional blood it needs during these times because the coronary arteries **dilate** (become wider).

## Electrical Conduction System

A network of specialized tissue capable of conducting electrical current runs through the heart. This electrical system is affected if part of the heart does not receive enough oxygen, or it is injured, or dies. Sometimes the injured part of the heart becomes irritable and begins to fire off uncoordinated electrical impulses. These impulses can start abnormal heartbeats called **premature ventricular contractions (PVCs).** If several PVCs occur close together, they produce a rhythm called **ventricular tachycardia (VT).** The heart in ventricular tachycardia continues to beat faster until its oxygen supply is exhausted. At this point the electrical impulses become completely uncoordinated and begin to fire off randomly. When this occurs the heart can no longer pump blood effectively. It then begins to quiver ineffectively in the chest. This state is called **ventricular fibrillation (VF).** The heart will be in VF for several minutes until it runs out of energy. Then all detectable electrical activity in the heart stops. This final state of complete electrical inac-

## FIGURE 16-1

The coronary arteries of the heart

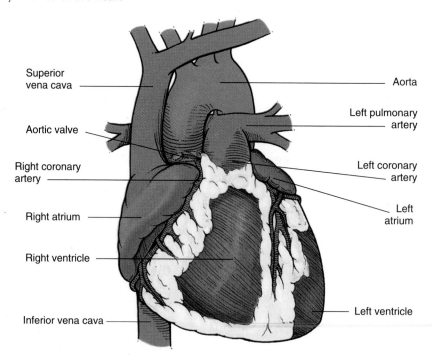

Superior vena cava

Aortic valve

Right coronary artery

Right atrium

Right ventricle

Inferior vena cava

Aorta

Left pulmonary artery

Left coronary artery

Left atrium

Left ventricle

tivity is called **asystole** (Figure 16-2). Your job as an EMT-B is to prevent a cardiac arrest before it happens, if possible. If it still occurs in spite of your best efforts, your job is to shock ventricular fibrillation before it becomes asystole.

## FIGURE 16-2

An ECG tracing of asystole

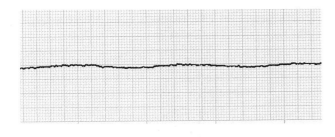

## THE BLOOD VESSELS

### Arteries

The arteries carry oxygen-rich blood from the heart to all body tissues. They branch into smaller arteries and then into arterioles. The arterioles, in turn, branch into smaller vessels until they connect to the vast network of capillaries.

Arteries contract to accommodate for loss of blood volume and also to increase blood pressure. Blood is supplied to tissues as they need it. Some tissues need a constant blood supply, especially the heart, the kidneys, and the brain. Other tissues, such as the muscles in the extremities, the skin, and the intestines, can function with less blood when at rest.

The aorta is the major artery that leaves the left side of the heart. It carries fresh,

oxygen-rich blood to the body. The aorta is found just in front of the spine in the chest and abdominal cavities. It has many branches that supply the heart, the head and neck, the arms, and many of the vital organs before it ends in the middle of the abdomen. The aorta divides at the level of the umbilicus into the two common iliac arteries that lead to the lower extremities (Figure 16-3a).

Once it passes through the network of capillaries, blood returns to the heart through

## FIGURE 16-3A

The major arteries of the body

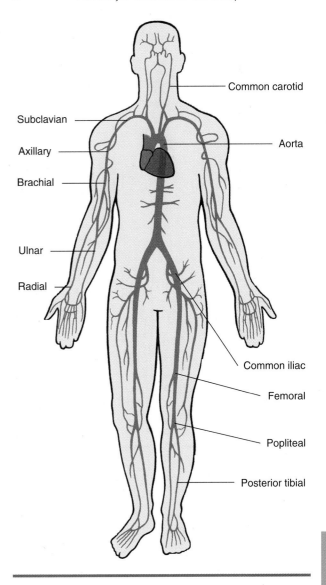

the veins. Capillaries empty into small venules that join to form veins. The veins become larger and larger and ultimately form two major vessels—the superior and inferior venae cavae (Figure 16-3b).

## FIGURE 16-3B

The major veins of the body

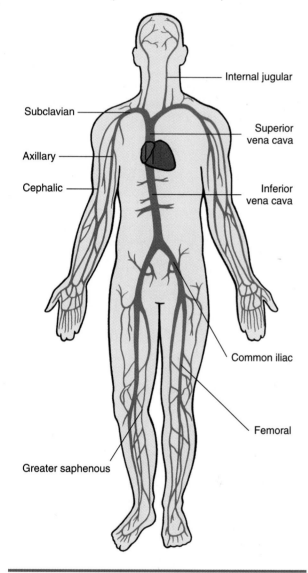

Internal jugular

Subclavian

Superior vena cava

Axillary

Cephalic

Inferior vena cava

Common iliac

Femoral

Greater saphenous

The venae cavae channel blood from the body and collect it just before it enters the heart. These two major vessels, part of the great vessels, are located in the midline, just to the right of the spine. Blood from the head,

neck, shoulders, and upper extremities passes through the superior vena cava. Blood from the abdomen, pelvis, and lower extremities passes through the inferior vena cava. The superior and inferior venae cavae join at the right atrium of the heart.

The right ventricle receives blood from the right atrium. Blood is then pumped from the right side of the heart. It travels through the pulmonary artery into the lung. Here it divides into right and left pulmonary arteries. These arteries divide until they form the pulmonary capillary system. In the capillaries, oxygen and carbon dioxide are exchanged. The newly oxygenated blood then collects in a network of combining veins and enters the four pulmonary veins. These veins unite at the left atrium. Blood then passes into the left ventricle and is pumped to the body and distributed by the arteries.

## CARDIAC COMPROMISE

### SIGNS AND SYMPTOMS

As an EMT-B, you may see a variety of signs and symptoms in a patient with acute ischemic heart disease. **Ischemia** occurs when the heart tissue does not receive enough blood flow. Therefore, the heart does not receive the oxygen and nutrients it needs. These signs and symptoms are as follows:

- sudden weakness
- nausea or vomiting
- sudden, unexplained sweating
- crushing, squeezing, or pressure-like chest pain, often radiating to one or both arms, the jaw, or the neck
- shortness of breath, with or without pain

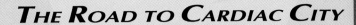

## THE ROAD TO CARDIAC CITY

YOU ARE THE EMT

You've just responded to an automobile accident that produced no injuries. You contact dispatch to inform them that you are available. Dispatch immediately sends you and your partner out for a "chest pain" call. On arrival, you find an 81-year-old woman who tells you that she has had chest pain for the past 4 hours. She has an extensive cardiac history and takes a number of medications. The patient is alert and oriented to person, place, and time. She describes the pain as being "like a heavy weight," and her skin is pale, cool, and slightly moist. Her lungs are clear. She has a blood pressure of 98/60 mm Hg, an irregular pulse of 112/min, and respirations of 18/min.

### For Discussion

1. Describe the relationship between airway management and the patient with a cardiac condition.

2. Why is preventing cardiac arrest in the prehospital setting a priority?

---

- epigastric (pit of the stomach) pain or indigestion
- anxiety, apprehension, or a feeling that the patient may die
- irregular heartbeat or sudden **arrhythmia** (abnormal heartbeat) with fainting
- pulmonary edema
- abnormal blood pressure and/or pulse

Unfortunately, the first sign of heart disease may be sudden death. About 40% of all patients who experience a severe heart attack never reach the hospital. Death is usually the result of cardiac arrest from ventricular fibrillation (VF). Remember, VF

occurs when the heart begins to quiver ineffectively in the chest and can no longer pump blood effectively. The chance to save a patient exists only if you can defibrillate the heart or begin CPR within 4 minutes of the event. Keep in mind that rapid BLS has successfully resuscitated many patients in cardiac arrest. Asystole may also be a cause of sudden death. This is a hard problem to detect because a patient in asystole appears the same as one in VF. Many ventricular arrhythmias can rapidly produce asystole if no treatment is given.

In general, patients in VF respond better to CPR than patients in asystole. More importantly, these patients need rapid defibrillation, as discussed in a later section. This is why early defibrillation is so important: it is critical to give the shock before the heart goes into asystole.

Most patients with a sudden ischemia of the heart who do not die will complain of sudden chest pain. This chest pain will be substernal (behind the breast bone) and will radiate to the lower jaw, to the left arm, to both arms, or to the epigastrium.

Remember that the severity of chest pain varies. There is less severe pain where the heart muscle has not been damaged, as with a condition called angina pectoris. There is also pain where damage to the heart has very likely occurred, as with a condition called acute myocardial infarction (AMI). Both conditions are described at the end of this chapter in the Atlas of Common Cardiac Conditions.

## ASSESSMENT FINDINGS

Your assessment findings of patients with heart ischemia will vary, depending on the extent and severity of damage to the heart. The most common findings are as follows:

- *Pulse.* Pulse rate normally increases in response to stress, fear, or an actual injury of the heart muscle. Arrhythmias are common with severe ischemia. With an arrhythmia, the patient may have an irregular pulse or no pulse. In some instances, **bradycardia** (an abnormal slowing of the heart rate or pulse) develops rather than **tachycardia** (an abnormally rapid heart rate or pulse).

- *Blood Pressure.* Blood pressure usually falls as a result of reduced cardiac output and decreased ability of the left ventricle to pump. However, if the heart has minimal damage, the blood pressure may actually rise.

- *Respiration.* Respirations are normal unless the patient has respiratory distress due to fluid in the lungs. In this case, the patient will have rapid, shallow respirations. Respirations may also be increased due to anxiety and/or pain.

- *General Appearance.* The patient appears frightened and is often in a cold sweat. The patient may feel nauseated and may vomit. The skin is often ashen as a result of poor cardiac output and inadequate skin perfusion. Occasionally, the patient may be cyanotic. When the heart is not pumping effectively, you may see that the patient has distended neck veins that do not collapse, even when the patient sits up.

- *Mental State.* One of the unexplained aspects of acute ischemia of the heart is that most patients have an almost overwhelming feeling of impending doom. They are convinced—almost resigned to the fact—that they are about to die.

## EMERGENCY MEDICAL CARE

Your work with a patient who has a cardiac condition begins immediately upon your arrival at the scene. As with all patients, your initial assessment should include reassuring the patient that you are there to help. Speak and act quickly, calmly, and professionally. Remember that all patients are frightened. Your professional attitude may be the single most important factor in making sure the patient cooperates. A patient who is anxious and agitated may actually have increased irregular or extra heartbeats. An arrhythmia may rapidly produce VF, asystole, and death. Apart from providing assurance and comfort, the calmness and poise with which you approach a patient may help prevent the patient's condition from becoming worse.

## DOWN AND OUT IN THE CORN

It's a hot August afternoon when a call comes in for a "man down." As you are heading out the door, your partner comments, "I hope this isn't a code, it's too hot to do CPR." It takes at least 10 minutes to make your way to the farm. On arrival, you are met by a very anxious looking woman. She tells you that she went looking for her husband when he didn't show up for lunch. She found him around the back of the barn slumped over, next to a running tractor. He was not responsive, and as best as she could tell, he did not have a pulse. You find the 62-year-old man in the position she described, pulseless and not breathing. His skin is warm and mottled. According to his wife, it's been about 25 minutes since she first found him.

### For Discussion

1. Describe the variables in the series of events that can result in an out-of-hospital cardiac arrest in which the patient does not survive.

2. Describe the similarities and differences of using an AED versus a manual defibrillator.

The next step is to perform a focused history and physical exam. Take a brief history from the patient, using OPQRST to determine the severity of pain. Friends or family members who are with the patient might have helpful information. As you take the patient's history, your partner should obtain and record the baseline vital signs. Note the exact time when the vital signs are taken. It is essential to monitor the vital signs closely, because a patient with acute heart ischemia is always at risk for sudden cardiac arrest.

Note: Should cardiac arrest occur, you must be ready to begin automatic defibrillation and CPR immediately. If the defibrillator is *immediately* available then place pads as you have been trained. Then analyze the heart rhythm and defibrillate if advised to do so. If the defibrillator is not immediately available, then do CPR until the defibrillator is available and can be applied. This treatment sequence is described in detail in the next section.

Next, place the patient in a comfortable position, usually sitting and well supported. Make sure the patient has no **dyspnea** (difficulty breathing) and has no airway obstruction. You are now ready to give the patient high-flow oxygen by nonrebreathing mask. Explain to the patient that you are giving oxygen before you position the nonrebreathing mask. Once the patient is on oxygen, reassess the vital signs. Remember that these steps occur quickly in the field.

Your next step is to report to medical control. Give the patient's history, vital signs, medications being taken, and the treatment you are giving. Consider giving nitroglycerin, if allowed by your medical director. Take care not to frighten the patient. Follow the instructions of medical control.

Proper emergency handling and prompt transport are critical. Some newer treatments for cardiac emergencies use drugs to dissolve blood clots. To be effective, this treatment must be started within 3 or 4 hours of the onset of the emergency. Alert hospital personnel about the patient's condition and your estimated time of arrival. Describe the patient's condition to hospital personnel on arrival and leave a copy of the ambulance report form for the patient's hospital records.

# OVERVIEW OF DEFIBRILLATION

## THE CHAIN OF SURVIVAL

The Chain of Survival shows the sequence of events that must occur to provide the best chance of survival from sudden, out-of-hospital cardiac arrest. The links in the Chain of Survival are as follows:

- recognition of early warning signs and early access and activation of EMS

- early BLS (within 4 minutes of cardiac arrest)

- early defibrillation (within 10 minutes)

- early ACLS, including intubation and IV medications (This means you

should consider early ALS or air medical transport if possible and appropriate, based on your local protocol.)

One of the four links of the Chain of Survival is early defibrillation. **Defibrillation** is the delivery of a direct current electric shock (or countershock) to the chest over the heart. This countershock should convert the heart from a rhythm that will not support life to one that will support life. Early defibrillation from an arrest caused by VF will provide a better chance that the patient can return to his or her previous life-style. However, delivering a countershock to a patient in arrest caused by a rhythm disturbance other than VF, or a very fast heart rate, is not likely to help. For example, a patient in asystole is generally not helped by a countershock.

The concept of early defibrillation is so important that the American Heart Association recommends it as a standard for BLS ambulance services. ALS personnel need not be present to perform this skill.

## TYPES OF DEFIBRILLATORS

### Fully Automated Defibrillators

Fully automated defibrillators were the first generation of defibrillators used by EMS personnel. This type of defibrillator is now uncommon. This device analyzes the heart rhythm and delivers a shock essentially without action from you. You only have to connect the machine through cables attached to the defibrillator pads to the patient and turn on the power. One major problem with this device is its sensitivity. If you touch or move the patient as the machine is analyzing the heart rhythm, the machine "sees" VF and shocks the patient. Semiautomatic defibrillators are much safer in this respect. The computerized rhythm analysis in the semiautomatic machines is also generally better.

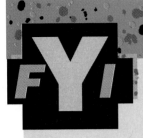

# Diseases of the Blood Vessels

The blood vessels can be damaged by disease and/or injury. A disease called **arteriosclerosis** can completely block the coronary arteries. As a result, oxygen and nutrients are cut off to that part of the heart. This lack of blood flow to a part of the body is called ischemia. Arteriosclerosis thickens and eventually destroys the walls of the arteries, due to a buildup of fatty deposits within them. This condition interferes with the ability of the coronary arteries to dilate and carry additional blood to the heart.

Arteriosclerosis involves other arteries of the body as well. The disease begins when a deposit of fatty material—cholesterol—begins to build up on the inside of an artery. Cholesterol may start building up in the arteries in individuals as young as age 18. As a person ages, more cholesterol is deposited. As a result, the inside diameter of the artery becomes smaller. As these cholesterol deposits grow larger, calcium deposits also form. The inner wall of the artery, which is normally smooth and elastic, eventually becomes narrowed, rough, and stiff.

Blood clots can form easily on the damaged walls of the arteries (Figure 16-4). Damage to the coronary arteries may become so severe that they cannot give the heart enough blood when it needs it the most. Therefore, during physical activity or emotional stress, the oxygen supply to the heart no longer meets the heart's needs.

## FIGURE 16-4

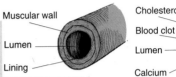

Muscular wall
Lumen
Lining

Cholesterol
Blood clot
Lumen
Calcium

A normal
coronary artery

A damaged
coronary artery

Heart disease most commonly affects people between the ages of 40 and 70. However, remember that serious heart-related symptoms can occur any time—from the teens to the 90s. A 28-year-old person with chest pain is not too young to have a heart attack.

## RISKS FOR HEART DISEASE

There are many factors that place a person at higher risk of heart disease. These are called risk factors and are divided into the following two groups:
1. Factors that can be controlled or modified
2. Factors that cannot be controlled or modified

Factors that can be controlled include cigarette smoking, high blood pressure, elevated cholesterol and triglyceride levels, lack of exercise, obesity, stress, and blood sugar levels associated with diabetes. Major risk factors that cannot be controlled include age, sex, race, heredity, and the presence of diseases such as diabetes.

## Semiautomated Defibrillators

Semiautomated or shock-advisory defibrillators (AED) are the most common type of basic defibrillator in use. The AED will shock VF or fast ventricular tachycardia (usually greater than 180 beats per minute) (Figure 16-5). The AED has an on-board computer chip that analyzes the heart rhythm in multiple (usually about seven) ways.

The AED will start to charge after the first few methods of analysis are complete. The other methods continue to verify that the patient has a shockable rhythm. If the AED waited to charge until the complete analysis were done, it would take much longer to charge and deliver the shock. The purpose of these multiple methods is to make sure that the patient's heart rhythm is one that you want to shock.

Do not touch the patient during rhythm analysis. This will create an artifact that may confuse the AED. As a result, the patient may receive an unnecessary shock or analysis may begin again, both of which may be dangerous or even deadly. If the patient's condition becomes worse during transport, you must pull over and stop the ambulance. However, you should not stop the engine. The AED cannot properly analyze the heart rhythm when the ambulance is moving.

Once the patient's heart rhythm is analyzed, the device will advise you by voice and/or words on a screen whether or not to shock the patient. If you are advised to shock, clear the patient, then push a button to give the shock. The shock is delivered through large adhesive defibrillator pads on the patient's chest. Most devices also have a manual control module for a physician or paramedic to use the machine as a manual defibrillator to shock other rhythms. In the semiautomatic mode, the AED is usually faster at delivering a shock than a paramedic with a manual defibrillator, usually in less than 1 minute.

## FIGURE 16-5

The semiautomated external defibrillator (AED)

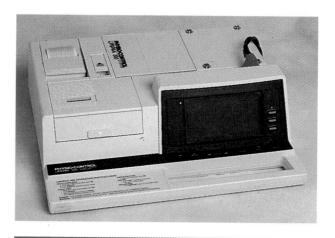

## Manual Defibrillators

Manual defibrillators are usually used by ALS services. With these devices, you must analyze and interpret the patient's heart rhythm (Figure 16-6). If you decide to deliver a countershock, you must push buttons either on paddles applied to the patient's chest, or through large adhesive patches applied to the chest. This is also called "hands-off defibrillation." Hands-off defibrillation is safer than using paddles. It is also more effective since the shock is delivered through a pad with a large surface area that closely adheres to the patient. These devices can be used to monitor and to treat rhythms other than VF or VT.

## Automatic Internal Cardiovertor Defibrillators

Automatic internal cardiovertor defibrillators (AICDs) are not devices used by EMT-Bs. They are devices implanted in the patient's chest. Thus, you are increasingly more likely to see patients with them. The AICD is implanted under the skin in the upper left abdomen and then connected to

## FIGURE 16-6

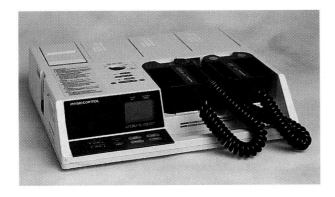

A manual defibrillator

pads on the outside of the heart. If the patient goes into VF or has a very fast rhythm, the device will shock the patient, usually up to five times. If a patient with an AICD is in cardiac arrest, treat him or her as any other patient. Apply the AED as usual to see if a shock is needed. Also try to determine if the AICD has "fired" already by asking the patient, family, or bystanders if the patient felt a countershock. They will often describe the firing as a "kick in the chest." This information will help hospital personnel to better assess the patient's situation. The AICD is not usually implanted in the area where you apply the defibrillator pads. However, you may wish to move the defibrillator pads slightly to avoid shocking through the implant. If the device fires while you are touching the patient, you will probably feel it, but it will not harm you.

## PERFORMING DEFIBRILLATION

You should attempt defibrillation only on unresponsive, pulseless patients who are not breathing (apneic). These are important criteria, as you must avoid delivering a shock to a patient who does not need one. You must strictly follow medical protocols and guidelines on the use of the AED to avoid problems.

## USING THE AED

The use of the AED must be a coordinated team effort. EMT-B #1 controls the AED. EMT-B #2 performs CPR, inserts airway adjuncts if needed, and gives oxygen when appropriate. If, in your system, you arrive at the scene alone with the defibrillator, your first priority is rhythm analysis and delivery of shock. This analysis should be done before CPR or before giving oxygen. You should call for additional help only after you have analyzed the heart rhythm and the AED advises one of the following:

- no shock
- shock, and you have delivered three stacked shocks

AEDs will often have a built-in event recorder, usually a removable computer module or tape microrecorder placed in the machine. This recorder allows later analysis and playback of the rhythms and shocks delivered at the scene for review and quality assurance purposes. AEDs may also have a voice recorder to allow you to record events by voice as they happen. If your AED has a voice recorder, make sure you turn it on now. It is a good habit to "think aloud" as you care for a patient in cardiac arrest.

For example, you may record the following:

CPR was in progress on arrival. It was stopped, and we confirmed the arrest, then restarted CPR. The machine was applied and it analyzed. Three shocks were initially delivered.

The patient started to have some spontaneous respirations, and started to become restless. His blood pressure was 100 over 60, 2 minutes out from the hospital.

The event recorder and the voice recorder provide a good source for review for the team at the scene, for members of the team who were not there, and for your medical director.

Thus, you must understand how the AED works, and more importantly, practice using it. Also remember that no defibrillator will work without properly functioning batteries. Check the batteries at the beginning of your shift and carry extra fully charged batteries in the unit, just to be sure. The most common cause of AED failure is low or dead batteries.

### Preparing to Defibrillate

As you are en route to a scene where a patient is in cardiac arrest, put on gloves and follow BSI techniques, as usual. Upon arrival, make sure that the scene is safe for you and your partner to enter. If bystanders or first responders are doing CPR, ask them to stop. Perform an initial assessment to verify that the patient is unresponsive, is not breathing, and has no pulse (Figure 16-7a). If the patient meets these criteria, your partner should resume one-rescuer CPR to support airway, breathing, and circulation (Figure 16-7b).

Next, you should prepare to use the AED. Attach the adhesive defibrillator pads to the patient and turn on the power (Figure 16-7c). One pad is marked "sternum." Apply this pad to the upper part of the right side of the chest at the base of the heart. Place the other pad at the apex of the heart over the lower part of the left side of the chest (Figure 16-7d). Pads provide much better contact with the patient, are safer, and deliver shocks more effectively than do paddles.

Once you have applied the pads and turned on the AED and the event recorder, have your partner stop CPR and clear the patient (Figure 16-7e). No one should touch the patient during the analysis or the shock period. Before delivering any shock, you must say, "Clear the patient." This will avoid injury to you or your partner. The artifact caused by touching the patient may fool the AED into reaching a false conclusion about the patient's heart rhythm. As a result, the AED may advise an unnecessary shock. Staying clear of the patient will avoid unneeded shocks to the patient and possible shock to you or your partner.

### Analyzing the Heart Rhythm and Delivering Shocks

The AED will now begin analysis of the patient's heart rhythm. After quickly using several different analysis methods to analyze the heart rhythm, the AED will then advise one of the following:

- press the button to shock the patient
- no shock is advised

**AED advises shock**  If the AED advises you to shock, clear the patient, press the shock button, then press the button to reanalyze (Figure 16-8a). During this initial phase (i.e., the first three countershocks), no one should touch the patient or do CPR. If the AED advises a second countershock, do so and then reanalyze the patient's heart rhythm. If the AED advises a third shock, then do so again.

The American Heart Association recommends that the first three shocks be delivered one right after the other. This series of three "stacked" shocks results in a better chance of defibrillation. They also recommend that AEDs be set to give sets of three shocks in a row. Many machines are programmed to do this without you even needing to press the analyze button in between

**FIGURE 16-7**

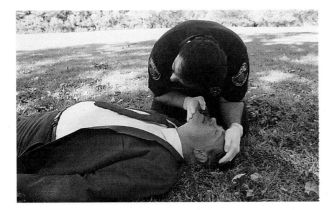

**A**    Assess for breathing and pulse

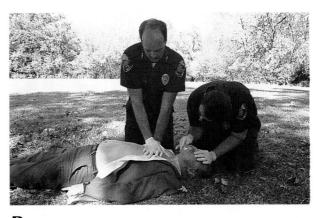

**B**    Resume CPR

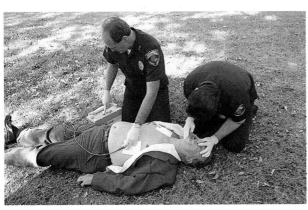

**C**    Apply defibrillator pads

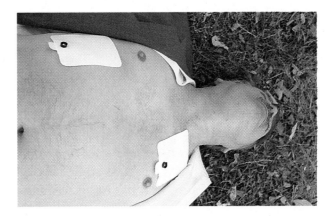

**D**    Proper positions for defibrillator pads

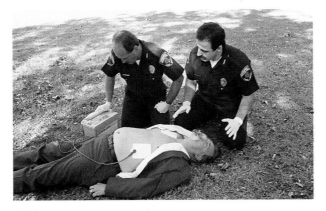

**E**    Clear the patient before giving the shock

shocks. After the third shock, the AED times a 60-second interval. After this interval has passed, the device recommends one of two things, as follows:

- check the patient
- push the analyze button and begin another set of three countershocks, as needed

If the patient has a pulse after the third countershock, check his or her breathing, to see if assisted ventilations are needed. You should not check the patient's pulse when the AED is analyzing the patient's heart rhythm. Typically, you will assess the pulse only after the third and sixth shocks (Figure 16-8b). If breathing is adequate, give the patient oxygen via a nonrebreathing mask. If the patient is not breathing adequately, assist ventilations with a BVM device or oxygen-powered breathing device. Begin packaging and transport of the patient and notify the hospital.

If the patient has no pulse after the third shock, then restart CPR (Figure 16-8c). After 1 minute of CPR, stop and have the AED reanalyze the heart rhythm. Repeat another cycle of up to three countershocks, as described above.

**AED advises no shock**    If the AED advises no shock after any rhythm analysis, then check the pulse. If the patient has a pulse, next check his or her breathing. If the patient is breathing adequately, give oxygen via a nonrebreathing mask and transport. If transport will be delayed, place the patient in the recovery position. If the patient is not breathing adequately, assist ventilations with high-concentration oxygen via a BVM device or oxygen-powered device.

If the patient has no pulse, restart CPR. After 1 minute of CPR, stop and have the AED reanalyze the heart rhythm. If the AED advises shock, deliver up to two sets of three stacked shocks, if needed. Perform 1 minute of CPR between each set of three

FIGURE 16-8

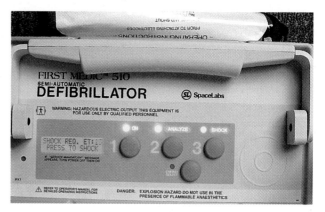

**A**    An AED screen showing shock advisory

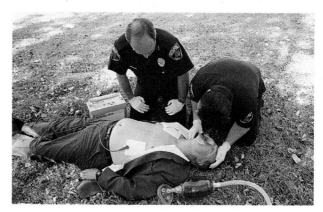

**B**    Reassess the pulse after shock delivery

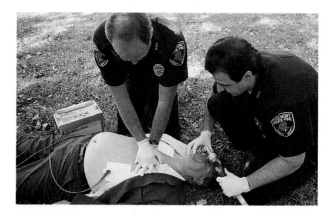

**C**    Resume CPR if no pulse

shocks. If the AED advises no shock, and the patient still has no pulse, restart CPR. After 1 minute of CPR, stop and have the

## COOPERATION OR CONFLICT

You are working on a 15-year-old girl who has been electrocuted and is now in cardiac arrest. Even though you are the defibrillator-certified EMT-B, your new partner, who won't even finish the EMT-B course for another 2 weeks, is not cooperating with you. As things go, he is challenging you and questioning your every move, especially on the use of the AED.

### For Discussion

1. Describe why proper sequencing of events is essential when using an AED.

2. How can equipment maintenance and daily checks of your unit impact management of cardiac arrest?

---

AED reanalyze the heart rhythm for a third time. If the AED advises shock, deliver up to two sets of three stacked shocks, if needed. Perform 1 minute of CPR between each set of three shocks. If the AED still advises no shock, restart CPR and transport.

Your approach depends on local protocol. Some medical directors may want transport after two sets of three countershocks. Others may want transport after three sets of three countershocks.

*Remember that no one should touch the patient during rhythm analysis or as you deliver the shock. This means no CPR! While it may seem like a long time, the 90 seconds needed to interrupt CPR and give the first three shocks are absolutely necessary. You should then restart CPR for 1 minute until you are ready to give the second set of three shocks.*

### PEDIATRIC CONSIDERATIONS

An AED should only be used with patients who are older than 12 years or weigh more than 90 lb. A shock from the AED at the usual energy settings will be too great for a young child or small person. In general, children go into arrest due to respiratory, not heart, problems. Thus, a child is not likely to respond to the AED anyway.

### TRANSPORTING THE PATIENT

You are now ready to transport the patient according to local protocol, as written by your medical director. Most medical directors will want you to provide transport after any one of the following events occur:

- the patient regains a pulse
- two sets of three stacked shocks are delivered
- the AED advises no shock three consecutive times

It may be in the best interest of the patient for you to transfer care to an ALS unit before you get to the hospital. This will allow more advanced procedures, such as administration of drugs or other interventions sooner. You may also wish to send for an air medical unit for quicker transport. These measures will improve the patient's chance of survival and perhaps later quality of life. However, depending on your local situation and geography, these options may not be practical or possible.

## SPECIAL TRANSPORT SITUATIONS

If you are transporting an unconscious patient, reassess the patient's pulse every 30 seconds while you are en route. This is to make sure that the patient is not in cardiac arrest. If the patient suddenly becomes unresponsive or has no pulse during transport you must stop the unit. The AED cannot analyze heart rhythms while the unit is in motion. Furthermore, it is not safe to defibrillate in a moving ambulance.

If the patient experiences loss of circulation and if the AED is not immediately ready, start CPR until it is ready. Once the pads have been applied and the power turned on, then push the analyze button as soon as the vehicle stops, and proceed with defibrillation as described above.

If you are transporting a conscious patient with chest pain, monitor the patient carefully en route. If the patient suddenly becomes unconscious, stops breathing, and has no pulse, you must stop the unit. As described above, prepare the patient for defibrillation. If the AED is not immediately ready, start CPR until it is ready. Once the

pads have been applied and the power turned on, then push the analyze button as soon as the unit stops, and proceed with defibrillation as described above.

Finally, if you are transporting a patient who suddenly has no pulse, but the AED advises no shock, you must start or restart CPR. You must also stop the unit so that you can reanalyze the heart rhythm. If the AED still gives three consecutive "no shock" messages, continue CPR and transport. However, if the AED advises you to shock, give up to six stacked shocks (two sets of three), or until the patient's pulse returns. Then continue transport.

## POSTRESUSCITATION CARE

After using the AED according to your local protocol, you must evaluate the patient for the following:

- the patient is still pulseless and no shock is recommended
- the patient is still pulseless and the AED advises you to shock
- the patient has a pulse

If the patient is still pulseless, and the AED is not recommending a shock, then what you do depends on local protocol. You should continue CPR, call on an ALS unit to meet you, or call on air medical for quicker transport.

If the patient has no pulse, but the AED advises a shock, then you have several options. First, you may call on an ALS unit or air medical transport. You may also consult with medical control to see if you should give more shocks, per your local protocol. You may also provide rapid transport, continuing CPR en route. The last option is least preferred because performing CPR in

## IS IT THE BIG ONE?

You have settled in for what you're hoping will be a long night's sleep. Your dreams of bliss fade away abruptly at 2 am, courtesy of your pager. Dispatch sends you and your partner down the road to a "possible heart." On arrival, you find a 59-year-old woman complaining that her "chest hurts." She tells you that the discomfort started about 11 pm, just before she went to bed. She states that she woke up about 1 am and tossed and turned for another hour. The pain got so bad that she finally decided to call 9-1-1. She is pale, cool, and clammy. She has a blood pressure of 102/66 mm Hg, an irregular pulse of 68/min, and respirations of 14/min. She takes no medications, has no allergies, and restates that she has never had pain like this before.

### For Discussion

1. What is the impact of denial on a patient having a myocardial infarction?

2. Describe the relationship between a slow pulse rate and blood pressure.

---

a moving ambulance is inadequate, difficult, and dangerous.

If the patient has a pulse, you should call on an ALS unit or air medical transport. These units can give medications to try to prevent another cardiac arrest. In any event the patient should be carefully watched, given oxygen or ventilated if necessary, and transported with a defibrillator in place. What you do will depend on your instructions from medical control and local protocol.

No matter what course of action you take, you should monitor the patient carefully and do the following:

- continue chest compressions
- ventilate the patient with high-flow oxygen, advanced airways, and suctioning, as needed
- leave the AED in place

Remember that you should give oxygen only after the first three countershocks or after the patient gets a pulse back. Use of airway adjuncts or invasive airway management also occurs after the initial three shocks. If successfully defibrillated, the patient may not need an airway adjunct, but will still need high-flow oxygen.

# DEFIBRILLATOR MAINTENANCE

Your service must keep a maintenance protocol for your AED (Figure 16-9). This protocol provides a systematic way for you to check and maintain the AED. The frequency with which you check the AED depends on how often you use the device and on the protocols written by your medical director. A very busy service may check the device every 8 hours, while a less busy service may do it once a day. The important thing is to document that the AED is checked methodically and regularly, including the batteries.

# MAINTAINING DEFIBRILLATION SKILLS

AEDs have revolutionized your ability to effectively treat patients in cardiac arrest. Your skills need to be maintained by refresher training at least every 3 months. In addition, the American Heart Association publishes a variety of guidelines and additional information on AEDs.

## *MEDICAL DIRECTION AND QUALITY IMPROVEMENT*

AEDs are medical devices. As such, both your state's laws and your medical director need to approve your service's use of the AED. An active medical director is also needed to monitor the quality of treatment given by your service. The medical director is also responsible for overseeing initial training and continuing education of AED operators at least twice a year.

Every incident in which the AED is used must be reviewed by the medical director or his or her designee. This is important to make sure that proper procedures are being followed. After each run is completed, download the event recorder, according to local protocol. Give a written report and the audiotape, depending on protocol, to the medical director or to his or her designee. Once you return to quarters, prepare the AED for its next use and put it on the charger. Remember that an AED will not work if the battery is not charged.

Each episode can then be reviewed with the team for positive reinforcement or constructive criticism, as needed. This is the basis for continuous monitoring of the quality of the defibrillation program. The medical director should review with the team the following events from each run in which the AED was used:

- the dispatch and response times
- whether prearrival instructions were given, if applicable in your area
- the sequence of actions at the scene, including the recording devices, the presence of correct criteria for applying the AED, the actions of the AED, proper use of oxygen, proper use of airway adjuncts, the written report, and postresuscitation care

# MEDICATIONS

Chest pain is treated with a medication called nitroglycerin. **Nitroglycerin** relaxes the smooth muscle of the blood vessel walls. This, in turn, dilates the coronary arteries and increases blood flow and the supply of oxygen to the heart muscle. Dilation of blood vessels also means that the heart pumps against less resistance. Therefore, the heart does not work as hard. Eventually this eases the chest pain. Nitroglycerin is the generic or chemical name of this med-

# FIGURE 16-9

AHA Daily Checklist for AED

## Automated Defibrillators: Operator's Shift Checklist

Date _____  Shift _____  Location _____

Mfr/Model No. _____  Serial No. or Facility ID No. _____

At the beginning of each shift, inspect the unit. Indicate whether all requirements have been met. Note any corrective actions taken. Sign the form.

| | OK as Found | Corrective Action/ Remarks |
|---|---|---|
| **1. Defibrillator Unit** <br> Clean, no spills, clear of objects on top, casing intact | | |
| **2. Cables/Connectors** <br> a. Inspect for cracks, broken wire, or damage <br> b. Connectors engage securely and are not damaged* | | |
| **3. Supplies** <br> a. Two sets of pads in sealed packages, within expiration date*    g. Spare charged battery* <br> b. Hand towel    h. Adequate ECG paper* <br> c. Scissors    i. Manual override module, key, or card* <br> d. Razor    j. Cassette tape, memory module, and/or event card plus spares* <br> e. Alcohol wipes* <br> f. Monitoring electrodes* | | |
| **4. Power Supply** <br> a. Battery-powered units <br>   (1) Verify fully charged battery in place <br>   (2) Spare charged battery available <br>   (3) Follow appropriate battery rotation schedule per manufacturer's recommendations <br> b. AC/battery backup units <br>   (1) Plugged into live outlet to maintain battery charge <br>   (2) Test on battery power and reconnect to line power | | |
| **5. Indicators*/ECG Display** <br> a. Remove cassette tape, memory module, and/or event card* <br> b. Power-on display <br> c. Self-test OK <br> d. Monitor display functional* <br> e. "Service" message display off* <br> f. Battery charging; low battery light off* <br> g. Correct time displayed; set with dispatch center | | |
| **6. ECG Recorder*** <br> a. Adequate ECG paper <br> b. Recorder prints | | |
| **7. Charge/Display Cycle** <br> a. Disconnect AC plug—battery backup units* <br> b. Attach to simulator <br> c. Detects, charges, and delivers shock for VF <br> d. Responds correctly to nonshockable rhythms <br> e. Manual override functional* <br> f. Detach from simulator <br> g. Replace cassette tape, module, and/or memory card* | | |
| **8. Pacemaker*** <br> a. Pacer output cable intact <br> b. Pacer pads present (set of two) <br> c. Inspect per manufacturer's operational guidelines | | |
| **Major Problem(s) Identified**    **(Out of Service)** | | |

*Applicable only if the unit has this supply or capability

ication. Common trade names include Nitro-bid, Nitrolingual, and Nitro-stat, along with many others. This medication comes in the following forms (Figure 16-10):

- a small white pill, about one half the size of an aspirin tablet
- a spray
- a paste
- a skin patch applied to the chest

The pill is not swallowed. Rather, it is placed under the tongue (sublingually) and allowed to melt. The spray is given on the mucosa inside of the cheek or under the tongue.

## INDICATIONS

Nitroglycerin should only be given to a patient having chest pain, if the patient has it prescribed, and/or your medical director authorizes you to give it. The way in which you use nitroglycerin, including when and how many tablets, and whether you need on-line medical control, depends on the protocols written by your medical director.

## PRECAUTIONS AND CONTRAINDICATIONS

Some precautions about nitroglycerin include the following:

- Make sure you do not get spray or melted tablet on your skin. If you do, you may get a headache, experience a decrease in your blood pressure, and increase in your pulse rate. It will have the same effects on you as it does on the patient. Thus you should be sure to wear gloves, as you should be doing anyway.
- If the patient has a nitroglycerin patch on the chest, and you need to use the defibrillator, take the nitroglycerin

## FIGURE 16-10

Nitroglycerin preparations

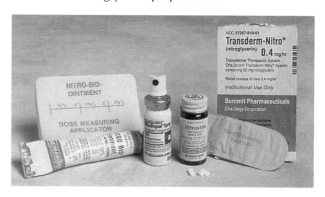

patch off the chest. Some of these patches have caught fire when the defibrillator goes off too close to them.

Contraindications include the following:

- hypotension or a systolic blood pressure of less than 100 mm Hg
- head injury
- infants and children
- patient has already taken three tablets before you arrive

## ACTIONS

Nitroglycerin relieves the pain of angina pectoris. It also relaxes and dilates blood vessels in the brain, sometimes causing a severe headache. Nitroglycerin usually works in seconds, but it may be 5 minutes until the full effect occurs. You should then recheck the blood pressure within 2 to 3 minutes and every 2 to 3 minutes after that. If the initial dose of nitroglycerin does not work, a second dose should be given after 3 to 5 minutes, if the blood pressure is above 100 mm Hg systolic and the patient still has chest pain. A third dose may be given 5 minutes after the second one. However, if there is no pain relief after three nitroglycerin tablets, then nitroglycerin is

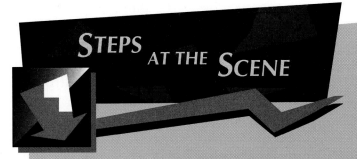

## STEPS AT THE SCENE

### GIVING NITROGLYCERIN

☐ Ask the patient, if possible, if he or she has taken nitroglycerin before and then ask about the effect on pain.

☐ Check the patient's systolic blood pressure to make sure it is above 100 mm Hg.

☐ Check the container to make sure that you are giving the nitroglycerin to the patient listed on the prescription label. Or, make sure that the patient fits the criteria for using nitroglycerin from the ambulance supply, per local protocol.

☐ Check the expiration date on the container.

☐ Make sure the patient is alert and understands what you are going to do. Explain how the nitroglycerin is given and what will happen once you give it.

☐ Tell the patient to raise his or her tongue and place the tablet under it, or tell the patient to place it under the tongue.

☐ Tell the patient to keep his or her mouth closed until the tablet is dissolved and absorbed. Advise the patient to avoid swallowing the tablet.

☐ Recheck the patient's blood pressure within 2 minutes.

☐ Reassess the patient, including the effect of nitroglycerin on pain.

☐ Remember that the side effects of nitroglycerin include hypotension (even to the point of fainting), headache, burning under the tongue, increased pulse rate.

---

not going to help. In these instances, the patient may have more severe heart ischemia or pain that is not related to the heart.

## ADMINISTRATION

Once you have completed the focused assessment and have decided that you want to give nitroglycerin, it is important to make sure that the patient's systolic blood pressure is greater than 100 mm Hg. Next, contact medical control for approval if you do not have standing orders.

Check the expiration date of the medication. If the nitroglycerin is older than 6 months, it may have lost its potency and

effectiveness. Good nitroglycerin tablets usually "burn" under the tongue or give the patient a headache, unless the patient is very accustomed to nitroglycerin. It may help to ask the patient how new nitroglycerin feels, if he or she has used it. If the nitroglycerin is old, you may have to ask the patient where a new bottle is, or use nitroglycerin from your unit, if state law and medical direction allow you to carry this medication.

When you give a patient nitroglycerin, you should have the patient lie down. If not, the patient may faint if the nitroglycerin substantially drops the patient's blood pressure. Before giving nitroglycerin, it is a good idea to determine how the patient reacted to it when and if he or she had it before. You need to be much more cautious if the patient has had an adverse reaction, such as fainting, to the medication.

It is helpful for hospital personnel if you try to determine the severity of the patient's chest pain. One popular method is to ask the patient to rate the pain on a scale from 1 to 10, where 10 is the worst pain that the patient has ever had and 1 is almost no pain. Ask the patient to rate the pain before giving the first dose of nitroglycerin and after each dose. This gives hospital personnel perspective on the pain, as far as what therapy they may want to proceed with next.

Remember improved blood flow to the heart will provide pain relief. This is the most important reason to give nitroglycerin. The sooner that pain is relieved, the more likely that damage to the heart will be prevented or minimized. You could even prevent a cardiac arrest. The battle cry of the cardiologist now is, "Time is myocardium." In essence, a "Golden Hour" has been established for ischemic heart disease, as it has been for trauma.

# Atlas of
# Common Cardiac Conditions

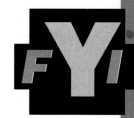

## ANGINA PECTORIS

If the heart does not have the oxygen supply to meet its needs for more than several seconds, severe chest pain will occur. The pain is often described as crushing—as it takes a patient's breath away. Some people describe it as "squeezing" or "like somebody standing on my chest." This pain is called **angina pectoris,** or simply angina. Angina pectoris indicates coronary artery disease. Thus, it is important for you to understand the pain and to recognize it.

The main symptom of angina is pain that occurs with exertion and is relieved by rest. This pain is usually felt under the sternum (behind the breastbone). The pain usually lasts from 3 to 8 minutes, but rarely longer than 10 minutes. However, physical exertion is not the only cause of angina. Emotional stress, a large meal, or anxiety may also trigger an attack.

Angina may be associated with shortness of breath (dyspnea), nausea, or sweating, and a feeling of weakness or tiredness. The pain goes away as soon as the heart gets enough oxygen to meet its needs. This happens as the patient relaxes or when oxygen is given. Although angina is painful, it does not mean death or even permanent heart damage. However, it does indicate that the patient has some degree of coronary artery disease.

There are other signs and symptoms of angina. Sometimes the patient will describe a "squeezing" sensation, tightness in the chest, or difficulty in breathing. The patient may also complain of pain in the lower jaw, the arms (especially the left arm), or the upper middle region of the abdomen. The patient may interpret these symptoms as indigestion or an ulcer. This is called referred pain. In fact, some people even go to see their dentist because of the jaw pain.

Angina is treated with nitroglycerin, as described in the chapter. This medication usually works in seconds, relaxing the muscle of the blood vessel walls. It also dilates the coronary arteries and increases blood flow and oxygen to the heart.

## ACUTE MYOCARDIAL INFARCTION

The coronary artery may be so severely damaged, or have a blood clot inside, that oxygen cannot reach the heart. This can result in death of the heart muscle. This condition is called **acute myocardial infarction (AMI).** The pain of an AMI is the same as that of angina. However, the pain of an AMI is more severe, lasts longer, and is not relieved by nitroglycerin.

### Signs and Symptoms

A patient with an AMI may not have chest pain. Instead, the patient may complain of pain in the lower jaw, the arms, or the neck. Shortness of breath, indigestion, or severe weakness or fatigue are also common complaints. This means that you must take all complaints of chest pain seriously. Your treatment may prevent angina from becoming an AMI. It may also make a developing AMI less serious.

AMI usually occurs in the left ventricle (Figure 16-11). This is the larger, thick-

## FIGURE 16-11

Acute myocardial infarction due to a blood clot

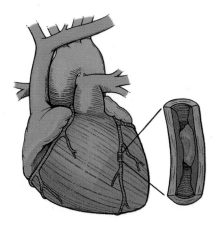

walled heart chamber that produces a higher systemic blood pressure. The left ventricle requires more blood and much more oxygen than the right ventricle. Therefore, the left ventricle suffers the most from a lack of oxygen.

### Consequences of AMI

AMI has three major and serious consequences, as follows:

1. Sudden death
2. Cardiogenic shock
3. Congestive heart failure (CHF)

### Sudden Death

Approximately 40% of all patients with AMI die before they reach the hospital. These deaths occur because of sudden abnormalities in the heart rhythm called arrhythmias. Arrhythmias prevent effective pumping action of the heart. The chance that an arrhythmia will occur after an AMI is greatest within the first hour. This risk becomes much smaller 3 to 5 days after an AMI. Arrhythmias may result in fibrillation or asystole (Figure 16-12). In either case, the clinical appearance of the heart is cardiac arrest. These patients require CPR.

AMI may result in a wide variety of arrhythmias, including the following:

- *Asystole.* This is complete absence of electrical activity of the heart.
- *Tachycardia.* This is rapid but regular beating of the heart.
- *Bradycardia.* This is an unusually slow but regular beating of the heart.
- *Ventricular fibrillation.* This is disorganized, ineffective quivering of the ventricles.

## FIGURE 16-12

Cardiac rhythms (top to bottom): ventricular tachycardia, ventricular fibrillation, asystole, bradycardia

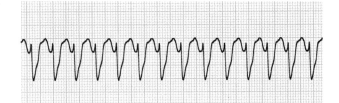

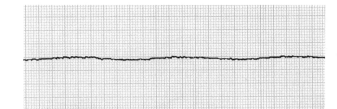

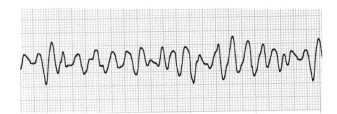

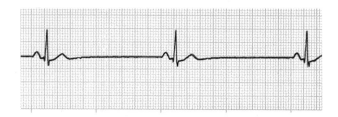

• *Ventricular tachycardia.* This is rapid, regular heart rhythm that results when several PVCs occur together.

## Cardiogenic Shock

Cardiogenic shock is a complication of AMI that occurs within 24 hours of the event. With this condition, damage is so severe that the heart is unable to sustain a normal systemic blood pressure. Thus, shock develops and may even result in death.

## Congestive Heart Failure

Just as the left ventricle can be damaged by coronary artery disease, it can be damaged by disease or chronic hypertension. When the heart muscle can no longer contract well enough, it attempts to maintain adequate cardiac output in other ways. One way is by beating faster. A second way is by increasing the size of the left ventricle. This is done in an attempt to increase the amount of blood pumped each minute.

When these adaptations can no longer make up for the decreased heart function, a condition called **congestive heart failure (CHF)** develops. It is called "congestive" heart failure because the lungs become filled (or congested) with fluid once the heart fails to pump the blood effectively. Blood tends to back up in the pulmonary veins. This increases the pressure in the capillaries of the lungs. When the pressure in the capillaries exceeds a certain level, fluid (mostly water) passes through the walls of the capillary vessels and into the alveoli. This condition is called **pulmonary edema.** Pulmonary edema may occur suddenly, as in AMI, or slowly over months, as in chronic congestive heart failure.

***Symptoms and Signs*** Once fluid passes from the capillaries to the alveoli, the patient has shortness of breath. The fluid tends

to make the lungs stiffer. Therefore, the patient has rapid, shallow respirations. The patient finds it harder to breathe lying down than standing or sitting. When the patient is lying down, the return of blood to the right ventricle and to the lungs increases and causes more congestion. Thus, the patient generally insists on sitting up. Other signs and symptoms include possible chest pain, greatly distended neck veins that do not collapse even when the patient is sitting up, and swollen limbs, particularly the feet (Figure 16-13).

---

## FIGURE 16-13

Pedal edema due to congestive heart failure

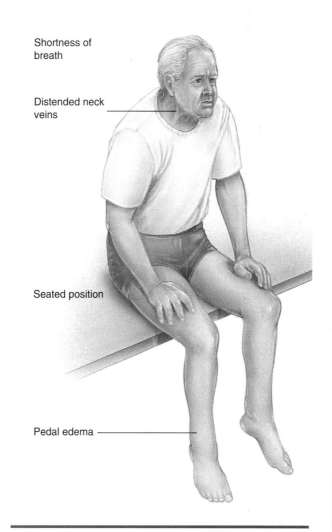

Shortness of breath

Distended neck veins

Seated position

Pedal edema

---

Patients with CHF usually have normal or somewhat high blood pressure, a rapid heart rate, and rapid, shallow respirations. As you listen to the back of the patient's chest, you may hear the sound of air bubbling through the fluid in the alveoli and bronchi. This sound is called **rales,** a sound like rattles or sand falling on an empty tin can. Rales are an abnormal sound that indicate a respiratory problem. You might also hear wheezing. In severe CHF, these sounds can be heard from the top to the base of the lung.

***Treatment*** Take the patient's vital signs, monitor the heart, and give oxygen. Allow the patient to remain sitting up with the legs down. It is important to reassure and calm the patient. Many patients with CHF will have prescribed medications. Make sure you take these patients to the hospital.

## PATIENTS WITH PRIOR HEART OPERATIONS AND PACEMAKERS

In the coronary artery bypass graft (CABG) operation, a vein from the leg or an artificial vessel is sewn directly from the aorta to a coronary artery beyond the point of the obstruction.

More recently, a different kind of operation, called an angioplasty or balloon angioplasty, has been used to widen the coronary arteries. In this operation, a tiny balloon is attached to the end of a long thin catheter. The surgeon introduces the balloon through the skin into a vein. Then, while watching an x-ray monitor, the surgeon threads the balloon into the coronary artery and then inflates it. The purpose of this operation is to dilate the coronary artery rather than bypass it. You will almost certainly have a patient with AMI or angina who has had such an operation.

Patients who have had a bypass graft will have a long surgical scar on their chests from the operation (Figure 16-14). Patients who have had an angioplasty will not. You should care for AMI in a patient who has had a bypass procedure or angioplasty the same way as one who has not. If CPR is required, carry it out in the usual way, regardless of the scar on the patient's chest.

### FIGURE 16-14

Patient with a long surgical scar after a bypass graft operation

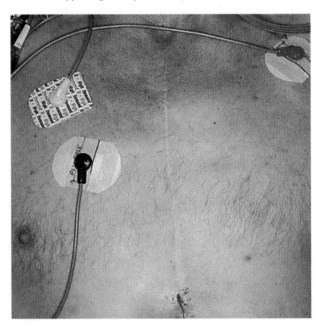

Many people with heart disease in the United States have cardiac pacemakers (Figure 16-15). These battery-powered devices maintain a regular cardiac rhythm and rate by delivering an electrical impulse through wires that are in direct contact with the heart. The generating unit is generally placed under a heavy muscle or a fold of skin. Pacemakers are inserted when the

## FIGURE 16-15

An X ray of an AICD implanted in a patient

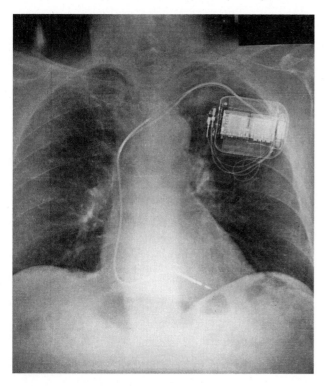

electrical control system of the heart is so damaged that it cannot function properly.

A patient with a pacemaker can be defibrillated just like any other. However, do not defibrillate through the pacemaker. A pacemaker implanted in the upper left chest will not interfere with pad placement. If the pacemaker is in the upper right chest, the pad at the base of the heart may be over the pacemaker. Therefore, before you defibrillate, you should move that pad down until you are not over the pacemaker.

If a pacemaker does not function properly, the patient may faint, or complain of dizziness, or weakness. The pulse ordinarily will be slow (35 to 45/min) and irregular. In this situation, the heart is beating without the stimulus of the pacemaker and without the regulation of its own electrical system. The heart tends to beat at a rate that is not fast enough to allow the patient to function normally. You should provide prompt transport for a patient with signs of a malfunctioning pacemaker.

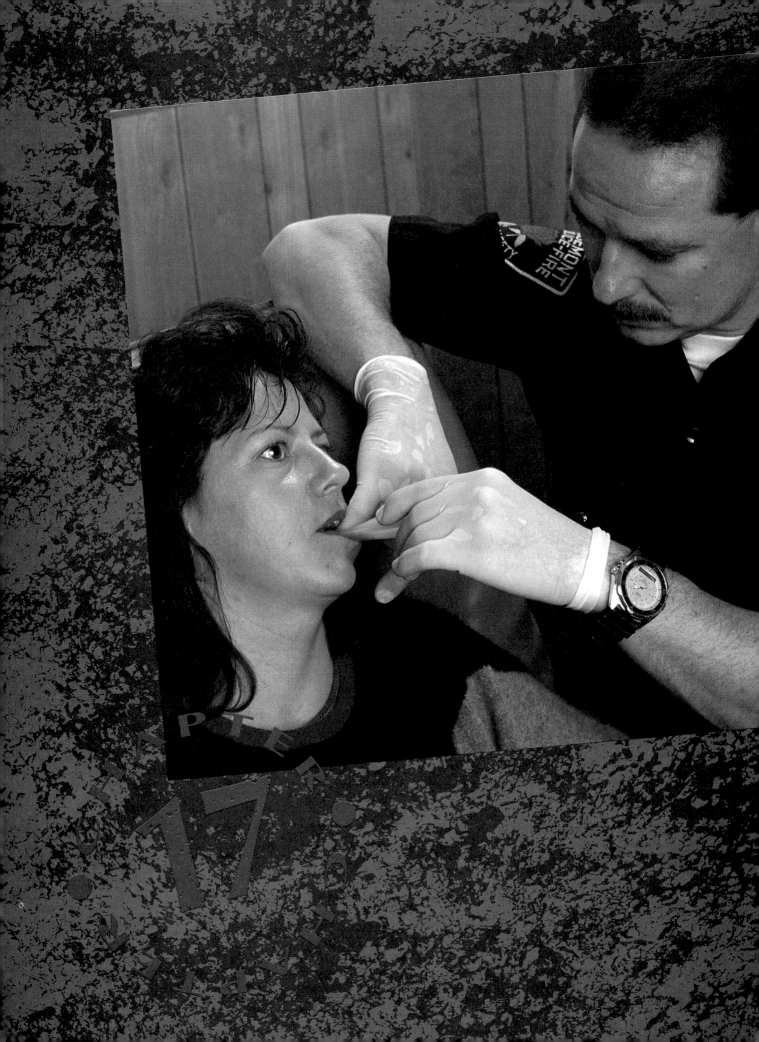

# Diabetic Emergencies

## Objectives

After you have read this chapter, you should be able to:

- Identify a patient on diabetic medications with altered mental status and the implications of a history of diabetes.
- Describe the emergency medical care of a patient who takes medication for diabetes and has an altered mental status and a history of diabetes.
- Establish the relationship between airway management and the patient with altered mental status.
- State the generic and trade names, medication forms, dose, administration, action, and contraindications for oral glucose.
- Evaluate the need for medical direction in the emergency medical care of a patient with diabetes.

## Overview

Diabetes mellitus is a serious disease that affects approximately 13 to 15 million people in the United States alone. Diabetes is caused by the lack of adequate amounts of insulin. Insulin is a hormone that enables glucose (sugar) to enter the cell where it can be used for energy metabolism. Diabetes is a progressive, permanent disease with many severe complications, including kidney failure, blindness, and damage to blood vessels and peripheral nerves. Most individuals with diabetes try to balance their food intake with their insulin therapy and do so quite well. Sometimes the balance shifts—either too much or too little food is ingested—or insulin levels change. As a result, problems develop. The patient's level of consciousness changes, resulting in disorientation, possible convulsions, or unconsciousness.

As an EMT-B, you must understand the basic problems associated with diabetes. This understanding is critical in order to make an accurate assessment of a diabetic emergency and give lifesaving treatment.

This chapter begins with a description of the signs and symptoms of a diabetic emergency. Step-by-step instructions for providing emergency medical care follow, along with a description of the use of oral glucose.

# Key Terms

**Diabetes**   Metabolic disorder in which the body cannot metabolize glucose, usually due to a lack of insulin.

**Glucose**   A simple sugar essential for cell metabolism in humans.

**Insulin**   An essential hormone produced by the pancreas that enables glucose to enter the cells of the body. Also manufactured to treat diabetes.

# UNDERSTANDING DIABETES

**Diabetes** is a metabolic disorder in which the body cannot metabolize glucose, usually due to a lack of insulin. **Glucose** is one of the basic sugars essential for cell metabolism in humans. **Insulin** is a hormone produced by the pancreas that enables glucose to enter the cells of the body (Figure 17-1). Diabetes is a disease with two distinct patterns. It may become evident when the patient is a child, or it may develop in later life—usually when the patient is in middle age. These two patterns have resulted in a great number of definitions concerning diabetes. You will likely hear or come to know some of these terms even though current medical practice discourages using many of them. A list of these common terms is provided in the FYI Glossary of Diabetes Terms.

Diabetes is also a disease of balance, which is important for you to remember. The body needs glucose for energy. However, to use glucose, the body must make and use insulin properly. Remember that a patient with diabetes may not have any insulin or may not have much working insulin. Thus, the patient must balance the need for glucose against his or her available insulin supply.

## TREATING DIABETES

Fortunately, diabetes can be treated. In fact, many methods of treatment exist. Each method must be tailored for the patient, depending on the severity of the disease. When the patient has no insulin, he or she may take a daily injection (or more) of insulin. These patients are called insulin-dependent diabetics. Most children with diabetes are insulin dependent. Not all adults who develop diabetes need to take insulin. Many adults with diabetes still produce insulin. However, the insulin is produced at a lower, and usually insufficient, level for the patient's regular diet and routine. In addition, the action of the insulin produced may be less effective. Therefore, many adults with diabetes can control their blood sugar levels with diet alone. For some, weight loss alone cures their diabetes. Others take pills that stimulate the pancreas to produce more insulin. Some adults also require small doses of insulin.

In the past, most patients checked their urine daily for the presence of sugar and

**FIGURE 17-1**

How insulin works

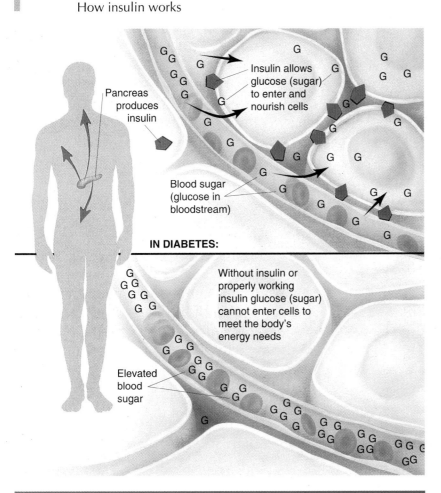

Pancreas produces insulin

Insulin allows glucose (sugar) to enter and nourish cells

Blood sugar (glucose in bloodstream)

**IN DIABETES:**

Without insulin or properly working insulin glucose (sugar) cannot enter cells to meet the body's energy needs

Elevated blood sugar

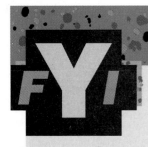

## Glossary of Diabetes Terms

**Diabetes mellitus**   Literally means "sweet diabetes." It refers to the presence of sugar in the urine and is the disease most people are referring to when the term "diabetes" is used.

**Juvenile-onset diabetes**   The form of the disease that first develops in childhood. Characterized by an absolute lack of insulin, which must be replaced daily for effective treatment. This term is no longer used medically, but you may still hear it. Now called type I diabetes.

**Adult-onset diabetes**   The form of the disease that develops as the patient ages. Characterized by a partial deficiency in insulin and does not usually require insulin for its treatment. This term is no longer used medically, but you may still hear it. Now called type II diabetes.

**Non-insulin-dependent diabetes**   The form of the disease that can be managed without using insulin. Measures such as weight loss, the use of oral medicines to stimulate insulin release, and diet are generally effective in its control.

**Insulin-dependent diabetes**   The form of the disease in which insulin must be used.

**Borderline diabetes**   Jargon used to characterize the patient whose blood glucose may be elevated on occasion or in whose urine sugar may be detected. It has little meaning and does not indicate the presence of the disease.

---

acetone. Now many patients monitor their own blood sugar level using special self-monitoring kits. With these kits, the patient can keep track of how much glucose (blood sugar) is currently in their blood. Monitoring blood glucose is a more direct and current assessment of their condition than detecting glucose in urine. Glucose in the urine may have been produced and stored in the bladder for several hours. These kits have devices for pricking the fingertip with a fine needle as well as standard tables for reading the strips (Figure 17-2a,b).

A more elaborate unit that provides a digital readout of the blood glucose levels is also available. In this unit, the test strip of paper exposed to the patient's blood is placed in the unit and analyzed automatically (Figure 17-2c).

It is important for you to understand that patients with diabetes are treated in different ways. You can then ask patients important questions about their condition. You may also see this equipment at the scene. This information or the presence of these kits will not change the way you treat the patient. However, you should record any information offered by the patient or family, based on data from these kits. This information could prove extremely valuable to medical control and hospital staff.

# DIABETIC EMERGENCIES

Diabetic emergencies can occur when a patient's blood glucose level gets too high or when it drops too low. Unfortunately, as you assess these patients in the field, the signs and symptoms for both conditions can appear the same.

## SIGNS AND SYMPTOMS

### Level of Consciousness

Too much blood glucose does not directly affect a patient's level of consciousness. However, when blood glucose levels become extremely high, they can have an indirect effect on level of consciousness. Remember that these patients do not have any or enough insulin, and glucose is not available for cells to use. These patients use fat for energy. Waste products from fat greatly increase the amount of acid in the blood and tissue. As a result, the cells do not work as they should and may eventually shut down. This, along with frequent urination, is what affects the patient's level of consciousness. Together, the presence of

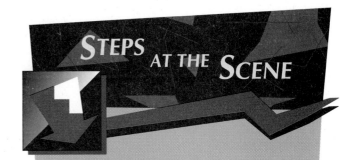

## STEPS AT THE SCENE

### GIVING ORAL GLUCOSE

☐ Verify that the patient's signs and symptoms are due to a diabetic emergency.

☐ Make sure that the patient is conscious and able to swallow.

☐ Squeeze an entire tube of glucose gel onto the bottom third of a tongue depressor.

☐ Place the tongue depressor between the cheek and gum, with the gel side toward the cheek.

☐ Allow the gel to dissolve, or instruct the patient to swallow it.

☐ Remove the tongue depressor and perform on-going assessment.

## FIGURE 17-2

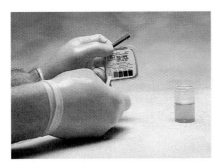

**A** Glucose test strips for urine

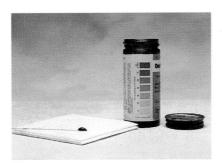

**B** Glucose test strips for blood

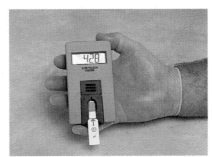

**C** Blood glucose self-monitoring unit

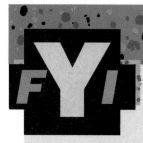

# Complications of Diabetes

Diabetes is a systemic disease that affects all tissues of the body. Thus, you will care for patients whose main problems are the complications of diabetes. The principal organs and structures damaged by diabetes over time include the kidneys, eyes, small arteries, and peripheral nerves. You may see patients who complain of visual disturbances or blindness. Others may have symptoms of kidney failure. You may also see ulcers or infections on the feet or toes.

Diabetes is also a risk factor for heart disease.

Although diabetes primarily affects the metabolism and the capacity of the body to use sugar for energy, no tissue escapes its effect. Patients with diabetes may be able to control their blood glucose levels with diet. These complications can also increase problems with management and control of the diabetes itself.

---

acid waste products in the blood and the loss of body fluid combine to affect level of consciousness.

Level of consciousness is also affected if the patient has taken too much insulin, has not eaten enough, or has exercised vigorously and used up all available glucose. Glucose is rapidly removed from the blood to supply energy to the cells. If this occurs, there is not enough glucose in the blood to provide the continuous supply needed by the brain. If blood glucose levels remain low, the patient may quickly lose consciousness, have permanent brain damage, or even die.

Therefore, when you are called to the scene of a diabetic emergency, you should ask the patient (or the family) the following questions:

- Have you taken your insulin today?
- Have you missed a meal today?

- Have you vomited after eating today?
- Have you done any strenuous exercise today?

Record the answers to these questions on the ambulance run report so that you can inform hospital personnel on arrival. You may also need to refer to the information later.

Changes in level of consciousness can also occur if the patient overeats and does not increase his or her insulin dose. In addition, stress, such as that from an infection, illness, overexertion, fatigue, or alcohol can cause problems even in a patient with well-controlled diabetes. However, these problems usually develop over a long period of time—hours or days.

## Other Signs and Symptoms

Patients experiencing a diabetic emergency may also have any one of the following signs and symptoms:

## SWEET, SWEET SHOCK

A college student comes home from his morning class to find his roommate unconscious and unresponsive. He immediately calls 9-1-1. On arrival, you find a 20-year-old woman dressed in a jogging outfit and running shoes lying on the couch in the living room. Her skin is cool and clammy, and she is unresponsive to any stimuli. The roommate states that she was fine an hour ago when they finished breakfast, and then he left to go to class. He states that she has no allergies, and does not take any medications except for her daily dose of insulin. He also states that she has just taken up jogging. The patient has a blood pressure of 94/52 mm Hg, a rapid, regular pulse of 126/min, and respirations of 28/min.

### For Discussion

1. Describe the relationship between food intake, physical activity, and insulin as they affect a person with diabetes.

2. Why should a patient with diabetes be given oral glucose at the scene? Why not wait until the patient reaches the hospital?

- rapid pulse
- normal or slightly low blood pressure
- dizziness, headache
- normal or rapid, deep sighing respirations
- sweet or fruity (acetone) breath odor
- sweating
- pale, moist (clammy) skin
- hunger
- anxiety, agitation, or lethargy
- intoxicated appearance
- aggressive or unusual behavior
- fainting, seizure, or coma
- frequent urination

Children who have diabetes pose special problems. Children are very active. As a result, they may rapidly exhaust their levels of glucose, even after a normal insulin injection. In addition, children are less likely to respond to the demands of eating correctly and on time. Signs and symptoms may develop very quickly.

### EMERGENCY MEDICAL CARE

Treating any patient with a significant decrease in level of consciousness as a result of a diabetic emergency is based on the timely administration of oral glucose.

Your first step in caring for the patient is to perform an initial assessment to verify that the airway is open. If the patient is not breathing or is having difficulty breathing, make sure you open the airway and assist ventilations, if necessary. Continue to monitor the airway as you provide care. Next, perform the focused assessment and detailed physical exam. At the same time, your partner should obtain the baseline vital signs and the SAMPLE history.

Next, confirm that the patient has a history of diabetes by asking the patient, the family, or by checking for medical identification. The patient may have a tag, bracelet, or card that identifies him or her as a diabetic. Inform medical control that you are at the scene of a diabetic emergency. At this point, you should also ask the patient or the family the questions listed above regarding last meal and insulin dose.

Before you can give the patient oral glucose, check to see if the patient can swallow. If so, give oral glucose, as described below, and according to local protocol.

## MEDICATIONS

Oral glucose is commercially available in gel form, which dissolves when placed in the mouth. The gel acts to increase blood glucose levels. The gel comes in toothpaste-type tubes in which one tube equals one dose (Figure 17-3). Trade names for oral glucose include Glutose and Insta-Glucose. You should give glucose gel to any patient with a decreased level of consciousness whose diabetes is controlled by medication. The only contraindication is inability to swallow or unconsciousness, since aspiration can occur. Giving this gel will not harm the patient, even if he or she does not really need it. Therefore, do not hesitate to give it.

## FIGURE 17-3

Oral glucose preparations

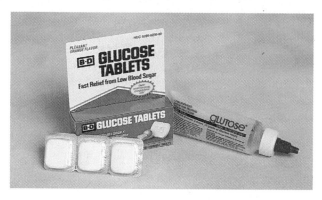

After you have confirmed that the patient is conscious and can swallow, you may give the glucose gel. First, squeeze the entire tube onto the bottom third of a tongue depressor (Figure 17-4a). As always, make sure you are wearing gloves before you place anything into the patient's mouth. Next, place the tongue depressor between cheek and gum, with the gel side next to the cheek (Figure 17-4b). Make sure

## FIGURE 17-4

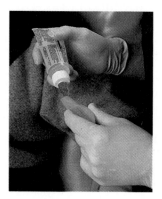

**A** Place oral glucose gel on a tongue depressor

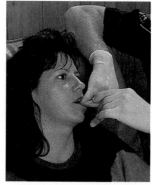

**B** Place gel between the cheek and gum

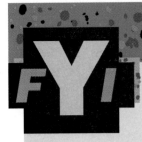

## Glucose and Insulin

Glucose is carried to all cells in the body by the blood in the arteries. Glucose provides the fuel or energy we need to live. When glucose is used for energy, the kidneys excrete carbon dioxide and water. Both of these waste products are easily excreted. However, glucose cannot enter a cell without insulin. Insulin is a hormone produced by special cells in the pancreas. Insulin helps glucose to enter cells (Figure 17-1). Without insulin, glucose cannot enter the cell, no matter how much glucose is available. Thus, a constant supply of insulin is absolutely necessary for our cells to function normally.

A patient with diabetes cannot use glucose normally for energy. This is because the patient does not have any insulin, or the insulin does not function properly. Without enough insulin, glucose cannot enter the cells. Thus, glucose remains in the blood and gradually accumulates. Once the amount of glucose reaches around two times normal, it is excreted by the kidney. This causes the patient to urinate large volumes of fluid frequently. This loss of water in such large amounts causes the classic symptoms of diabetes, as follows

- frequent, large volume urination (polyuria)
- frequent drinking to satisfy continuous thirst (polydipsia).

Because glucose cannot supply energy without insulin, the body must find other fuel sources. In most people, fat is a readily available resource. When fat is used for energy instead of glucose, the waste products change. With fat, acetone and other chemicals, called ketones and fatty acids, are formed as waste products. These substances are not easily excreted and can be detected in the urine and the blood. As they accumulate in blood and tissue, they can trigger a dangerous condition called ketoacidosis. Signs and symptoms of this condition include vomiting, abdominal pain, and deep, rapid breathing. When the acid levels of the body become too high, individual cells cannot live and will cease to function. If the patient is not given proper fluid and insulin, diabetic coma and eventually death can result.

that the gel is placed on the mucous membranes. Remove the tongue depressor once the gel is dissolved, or if the patient loses consciousness or has a seizure.

Make sure you reassess the patient regularly after giving glucose, even when you see rapid improvement in the patient's condition. Watch for possible airway problems, sudden loss of consciousness, or seizures to develop. Provide prompt transport to a medical facility for examination. Do not delay transport to give oral glucose.

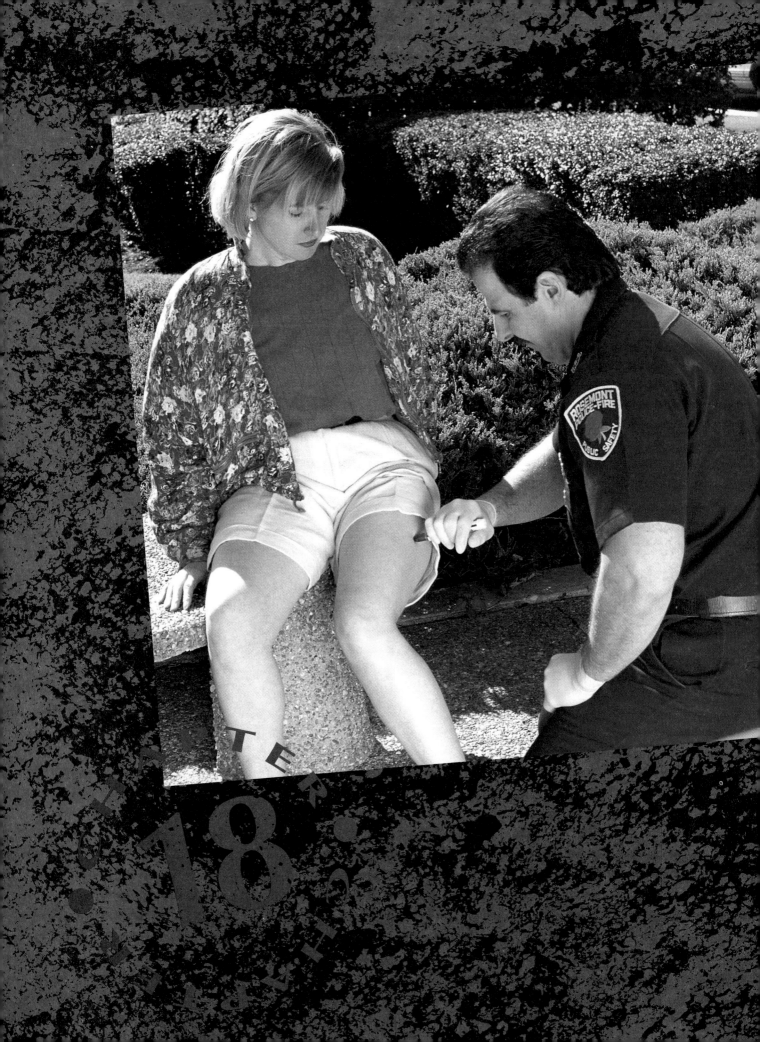

# Allergies and Poisoning

## Objectives

After you have read this chapter, you should be able to:

- Recognize a patient having an allergic reaction.
- Describe the emergency medical care of a patient having an allergic reaction.
- Describe the mechanisms of allergic response and the importance of airway management in a patient having an allergic reaction.
- State the generic and trade names, medication forms, dose, administration, actions, and contraindications for the epinephrine auto-injector.
- Distinguish between patients having an allergic reaction and those having a reaction that requires immediate care, including use of an epinephrine auto-injector.
- List various ways that poisons enter the body.
- List the signs and symptoms associated with poisoning.
- Discuss the emergency medical care for suspected poisoning and overdose victims.
- Establish the relationship between the patient suffering from poisoning or overdose and airway management.
- State the generic and trade names, indications, contra-indications, medication form, dose, administration, side effects, and reassessment strategies for activated charcoal.
- Recognize the need for medical direction in caring for the poisoned or overdosed patient.

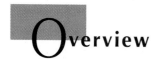

# Overview

Life-threatening allergic reactions can occur in response to almost any substance that a patient may encounter. Some of the more common allergens include food and medications. Reactions can range from mild with itching, redness, or tenderness, to severe with shock and respiratory failure. Recognizing and managing the many signs and symptoms of allergic reactions may possibly be the only thing standing between a patient and imminent death.

Every year, about 5 million children and adults swallow, inhale, inject, or absorb poisonous substances. These poisonings are usually accidental, although intentional poisonings and suicides also occur. In dealing with poisoning cases, you have many responsibilities, ranging from identifying a toxic substance to treating various types of poisonings. This chapter explores these responsibilities.

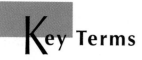

# Key Terms

**Allergens** Substances that cause allergic reactions.

**Allergic reaction** Reaction that occurs when the body has an immune response to an agent that is introduced either on the surface of or into the body.

**Anaphylaxis** An extreme allergic reaction.

**Ingestion** Swallowing; taking a substance by mouth.

**Poison** Substance whose chemical action could damage structures or impair function when introduced into the body in a relatively small amount.

**Stridor** Noisy respirations resulting from a large partial blockage of the upper airway.

**Toxin** A poison or harmful substance, produced by bacteria, animals, or plants.

**Urticaria (hives)** Small areas of generalized itching, burning that appear as multiple raised, reddened areas on the skin.

**Vomitus** Vomited material.

**Wheezing** An audible high-pitched breath sound usually resulting from a small airway blockage.

# ALLERGIC REACTIONS

An **allergic reaction** occurs when the body has an immune response to an agent that is introduced either on the surface of or into the body. An extreme allergic reaction is called **anaphylaxis.** Allergic reactions most often occur in response to one of the following four stimuli:

1. *Insect bites and stings.* A sting is an injection of a specific venom. The sting of a honeybee, wasp, yellow jacket, or hornet can cause severe immediate allergic reactions in people allergic to these toxins. **Toxins** are poisons or harmful substances, produced by bacteria, animals, or plants. The speed of these reactions is similar to that of reactions to injected medications.

2. *Medications.* Injection of drugs such as penicillin may cause an immediate and severe allergic reaction. Reactions to other medications such as oral penicillin may be slower but equally severe.

3. *Food.* Eating certain foods, such as shellfish or nuts, may result in slower, yet equally severe, allergic reactions.

4. *Plants.* Inhaling dusts, pollens, or other plant materials to which the patient is sensitive may result in a rapid and severe allergic reaction.

## ASSESSMENT FINDINGS

Allergens and the symptoms they cause can be wide ranging. **Allergens** are substances that cause allergic reactions. Your assessment should include evaluations of the patient's skin, respiratory system, circulatory system, and mental status. You will also be looking for general findings, such as watery eyes or a runny nose. A reaction to food or medication often only causes itching or a rash. In some instances, it may produce life-threatening reactions. Other allergens can cause severe reactions. A person with an allergy to bee venom may react violently to a sting and develop a hypersensitivity reaction called anaphylaxis or anaphylactic shock.

### Skin

Flushing, itching, or burning of the skin is common, especially over the face and upper chest. Hives may spread over large areas of the body. **Hives (urticaria)** are characterized by generalized itching and burning and appear as multiple raised, reddened areas on the skin (Figure 18-1). Swelling, especially of the face, neck, hands, feet, and/or tongue may occur. Also look for swelling and cyanosis or pallor around the lips. The patient's skin may also appear flushed.

### Respiratory System

At first, the patient may sneeze or have an itchy, runny nose. Tightness in the chest may then develop, along with an irritating, persistent dry cough. The patient's respirations may become rapid or labored. The patient may then begin wheezing or begin to

## FIGURE 18-1

Hives (urticaria)

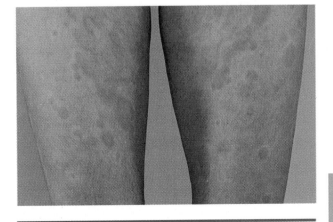

have noisy respirations (stridor). **Stridor** is characterized by noisy respirations that result from a large partial blockage of the upper airway. **Wheezing** is an audible high-pitched breath sound that usually results from a small blockage of the upper airway. These changes in respirations occur because fluid and mucus are secreted into the bronchial passages and alveoli in reaction to the allergen. The patient then tries to cough up the fluid and mucus.

Exhalation, which is normally the passive, relaxed part of breathing, suddenly becomes forced and requires effort. The fluid in the air passages and the constricted bronchi result in this characteristic wheezing as the patient works hard to exhale. Breathing rapidly becomes more difficult, and the patient may even stop breathing. Prolonged respiratory difficulty can cause rapid heartbeat (tachycardia), shock, and even death.

### Circulatory System

The patient's pulse may initially increase. However, as the peripheral blood vessels dilate, the patient's blood pressure will ultimately decrease. Eventually, the pulse will be weak and barely palpable. The patient may turn pale and become dizzy as the vascular system fails. Fainting and coma may follow.

### Other Findings

A patient having an allergic reaction will often be anxious and even have a sense of impending doom. The patient may also experience abdominal cramps, headache, and itchy, watery eyes.

## EMERGENCY MEDICAL CARE

If the patient seems to be having an allergic reaction, you should give oxygen as you

**FIGURE 18-2**

EpiPen (right), AnaKit (left)

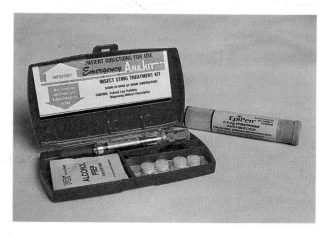

complete the initial assessment. Next, obtain a baseline vital signs and a SAMPLE history. Inform medical control about the patient's condition, and then find out whether the patient has any prescribed preloaded medications for allergic reactions. With the consent of medical control, you may give the patient the medication.

### Giving Epinephrine = adrenaline (same thing)

Patients who have a history of severe allergic reactions may have kits that contain prescribed epinephrine to combat allergic reactions or anaphylaxis (Figure 18-2). Some medical directors may authorize you to give the patient his or her own medication. Your medical director may also authorize you to carry an epinephrine auto-injector (EpiPen). This device has epinephrine (Adrenalin) that can be used if medical control believes that the patient's signs and symptoms indicate a severe allergic reaction. This liquid is administered via an automatic needle and syringe system. The adult system delivers 0.3 mg of epinephrine whereas the infant/child auto-injector delivers 0.15 mg.

Epinephrine is a rapidly acting agent that produces bronchodilation to reverse the effects of the allergen on the airway. It acts rapidly to constrict the blood vessels and to produce acute relief. Most kits also contain some oral or IV antihistamine. These various agents are specific to counter the production of histamine. Histamine is believed to be the specific substance produced by the body responsible for the attack. Usually, antihistamines are slower in onset of action and effective over a longer period of time than epinephrine.

Once you have confirmed that the patient has a prescribed auto-injector, consult medical control for an order to give the medication. If the patient is able to use the auto-injector himself, help him do so. However, before you give the medication or help the patient to self-inject, make sure you are following BSI techniques. Check the kit to see that it was prescribed for the patient. If it was not, you cannot give the medication. If this is the case, inform medical control and then provide immediate transport. If the kit was prescribed for the patient, next check to make sure that the medication is not discolored or expired.

You are now ready to give the medication. First, remove the safety cap from the auto-injector and wipe the patient's thigh with alcohol (Figure 18-3a). Place the tip of the auto-injector against the lateral part of the patient's thigh, midway between the patient's waist and the knee (Figure 18-3b). Next, push the injector firmly against the thigh until the injector activates, about 5 to 10 seconds. This helps prevent the "kick" the spring-loaded syringe causes when the needle is pulled from the injection site too soon. Hold it in place until the medication is injected (Figure 18-3c). Remove the injector from the patient's thigh and dispose of it in the proper biohazard container.

Make sure you record the time and dose of injection on your run sheet. Remember

## FIGURE 18-3

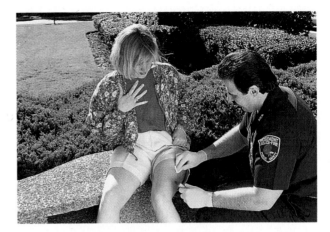

**A**    Prepare the leg for injection

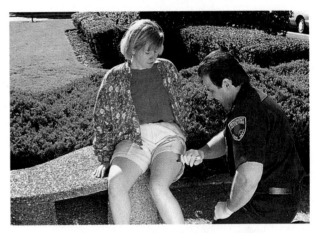

**B**    Place tip of the EpiPen against the thigh

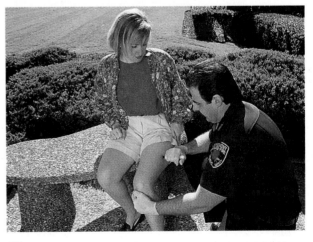

**C**    Push the EpiPen against the thigh until activated

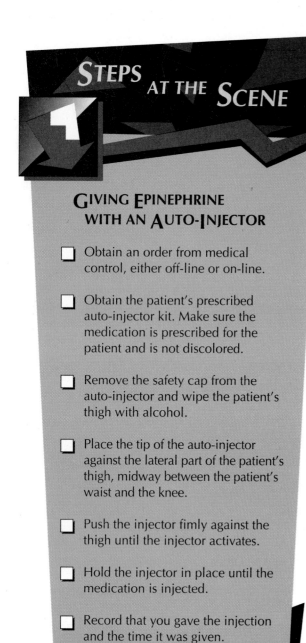

## GIVING EPINEPHRINE WITH AN AUTO-INJECTOR

☐ Obtain an order from medical control, either off-line or on-line.

☐ Obtain the patient's prescribed auto-injector kit. Make sure the medication is prescribed for the patient and is not discolored.

☐ Remove the safety cap from the auto-injector and wipe the patient's thigh with alcohol.

☐ Place the tip of the auto-injector against the lateral part of the patient's thigh, midway between the patient's waist and the knee.

☐ Push the injector fimly against the thigh until the injector activates.

☐ Hold the injector in place until the medication is injected.

☐ Record that you gave the injection and the time it was given.

☐ Dispose of the auto-injector in the proper biohazard container.

to closely monitor the patient's vital signs. Epinephrine will dilate the bronchioles and make it easier for the patient to breathe. It also constricts blood vessels. Thus, the patient's blood pressure may rise significantly.

Some other side effects include tachycardia and pallor (caused by vasoconstriction of the skin). Epinephrine commonly causes dizziness, chest pain, headache, nausea, and vomiting. All of these effects may cause the patient to feel anxious or excited.

If the patient has one of these devices, it is important to reassess and record vital signs 2 minutes after use. If no epinephrine auto-injector is available, the patient should be transported immediately. If your initial assessment revealed no evidence of an allergic reaction, you should not give epinephrine.

## REASSESSMENT STRATEGIES

Provide rapid transport for any patient who may be having an allergic reaction. Continue to reassess the patient's vital signs as described above en route. You must also closely monitor the patient's airway, breathing, and circulation. If the patient's condition becomes worse, you may need to give more than one injection of epinephrine. However, before you give another injection, consult medical control for approval. As with any patient you are transporting, be prepared to treat the patient for shock, begin BLS measures, or use the AED if necessary.

## POISONS

A **poison** is a substance whose chemical action could damage structures or impair function when introduced into the body in a relatively small amount. A substance is a poison regardless of whether it is swallowed, inhaled, injected, or absorbed. Notice that, by definition, very small amounts of poisonous substances can cause injury or death. The mechanism of injury is

## PESTICIDE PREDICAMENT

A loud crash in the area of the chemical shed at Bob's Garden Center prompts Bob's wife to see what her husband has done. She finds him in an angry state as he is trying to clean up the 5 gallons of pesticide from the container he dropped. The smell is overwhelming. She notices that her husband is acting somewhat strangely, so she decides to call 9-1-1. While they are waiting for the ambulance, she convinces him to abandon the clean-up efforts. They go outside where he can get some fresh air, and she rinses him off. On arrival, you find the wife hosing her husband down. He is complaining of having a "pounding headache," and is alert only to person and place. He says that both his legs and his groin are "burning."

### For Discussion

1. Why is it essential to remove the patient's clothing before placing him in the ambulance?

2. Whenever possible, why is it beneficial to take the chemical container to the hospital?

also a critical qualifier. A poison's damage is due to a chemical rather than a biological or physical process. Poisons either change the cells' normal metabolism or destroy them outright.

Poisoning deaths are rare and, among children, have decreased since the 1960s, probably due to safety caps on drug containers. However, there has been an increase in poisoning deaths in adults. About two of every three poisoning fatalities today are due to the use of illegal drugs.

Aggressive treatment for poisons, especially those that are ingested, can save lives. Your role, therefore, is to provide immediate care and prompt transportation.

## EMERGENCY MEDICAL CARE

As an EMT-B, your primary responsibility is to recognize that a poisoning has occurred. If you have the slightest suspicion that the patient has taken a poisonous substance, contact medical control immediately and begin emergency medical treatment. It is critical to consult medical control before you treat any poisoning victim.

Common signs and symptoms of poisoning include the following:

- history of ingestion or other exposure
- nausea or vomiting
- abdominal pain

- diarrhea
- dilation or constriction of the pupils
- excessive salivation
- sweating
- difficulty breathing or decreased respirations
- cyanosis
- unconsciousness or altered level of consciousness
- convulsions

The following are important considerations when caring for a patient believed to have ingested or been exposed to a poison:

- the type of substance
- the time of ingestion/exposure
- the amount of substance ingested
- the amount of time exposed
- the weight of the patient

Some chemicals irritate or burn the skin or mucous membranes, producing redness, blistering, or even severe burns. The presence of such injuries around or in the mouth strongly suggests the patient has ingested poison.

If you suspect poisoning, try to identify the poison. Look for overturned bottles, scattered pills, chemicals, or damaged plants. Examine the remains of any food or drink. Place suspicious material in a plastic bag and bring it to the hospital. If the patient vomits, collect the **vomitus** (vomited material) as well. Labeled containers can be particularly helpful. Labels often include the drug's name, ingredients, concentration, and quantity. Bringing this information to the hospital with you may be the most important thing you do after resuscitating and treating a patient.

External decontamination is also important. Remove tablets or fragments from the patient's mouth. Wash any poisons off the skin. Monitor the patient for signs of breath-ing difficulty. Your treatment will likely focus on support—on assessing and maintaining the patient's ABCD.

## Ingested Poisons

About 80% of all poisonings involve **ingested** (swallowed) poisons. These include drugs, alcohol, household products, contaminated foods, and plants. Among adults, drugs are the most commonly ingested poisons. But about a third of adult poisonings involve other substances, such as cleansers, soaps, insecticides, acids, or alkalis. Plant poisonings are common among children, who often bite the leaves of various plants.

In assessing the potential for ingested poisons, be alert for an unusual breath odor. This is a common finding with this type of poisoning. In treating a patient who has ingested poison, remove any remaining poison from the mouth and administer activated charcoal. Be sure to contact medical control.

If the ingested substance is an opiate, sedative, or barbiturate, expect depression of the CNS, especially respiratory depression. You may need to provide aggressive ventilatory support and even CPR. These patients need rapid transport.

## Inhaled Poisons

Patients who have inhaled a poison (natural gas, aerosols, pesticides, carbon monoxide, chlorine, or another gas) may have the following signs and symptoms in addition to those listed previously:

- respiratory distress
- cough
- chest pain
- hoarseness
- dizziness

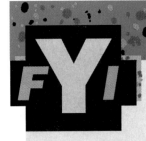

# Food Poisoning

Food poisoning is almost always caused when food is contaminated with bacteria. The food itself can appear perfectly good—without any obvious decay or odor. There are two types of food poisoning: 1) when the bacteria themselves cause disease, and 2) when the bacteria produce toxins that cause disease.

Most of the bacteria that directly cause disease are *Salmonella* bacteria. The resulting condition, called salmonellosis, is characterized by severe gastrointestinal symptoms—nausea, vomiting, abdominal pain, and diarrhea—for up to 72 hours after ingestion. In addition, patients may have fever and generalized weakness. Kitchen cleanliness usually prevents contamination, while proper cooking kills *Salmonella* bacteria.

Food poisoning is more commonly due to the ingestion of bacterial toxins. The symptoms are not caused by the bacteria themselves, but rather by powerful toxins the bacteria produce. The *Staphylococcus* bacterium is a common culprit. This type of food poisoning is often the result of advance preparation.

If food, particularly mayonnaise, is left warm for many hours, the bacteria have a chance to grow and produce toxins. Usually, staphylococcal food poisoning produces violent gastrointestinal symptoms (nausea, vomiting, and diarrhea) within 1 to 3 hours of ingestion. In general, the symptoms end 6 to 8 hours later.

The most severe form of toxin ingestion is botulism. Frequently fatal, this disease occurs when someone ingests the toxins produced by *Clostridium* bacteria, usually found in improperly canned food. The symptoms of botulism are neurologic: blurred vision, weakness, and difficulty speaking and breathing. Symptoms develop as long as 24 hours after ingestion.

In general, you should not try to diagnose acute gastrointestinal problems. Rather, you should transport the patient promptly. If you suspect botulism, be prepared to assist ventilations and provide BLS. If two or more people in a group are obviously suffering from food poisoning, bring along some of the suspected food.

- confusion
- headache
- stridor or wheezing

Some inhaled poisons, such as carbon monoxide, are odorless and produce profound hypoxia without irritating or damaging the lungs. Others, such as chlorine, are very irritating and result in airway obstruction and pulmonary edema. The patient may have difficulty breathing and chest pain. Some inhaled toxins may cause severe coughing, hoarseness, and dizziness.

# WHEN DEPRESSION SETS IN

You've had an easy day of transferring patients between facilities when you are dispatched to a "possible suicide." The address is just around the corner, so you're on scene quickly. As you pull up, a distraught woman tells you she thinks her husband has just tried to kill himself. As you grab your gear, the woman says her husband lost his job about 2 months ago and has been unable to find work. He has been very depressed. Inside, you find a conscious 43-year-old man slumped against the couch. On the floor, there's an empty bottle of sleeping pills and a bottle of Tylenol. You also note two empty wine bottles nearby.

## For Discussion

1. Describe the actions of activated charcoal when given to a patient who has swallowed a poison or taken an overdose.

2. Describe your steps in airway management of a patient who has swallowed a poison.

When treating a patient who has inhaled a poison, the patient must be moved into the fresh air. If the situation involves hazardous materials, the HazMat team should move the patient. *Do not enter a hazardous materials scene without the proper protective equipment and the proper training.* An injured or dead EMT-B is of little use to the patient. Always use a self-contained breathing apparatus (SCBA), if trained, to protect yourself from inhalation poisoning.

You may need to give high-flow oxygen via nonrebreathing mask and begin BLS measures. Administer oxygen whenever the patient has hypoxia, pulmonary edema, or an airway obstruction. Make sure a suctioning unit is readily available in the event that the patient vomits. Provide rapid transport for these patients. Some inhaled poisons cause progressive lung damage, even after the patient is removed from direct exposure. Many times, these patients may require 2 or 3 days of intensive care before their lungs perform normally again.

### Toxic Injections

Poisoning by injection is almost always the result of deliberate drug overdose. Another common source of injected poisons is an insect sting or animal bite. Stings and animal bites are discussed in chapter 19, Environmental Emergencies.

After a toxic injection, the patient may complain of weakness, dizziness, fever, or chills. In general, injected poisons are impossible to dilute or remove. The emergency medical care is, therefore, supportive. Make sure the patient's airway is open. Provide high-flow oxygen. Always be alert for nausea and vomiting, which could obstruct the airway. Be prepared to provide BLS, which might be necessary if the poison is rapidly absorbed.

If the area around the site of an injection starts to swell, remove all rings, watches, or bracelets. In some instances, an ice pack or cold pack may be ordered to decrease local pain and swelling about the injection. In other cases, medical control may advise you to apply a constricting band above and below the site of the injection. Tighten it just enough to block the flow of blood through the veins. This is called a venous tourniquet. Do not cut off arterial flow. Make sure the patient's pulse is still palpable distal to the constricting band. Care of snakebite injuries is discussed in chapter 19, Environmental Emergencies.

Sometimes, poisonings severely injure the tissues around the injection site. This may require complex surgical procedures to correct. Thus, prompt transport is necessary. Remember to bring a sample of the injected substance, if one has been found.

### Absorbed Poisons

Many corrosive substances damage the skin, mucous membranes, or eyes upon direct contact. Acids, alkalis, and some petroleum and benzene products are very destructive. In assessing the potential for an absorbed poison, look for traces of powder or liquid on the patient's skin. Absorbed poisons can cause inflammation, chemical burns, or specific rashes and lesions. Other common signs and symptoms include intense burning, itching, and irritation as well as a redness on the exposed surface.

The emergency treatment for contact poisoning is to remove any residue of the irritating or corrosive substance as soon as possible. Remove any clothing that has been contaminated. Use care to avoid contaminating yourself or members of your team, bystanders, or other medical personnel while doing this.

If the absorbed poison was a liquid, irrigate the exposed area for at least 20 minutes. If it was a dry material, thoroughly brush the chemical off and then wash the affected area with soap and water or flood the exposed part for at least 20 minutes. If the patient has been exposed to a large amount of poison, flooding may be the most rapidly effective treatment.

Do not spend time trying to chemically neutralize substances that have contacted a patient's skin. Rather, wash the substance off immediately with water. This procedure is faster and more effective than attempting to neutralize a substance chemically.

If the chemical has contacted the patient's eyes, irrigate the eyes rapidly with a large volume of water. You should irrigate the eyes for at least 20 minutes.

The only time you should not irrigate the contact area with water is when the poison reacts violently with water. For example, phosphorus and elemental sodium are dry, solid chemicals that catch on fire when they touch water. Fortunately, people are rarely exposed to these substances. If you do encounter this situation, begin as you do with other dry chemical poisonings. Brush the chemical off the patient and remove contaminated clothing. Then apply a dry dressing to the burn area. Wear gloves and the proper protective clothing and be especially careful to avoid contaminating yourself. Transport the patient promptly.

## JUST SAY NO TO SEAFOOD

You are called to the state fairgrounds for a woman having "difficulty breathing." You clear the security gate and are directed to the first aid station where you find a 33-year-old woman sitting hunched over in obvious respiratory distress. As you try to obtain a history, she only answers you in one- to two-word bursts. She manages to tell you that she was eating at the food circle. She thinks her salad must have had seafood in it. She is allergic to seafood and has had this type of problem before, but never this severe. She also tells you there is an EpiPen in her purse. Her voice seems to be getting more hoarse as she speaks. Her skin is flushed, and she is starting to show some generalized hives. She has a blood pressure of 96/66 mm Hg, a pulse of 132/min, and respirations of 40/min.

### For Discussion

1. How does the "allergic reaction" affect the patient's respiratory and circulatory systems? What happens to produce the symptoms?

2. Explain why epinephrine is the drug of choice for treating signs and symptoms of allergic (anaphylactic) reaction.

## MEDICATIONS

### Activated Charcoal

Activated charcoal is a finely ground charcoal that adsorbs (sticks to) many commonly ingested poisons. You should avoid using the powdered form of this medication in the field. However, many suspensions are available (Figure 18-4). Some common trade names for this mixture are InstaChar, Actidose, and LiquiChar. Most of these suspensions come in plastic bottles, each containing up to 50 g of activated charcoal.

You should give activated charcoal to any patient you suspect has ingested a poisonous substance. However, you should not administer this medication if the patient ingested an acid or alkali, has an altered level of consciousness, or cannot swallow.

The usual dosage for an adult or child is 1g of activated charcoal per kilogram of body weight. Therefore, the usual adult dose is 25 to 50 g. The usual pediatric dose is 12.5 to 25 g.

Before giving a patient activated charcoal, you should check with medical direction. If the treatment is approved, shake the bottle vigorously to mix the suspension. Try to cover the outside of the container, and ask the patient to use a straw so the fluid is not visible. Because the medication looks like mud, you may need to persuade the patient to drink it. In particular, a child may be afraid to swallow the inky, messy fluid. However, you should never force the liquid into someone's mouth. If the patient takes a long time to drink, shake the container frequently to keep the medication mixed. After giving the patient the activated charcoal, document your activity and time.

Activated charcoal works by binding to the poison, preventing the toxin from being absorbed. Some brands bind more poisons than others. Your medical director will likely decide the brand you will carry on your unit.

The major side effect of ingesting activated charcoal is black stools. If the patient has ingested a poison that causes nausea, the patient may vomit after taking activated charcoal. If so, you should repeat the dosage. Thus, as you reassess the patient, be prepared for vomiting, nausea, and possible airway problems.

## FIGURE 18-4

Activated charcoal preparations

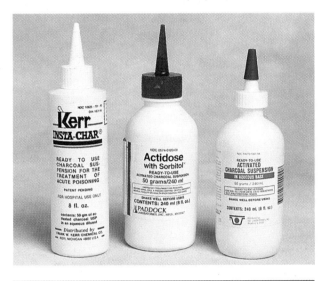

# Atlas of
# Substance Abuse

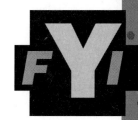

Substance abuse is a national problem. Most injured patients seen in our urban medical and trauma centers today are somehow connected to or the result of alcohol and/or abuse of other dangerous drugs. In fact, this problem has become so widespread and expensive that it has forced many inner city hospitals to close.

As an EMT-B, you need to understand the role you play in caring for this type of patient. Recognize that along with the abuse problem, these patients may have various injuries. Providing BLS care often means the difference between life and death in a severely injured or ill substance abuse patient. Of course, you cannot resolve the patient's substance abuse problem. Your responsibility, as with all patients, is to provide lifesaving care. Remember, though, that the substance abuse problem will have an effect on how you handle the patient.

This FYI focuses on two major forms of substance abuse: alcohol abuse and abuse of various types of drugs. Substance abuse is defined, along with issues of EMT-B safety in handling substance abuse patients. The symptoms of alcoholism, the effects on the body of too much alcohol, and the treatment of intoxicated patients are then discussed. The next section on drug abuse is much broader. This section begins with a description of the various types of drugs that are abused. Specific problems of drug abuse and the emergency medical care are then discussed.

## WHAT IS SUBSTANCE ABUSE?

In the past, the term **substance abuse** generally meant a specific drug addiction. Even though drug use and addiction are major problems in the United States, they are not the only forms of substance abuse. Other substances are commonly abused, as follows:

- alcohol
- food
- laxatives
- emetics
- over-the-counter medications, such as aspirin and vitamins

With substance abuse, the user takes an agent or agents for certain desired effects. The user often does not have a doctor's order, nor takes the proper dose of the agent. In fact, the user often has no medical need to use the agent. As time passes, the user often loses control over the amount of substance he or she is taking. However, over time and with continued use, the user does need increasing amounts of an agent used to achieve the same result. This is called developing a **tolerance** to an agent. Increasing tolerance can lead to **addiction.**

### Safety Issues

As an EMT-B, you are trained to put your safety and the safety of your team first at every incident. You must be especially careful in dealing with the population of substance abusers. Although patients whose problems involve food, vitamins, aspirin, steroids, or laxatives usually pose little health threat, patients with drug and alcohol abuse problems are a different story.

Patients who are known drug abusers have a fairly high incidence of serious and unrecognized infections, such as AIDS and/or hepatitis. These patients may also bite, hit, or otherwise injure you. They often have open and draining wounds as a result of their drug use. Severe bleeding, especially in patients with alcohol abuse problems, is also common. As a result, virtually every avenue is open for contact with the blood and body fluids of an infected patient. Thus, the importance of BSI techniques cannot be stressed enough. Wear the proper protective equipment for the situation.

Even though a substance abuse patient may be frightened or aggressive, your treatment should be the same as that for a patient with any chronic disease. Your approach should be calm and professional. How you handle the patient can calm fear and panic and actually defuse frightening situations. Expect the unexpected with these patients and always keep your safety in mind. Remember that the drugs used generally pose no great threat to you. However, the drug user can.

## ALCOHOL ABUSE

The most commonly abused drug in the United States is alcohol. It affects people from all walks of life and kills more than 200,000 people each year. Alcoholism is the third greatest national health problem after heart disease and cancer.

Alcohol is a powerful central nervous system (CNS) depressant. It interferes with the capacity of the individual to think, function, and face situations rationally. More than 50% of all traffic fatalities or injuries, 67%

of murders, and 33% of suicides are alcohol related.

### Effects of Alcohol

In general, alcohol dulls the sense of awareness, slows reflexes, and increases reaction time. It is important for you to remember that a patient who is intoxicated may also be ill or injured. Look for signs of head trauma, toxic reactions, or uncontrolled diabetes in patients who are under the influence of alcohol. All intoxicated patients are suffering from a drug overdose and must be examined thoroughly. Remember, it is impossible for you to know if alcohol is the patient's only problem. Thus, it is critical for you to transport the patient for evaluation by a physician. In most states, intoxicated patients cannot refuse transport.

Intoxication has many signs and symptoms, such as aggressive and inappropriate behavior and lack of coordination. Injuries are common and often not perceived by the patient. Thus, you must carefully assess the patient for injuries. A patient may have consumed so much alcohol that signs of serious CNS depression appear. In such cases you must provide complete respiratory support. This excessive ingestion of alcohol can result in death.

Large amounts of alcohol irritate the stomach. A patient who has consumed too much alcohol may have forceful vomiting. Sometimes these patients will vomit blood (hematemesis). You should also suspect internal bleeding in an intoxicated patient who appears to be in shock (hypoperfusion). Prolonged alcohol abuse eventually results in such poor liver function that blood does not clot effectively. This results in the patient experiencing severe bleeding after any type of trauma or after a needle stick.

A patient in alcohol withdrawal may experience alcoholic hallucinations or delirium tremens (DTs). These conditions may develop if a patient is cut off from his or her daily source of alcohol. Hallucinations can be visual or auditory. A patient with an otherwise fairly clear mental state may see fantastic shapes or figures or hear odd voices. Hallucinations may be frightening, but they come and go. They often precede DTs, which is a much more severe complication.

DTs may develop 1 to 7 days after alcohol withdrawal. Patients with DTs are extremely ill and must be transported immediately. Patients will often experience one or more of the following signs and symptoms:

- agitation and restlessness
- fever
- sweating
- confusion and/or disorientation
- delusions and/or hallucinations
- seizures

### Emergency Medical Care

Given the widespread use of alcohol, you are not likely to be called to care for a patient who has signs of intoxication alone. You will usually care for patients who are seriously ill or injured due to intoxication. Provide prompt transport for these patients after you have completed your assessment and given necessary care. Watch for breathing problems and vomiting with these patients.

As stated above, patients experiencing hallucinations or DTs are extremely ill. Hallucinations and restlessness may develop before seizures and complete delirium. Should seizures develop, you should treat them as you would any other seizure. The patient should not be restrained, although you must protect the patient from self-injury. Give the patient oxygen and watch carefully for vomiting.

Hypovolemia may develop due to sweating, fluid loss, insufficient fluid intake, or vomiting associated with DTs. Should signs of hypovolemic shock develop, you should provide prompt transport. Elevate the patient's feet slightly, clear the airway, and turn the head to one side to minimize the chance of aspiration during transport. Generally, these patients may not respond appropriately to suggestions or conversation. However, they are often frightened. Thus, your approach should be calm and relaxed. Reassure the patient and provide emotional support.

## DRUG ABUSE

### Types of Drugs

Aside from alcohol, drugs that are commonly abused include the following:

- opium compounds
- CNS depressants
- CNS stimulants
- nicotine
- marijuana
- hallucinogens
- inhalants

**OPIUM COMPOUNDS**  The opium analgesics (pain relievers) are natural or synthetic derivatives of opium from poppy seeds. They include heroin, morphine, Demerol, Dilaudid, methadone, and others. Codeine is also in this group. These drugs are all pain relievers and have a wide range of legitimate use. Individuals may have started using these agents with an appropriate medical prescription or as a recreational venture.

**CNS DEPRESSANTS**  The barbiturates and other hypnotic (sleep-inducing) drugs are CNS depressants. These agents have effects much like alcohol. They do not relieve pain, nor do they produce a specific "high." They are often used with alcohol or with opium analgesics to increase the effects of another agent.

*Inhalants*   Inhalants are CNS depressants that produce effects remarkably similar to those of alcohol. These agents include acetone or toluene that are found in glues, cleaning compounds, and lacquers. Also included are gasoline, various halogenated hydrocarbons used as propellants in aerosol sprays, and Freon. None of these agents is a medication.

The effects of a CNS depressant range from mild drowsiness to coma. Other signs and symptoms include vomiting and aspiration, respiratory depression or arrest, and self-injury. Sometimes, patients fall asleep in odd positions, with an arm or leg curled under their body or hanging over a chair or couch. The result is compression of blood vessels, which reduces circulation in the extremities, sometimes for hours. The decreased blood flow can result in permanent damage and even loss of the limb. Nerves can be compressed, causing paralysis. Sometimes patients fall and injure themselves without knowing it. These injuries may be neglected for long periods of time.

**CNS STIMULANTS**   The effect of CNS stimulants depends on the route of administration, the drug, its dose, and the circumstances. Amphetamines are commonly taken orally to make the user "feel good," improve task performance, suppress appetite, or prevent sleepiness. They may just as easily produce irritability, anxiety, and lack of effective concentration. Common examples include amphetamine, methamphetamine, and Benzedrine. Caffeine, certain antiasthmatic drugs, and nasal decongestants are all mild stimulants.

CNS stimulants will cause rapid heart rate, increased blood pressure, rapid breathing, an excited state, agitation, headaches,

sleeplessness, and a sense of euphoria or well-being. Seizures may occur with abuse of some stimulants. Disorganized behavior may also accompany the use of these agents. Taken as prescribed for specific medical problems, they can be beneficial. When they are used in an uncontrolled fashion, they can become addictive.

Stimulants make the user restless and sometimes very anxious. You may be called to care for a patient who is so frightened that he or she may appear paranoid or have totally wrong thinking. A patient who has suddenly stopped using stimulants may be severely depressed.

*Cocaine*   Cocaine should be considered separately, even though it is in the family of CNS stimulants. Cocaine may be taken in a number of different ways. Classically, it is inhaled into the nose and absorbed through the nasal mucosa. This route of use damages the tissue, causes nosebleeds, and ultimately destroys the nasal septum. It can also be injected IV or "popped" SC. Cocaine can be absorbed through all mucous membranes and even across the skin. The duration of action for a given dose is less than 1 hour.

Crack is pure cocaine in crystal form. It melts at 93°F and vaporizes at a slightly higher temperature. Thus, crack is easily mixed with tobacco and smoked or smoked alone. In this form, it reaches the vast capillary network of the lung and can be absorbed in seconds. The immediate outflow of blood from the heart spreads the drug to the brain promptly, and its effect is felt almost at once. Obviously, smoked crack produces the most rapid means of absorption possible and hence the most potent effect.

*Nicotine*   Nicotine is a mild CNS stimulant. In fact, it is the agent that contributes to the continuing use of cigarettes. While nicotine is usually not a cause for an emergency call, you will likely care for many problems associated with smoking.

**MARIJUANA**    Inhaling marijuana smoke from a cigarette produces euphoria, relaxation, and drowsiness. The drug impairs short-term memory and the capacity to do complex work. In some people, the euphoria progresses to depression and confusion. An altered perception of time is common, and anxiety and panic can occur. With very high doses, patients experience hallucinations.

**HALLUCINOGENS**    Hallucinogens (psychedelic agents) alter an individual's sense of perception. These agents induce hallucinations, intensify what the user sees and hears, and generally separate the user from reality. The user, of course, expects that the altered sensory state will be pleasurable. However, this often is not the case. The induced hallucination may be terrifying. At some time, you are almost certain to be called to care for a patient who is having a "bad trip."

### Routes of Administration

Many agents are taken by mouth and usually pose no particular problem for the patient. Other agents are injected by needle, either IV, SC, or IM. Obviously, most agents taken this way are not prepared in the same way as an injection you would receive from your doctor. These agents are often "cut" or diluted by agents such as sugar or other drugs.

Addicts are often willing to take any drug by any route to experience a new "high." Thus, many agents not designed for injection are being given by needle. A group of addicts will often share the same needle. Usually, one user will reuse a single needle for several injections.

The results of this practice can be devastating. Tissue can be destroyed by the direct action of the injected material on it. Bacteria with resulting infection can be introduced into a vein, tissue, or muscle at each injection. Even more lethal are the severe systemic infections, hepatitis, and HIV that can be transmitted through direct blood contact. When many users share one needle, they are at a high risk for contracting any of these diseases.

### Emergency Medical Care

When you suspect drug use is part of your patient's problem, look for signs that will identify the agent. Try to identify the agent and collect a sample to take to the hospital. This information is absolutely necessary for the physician.

Examination of the patient may reveal further clues. The sections below provide a general picture of common signs and symptoms associated with drug use. Also given are appropriate measures of supportive care.

**CNS DEPRESSANTS**    A patient who has a decreased level of consciousness after taking a CNS depressant should be gently stimulated. A patient who is unconscious may go into respiratory arrest. Thus, you should try to keep the patient awake during transport. Talk to the patient, gently pinch, or lightly shake the patient to try to rouse him or her. Be ready to assist ventilation and watch for vomiting. Give the patient oxygen. Do not induce vomiting, even if you are sure that the agent was taken by mouth. Provide prompt transport and report any information about the agent to hospital staff.

**CNS STIMULANTS**    A patient who is anxious, excited, or paranoid as a result of taking a CNS stimulant should be handled in a calm, professional manner. Often a quiet attitude and gentle approach will be most successful. Gaining the patient's confidence with a pleasant manner often works. Using restraints will increase a patient's anxiety and fear. Thus, you should not use restraints unless the patient is likely to injure you, your team, or himself or herself. Remember that law enforcement officers should be at the scene to restrain the patient, if necessary. Do not leave the patient alone during transport or even placed alone in the ambulance where difficult behavior cannot be controlled.

If the patient is having a seizure, you must protect him or her from self-injury. Give the patient oxygen and have a suctioning unit readily available. Provide prompt transport, as the patient needs hospital care.

Occasionally, a patient who is taking stimulants will experience severe depression if he or she stops taking the drug for some reason. Withdrawal symptoms usually include listlessness, apathy, and hunger. The patient may go into a coma, and respiratory depression requiring full life support may be needed.

**HALLUCINOGENS**    You should care for a patient experiencing a bad reaction from a hallucinogenic agent the same as you would a patient on a CNS stimulant. Use a calm, professional manner and provide emotional support. Do not use restraints unless you or the patient are in danger of injury. Remember the guidelines for using restraints. Hallucinations or odd perceptions can occur suddenly. Therefore, you should never leave the patient alone. Patients have been known to leap from vehicles or windows under the influence of various agents. Thus, you must watch the patient carefully en route.

**INHALANTS**    Inhalants may be contained in an aerosol can, a bottle of glue, or a tin of gasoline. A patient in severe respiratory distress from an inhalant is usually hypoxic. Hypoxia is often caused by the device used to inhale the active vapors. These substances are commonly inhaled from within a closed plastic bag that collapses and may obstruct the airway. Your care of the patient must focus on supporting ventilation. Give oxygen, artificial ventilation, and even CPR, as needed. These patients need prompt transport. You should expect the patient to vomit. If the patient does not have severe hypoxia, you should provide the same care as that for any other CNS depressant.

Try to identify and/or bring the agent to the hospital. Take care to avoid needless exposure of medical personnel. Some agents, such as glycols, have very specific tissue toxicity (kidney or liver). Rapid identification at the hospital may help start treatment to protect these organs.

### Other Effects of Substance Abuse

**INJURIES**    Rapid assessment of the drug user is absolutely essential. If you do not look for injuries, you are not likely to find them. The patient is not likely to complain of pain or show some of the usual signs and symptoms of injury. Care for injuries in the same way you would for any other patient. A swollen cyanotic limb that has been compressed must be splinted and positioned as naturally and comfortably as possible. Head injuries must be recognized promptly because their effects often mimic drug use and vice versa. Provide prompt transport for the drug user who has an injury.

**INFECTIONS**    In addition to the effects of the drugs, the drug user may develop major systemic or local infectious problems. As a result, you must follow BSI techniques any time you may come into contact with body fluids. The local problems are almost always abscesses or cellulitis. Cellulitis is characterized by redness, swelling, warmth, and tenderness around the soft tissue. It usually occurs in an extremity at an injection site. You should splint the infected limb and provide prompt transport. Abscesses, especially if they have ruptured and are draining, should be dressed with sterile bandages.

The drug user with a major systemic infection usually shows signs of that problem. Seizures, coma or other neurologic problems, and fever occur with a brain abscess. Jaundice is a classic sign of hepatitis. These patients require prompt transport to the hospital.

**MULTIPLE DRUG USE**    A drug user may have used as many as three or four different agents at a time. The use of drugs in conjunction with alcohol is also common. When the drugs complement one another, the effects are generally much greater than when each drug is used alone. Sometimes, users take drugs with opposite effects. In general, the opposing effects do not cancel each other. They usually result in panic reactions or profound depression.

Unfortunately, multiple drug use is quite common and results in a complex clinical picture, which makes identifying agents difficult.

**DRUG WITHDRAWAL**    Patients who are addicted to drugs usually experience a severe reaction when the drug is withdrawn. Signs and symptoms of withdrawal include the following:

- anxiety
- nausea and vomiting
- seizures
- delirium and hallucinations
- profuse sweating
- rapid heart rate
- severe abdominal cramps

Ordinarily, you will not be called to care for a patient in acute withdrawal. But if you do, the patient may be able to tell you the exact situation.

Patients experiencing acute withdrawal are as urgently ill as those suffering from a drug overdose. You should provide prompt transport to the hospital where they can receive proper treatment.

## OTHER FORMS OF SUBSTANCE ABUSE

Virtually anything that can be taken as an agent, eaten or drunk, has been used to excess. There are compulsive water drinkers, steroid abusers, over-the-counter "pill poppers," and abusers of a variety of agents and foods. You will undoubtedly meet people with this type of behavior. Generally, you should try to identify the abused substance and provide supportive care as described above.

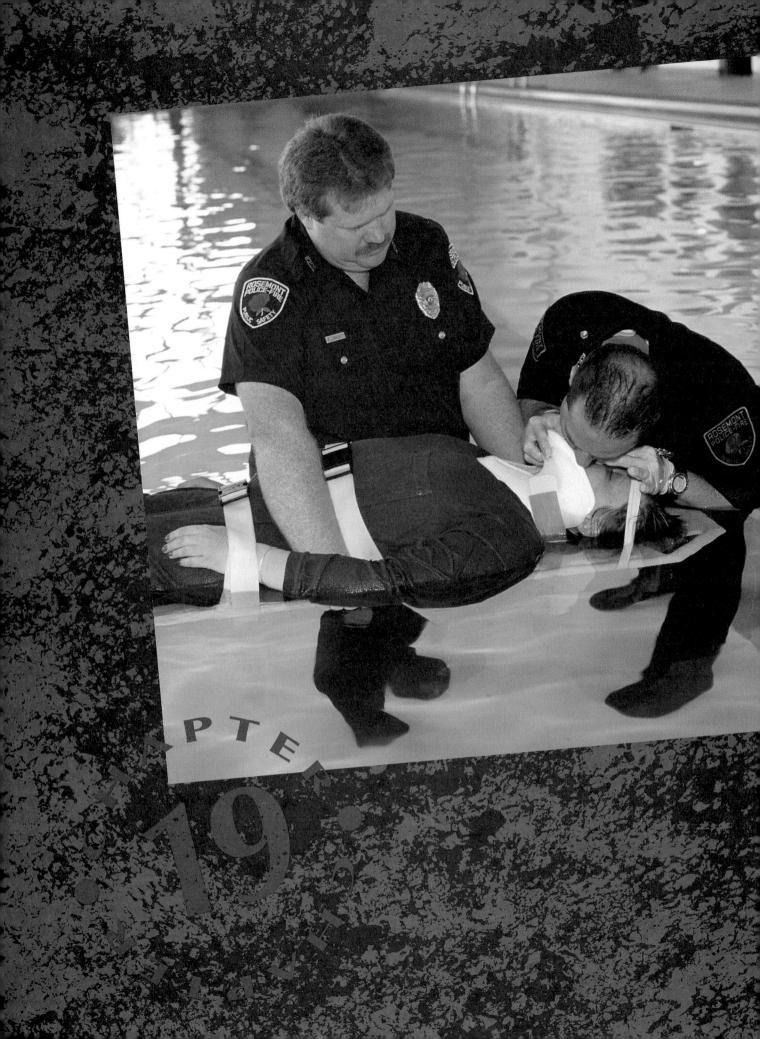

# Environmental Emergencies

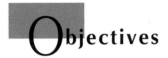

## Objectives

After you have read this chapter, you should be able to:

- Describe the various ways that the body loses heat.
- List the signs and symptoms of exposure to cold and heat.
- Describe the steps in providing emergency medical care to a patient exposed to cold or heat.
- Recognize the signs and symptoms of water-related emergencies.
- Describe the complications of near drowning.
- Discuss the emergency medical care of bites and stings.

## Overview

Environmental emergencies can occur in any part of the country and at any time of year. Emergencies involving exposure to heat and cold affect individuals in many different settings. The greatest number of cases of hypothermia occur in the urban setting, many involving the elderly. Heat-related emergencies can range from the very minor to life-threatening conditions.

The increased popularity of water sports has increased the number of water-related emergencies. Each year in the United States, water accidents claim about 9,000 lives. Most often you will be called to near-drowning emergencies.

Knowing how to start artificial ventilation in the water, prevent further injury to the spine, and begin CPR will increase the patient's chance of survival.

Insect bites and stings, though painful, are usually not serious. However, bites can occur from poisonous snakes, spiders, or ticks. You must be prepared to identify the symptoms of serious reactions to bites and stings. It is also helpful if you are familiar with the most common types of poisonous snakes and spiders in your area.

## Key Terms

**Ambient temperature**   The temperature of the environment.

**Conduction**   The loss of body heat by touching a colder object.

**Convection**   The loss of heat through moving air, from the body surface to a colder area.

**Diving reflex**   Slowing of the heart rate caused by submersion in cold water.

**Drowning**   Death from suffocation by submersion in water.

**Envenomation**   Deposit of venom into a wound.

**Evaporation**   The loss of body heat as a result of water changing from a liquid to a gas.

**Hyperthermia**   A condition in which the body gains or retains more heat than it loses, usually 101°F or higher.

**Hypothermia**   A condition in which the body loses more heat than it produces, usually 95°F or lower.

**Near drowning**   Survival, at least temporarily, after suffocation in water.

**Radiation**   The loss of body heat as a result of being in a colder environment.

**Shivering**   An involuntary response to generate more body heat through muscular activity.

# Hypothermia

Our normal body temperature of 98.6°F (37°C) is maintained by a set of complex mechanisms. Our internal temperature tries to remain constant, regardless of the **ambient temperature,** or temperature of the environment.

When the body loses more heat than it retains or gains, the result is called **hypothermia,** or a low body core temperature. A patient with hypothermia usually has a core body temperature of 95°F (35°C) or lower. Hypothermia can develop quickly, as when someone is immersed in cold water. However, it can also develop more gradually, as when an individual is exposed to a cold environment for several hours or more. Hypothermia does not always occur in rural or remote areas. It is a problem in urban areas as well. Nor does the temperature have to be below freezing for it to occur. In the winter, homeless persons and those who lack heating for their homes may develop hypothermia. Hypothermia may also occur in the summer, as when a swimmer remains in the water too long.

Internal body temperature can decrease a few degrees, and the body will tolerate the change. **Shivering** is an involuntary response to generate more body heat through muscular activity. However, when the core or inner temperature drops, the body loses its ability to regulate temperature and to generate body heat. The body then begins to gradually lose body heat. The body loses heat in the following five ways:

1. **Conduction.** This is a loss of body heat as a result of touching a colder object.

2. **Convection.** This is heat transfer, as when air moves across the body surface to a cooler area. An individual wearing light clothing who is standing outside loses heat by convection.

3. **Evaporation.** This is the loss of body heat as a result of water changing from liquid to a gas. Heat is removed from the body when sweat or water evaporates from the skin.

4. **Radiation.** This is the loss of body heat as a result of being in a cooler environment. An individual standing in a cold room will lose heat by radiation.

5. **Respiration.** This allows the warm air in the lungs to be exhaled, releasing body heat.

A sick or injured person who has been exposed to a cold environment may develop hypothermia. In fact, a sick or injured person is more susceptible to cold injury than a healthy person. Remember that *all* patients with severe, multiple injuries are likely to have some degree of hypothermia. If you work in a cold environment, you may carry a hypothermia thermometer (Figure 19-1). Regular thermometers do not register temperatures as low as those on hypothermia thermometers.

## FIGURE 19-1

A hypothermia thermometer

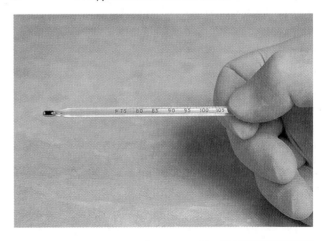

## COLD-RELATED EMERGENCIES

A cold emergency, or generalized hypothermia, has four main predisposing factors, as follows:

1. Environment
2. Age of the patient
3. Medical condition of the patient
4. Ingestion of drugs or poisons

When the body or part of the body is in water colder than 98°F (37°C), heat passes directly from the body to the water. This heat loss through conduction is called an immersion injury. An unconscious patient lying on a cold metal platform may also develop hypothermia by conduction.

Patient age is also a factor in hypothermia. It is more common in the elderly and the very young. The very young cannot put on or take off clothes to protect against the cold. They are also small with a large surface area and have less body fat. Due to their small muscle mass, children do not shiver as effectively as adults, and infants cannot shiver at all.

Patients with injuries or illnesses, such as shock, head injury, burns, generalized infection, injuries to the spinal cord, diabetes, and hypoglycemia are more prone to hypothermia. Drugs and poisons also can contribute to an individual's inability to adapt to temperature extremes.

### Signs and Symptoms

Signs and symptoms of hypothermia gradually become more severe as core temperature falls. It is important for you to recognize these signs and symptoms as they progress. This will help you to assess whether the patient has mild or more severe hypothermia. Thus, as you begin your assessment, you need to assess the patient's general temperature. Place the back of your hand between the patient's clothing and the patient's abdomen. Does the abdomen feel cool to touch? If the abdomen feels cool, the patient is likely experiencing a generalized cold emergency.

Mild hypothermia occurs when the core temperature is between 90° and 95°F (32° and 35°C). The patient is usually alert and shivering. The patient may also jump up and down and stamp the feet in an attempt to produce more heat. With mild hypothermia, the pulse rate and respirations are usually rapid. The skin may appear red at this point, but may eventually appear cyanotic.

More severe hypothermia occurs below 90°F (32°C). Shivering stops, and muscular activity decreases. Small, fine muscle activity, such as coordinated finger motion will stop first. Later, as the core temperature falls further, all muscle activity stops.

As the core temperature drops to 85°F (29°C), the patient becomes lethargic. Level of consciousness decreases, and the patient may lose interest in trying to stay warm. In fact, the patient may even try to remove his or her clothes. Poor coordination and memory disturbances follow, along with reduced or complete loss of sensation, mood changes, and impaired judgment. The patient becomes less communicative, complains of dizziness, experiences joint or muscle stiffness, and has trouble speaking. The patient may still be shivering, or shivering may stop. The muscles become rigid, and the patient begins to appear stiff or rigid.

If the temperature continues to fall to 80°F (27°C), the vital signs begin to decrease. The rapid pulse slows down and becomes weaker. At this stage, it may be barely palpable and irregular, or completely absent. Early, rapid respirations slow to shallow, or even absent respirations. Cardiac arrhythmias may occur as the blood pressure decreases or disappears. The skin becomes pale, then cyanotic, and finally stiff and hard. Below 80°F, the patient may have no heartbeat or pulse, and pupillary reaction is slow. At this point, the patient may appear dead.

## THE HUNT FOR THE HUNTER

The search and rescue team has been looking for a lost hunter for the past 2 days. EMS has kept an ambulance posted at a nearby ranger station in case the hunter is found alive. Countless hours later, the radio crackles to life. The hunter has been found! You respond, driving to the Gaston River bridge. The hunter is lying beside the bridge's pilings. An empty thermos jug beside him smells suspiciously of liquor. He has no coat and is wearing a wet flannel shirt. He does not appear to be shivering even though it is a cold day with a temperature in the mid-30s. He seems sleepy and can barely answer your questions. As you attempt to move him onto the stretcher, you note that he feels stiff, as if his muscles are rigid. When you try to take a blood pressure, you get no reading.

### For Discussion

1. What is the significance of finding this patient in a flannel shirt as it relates to his level of hypothermia?

2. Describe the impact of alcohol on hypothermia.

No matter how serious the cold injury, you must continue to care for the patient. Remember that a patient who appears dead may be very much alive. Also remember that even though the patient may not respond to your questions, he or she may be able to hear you.

### Emergency Medical Care

Even mild hypothermia can have serious complications. All patients with hypothermia should be transported to the hospital for evaluation. Your focus in caring for these patients in the field is threefold: 1) stabilize the vital functions, 2) prevent further heat loss, and 3) provide prompt transport.

Thus, your first step is to move the patient from the cold environment to prevent further heat loss. Do not allow the patient to walk, as this may further damage the feet. Next, remove any wet clothing and cover the patient with a dry blanket. Make sure you handle the patient gently, so that you will not cause any pain or possibly further injury to the skin. Do not massage the extremities. Do not allow the patient to eat, drink, or use any stimulants, such as coffee, tea, or cola. In addition, the patient should not be allowed to smoke or chew tobacco.

Give the patient warm, humidified oxygen, if you have not already done so as part of the initial assessment. Next, assess the patient's pulse for 30 to 45 seconds before starting CPR. If the patient has no pulse and is not breathing, begin BLS measures and passive rewarming. This means covering the patient with blankets and turning up the heat in the patient compartment of the unit.

However, if the patient is alert and responds appropriately, begin active rewarming. This means wrapping the patient in blankets and applying heat packs or hot water bottles to the groin, axillary, and cervical regions. Turn the heat up high in the patient compartment of the ambulance.

## LOCAL COLD INJURIES

Most injuries from the cold affect only specific parts of the body, such as the ears, nose, and face, that have been exposed to the cold. The extremities, particularly the feet, are especially vulnerable to cold injury (Figure 19-2). There are three important environmental factors that determine the severity of a local cold injury, as follows:

1. The amount of time exposed
2. The temperature to which the body part was exposed
3. The velocity of the wind during exposure

The following factors may make an individual more susceptible to localized cold injury:

- poor or inadequate insulation from the cold or wind
- impaired circulation from tight clothing or shoes
- circulatory disease
- fatigue
- poor nutrition
- alcohol or drug abuse
- cigarette smoking
- hypothermia
- exposure to wet conditions

In hypothermia, blood is shunted (or blocked) away from the extremities and redirected to the body core. Blood is redirected in an attempt to maintain the temperature of the body core. However, it also increases the risk of local cold injury to the extremities, ears, nose, and face. As a result, a patient with hypothermia should be assessed for local cold injuries, and vice versa. Remember that both local and generalized problems can occur in the same patient as a result of cold exposure.

## FIGURE 19-2

Frostbite of the foot

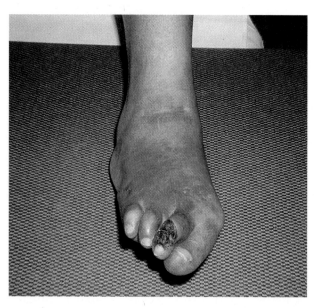

**Signs and Symptoms**

**Early or Superficial Injury** Superficial cold injury occurs after prolonged exposure to the cold. These injuries most commonly affect the ears, fingers, and nose. With this type of local injury, the skin may freeze, but not the deeper tissues. Superficial injuries are usually not painful. In fact, the patient often is not aware that a cold injury has

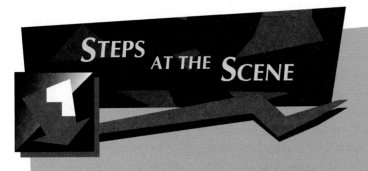

## STEPS AT THE SCENE

### CARING FOR A SUPERFICIAL COLD INJURY

☐ Move the patient from the environment to prevent further exposure to the cold.

☐ Do not allow the patient to stand or walk on an injured extremity.

☐ Handle the injured area gently to protect it from further injury.

☐ Never rub or massage the injured area. Rubbing injured tissues causes further damage.

☐ Give the patient oxygen, if you have not already done so as part of the initial assessment.

☐ Remove any wet or restricting clothing.

☐ Splint the extremity and cover it loosely with a dry, sterile dressing.

☐ Assess for signs and symptoms of generalized hypothermia. Make sure the patient is not re-exposed to the cold.

☐ Support the patient's vital functions and provide rapid transport.

---

occurred. At this stage, the skin turns pale (blanches), and normal color does not return after palpation of the skin. The patient complains of loss of feeling and sensation in the injured area, but the skin remains soft. During rewarming, the affected part will tingle and become red.

**Late or Deep Injury** A deep injury is the most serious type of local cold injury because the tissues are actually frozen. As the tissues freeze, cells are permanently damaged. Ice crystals within the cells may cause physical damage to them. The change in the water content in the cells may also change the concentration of electrolytes. This results in permanent changes in the chemistry of the cell. When the ice thaws, other chemical changes occur in the cell. As a result of

these changes, damaged cells die and gangrene occurs, or the cells are permanently damaged. If gangrene occurs, the dead tissue turns black and must be surgically removed, sometimes by amputation. If less severe damage occurs, the injured part will change permanently. The part may remain red, tender to touch, and/or unable to tolerate further exposure to cold. This type of injury is commonly called frostbite.

A late or deep injury is characterized by white, waxy skin. The part feels firm to frozen as you gently touch it. Much like a burn, the depth of skin damage varies. Blisters and swelling may be present. If a deep injury has thawed or is partially thawed, the skin may appear red with areas of purple and white, or it may appear mottled and cyanotic.

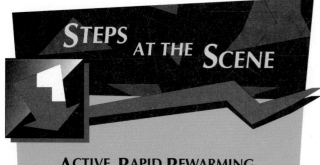

## STEPS AT THE SCENE

### ACTIVE, RAPID REWARMING OF A LOCAL COLD INJURY

- ☐ Immerse the affected part in a warm water bath. The water temperature should be between 100° and 112°F (38° and 44.5°C).

- ☐ Monitor the water temperature so that it does not cool from the frozen part.

- ☐ Continuously stir the water.

- ☐ Keep the affected part in the water until it feels soft and the color (redness) and sensation return.

- ☐ Cover the area with dry, sterile dressings. With the hands and feet, place dressings between the fingers or toes.

- ☐ Protect the thawed area from refreezing.

- ☐ Expect the patient to complain of severe pain.

When caring for a deep cold injury, you should include the following four steps in addition to those listed previously:

1. Remove the patient's jewelry.

2. Cover the injured area with dry cloth or dressings.

3. Avoid breaking any blisters.

4. Do not apply heat or try to rewarm the area.

Occasionally, you may be in a situation where prompt hospital care is not available. In a wilderness situation, or when an extremely long or delayed transport cannot be avoided, you should attempt active, rapid rewarming. However, if you rewarm the patient's feet, be prepared to carry the patient out of the area. Do not allow the patient to walk.

## HYPERTHERMIA

Ordinarily, the heat-regulating mechanisms of the body work very well. However, we will become ill when our body is exposed to more heat energy than it can handle. When the body gains or retains more heat than it loses, the result is called **hyperthermia,** or a high core temperature, usually 101°F (30.3°C) or higher.

The body uses several mechanisms to decrease body heat. The most efficient mechanisms are sweating (and evaporation of the sweat), and dilation of blood vessels in the skin. Dilation brings blood to the skin surface. This, in turn, increases the amount of radiation of heat from the body. As we feel hot, we generally remove clothing and move to a cooler place. This helps us to radiate body heat even more.

### HEAT-RELATED EMERGENCIES

When the body is in a hot environment, or when too much body heat is produced by vigorous physical activity, the body will attempt to rid itself of the excess heat. The body's most efficient mechanisms are sweating (and evaporation of the sweat) and dilation of skin blood vessels. Dilation of the blood vessels brings blood to the skin surface. This increases the rate of radiation of heat from the body.

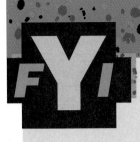

# Glossary of Environmental Emergencies Terms

**Chilblains** Chilblains is a form of cold exposure where exposed parts of the body become very cold but not frozen. It is characterized by redness and swelling.

**Frostbite** Frostbite is the most serious local cold injury because the tissues are actually frozen. The affected tissues are hard and cold to the touch. The skin is usually white, yellow-white, or blue-white.

**Frostnip** Frostnip is a form of cold exposure that occurs after prolonged exposure to the cold. The skin may be frozen, but freezing of the deeper tissues has not occurred. The skin becomes pale (blanched). Exposed parts of the body such as the ears and nose are commonly affected.

**Heat Cramps** Heat cramps are painful muscle spasms that occur after vigorous activity. They usually occur in the leg or abdominal muscles. The exact cause of heat cramps is not well understood. A change in the body's electrolyte balance and dehydration may play a role in the development of muscle cramps.

**Heat Exhaustion** Heat exhaustion, also called heat prostration or heat collapse, is the most common serious illness caused by heat. It occurs when the body loses so much water and electrolytes through very heavy sweating that fluid depletion occurs. Patients who develop heat exhaustion are in mild hypovolemic shock. The skin is usually cold and clammy and the face gray. The patient may also complain of feeling dizzy, weak, or faint, with accompanying nausea or headache. The vital signs may be normal, although the pulse is often rapid. The body temperature is usually normal or slightly elevated, but on rare occasions it may be as high as 104°F (40°C). If not treated, heat exhaustion can develop into heatstroke.

**Heatstroke** Heatstroke is the least common but most serious illness caused by heat exposure. Left untreated, heatstroke will always result in death. When the body is subjected to more heat than it can handle and the normal mechanisms for releasing excess heat are overwhelmed, the body temperature can rise rapidly up to 106°F (41°C) or more. The skin is usually hot, dry, and flushed because the sweating mechanism has been overwhelmed. However, early in the course of heatstroke, the patient may still be sweating and the skin may be moist or wet. As the body core temperature (the temperature of the heart, lungs, and vital organs) rises, the patient's level of consciousness falls. As the patient becomes unresponsive, the pulse becomes weaker and the blood pressure falls.

**Immersion Foot** Immersion foot, also called trench foot, occurs after prolonged exposure to cold water. It is common in hikers or hunters who stand for a long time in cold water. The skin of the foot is wrinkled, pale, and cold to the touch.

When these mechanisms are overwhelmed and the body is no longer able to tolerate the excessive heat, we become ill. Climate becomes a factor when high air temperature reduces our ability to lose heat by radiation, and high humidity reduces our ability to lose heat through evaporation. Another contributing factor is vigorous exercise. During activity, the body can lose more than 1 L of sweat per hour. This causes a loss of fluid and electrolytes.

People who are at greatest risk for heat illnesses include the elderly and children. The elderly are often on medications, lack mobility, and do not adjust well to the heat. Newborns and infants also exhibit poor thermoregulation, lack mobility, and often wear too much clothing.

Medical conditions, such as heart disease, COPD, diabetes, dehydration, and obesity, are predisposing factors. Fatigue and infections or other conditions causing fever are also predisposing factors. You should be especially observant for persons with neurologic impairment and those with limited mobility.

Certain drugs, when taken for other conditions, may make a person susceptible to heat illness as well. Alcohol and medications that decrease the ability of the body to sweat can cause an individual to be more prone to heat illness. Thus, you should always obtain a history on the use of drugs and/or medications when you are treating a patient for a heat illness.

### Signs and Symptoms

The signs and symptoms of exposure to heat include the following:

- muscle cramps
- weakness or exhaustion
- dizziness or faintness
- altered level of consciousness
- unresponsiveness
- rapid heart rate

- moist, pale skin that is normal to cool
- hot, dry or moist skin

### Emergency Medical Care

As you assess a patient with a heat-related emergency, you will notice that the patient's skin will either be hot or normal to cool. Therefore, as you plan your care of the patient, you must evaluate both the skin temperature and the patient's other signs and symptoms.

In all cases, you should move the patient from the hot environment. Ideally, you should move the patient to the back of an air-conditioned ambulance. Next, you should give the patient oxygen if you have not already done so as part of the initial assessment. Third, you should loosen or remove layers of clothing to help cool the patient.

For patients with moist, pale, and normal to cool skin, you should next do as follows:

- place the patient in a supine position with the legs elevated
- fan the patient
- give the patient water to drink, only if the patient is responsive and not vomiting (If the patient is unresponsive or is vomiting, provide BLS care as needed and transport.)

For patients with hyperthermia and hot, dry or moist skin, you should next do as follows:

- fan the patient aggressively and run the air conditioner in the patient compartment on high
- apply cool packs to the neck, groin, and armpits
- apply water with a sponge or wet towel to keep the skin wet
- provide immediate transport, as this is a life-threatening emergency

## WATER-RELATED EMERGENCIES

**Drowning** is death due to suffocation in water. **Near drowning** is defined as survival, at least temporarily, after suffocation in water. Drowning usually results from a cycle of events that results in panic in the water (Figure 19-3). Panic can set up a cycle that will end in death. Even someone who is submerged in water for a short period of time can panic. The person struggles to the surface or the shore and becomes fatigued or exhausted. This panic-driven effort only causes the person to sink deeper into the water.

Drowning may also result from a breath-holding blackout. Swimmers who want to stay underwater for a long period of time breathe rapidly and deeply before entering the water. This hyperventilation lowers the carbon dioxide level in the bloodstream while increasing the oxygen level. As the person swims underwater, the oxygen is consumed. The carbon dioxide, much of which has been blown off by the hyperventilation, does not build up to a high enough level to trigger breathing. An elevated level of carbon dioxide in the blood is the strongest stimulus for breathing. Without this stimulus, the swimmer will not feel the need to breathe even though all of the oxygen in the lungs has been used. The person will then lose consciousness and may drown.

**EMT**

### THROUGH THE ICE ISN'T NICE

**YOU ARE THE EMT**

You and your partner are called to a lake where a snowmobile has gone through the ice. On arrival, you see one snowmobiler lying on the ice. The other victim is submerged, but the person on the ice is holding on to the other victim by one arm. A witness says the accident occurred about 10 minutes ago. At first, the victim in the water was floating with his head clearly in sight. Several times he tried to climb onto the ice, but the edge kept breaking away. About 3 or 4 minutes ago, he began to tire and started to sink. The witness says the person on the ice could no longer hold the other victim's head above water, but at least he managed to keep him from totally sinking.

### For Discussion

1. Explain the reasons for continued CPR on a patient in cardiac arrest after drowning in very cold water.

2. If you suspected a near-drowning victim had a spinal injury, how would you modify patient care?

## Figure 19-3

Effect of panic in water-related accidents

Something goes wrong

Swallowing of water
Fatigue
Unable to cope with currents
Injuries
Cold
Entanglement in kelp
Loss of orientation
Nitrogen narcosis

Panic
(loss of control)

Cardiac arrest

Inefficient
breathing
$CO_2$ retention
$O_2$ deprivation

Exhaustion

Decreased
buoyancy

## Rescuer Safety

You must ensure the safety of you and your team before a water rescue can begin. You must have a prearranged plan, which includes access to and cooperation with local rescuers who are trained and skilled in water rescue. Work with them in developing a protocol for water rescue. Immediate access to life jackets and other rescue equipment is vitally important. The success of any water rescue depends on how rapidly the patient is removed from the water and proper ventilation procedures are started.

You and your partner should always attempt a land-water rescue first. If the patient is conscious and still in the water, throw a rope, life preserver, or any available object that will float to the patient. Many items can be floated out to the patient. For example, an inflated spare tire, rim and all, will float well enough to support two people in the water.

Do not attempt a swimming rescue unless you have been trained and are experienced to do so. When you attempt a swimming rescue, always wear a personal flotation device (PFD). Well-meaning, inexperienced people have found themselves in trouble while attempting a swimming rescue. The basic rule of water rescue is, "Throw, tow, row, and only then go!"

## Resuscitation Efforts

You should never give up on resuscitating a drowning patient. When a person is submerged in water colder than body temperature, heat will be conducted from the body to the water. This lowers the body temperature. Patients submerged in water colder than 70°F (21°C) will develop hypothermia. This protects the vital organs from the lack of oxygen. Sometimes exposure to cold water will induce certain reflexes. These reflexes may preserve the patient's basic body functions for a long period of time.

One of these reflexes is called the **diving reflex.** When an individual dives or jumps into very cold water, a sudden reflex involving the vagus nerves can occur. This reflex causes the heart rate to decrease. At this point, the person may lose consciousness and drown. However, because of hypothermia and a lowered metabolic rate, the person may be able to survive for an extended period of time underwater. Therefore, you should always begin full resuscitation efforts, even if the patient has been underwater for an hour or more. Provide transport to the hospital for evaluation by a physician.

If the patient is submerged in warm water, begin resuscitation efforts as you would for any patient who is not breathing and has no pulse. Remember you must provide transport of all patients involved in near-drowning accidents. Even if initial resuscitation in the field appears completely

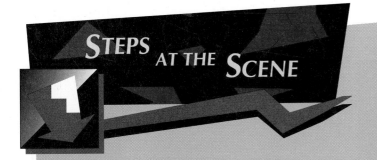

- [ ] Rotate the entire upper half of the patient's body as a unit. Twisting the head may only aggravate any injury to the cervical spine.

- [ ] EMT-B #1 should support the head and trunk.

- [ ] EMT-B #2 should open the airway and begin artificial ventilation.

- [ ] Give mouth-to-mask ventilations (or other means) as soon as the patient is faceup in the water. Immediate ventilation is the primary treatment of all drowning and near-drowning patients.

- [ ] Float a buoyant spine board under the patient.

- [ ] EMT-B #1 should secure the head and trunk to the board. ***Do not remove the patient from the water until he or she is secured to the spine board.***

- [ ] Remove the patient from the water on the spine board.

- [ ] Check the pulse immediately after you remove the patient from the water. It may be difficult to find due to peripheral vasoconstriction and low cardiac output. If the patient has no pulse, start CPR immediately. Remember that full CPR cannot be done in the water.

- [ ] Cover the patient with blankets to prevent further heat loss and then provide immediate transport. Give the patient oxygen or continue CPR en route, if necessary.

successful, the patient can still aspirate fluids. This may result in complications that last for days or weeks.

## EMERGENCY MEDICAL CARE

Your focus is to get these patients breathing again as soon as possible. Thus, you should begin mouth-to-mask ventilation as soon as possible, even before you remove the patient from the water. First, place the patient's head in a neutral position. Next, open the airway with the jaw-thrust (for patients with possible spinal injury) or chin-lift maneuver. If the patient does not have a possible spinal injury, turn him or her to the left side to allow water, vomitus, and secretions to drain from the upper airway. Have a suctioning unit ready so that you can remove vomitus, water, and secretions from the mouth, if necessary. Give the patient oxygen once you have removed him or her from the water.

If the patient has an upper airway obstruction by a foreign object, remove the obstruction manually, by suction, or by abdominal thrust. Continue to assist ventilation.

If gastric distention interferes with ventilation, place the patient on his or her left side. Next, place your hand over the epigastric

## FIGURE 19-4

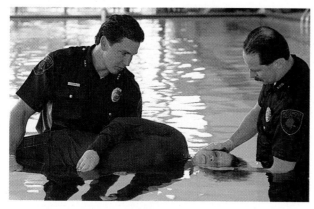

**A**   Support the head and neck

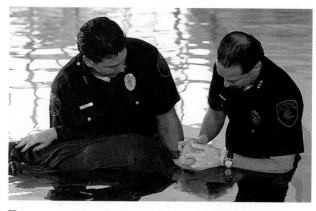

**B**   Open the airway and begin artificial ventilation

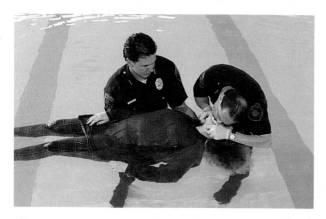

**C**   Give mouth-to-mask ventilations

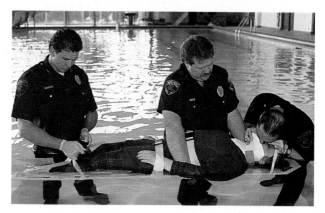

**D**   Secure the head and trunk to the spine board

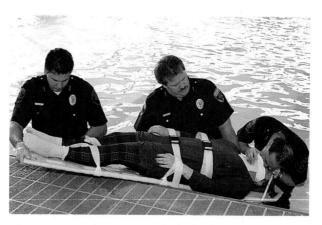

**E**   Lift the patient out of the pool

area of the patient's abdomen. Apply firm pressure to relieve the distention. Make sure there is a suctioning unit available in case the patient vomits. You should only do this if gastric distention interferes with your ability to ventilate the patient effectively.

Always assume that there is a spinal injury if the patient is involved in a diving accident, is unconscious, or is conscious but complains of weakness, paralysis, or numbness in the arms or legs. Most spinal injuries that result from diving accidents affect the cervical spine. When you suspect a spinal injury, you must protect the neck from further injury. Thus, you must immobilize the neck while the patient is still in the water. To do this properly, two EMT-Bs are needed to turn the patient. It is helpful to have three EMT-Bs remove the patient from the water so that artificial ventilation does not have to be interrupted.

### Caring for a Diving Accident Patient

1. Rotate the entire upper half of the patient's body as a unit. Twisting the head may only aggravate any injury to the cervical spine.

2. EMT-B #1 should support the head and neck. EMT-B #2 supports the body as the patient is turned (Figure 19-4a).

3. EMT-B #1 should open the airway with the jaw-thrust maneuver and begin artificial ventilation. EMT-B #2 supports the head and neck by holding the head and neck (Figure 19-4b).

4. Give mouth-to-mask ventilations (or other means) as soon as the patient is faceup in the water (Figure 19-4c). Immediate ventilation is the primary treatment of all drowning and near-drowning patients. Move to shallow water, if possible.

5. EMT-B #3 floats a buoyant spine board under the patient.

6. EMT-B #1 should continue artificial ventilations. EMT-B #3 applies the cervical collar and secures the head and trunk to the board (Figure 19-4d). *Do not remove the patient from the water until he or she is secured to the spine board.*

7. Remove the patient from the water on the spine board (Figure 19-4e).

8. Check the pulse immediately after you remove the patient from the water. It may be difficult to find due to peripheral vasoconstriction and low cardiac output. If the patient has no pulse, start CPR immediately. Remember that full CPR cannot be done in the water.

9. Cover the patient with blankets to prevent further heat loss and then provide immediate transport. Give the patient high-flow oxygen or continue CPR en route, if necessary.

Occasionally, you will find that a patient's lungs cannot be ventilated due to a spasm of the larynx muscles. When very small amounts of water are inhaled, it severely irritates the larynx. This makes the muscles of the larynx and the vocal cords spasm. These spasms are called laryngospasm. Laryngospasm prevents more water from entering the lungs. As a result, the patient does not receive enough oxygen to the brain and eventually loses consciousness. At this point, the spasm relaxes, and rescue breathing becomes effective.

## BITES AND STINGS

Although many stings and bites are painful, most are usually not serious. However, these injuries may result in an ambulance call. Spiders are numerous and widespread in the United States. Two species—the black widow spider and the brown recluse spider—give serious, sometimes even life-threatening bites. Many other spiders bite, but these injuries do not produce serious complications.

Bites from snakes are sometimes serious. Of the approximately 150 different species of snakes in the United States, only four are poisonous: the rattlesnake, the copperhead, the cottonmouth (water) moccasin, and the coral snake. When you respond to a snake bite, you must identify whether envenomation has occurred. **Envenomation** is deposit of venom into the wound.

Insects, scorpions, and marine animals also have painful stings. Some of these injuries are potentially dangerous. Some people are highly allergic to bee stings. Your care for these allergic reactions is described in chapter 18, Allergies and Poisoning.

## SIGNS AND SYMPTOMS

As you assess a patient with a bite or sting, you should try to obtain a complete history of the injury. If the injury was a bite, try to determine exactly what type of spider or snake was involved. Information to obtain from the patient about an insect, reptile, or animal bite or sting should include the following:

- size
- color
- markings
- shape of the head
- location of the event
- how it happened
- if the spider or snake was captured or could be
- if the insect, scorpion, or marine animal was captured

Your next step is to perform an initial assessment. As you move to the detailed physical exam, look for the following signs and symptoms:

- redness and heat
- pain
- swelling
- weakness or decreased use of a part of the body

- bite marks or a stinger
- generalized weakness
- dizziness
- chills
- fever
- pallor
- nausea and vomiting

## EMERGENCY MEDICAL CARE

Your first step in caring for any patient with a bite or sting should be to calm and reassure the patient. Remind the patient that stings and bites are usually not life threatening. Next, place the patient in a supine position. This will decrease the spread of any venom.

### Care of Insect Stings

For a patient with a sting, your next step is to remove the stinger. The best way to remove a stinger is to scrape it off the surface of the skin with the edge of a card. Do not use a tweezers or forceps, as squeezing the stinger may only inject more venom into the wound. Next, gently wash the area with soap and water or a mild antiseptic. Remove jewelry from the area, if possible, before swelling begins.

You should now place the injected site in a position slightly below the level of the patient's heart. Apply ice or cold packs to the area, but not directly on the skin. Cold may help relieve the pain and slow the absorption of the toxin. However, you do not want to freeze the tissue.

As you prepare the patient for transport, be alert for vomiting. Anxiety as well as the toxin can have this effect. Also watch for any signs of developing shock or allergic reaction. Do not give anything by mouth, especially alcohol. Place the patient in a shock position and give oxygen, if needed. Check the patient's vital signs and continue to monitor them. Be prepared to provide BLS measures, if needed.

### Care of Spider Bites

For a patient with a spider bite, you should next gently wash the area with soap and water or a mild antiseptic. Remove jewelry from the area, if possible, before swelling begins. Apply cold to the area, as with insect bites. Again, make sure you do not place ice directly on the skin.

As you prepare the patient for transport, be alert for signs of respiratory distress. Provide BLS measures, if needed. Also, try to identify the type of spider and bring it with you to the hospital

### Care of Snake Bites

For a patient with a snake bite, you should first inform medical control that the patient has a snake bite and, if possible, describe the snake. At this point, you will need to discuss with medical control the use of venous tourniquets. After consulting with medical control, lightly place venous tourniquets above and below the bite. The tourniquets should not be so tight that they cut off arterial blood flow. Make sure that the patient's pulse is still palpable distal to the tourniquet.

Once the venous tourniquets have been applied, splint the extremity to minimize movement and the spread of venom at the site. ***Do not apply cold to snake bites.*** Occasionally, a patient will have a bite on the trunk rather than on the extremity. This makes the use of tourniquets and splinting impossible. As you prepare the patient for transport, be alert for signs of a developing allergic reaction. Provide BLS measures, if needed. Keep the patient supine, as quiet as possible, and transport promptly.

If the snake has been killed, put it in a bag and bring it with you to the hospital. Identifying the snake is extremely important to hospital personnel so that they can give the correct antivenin.

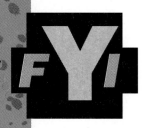

# Atlas of Specific Types of Bites and Stings

### BLACK WIDOW SPIDER

The black widow spider has a glossy black body and a distinctive, bright red-orange marking in the shape of an hourglass on its abdomen. These spiders prefer dry, dim places around buildings, in woodpiles, and among debris. The danger of a black widow spider bite is that the venom is poisonous to nerve tissue. The venom directly attacks spinal nerve centers and causes systemic symptoms. Severe cramps, rigid abdominal muscles, tightness in the chest, and difficulty breathing occur over 24 hours. Other signs and symptoms include dizziness, sweating, vomiting, nausea, and skin rash.

### BROWN RECLUSE SPIDER

Dull brown in color, the brown recluse spider has a dark violin-shaped mark on its back, which can be easily seen from above. It tends to live in dark areas, corners, old unused buildings, under rocks, and in woodpiles. It is also found indoors in cooler areas and lives in closets, drawers, cellars, and old piles of clothing. The venom of this spider causes severe local tissue damage, producing a large, nonhealing ulcer if not treated promptly. The bite area becomes red, swollen, and tender, and develops a pale, mottled cyanotic center. A small blister may form. Several days after a bite, a large scab of dead skin, fat, and debris develops and deepens to produce a large ulcer.

### PIT VIPERS

Rattlesnakes, copperheads, and cottonmouth (water) moccasins are considered pit vipers. Rattlesnakes can usually be identified by the rattle on the tail. Rattlesnakes have many patterns of color, often with a diamond pattern. Copperheads are reddish or coppery with brown or red cross bands. Cottonmouth moccasins, also called water moccasins, are olive or brown, and have black cross bands and a yellow undersurface. They are water snakes and tend to be aggressive.

The signs of envenomation by a pit viper are severe burning pain at the site of the injury, followed by swelling and discoloration. These signs are evident within 5 to 10 minutes after the bite has occurred and spread slowly over the next 36 hours. Bleeding under the skin causes ecchymosis. Other signs may include weakness, sweating, fainting, and shock.

The venom of the pit viper causes localized destruction of all tissues. It can also interfere with the body's clotting mechanism and cause bleeding elsewhere in the body. Tissue destruction locally starts from the moment of envenomation. If 1 hour has passed from the time the patient was bitten and there is no swelling, discoloration, or severe local pain, you can assume that envenomation has not occurred.

### CORAL SNAKE

The coral snake is a rare, small, colorful reptile with a series of bright red, yellow, and black bands that completely encircle its body. It lives primarily in Florida and in the desert Southwest. Many harmless snakes have coloring similar to the coral snake. The difference is that the red and yellow bands of the coral snake are next to one another, completely encircling the body.

The coral snake is not a pit viper. The head is not triangular, there are no pits, and no projecting fangs. The coral snake usually bites its victims on a small part of the body, especially a finger or toe. However, its venom is a powerful toxin that causes paralysis of the nervous system. Usually, there are minimal or no local symptoms of a coral snake bite. However, within a few hours the patient may begin acting strange. This is followed by progressive paralysis of eye movements and respirations. If the bite is from a coral snake, inform medical control immediately. The hospital may have to order this special antivenin from a central supply source.

## BEE, WASP, HORNET, YELLOW JACKET, AND ANT STINGS

The stinging organ of most bees, wasps, or hornets is a small hollow spine that projects from the abdomen. Venom can be injected through this spine directly into the skin. The stinger of the honeybee is barbed so that the bee cannot withdraw it and must leave a part of its abdomen imbedded with the stinger when it flies away. Because of this, the honeybee can only sting once. However, this stinging organ with its attached muscle can continue to inject venom for up to 20 minutes.

Honeybee venom is a common allergen. As such, it may cause a violent hypersensitivity reaction called anaphylaxis or anaphylactic shock. Signs and symptoms are described in chapter 18, Allergies and Poisoning. If untreated, anaphylactic shock can result in death. You should assist the patient with prescribed epinephrine, or provide BLS measures and rapid transport.

Wasps or hornets, with unbarbed stingers, can sting repeatedly. Identifying a stinging insect is often impossible, because

it tends to fly away immediately after the injury.

Some species of ant, especially the fire ant, can bite repeatedly and often inject an irritating toxin at the bite site. These bites usually occur on the feet and legs. It is not uncommon for the patient to sustain many bites within a very short period of time.

Symptoms associated with insect stings or bites usually occur at the site of injury. Local symptoms of stings and bites may include sudden pain, severe swelling, heat, and redness about the affected area. Sometimes a wheal (whitish firm elevation of the skin) may occur, with itching.

## SCORPION STINGS

Scorpions are rare. They are found primarily in the Southwest and in deserts. Scorpions have a venom gland and a stinger at the end of their tail. These injuries are ordinarily very painful but not dangerous. Local swelling, pain, and discoloration result from a scorpion sting. The more dangerous Arizona scorpion injects a venom that may produce a severe systemic reaction including circulatory collapse, severe muscle contractions, excessive salivation, hypertension, convulsions, and cardiac failure. If the patient has been stung by an Arizona scorpion, notify medical control. Provide BLS measures and rapid transport.

## MARINE ANIMALS

With the exception of the shark and barracuda, most marine creatures are not aggressive and will not deliberately attack a human. The most common injuries occur when an individual swims into the tentacles of a jellyfish, a Portuguese man-of-war, anemones, corals, or hydras. Stepping on the back of a stingray, or falling or stepping on a sea urchin also results in injuries.

Some sea animals, such as nonpoisonous water snakes, may cause injuries by minor bites. Many fish are poisonous if eaten. Other rare conditions include shocks from electric eels or skin rashes from marine parasites.

For stings from marine animals, remove the patient from the water and pour rubbing alcohol on the affected area. Then sprinkle the area with meat tenderizer and dust the area with talcum powder to inactivate the poison. Injuries from the spines of marine animals can be treated by soaking the affected area in hot water for 30 minutes.

## DOG BITES AND HUMAN BITES

### Dog Bites and Rabies

Dog bites are potentially serious problems. The animal's mouth is heavily contaminated with bacteria, and serious infection may result from a bite. You should consider all dog bites as contaminated and potentially infected wounds.

A patient who has been bitten is often extremely upset and frightened. Most dog bites are not serious; therefore, calm reassurance on your part is extremely important. The prehospital treatment for dog bites of any severity is to place a dry, sterile dressing over the wound and promptly transport the patient to the emergency department.

A major concern with dog bites is the spread of rabies. Rabies is an acute, usually fatal viral infection of the central nervous system. The virus is present in the saliva of an infected animal and is transmitted by licking an open wound or biting. All warm-blooded animals can be affected. Although rabies is extremely rare today, particularly with the widespread inoculation of pets, it still exists. Stray dogs may not have been inoculated and could be carriers of the disease. Certain other animals such as squirrels, bats, foxes, skunks, and raccoons may

also carry rabies. A rabid animal may act perfectly normal or it may appear vicious or wild, salivate excessively, or show some other form of unusual behavior. You cannot tell whether an animal is rabid by its behavior.

The vaccine that is used to prevent rabies in pets is very effective. If an animal has been inoculated against rabies, it ordinarily will be wearing a tag on its collar. It is very important to identify this fact if the animal can be located. If the animal does not have a rabies tag, it should be captured (not killed) by an animal control officer and turned over to the health department for observation. Unless you are specially trained in handling animals, you should not attempt to handle a strange dog or wild animal but instead call the local animal control officer. If the animal is then suspected of having rabies, it is killed and the brain studied to determine whether the animal was rabid. When the animal cannot be found or identified, the patient usually is treated with rabies inoculations. If started early enough, these inoculations will prevent rabies from developing.

On occasion, you will be called to treat a child who has been attacked by a dog. The dog may be a stray, or it may even be a family pet. These dogs are not always vicious or rabid; sometimes the child unknowingly provokes the dog. Even though the dog may not appear rabid or vicious, you must assume that it may turn on you and attack. Therefore, do not enter the scene until the animal has been secured by either the police or the animal control officer. Then, carry out the necessary emergency care and transport the child to the emergency department promptly.

### Human Bites

The human bite is relatively uncommon but potentially one of the most severe injuries seen today. The human mouth contains an exceptionally wide range of virulent bacteria, more so than the mouth of a dog. For this reason, any human bite that has penetrated the skin must be regarded as a very serious injury. A laceration caused by a human tooth, such as may result on a hand from punching someone in the mouth, can result in a serious, spreading infection. The emergency treatment for human bites is prompt immobilization of the area with a splint or bandage, application of a dry, sterile dressing, and transport to the emergency department for surgical cleansing of the wound and antibiotic therapy. Remember when you are treating someone who has been punched in the mouth that the person who delivered the punch may also need treatment.

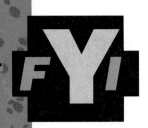

# Atlas of
# Scuba Diving Emergencies

With over 3 million SCUBA sport divers in the United States and 200,000 new divers trained annually, SCUBA diving emergencies are becoming more common. These emergencies usually occur in one of the three phases of the dive: descent, bottom, and ascent.

## DESCENT PROBLEMS

Descent problems are usually due to the sudden increase in pressure on the body as the diver goes deeper into the water. Structures such as the lungs, sinus cavities, middle ear, teeth, and the area of the face surrounded by the diving mask cannot adjust to the increased external pressure of the water. This can cause severe pain, forcing the diver to return to the surface to equalize the pressures. If the diver continues to have pain, particularly in the ear, after returning to the surface, he or she should be transported to the hospital. A diver with a ruptured eardrum risks cold water entering the middle ear. The diver may then lose his or her balance and orientation, shoot to the surface, resulting in ascent problems.

## BOTTOM PROBLEMS

Bottom problems are rare. Most are due to faulty connections in the diving gear. Occasionally, a diver becomes disoriented, lost, or tangled in a kelp forest and begins to panic. All of these situations can cause drowning or rapid ascent. All require emergency resuscitation and transport.

## ASCENT PROBLEMS

Most serious injuries associated with diving are related to ascending from the bottom. The ascent may be too rapid or without decompression stops, or the result of panic from a descent or bottom problem. These emergencies usually require resuscitation. Two dangerous medical emergencies as a result of ascent problems are air embolism and decompression sickness, or the bends.

### Air Embolism

The most common and most dangerous emergency in SCUBA diving is air embolism. Air embolism results when the diver holds his or her breath during a rapid ascent. The air pressure in the lungs remains at a high level while the external pressure on the chest decreases. The air inside the lungs then expands rapidly, causing rupture of the alveoli. The air released from this rupture may enter one of the following:

- the pleural space, resulting in a pneumothorax
- the mediastinum, resulting in pneumomediastinum
- the bloodstream, resulting in air bubbles called air emboli

Pneumothorax and pneumomediastinum both result in pain and severe breathing problems. An air embolus in the bloodstream will act as a "plug" and prevent the normal flow of blood and oxygen to parts of the body. The brain or spinal cord are most severely affected because they require a constant supply of oxygen.

The following are signs and symptoms of air embolism:

- mottling of the skin
- pink or bloody froth at the nose and mouth
- severe pain in the muscles, joints, or abdomen
- difficulty breathing and chest pain
- dizziness, nausea, and vomiting
- dysphasia
- vision problems
- paralysis and coma

### Decompression Sickness

Decompression sickness (the bends) also results from too rapid an ascent. However, the mechanism of injury is different. During the dive, nitrogen that is being breathed dissolves in the blood. When the diver ascends rapidly, the external pressure is decreased. The dissolved nitrogen forms small bubbles around and within the blood vessels. These bubbles cause pain, swelling, decreased blood flow, and blockages in blood vessels. The most striking symptom is abdominal and joint pain so severe that the patient literally doubles up or "bends."

Often it is difficult to distinguish between air embolism and decompression sickness. As a general rule, air embolism occurs immediately on return to the surface. The symptoms of decompression sickness may not occur for several hours or days.

## EMERGENCY MEDICAL CARE

Your assessment of a SCUBA diving emergency should include a detailed dive history, recording the hour, times, number, depths, and order of the dives. Determine how much compressed air was actually used and how the tanks were filled, if possible. Assess any event that may have led to a rapid, uncontrolled ascent. Ask other divers or bystanders about the patient's complaints and possible mood or personality changes, especially if the diver is unresponsive.

Your care of a patient who has an air embolism or decompression sickness without a spinal injury should begin by removing the patient from the water. Keep the patient calm and use blankets to prevent hypothermia. Next, begin BLS measures and give the patient oxygen.

Turn the patient onto his or her left side, with the head lower than the feet. This position will decrease the chance of an air embolism traveling to the brain. Listen to the chest for absent or decreased breath sounds that would indicate a pneumothorax. Assess and monitor the patient's level of consciousness using the AVPU scale. This information will assist the hospital personnel in selecting the correct treatment program.

Provide prompt transport to the nearest facility equipped with a recompression chamber. Continue to give oxygen en route. If facilities are available, the patient's SCUBA tank should be analyzed for the amount of air and other gases remaining in it. Transport the tank and gear with the patient.

Injury from decompression sickness is usually reversible with recompression treatment. However, if the bubbles block the critical blood vessels that supply the brain or spinal cord, permanent central nervous system injury may result. Therefore, the key in emergency management of these serious ascent problems is to begin BLS measures, give oxygen, and arrange for recompression as rapidly as possible.

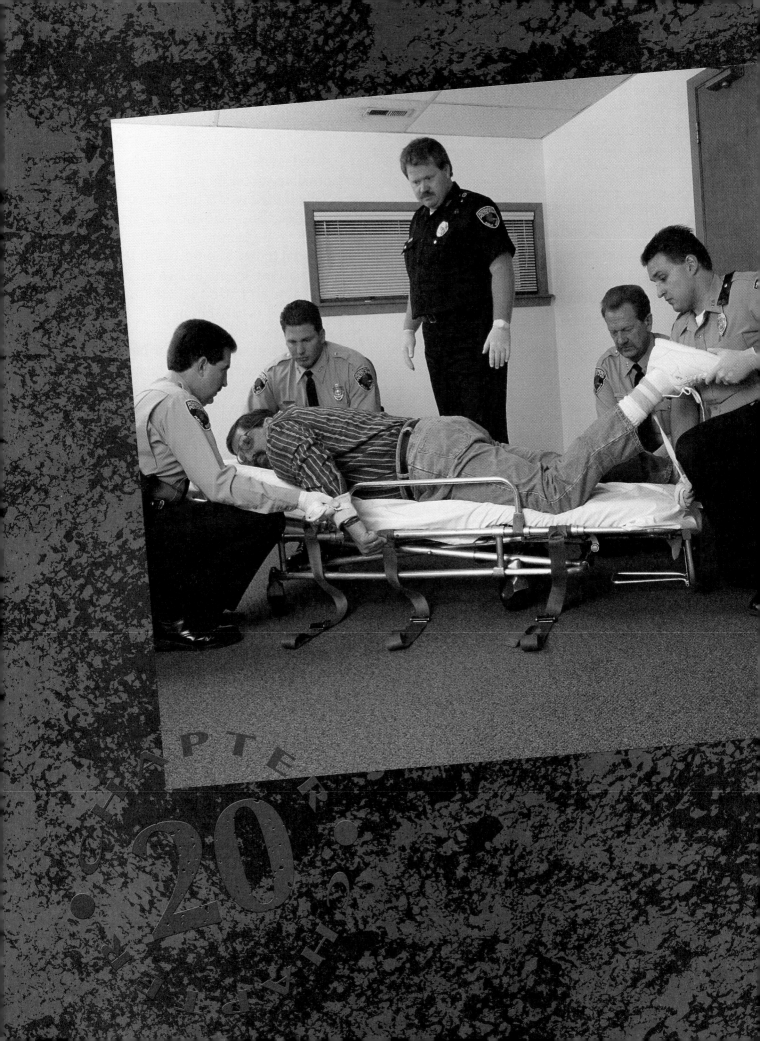

# Behavioral Emergencies

After you have read this chapter, you should be able to:

- Define behavioral emergencies.
- Discuss the various reasons that may cause a psychological crisis or an altered behavior.
- Discuss the special medicolegal considerations of managing behavioral emergencies.
- Discuss the special considerations for assessing a patient with behavioral problems.
- Discuss the behavioral characteristics that suggest a patient is at risk for suicide or violence.
- Discuss methods to calm behavioral emergency patients.

## Overview

Any emergency medical situation, whether sickness or injury, may become a crisis in the patient's mind. A crisis is a state of emotional confusion or turmoil that may develop suddenly or over a long period of time. It may be caused by a sudden, stressful situation that the patient sees as a critical turning point in his or her life. No matter what the cause, all emergency situations create stress in the patient, the patient's family, and the EMT-B at the scene. The most important aspect of your initial assessment and treatment in these situations is your common sense, along with your ability to communicate with the patient. It is important for you to be able to handle patients with emotional or physical problems that cause behavioral changes. Their behavior could affect the early assessment process.

Whenever you encounter a behavioral emergency, you need to protect yourself, your partner, the patient, and any others on the scene. You and your partner may be at risk if the patient becomes violent. Always inform medical control and contact law enforcement whenever you are faced with a potentially disruptive situation.

# Key Terms

**Behavior**   Manner in which a person acts. Pertains to any or all activities, including physical and mental.

**Behavioral emergency**   A situation in which the patient acts abnormally in a way that is unacceptable or intolerable to the patient, family, or community.

**Depression**   A state in which the patient may not want to do anything, even move, and may not cooperate or answer questions.

**Disruptive behavior**   Behavior that puts the patient or others in danger or delays treatment.

**Mania**   A state in which the patient may be severely agitated (manic), moving around frantically and speaking rapidly, but never finishing a sentence or a complete thought.

**Paranoia**   A state in which the patient may believe that people (including you) are plotting to harm or kill him or her.

**Suicidal act**   A situation in which a patient may be threatening to kill himself or herself or may have already made an attempt.

# BEHAVIORAL EMERGENCIES

**Behavior** is the manner in which a patient acts or performs in response to the environment. This includes any or all activities—both physical and mental. **A behavioral emergency** exists when the patient acts abnormally in a way that is unacceptable or intolerable to the patient, family, or community. The behavioral change may be due to an emotional, psychological, or physical condition. Common physical causes include a lack of oxygen, head injury, or low blood sugar as in a diabetic patient.

People experiencing behavioral emergencies may delay treatment or become violent, either to themselves or to others. This is referred to as **disruptive behavior.**

## PHYSICAL CAUSES

There are many potential causes for a change in behavior, including several physical and medical conditions. Excessive heat or cold, for example, can lead to changes in a person's behavior. A lack of oxygen or an inadequate blood flow to the brain can produce the same effect.

Head injuries or strokes can also lead to disruptive behavior. With a concussion, the patient may behave abnormally immediately after the injury. However, abnormal behavior can also occur 2 to 3 weeks after the injury. This is usually due to a chronic subdural hematoma. Whenever a patient's family reports a significant personality change, consider the possibility of a head injury or stroke.

Alcohol or drug abuse can produce disruptive behavior. Look for evidence of substance abuse—drug paraphernalia or an empty liquor bottle. Even if you find such clues, bear in mind that there may be other causes of behavioral changes. Do not "write off" the unruly or abusive patient as "just another drunk."

Certain metabolic disorders, such as high or low blood sugar, may lead to disruptive behavior. Other endocrine disorders (especially thyroid disease) can produce wide ranges of abnormal behavior—from extreme agitation to marked lethargy. Try to determine if a patient who is acting abnormally has a history of a metabolic disorder. Ask the patient or family if similar reactions occurred before or if the patient is taking any prescribed medication.

Neurologic diseases, particularly organic brain syndrome, may also lead to disruptive behavior. The vast majority of patients with organic brain syndrome are elderly. As the disease progresses, they experience a gradual loss of function. Frequently, the first sign of this disease is a personality change. The family, and sometimes even the patient, will be aware of the change. Patients with organic brain syndrome are often disoriented. They do not know where they are. They may not know the date or be able to answer a simple question, such as "Who is the President of the United States?"

## PSYCHOGENIC CAUSES

Many different forms of psychiatric illness also cause disruptive behavior. Many psychiatric disorders produce a wide range of behavioral problems. Psychiatric patients may also exhibit great variations in their behavior over a short time. They often experience wide mood swings—calm one minute and violent the next. They are often agitated or easily panicked. Their thinking or behavior may appear bizarre. These patients often represent a danger, either to themselves or to others on the scene. The following are just four of the common presentations of psychiatric illness:

1. **Paranoia.** A patient may believe that people (including you) are plotting to harm or kill him or her.
2. **Mania.** A patient may be severely agitated (manic), moving around frantically and speaking rapidly, but never finishing a sentence or a complete thought.
3. **Depression.** A patient may not want to do anything, even move, and may not cooperate or answer questions.
4. **Suicidal act.** A patient may be threatening to kill himself or herself or may have already made an attempt.

## SUICIDE

You must recognize self-destructive behavior before a patient commits suicide. Look for warning signs. People who are alone, without support, are often at risk. If they are alcoholic or depressed, the risk of suicide is even higher.

The signs of depression that often accompany suicide attempts include a sad, tearful demeanor, and thoughts of death. The patient may not feel like doing anything. Some of these patients may not cooperate or answer questions.

You should be concerned if the patient verbalizes a defined plan of action. This is especially true if the patient has gathered destructive articles, such as a gun or a large volume of pills.

Another risk factor is a past history of self-destructive behavior. Also consider any recent bad news the patient may have received, such as the diagnosis of a serious illness or the loss of a significant loved one. Has the patient been arrested, imprisoned, or lost a job? Any of these environmental stresses could cause a change in a person's mental status.

## EMERGENCY MEDICAL CARE

Before you can begin caring for a patient in a behavioral emergency, assess the scene to make sure it is safe for you and your partner to enter. Unless the patient is in danger, always consider your own and your partner's safety before making contact.

Look for a possible cause for the behavioral change. Is there a head injury? Has the patient been ill recently? Are there signs of drug or alcohol use? Is there a history of similar behavior or psychiatric illness? Get a history of the behavior. Did it come on suddenly or gradually? The family may be able to help if the patient is calm and trusting. Question the family about past aggressiveness, combativeness, or self-destructive behavior.

Never turn your back on a disturbed patient. Always keep your eyes focused on the patient. Be alert for any obviously aggressive behavior. Even people small in stature can be dangerous if they are severely agitated. If the patient has a knife or gun, stay clear. Do not become a casualty yourself. Initial management of these patients is a job for law enforcement.

Never leave the patient alone. Firmly establish yourself as a professional responsible for helping the patient. Act confidently and decisively. Your mood, as well as your words and body language, will help keep the patient calm. Always tell the patient what you are going to do before you do it. Keep your movements slow and deliberate, and speak in a calm, reassuring voice. Maintain a comfortable distance between you and the patient.

Encourage the patient to talk. Ask questions and let the patient tell you what happened. Prove you are listening by rephrasing or repeating portions of the patient's tale.

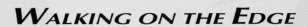

## WALKING ON THE EDGE

The "off-going" crew has just finished giving you a report when you are dispatched to the bridge over the Fowler River for a "jumper." You arrive a few minutes later and find that law enforcement has secured the bridge. The patient is perched in the middle of the span. He shouts, "If you get too close, I'll jump and take you with me." He says he lost his job 2 months ago. Since then, his wife left him and moved back in with her parents. He says he has nothing left to live for and has planned this for the past week. He started drinking this morning, he adds, but now "it's time to go."

### For Discussion

1. Name at least two medical conditions that can result in altered mental status. How can you determine the cause of a patient's behavioral emergency?

2. Describe how to evaluate mental status in your initial assessment and detailed focused exam.

Acknowledge the patient's feelings of anger or despair.

Answer any questions honestly; do not lie. And never challenge or argue with a disturbed patient. Use direct eye contact, but avoid any unnecessary physical contact. Do not "play along" with the patient if he or she sees or hears things that are not real. Emphasize that you are there to help. You should be willing to remain at the scene for an extended time, if necessary. Ask trusted family members or friends to help, if possible.

Assess the patient's mental status. Look for clues in the patient's appearance, activity, and speech. Is there any disorientation regarding time, place, or identity?

Once you secure the patient, provide transport to the hospital. Bring with you any medications or drugs that the patient may have been using.

Throughout your assessment and treatment, remain alert for signs of potential violence. Clenched or tensed fists or a combative posture are early warning signs. The patient may be yelling or verbally threatening himself or others. Always be wary if the patient comes toward you or is moving with quick, irregular motions. Be exceedingly cautious if the patient is carrying heavy or threatening objects. And be aware of nearby objects, as they may be potentially dangerous weapons.

## MEDICOLEGAL CONSIDERATIONS

When dealing with emotionally disturbed patients, the best legal situation is to obtain the patient's consent to medical treatment. This may be difficult, since these patients often resist treatment. They may even threaten you and your partner or others at the scene. If the patient presents a threat to self or others, you can legally care for, and even restrain, the patient against his or her will.

### RESTRAINING A PATIENT

You should always try to transport a disturbed patient without restraints, if possible. However, if you believe a patient will injure himself, herself, or others, you can legally restrain him or her. Always consult medical control and contact law enforcement for help before restraining a patient.

Once the decision has been made to restrain a patient, carry it out quickly. Be aware of BSI considerations. If the patient is spitting, place a surgical mask over his or her mouth. To safely restrain a patient, make sure you have adequate help. Whenever possible, ask that law enforcement physically restrain the patient. There should be at least four officers present. Each should be responsible for one extremity. Before you begin, discuss the plan of action. As you prepare to restrain the patient, stay outside the patient's range of motion.

In subduing a disturbed patient, use the minimum force necessary to restrain the patient. That amount will vary, depending on a number of factors. One significant factor is how much force is necessary to keep

## FIGURE 20-1

Proper restraint of a patient by law enforcement officers

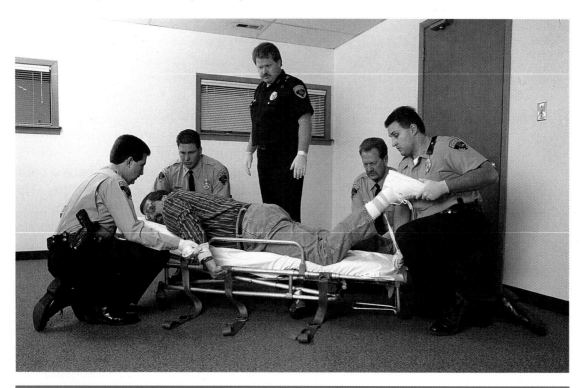

the patient from injuring himself, herself, or others. A patient's sex, size, strength, and mental status all affect the amount of force you can use. The type of abnormal behavior the patient is exhibiting and the type of restraints you will be using are two final factors. You should use soft, wide leather or cloth restraints, not police-type handcuffs.

Acting at the same time, the police officers should secure the extremities with equipment approved by medical control (Figure 20-1). Somebody, preferably you or your partner, should continue to talk to the patient throughout the process. Remember to treat the patient with dignity and respect at all times.

Place the patient facedown on a stretcher and secure the patient with multiple straps (Figure 20-2). Assess the airway and circulation frequently while the patient remains restrained. Document the reason for the restraint and the technique that was used. Be especially careful if a combative patient suddenly becomes calm and cooperative. This is not the time to relax but to secure the situation. The patient may suddenly become combative again and injure himself or you. However, you can use reasonable force to defend yourself against an attack by an emotionally disturbed patient.

To protect yourself against false accusations, promptly document the patient's abnormal behavior. When transporting the patient, ask a witness, usually a police officer, to ride in the vehicle. Disturbed patients commonly accuse EMS personnel of sexual misconduct. If available, an EMT-B of the same sex riding with the patient can help avoid a situation in which false accusations may occur.

## FIGURE 20-2

Check the distal pulses of a patient in restraints

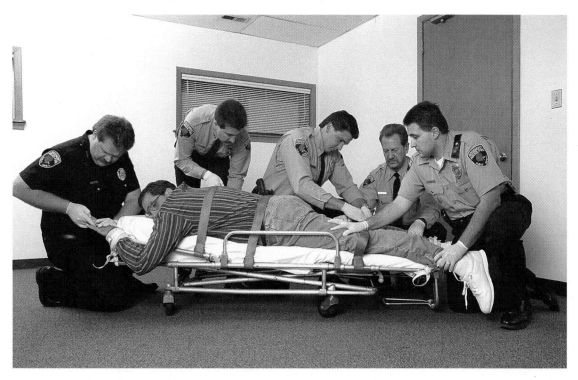

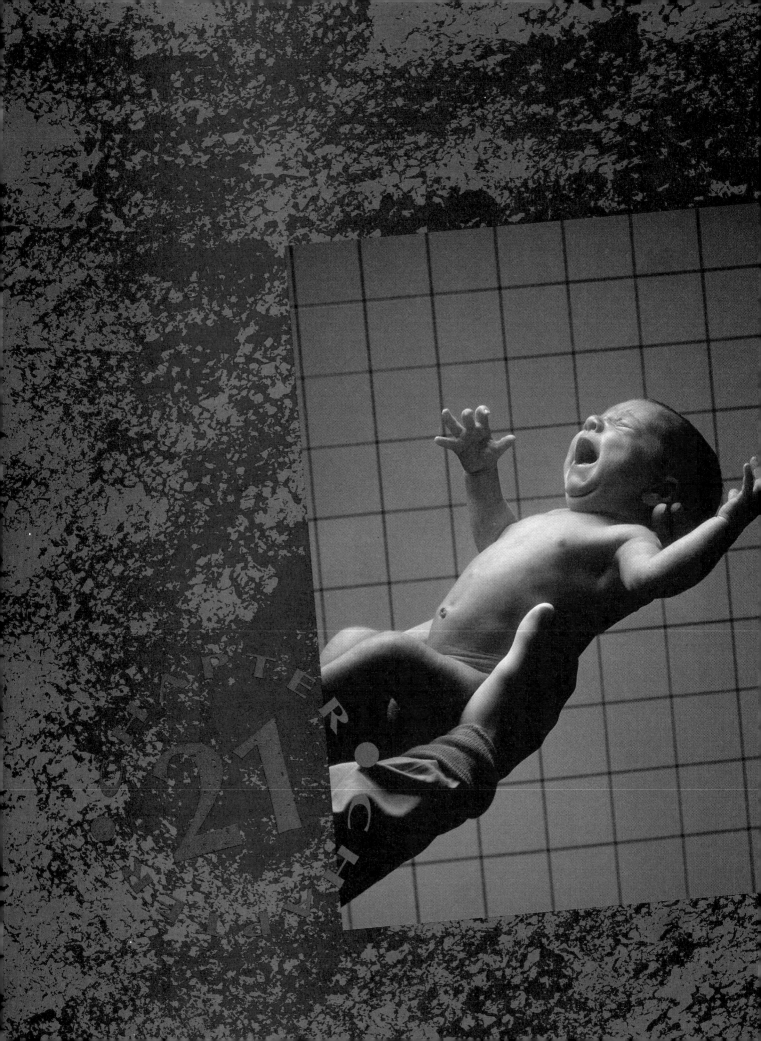

# CHAPTER 21

# Obstetrics and Gynecology

## Objectives

After you have read this chapter, you should be able to:

- Identify the following structures: uterus, vagina, fetus, placenta, umbilical cord, amniotic sac, perineum.
- Identify and explain the use of the contents of an obstetrics kit.
- Identify predelivery emergencies.
- State indications of an imminent delivery.
- Differentiate the emergency medical care provided to a patient with predelivery emergencies from a normal delivery.
- State the steps in the predelivery preparation of the mother.
- Establish the relationship between body substance isolation and childbirth.
- State the steps to assist in the delivery.
- Describe the care of the baby as the head appears.
- Describe how and when to cut the umbilical cord.
- Discuss the steps in the delivery of the placenta.
- List the steps in the emergency medical care of the mother after the delivery.
- Summarize neonatal resuscitation procedures.
- Describe the procedures for the following abnormal deliveries: breech birth, prolapsed cord, limb presentation.
- Describe special considerations during delivery, including multiple births, meconium, and premature births.
- Discuss the emergency medical care of a patient with a gynecologic emergency.

# Overview

Most babies in the United States are born in hospitals. You will rarely be called to care for a pregnant woman who is so far along in the delivery process that there is not time to get her to a hospital. However, it does happen. Therefore, you must be prepared to move quickly and efficiently. You will need a sterile emergency delivery pack, and you must watch for a number of potential problems. The umbilical cord could be wrapped around the baby's neck. The baby could have difficulty breathing. The mother might have excessive bleeding. Fortunately, most emergency births are trouble free. However, you must understand and be familiar with the delivery process.

This chapter begins with an anatomy review of the pregnant woman. Next, the signs of labor are described, as are predelivery emergencies. The middle section of the chapter explains how you should prepare for a delivery. The proper equipment and positioning of the patient are emphasized. A step-by-step discussion of the delivery process is presented next, including possible complications. Sections on postdelivery care, neonatal resuscitation, abnormal deliveries, and multiple births are also presented. The chapter concludes with a brief discussion of other gynecologic emergencies and care of sexual assault victims.

# Key Terms

*Handwritten note: Bloody Show = stringy type of mucous (maternal) discharged through birth canal when active labor comes*

**Amniotic sac**  The fluid-filled, bag-like membrane that grows around the developing fetus, inside the uterus.

**Birth canal**  The vagina and lower part of the uterus.

**Bloody show**  A small, bloody mucous plug from the cervix that comes out of the vagina, often signaling the beginning of labor.

**Breech presentation**  Delivery in which the baby's buttocks, rather than the head, appears first.

**Cervix**  The opening or mouth of the uterus.

**Crowning**  The appearance of the baby's head at the cervix during labor.

**Fetus**  The developing baby in the uterus (womb).

**Fontanels**  Two soft areas on the baby's head, one near the front and one near the back.

**Labor**  A three-stage process that begins with the first regular uterine contractions, includes delivery of the baby, and ends with delivery of the placenta.

**Meconium**  Sterile fecal material released from the baby's bowels before birth.

**Miscarriage**  Delivery of the fetus and placenta before 20 weeks gestation, for any reason.

**Placenta**  Afterbirth that develops on the wall of the uterus and is

*[handwritten: organ that which fetus ___ waste products during pregnancy]*

connected to the fetus by the umbilical cord.

**Premature**  Any baby that delivers before 8 months gestation or weighs less than 5½ lb.

**Umbilical cord**  The tissue that connects the placenta with the fetus.

**Uterus**  The womb. The hollow organ inside the female pelvis where the fetus grows.

**Vagina**  The outermost part of a woman's reproductive system. Forms the lower part of the birth canal.

*[handwritten: Perineum = skin between birth canal & anus]*

*[handwritten: Crowning = bulging out of vaginal opening as fetuses head or part presses against it.]*

## ANATOMY REVIEW

The **fetus** is the developing unborn baby that grows inside the mother's uterus (womb) for 9 months. The **uterus** is the muscular organ where the fetus grows. It is responsible for contractions during labor, and ultimately, helps to push the baby through the birth canal. The **birth canal** is made up of the vagina and the lower part of the uterus. The **vagina** is the outermost cavity of a woman's reproductive system and forms the lower part of the birth canal.

During the 9 months of gestation, the mother's abdomen grows larger as the uterus enlarges with the growing fetus. As the fetus grows, it requires more and more nourishment. Through the placenta, oxygen and other nutrients cross from the mother's circulation along the umbilical cord to help the fetus grow. The **placenta** (sometimes called afterbirth) develops on the wall of the uterus and is connected to the fetus by the umbilical cord. The **umbilical cord** is made of tissue and connects the placenta with the fetus. The fetus develops inside a fluid-filled, bag-like membrane called the **amniotic sac** (Figure 21-1).

## THE BEGINNING OF LABOR

The onset of labor is the beginning of the delivery process. **Labor** is a three-stage process that begins with the first regular uterine contractions, includes delivery of the baby, and ends with delivery of the placenta. It begins with the contractions (tightening) of the muscles of the uterus. These are sometimes called labor pains. The first stage begins with the first contraction of the uterus, and ends when the cervix is fully dilated (opened). The second stage begins when the cervix is fully dilated and ends when the baby is born. The third stage begins with the birth of the baby and ends

**FIGURE 21-1**

Anatomy of a pregnant woman

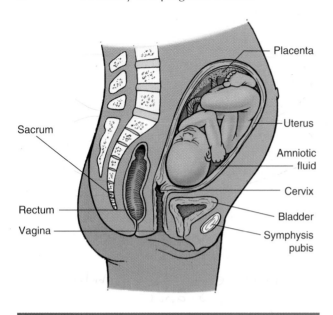

During the second stage, you will have to make a decision about helping the mother to deliver at home or providing transport to the hospital. As delivery nears, crowning occurs, the **cervix** (opening) of the uterus dilates, and the baby's head and body pass through into the vagina. **Crowning** occurs when the top of the baby's head is visible at the cervix (Figure 21-2). At this point, delivery can happen immediately. Contractions become stronger and more regular as the baby begins to move down the vagina. The mother will feel increasing pressure in her lower abdomen. She may also feel that she has to move her bowels. This sensation is normal and means that the baby's head is pressing on the rectum.

The third stage begins once the baby has been born. In this stage the placenta is usually delivered, within 30 minutes after the delivery of the baby. You will not usually transport the mother during that time. It is important that you follow BSI techniques in all stages of labor.

with the delivery of the placenta. The total time of labor varies greatly, but it is usually longer in a woman who is having her first baby (called a primigravida). Labor is usually shorter in women who have already had a baby (called a multigravida).

Other signs that labor has started include the following:

- **Bloody show** This is a small plug of blood-stained mucus that forms in the cervix. It comes out of the vagina as labor begins.

- **Rupture of the amniotic sac** This is typically a gush of clear fluid that comes from the uterus out through the vagina. Typically, there is about 1 L of amniotic fluid. However, the fluid does not always come out in one large amount. Any loss of amniotic fluid is a sign that labor is about to begin.

Remember that these signs may occur even before contractions begin.

You will usually have time to transport the mother during the first stage of labor.

**FIGURE 21-2**

Crowning

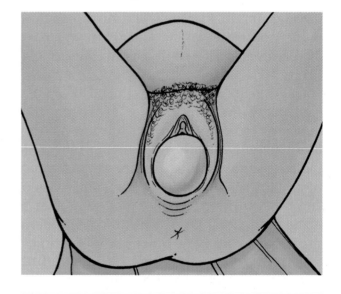

## HERE COMES THE STORK

You and your partner respond to a private residence for a woman having a baby. On arrival, you find a 19-year-old woman lying on the bathroom floor with a small puddle of blood-tinged fluid on the floor. There is a 1-year-old infant crying in a playpen nearby. The patient is having contractions every 2 minutes. She tells you that she has not seen a physician since she became pregnant about 8 months ago. On examination, you see what appears to be part of the baby's head showing from the vagina. Your partner has obtained the vital signs while you were talking to the patient. The patient has a blood pressure of 138/84 mm Hg, a pulse of 120/min, and respirations of 20/min. The hospital is approximately 20 minutes away.

### For Discussion

1. Describe the difference between patient care in a predelivery emergency and patient care during a normal delivery.

2. Describe the relationship and importance of BSI techniques during childbirth.

## PREDELIVERY EMERGENCIES

Most pregnant women are healthy, but some may have other medical conditions along with being pregnant. You must be able to recognize these conditions should they occur.

### MISCARRIAGE

Delivery of the fetus and placenta before 20 weeks is called a **miscarriage** or a spontaneous abortion. Miscarriage often occurs very early in a pregnancy. Thus, the mother may not even know she is pregnant. Early miscarriage is often discovered only when problems such as persistent bleeding or infection develop.

The most serious complications of miscarriage are bleeding and infection. Bleeding usually occurs as a result of the following:

- portions of the fetus or placenta are left in the uterus
- injury to the wall of the uterus, such as tearing of the uterus and possibly the bowel or bladder

Infection can result from tearing of the uterus. A woman may also have persistent bleeding and infection after a planned abortion. Planned abortions are usually done in the hospital or in a clinic. However, a woman may attempt to end a pregnancy herself. Thus, bleeding and infection can occur from unsterile instruments or a complication of the abortion.

### Emergency Medical Care

Your first steps in caring for a woman having a possible miscarriage are the same as any other medical emergency involving heavy bleeding. First, make sure the scene is safe for you to enter and follow BSI techniques. Next, do an initial assessment. Is the woman's airway open? Is she having any difficulty breathing?

The history and physical exam should follow. Ask the woman if she is pregnant. If she does not know, ask her the date of her last menstrual period. Remember, if this is an early miscarriage, she may not know. Inform medical control about the situation. Obtain the baseline vital signs, looking for signs of possible shock.

Gently cover the vagina with sterile pads to control the bleeding. If possible, collect any tissue that passes through the vagina and bring it to the hospital. *Never* try to pull any tissue out of the vagina. Rather, cover this material with a sterile pad as well. In rare instances, massive bleeding may occur, causing severe hypovolemic shock. Consult medical control for instructions and provide prompt transport.

## SEIZURES

One of the most alarming predelivery problems involves sudden seizures or convulsions in the mother. These seizures are usually related to severe high blood pressure. This condition is called eclampsia. Your care of the mother includes performing your usual assessments and obtaining a history and baseline vital signs. Inform medical control of your findings, particularly the mother's blood pressure. Place her on her

left side for transport and keep her as quiet as possible. Monitor the airway and give her oxygen. Be ready to suction the airway if she vomits. Provide prompt transport, monitoring the airway and vital signs en route.

## VAGINAL BLEEDING

Vaginal bleeding that occurs before labor begins may indicate a very serious condition. As discussed above, bleeding in early pregnancy may be a sign of miscarriage. In the later stages of pregnancy, bleeding may indicate problems with the placenta. The placenta may separate prematurely from the wall of the uterus. This is called placenta abruptio. The placenta may also grow and develop over the opening of the uterus or cervix. This is called placenta previa. It is important for you to remember that any vaginal bleeding in a pregnant woman is a potentially serious sign. Prompt transport with any type of vaginal bleeding is a must.

hypotension of mother

### Emergency Medical Care

Before you begin caring for the patient, be sure you follow BSI techniques. If there is massive bleeding, you may want to double glove. Perform the initial assessment. Is the patient having any difficulty breathing? As you obtain the history and perform the physical exam, ask the patient if she has any pain. Inform medical control, as this information will be helpful to hospital personnel. Next, obtain the baseline vital signs, looking for signs of possible shock. If the patient shows signs of shock, place her on her left side during transport. A pregnant woman is usually more comfortable lying on her side than on her back. This position also helps keep her circulation from the legs to the heart working properly. The weight of the enlarged uterus may cause circulation problems if the woman is lying on her back.

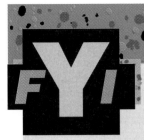

## Delivery Without Sterile Supplies

On rare occasions, you may have to deliver a baby without a sterile emergency delivery pack. If you can, use clean sheets and towels to create a "sterile field" between the mother's legs. Make sure that you are wearing gloves and eye protection and that you follow BSI techniques.

Carry out the delivery as if sterile supplies were on hand. As soon as the baby is born, you should wipe out the inside of its mouth with your gloved finger to clear the mouth of blood and mucus. Without the delivery pack, you should not cut or tie the cord. Instead, as soon as the placenta is born, wrap it in a clean towel or put it in a plastic bag and transport it with the baby. Always keep the placenta and the baby at the same level, so blood does not drain from the baby into the placenta. Keep the baby warm, and provide prompt transport.

Next, place a sterile pad or sanitary napkin over the vagina and replace it as often as necessary. Save the pads so that the hospital personnel can estimate how much blood has been lost. Do not put anything into the vagina or pack the vagina. Save any tissue that may be passed from the vagina.

### TRAUMA

Trauma to a pregnant woman and unborn fetus can be very serious. Severe bleeding may occur from injuries of the uterus. The result can be severe injury to the fetus due to a lack of oxygen. A pregnant woman who has traumatic injuries should be treated as any other trauma patient. Remember to place the patient on her left side, rather than on her back. Maintain the airway, give the patient oxygen, and control external bleeding. This will relieve the pressure of the uterus on the aorta, the venae cavae, and other organs in the abdomen.

## PREPARING FOR DELIVERY

When a woman is in labor, you must determine if she is going to deliver at the scene, or if you have time to transport. Thus, you must keep medical control informed about the patient's condition. Consider delivery at the scene if any of the following conditions have occurred:

- When delivery can be expected within a few minutes
- When the hospital cannot be reached due to a natural disaster, weather, or traffic conditions
- When no transport is available

To determine whether the delivery is imminent, you will need to ask the patient a series of questions, as follows:

- Are you pregnant?
- How long have you been pregnant?

- Is this your first baby?
- Are you having contractions or pain?
- How many minutes apart are your contractions?
- Are you bleeding?
- Have you had any kind of discharge?
- Did your water break?
- Do you feel like you need to push? Move your bowels?

Then look for crowning. To do this, gently spread the mother's legs apart. Reassure her that you are looking for crowning so that you know whether delivery at the scene is necessary. Do not touch the vaginal area except during delivery. Ask the patient if she has had a baby before. If so, she may be able to tell you if she is about to deliver. If she says yes, prepare for delivery. If she feels like her bowels have to move, the baby's head is pressing on the rectum. In this case, delivery is about to occur. Feel her abdomen. If it feels hard, then she is about to deliver.

Once labor has begun, there is no way it can be slowed down or stopped. Never attempt to hold the patient's legs together. To do so would only complicate the delivery. Do not let her go to the bathroom. Instead, reassure her that this feeling is normal and that it means she is about to have the baby.

If the baby is crowning, consult with medical control about delivering at the scene. Once the decision to deliver at the scene has been made, move quickly but calmly. Make sure that you follow BSI techniques. Delivery usually requires two people. If you are alone, ask a nurse, a police officer, or a family member or neighbor to help you.

Never leave the patient once the decision has been made to deliver at the scene. Ask someone else to get help if it is needed. Remember, the patient, not you, delivers the baby. Your part is to help, guide, and support the baby as it is born.

Your emergency vehicle should always be equipped with a sterile emergency delivery pack containing the following items (Figure 21-3):

- 1 pair of surgical scissors
- 3 hemostats or special cord clamps
- Umbilical tape or sterilized cord
- Small rubber bulb syringe
- 5 towels
- 1 dozen 2" × 10" gauze sponges
- 3 or 4 pairs of sterile gloves
- 1 baby blanket
- Sanitary napkins
- Plastic bag

**FIGURE 21-3**

Emergency delivery pack

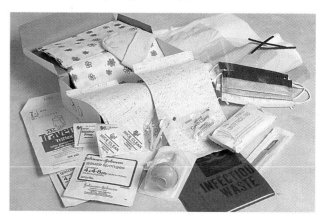

## POSITIONING AND SUPPORTING THE PATIENT

The way you position the patient for delivery depends on where you and the patient are located. However, before you begin, make sure you follow BSI techniques. You will find it easier to help the patient deliver if she is lying on a flat, sturdy surface. In fact, you will find it easier to work there than if the patient is in bed. Thus, if you are going to help the patient deliver at her home, move her to a spine board or to the floor. Pad the board or the area with blankets, folded sheets, or towels. Put a pillow under her hips. Sometimes it is better to put the pillow under one hip to allow her to turn to one side. This also may make suctioning the baby easier when it is born.

Next, flex her hips and knees and spread her legs apart. Support her head with one or two pillows (Figure 21-4). Place newspapers or sheets on the floor around the delivery area. This will help soak up the fluid when the amniotic sac ruptures.

In very rare cases, a patient will deliver in an automobile. If this is the case, help the patient to lie on the seat, with one foot on the floor and the other on the seat, with the knee and hip bent.

Your partner should be kneeling at the patient's head to comfort and reassure her during delivery. The patient may want to grip someone's hand. She may have to vomit. In that case, make sure your partner turns her head to the side. This makes it easier for her mouth and airway to remain clear. You should kneel next to the patient's

right side if you are right-handed or at her left side if you are left-handed.

## DELIVERING THE BABY

Place the emergency delivery pack close to the patient so that you can reach it easily. Open the pack carefully so that its contents remain sterile. Then, place one sterile, folded towel under the patient's buttocks. Place another sterile towel between her legs, just below the vagina. Spread a third towel across her abdomen (Figure 21-5). This is called creating a sterile field around the vagina.

Make sure that you can see the vagina at all times. Time the contractions from the beginning of one to the beginning of the next. Remind the patient to take quick, short breaths during each contraction. In between contractions, encourage the patient to rest and breathe deeply through her mouth. Also remind her not to strain with the contractions.

### FIGURE 21-4

Positioning the patient for delivery

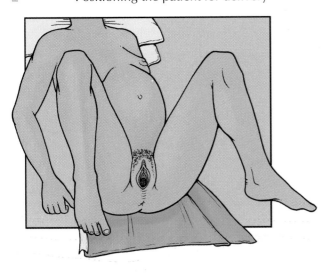

### FIGURE 21-5

Creating a sterile delivery area

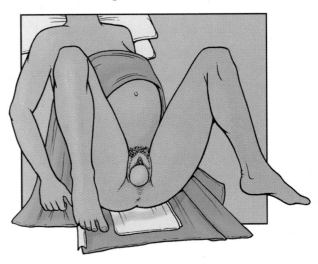

## DELIVERING THE HEAD

Watch the head as it is crowning and then as it exits the vagina. Once you see that the head is coming out farther with each contraction, place your right hand (or your left hand if you are left-handed) over the head (Figure 21-6). Place the flats of your fingers on the bony part of the skull and exert very gentle pressure on it. This will allow the head to come out smoothly. It also prevents the baby's head and body from suddenly popping out during a strong contraction, possibly causing injury. You may want to move to the patient's feet so that you are between the patient's legs during the delivery.

As the head emerges, you will see that it is usually tilted to the side rather than straight up and down. A baby's head has two soft areas—one near the front of the head and one near the back of the head. These areas are called the **fontanels.** The brain is covered only by skin and membranes at these places. Thus, you must be careful not to push your finger or thumb into one of the fontanels. As the head emerges, hold it carefully in your palm. Make sure that you do not touch the baby's face or the fontanels. Maintain gentle pressure during contrac-

tions and decrease the pressure slightly between contractions. It may take several contractions for the head to be completely delivered (Figure 21-7).

### Unruptured Amniotic Sac

Usually, the amniotic sac will break or rupture at the beginning of labor. The sac may also rupture during contractions. In rare cases, it will not rupture at all. In this instance, the baby's head will emerge from the vagina still covered by the sac. This situation is serious, as the sac will suffocate the baby if it is not removed. Therefore, you should puncture the sac with a clamp, away from the baby's face. Be very careful not to injure the baby. As the sac is punctured, amniotic fluid will gush out. Move the sac away from the baby's face. Clear the baby's mouth and nose immediately, using the bulb syringe and gauze sponge.

### Umbilical Cord Around the Neck

As the head emerges from the vagina, be sure to support it with the palm of your hand. As you are supporting the head with one hand, use the index finger of your other

### FIGURE 21-6

Supporting and delivering the head

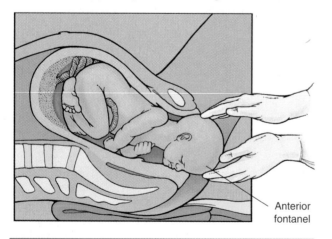

Anterior
fontanel

### FIGURE 21-7

The head completely delivered

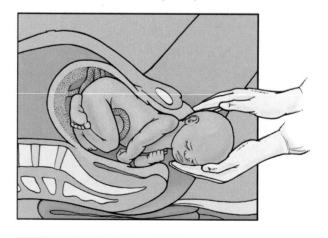

## FIGURE 21-8

Releasing the umbilical cord from the baby's neck

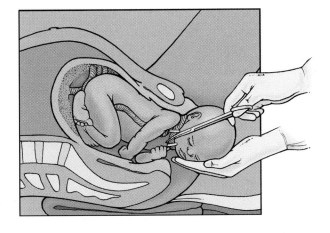

## FIGURE 21-9

Suctioning the mouth and nose

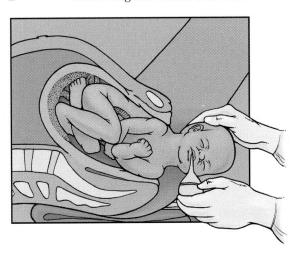

hand to feel whether the umbilical cord is wrapped around the neck. Usually, the cord is not wrapped around the baby's neck and does not have to be cut until after the birth. However, a cord wound tightly around the neck could strangle the baby. Therefore, the cord must be released from the neck immediately (Figure 21-8). Usually, you can slip it over the baby's shoulder. If you cannot, and if the cord feels tightly wound around the neck, you must cut it.

To cut the umbilical cord, first place two clamps on the cord, about 2" apart. Cut the cord between the clamps. Then you can unwrap it from around the neck. The cord is fragile and easily torn. Thus, you must handle it very carefully. Do not take the clamps off the ends of the cord. The clamps can be removed only after the ends of the cord have been tied. This is discussed later in the chapter.

Once the head is delivered, the baby's face will turn sideways. Suction the baby's mouth and nose when the whole face is visible. Squeeze a bulb syringe and gently insert it into the mouth about 1½". Make

sure the syringe does not touch the back of the baby's mouth. The syringe will remove any mucus, blood, water, or amniotic fluid from the mouth. Empty the syringe onto the towel across the mother's abdomen. Suction the mouth two or three times and suction each nostril two or three times (Figure 21-9). A baby breathes from his or her nose, so it is important that you clear the nostrils.

## DELIVERING THE BODY

By the time you finish suctioning the mouth and nose, you should be able to see the upper shoulder in the vagina. The baby's head is the largest part of the body. Thus, the rest of the baby usually delivers easily. Support the head and upper body as the shoulders deliver. Then the rest of the body will appear and be delivered. Grasp the feet as they emerge. Once the baby is born, make sure you support it with both your hands. Handle the baby firmly but carefully. It will be slippery. Make sure you do not squeeze the neck or chest (Figure 21-10).

**FIGURE 21-10**

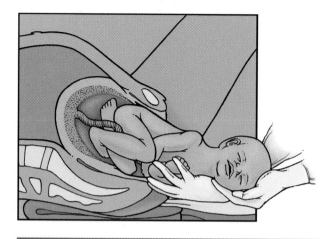

Delivering the body

## POSTDELIVERY CARE

### INITIAL CARE OF THE BABY

As soon as the baby is born, place it immediately on a towel or in a blanket on its side. Wrap the baby so that only the face is exposed, but make sure the top of the head is covered. Also make sure that the baby's neck is in a neutral position so the airway remains open. Newborn babies are very sensitive to cold, so if it is at all possible, you should keep the blanket warm before you use it. Keep the baby's head slightly lower than the rest of its body and turn it slightly to one side. Use a sterile gauze pad to wipe blood and mucus from the baby's mouth and nose and then suction again. Suctioning the nose is particularly important since babies breathe through their noses (Figure 21-11). You can cradle the baby in one arm while you are suctioning the nose and mouth. The baby does not need to be on a flat surface for suctioning. By now the baby should be pink and breathing on its own. If the baby is not breathing

on its own, you should begin steps for neonatal resuscitation, as described in a later section.

Keep the baby at the same level as the mother's vagina until you cut the umbilical cord. If the baby is higher than the mother's vagina, blood will move from the baby through the umbilical cord back into the placenta. Your partner or helper should monitor the baby and handle postdelivery care.

### Cutting the Umbilical Cord

Once the baby is born, the umbilical cord is of no further use to either the mother or the baby. Postdelivery care of the umbilical cord is important, as infection is easily transmitted through the cord to the baby. Thus, your next step is to clamp, tie, and cut the umbilical cord. Use the two clamps in the emergency kit. Clamp the cord about four fingers width from the baby. Place the clamps about 2" to 6" apart. Once they are firmly in place, cut the cord between them using the sterile scissors.

**FIGURE 21-11**

Positioning the newborn

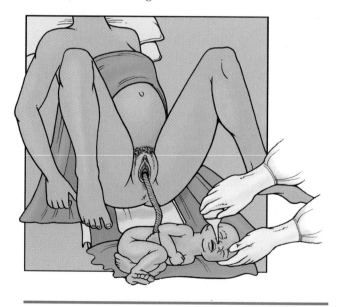

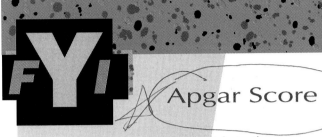

# Apgar Score

A rough and rapid guide to the status of a newborn can be quickly obtained by calculating the Apgar score. The following five indicators are combined into the Apgar score:

1. Appearance
2. Pulse
3. Grimace or irritability
4. Activity or muscle tone
5. Respiration

Each of the five areas is given a score from 0 to 2. The higher the score, the better the baby is doing. A perfectly healthy, normal baby will have a total score of 10. The Apgar score is calculated at 1 and 5 minutes when births occur in the hospital and can be calculated in the field as well.

## Appearance

Note the appearance and color of the baby's skin. The skin should turn pink shortly after birth in Caucasian children, and there should be no central cyanosis. In deeply pigmented children, assess the mucous membranes. These should also turn pink quickly when oxygenation is adequate.

## Pulse

Pulse rate should be over 100 beats/min. You should be able to measure this with a stethoscope or by pulsations in the umbilical cord, which are usually easily felt. If a pulse is absent this indicates the need for immediate CPR.

## Grimace

Grimacing, crying, or withdrawing in response to stimuli is normal in a newborn and indicates that the baby is doing well. You can test this by snapping a finger against the sole of the baby's foot. If the baby cries or withdraws the foot, this is considered a normal response.

## Activity

Activity or muscle tone can be assessed by checking the baby's hips and knees. Usually these are held flexed, with some resistance or muscle tone when attempts are made to straighten the legs. A child should not be floppy and limp.

## Respirations

Normally a newborn's respirations are regular and rapid, with a good strong cry. If respirations are shallow, labored, or the cry is weak, you should assist ventilations. Absence of respirations or crying is a serious sign and indicates the need for assisted ventilations and possibly full CPR.

Do not hurry this step, as the point between the cord and the baby is fragile and easily torn. If it is handled too roughly, it could be torn from the baby's abdomen, resulting in severe bleeding and possibly death.

Once you have cut the cord, you should tie the end coming from the baby. You may have cut the cord earlier to remove it from around the baby's neck as the head was being delivered. If this was the case, now is the time to tie it. The emergency kit contains special umbilical tape for tying the cord. Do not use ordinary string or twine, as it will cut through the soft, fragile tissues of the cord. Place a loop of the tape around the cord, about 1" nearer to the baby than the clamp. Tighten the tape slowly so that it does not cut the cord and then tie it firmly with a square knot. Cut the ends of the tape but do not remove the clamp. Do not remove the clamp on the end of the cord coming out of the mother's vagina. This part of the cord is attached to the placenta and will be delivered when the placenta delivers (Figure 21-12).

## DELIVERY OF THE PLACENTA

You should now watch for delivery of the placenta. The placenta is attached to the end of the umbilical cord that is coming out of the vagina. The placenta, like the baby, delivers itself. The placenta usually delivers

## FIGURE 21-12

Cutting the umbilical cord

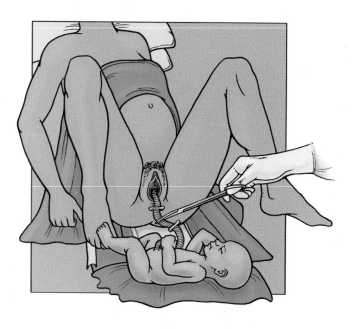

itself within a few minutes of the baby's birth, but it may take as long as 30 minutes.

You should expect bleeding, usually less than 250 mL, before the placenta delivers. The mother can tolerate up to 500 mL of blood loss after delivery. However, once the placenta delivers, the bleeding, except for a few drops, should stop. You should give oxygen and provide prompt transport if any of the following occur:

- 30 minutes go by and the placenta has not delivered

- 250 mL of bleeding occurs before delivery of the placenta

- significant bleeding occurs after the delivery of the placenta

You may speed up delivery of the placenta by gently massaging the lower abdomen with a firm, circular motion. This massage is much like kneading. Your fingers should be fully extended and located over the pubic bone as you massage. The abdominal skin will be wrinkled and very soft. You should be able to feel a firm, grapefruit-sized mass in the lower abdomen. This is the uterus, with the placenta inside. As the uterus is massaged, it will contract and become firmer.

If the baby is breathing well and is in good condition, place it at the mother's breast and allow it to nurse. This will also stimulate the uterus to contract and help to deliver the placenta. *Never pull on the end of the umbilical cord in an attempt to speed delivery of the placenta.* You may tear the cord, or the placenta, or both. This will result in serious, even life-threatening, bleeding.

Once the placenta delivers, inspect it carefully. The normal placenta is round, measures about 7" in diameter, and is about 1" thick. One surface is smooth and covered with a shiny membrane. The other surface is rough and lobe like (Figure 21-13). Wrap the placenta in a towel, place it and the cord in a plastic bag and bring them to the hospi-

## FIGURE 21-13

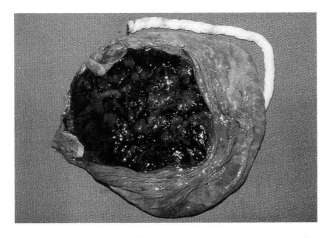

Anatomy of the placenta

tal. Hospital personnel will examine the placenta. This is to make sure that the entire placenta has been delivered and that no part is still in the mother's uterus. If a piece of the placenta is in the uterus, it could result in constant bleeding or infection.

Before you transport the mother and baby, place a sterile pad or sanitary napkin over the vagina and lower the mother's legs. Never put anything into the vagina. Monitor the mother's vital signs and give her oxygen, if needed. As you prepare to transport the mother and the baby, thank anyone who assisted, congratulate the mother, and record the time of birth for the record-of-live-birth form.

# RESUSCITATION OF THE NEWBORN

A newborn will usually begin breathing on its own within seconds after birth. If it does not, you should gently tap or flick the soles of the feet to stimulate it. You may also gently rub its back. However, if after 10 or 15 seconds, the baby is still not breathing,

you must begin resuscitation efforts. Resuscitation efforts should follow the 1994 guidelines established by the American Heart Association (Figure 21-14).

## ASSESSING THE BABY

Suctioning and stimulation should result in an immediate increase in respirations. If they do not, you must begin artificial ventilation, as described below. If the baby is breathing well, you should next check the heart rate by feeling the brachial pulse. The heart rate should be at least 100/min. If it is not, begin artificial ventilation. Reassess respirations and heart rate every 30 seconds.

Your next step is to assess the baby's skin color. If the baby is cyanotic all over, a condition called central cyanosis, you should give oxygen. Babies often have cyanosis in the extremities after birth. You are looking for overall or central cyanosis. If the baby has adequate ventilations and heart rate, but is still cyanotic, give oxygen at 10 to 15 L/min via oxygen tubing held as close as possible to the baby's face. There is no danger in

## FIGURE 21-14

Resuscitation process for the newborn

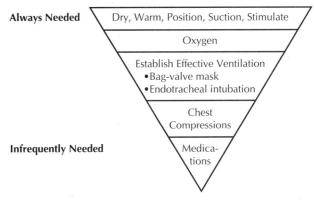

**Assess and Support:** Temperature (warm and dry)
**A**irway (position and suction)
**B**reathing (stimulate to cry)
**C**irculation (heart rate and color)

**Always Needed** — Dry, Warm, Position, Suction, Stimulate

Oxygen

Establish Effective Ventilation
•Bag-valve mask
•Endotracheal intubation

Chest Compressions

**Infrequently Needed** — Medications

Reproduced with permission. *Textbook of Pediatric Advanced Life Support*, 1994 © Copyright American Heart Association.

giving high concentrations of oxygen, if it is given over a short period of time.

## PROVIDING ARTIFICIAL VENTILATION

In situations where assisted ventilations are needed, you should use a BVM device. Cover the baby's nose and mouth with the mask and begin respirations at a rate of 40 to 60 breaths/min. Make sure you have a good face-to-mask seal. Use enough gentle pressure to make the chest rise with each breath. It may be necessary to bypass the pop-off valve in order to ventilate initially. After the initial resistance, the pressures needed to inflate the chest should be 30 to 40 cm $H_2O$. The volumes required are 6 to 8 mL/kg (Figure 21-15).

Assisted ventilation has been successful if you see bilateral chest wall expansion and hear breath sounds. If the baby starts to breathe on its own, attach an oxygen tubing to the mask and let the baby breathe until it becomes pink. After 15 to 30 seconds of adequate respirations, assess the heart rate. If the heart rate is at least 100 beats/min

## FIGURE 21-15

Providing ventilations with a BVM device

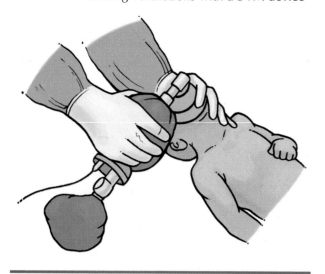

and the baby is breathing on its own, you may stop assisted ventilations. Before you stop, gradually decrease the rate and pressure of the assisted ventilation. You may also begin to gently rub the baby to help it maintain respirations. However, if the baby is still not breathing on its own, you must continue assisted ventilation.

## PROVIDING CHEST COMPRESSIONS

If the heart rate is less than 60 beats/min, or between 60 and 80 beats/min and not rising, you should continue assisted ventilation and begin chest compressions. If the heart rate is between 60 and 80 beats/min and rising, you should continue assisted ventilation, but chest compressions are not necessary.

There are two ways to give chest compressions to a baby. You should know how to do both. The first and preferred way is to place both your thumbs on the middle third of the sternum, with the rest of your fingers encircling the chest (Figure 21-16a). In very small babies, you may have to place one thumb over the other to perform chest compressions (Figure 21-16b). Your thumbs should be placed just below an imaginary line drawn between the nipples on the middle third of the sternum. Select a point in the midline of the sternum one finger breadth below the line between the nipples (Figure 21-16c). Press the two thumbs gently against the lower half of the sternum. The sternum and rib cage of the newborn are flexible and easily compressed. Use only enough force to compress the sternum ½" to ¾".

If your hands are too small to encircle the baby's chest, you should use your middle and ring fingers of one hand to provide chest compressions. In this situation, your other hand should support the baby's back.

Assisted ventilation is done during a pause after every third compression. You

**FIGURE 21-16**

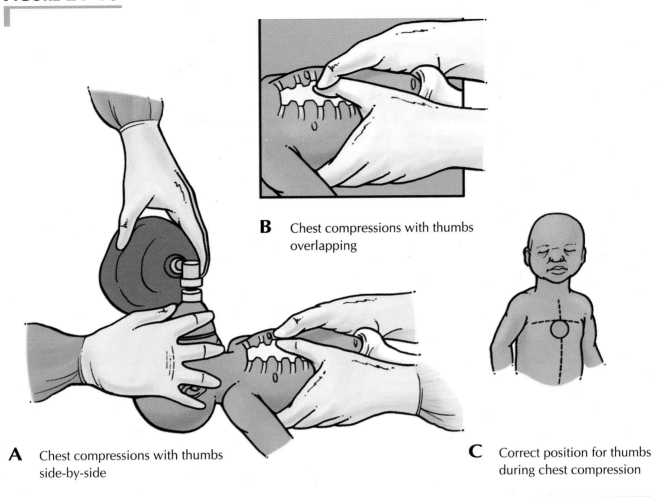

**B** Chest compressions with thumbs overlapping

**A** Chest compressions with thumbs side-by-side

**C** Correct position for thumbs during chest compression

should perform a combined total of 120 ventilations and compressions per minute, or 90 compressions to 30 ventilations/min. Remember that ventilation is as absolutely vital in performing CPR in the newborn as it is in the adult.

## TRANSPORT CONSIDERATIONS

If the baby does not begin breathing on its own or have an adequate heart rate, you must continue CPR en route to the hospital, if necessary. Ask for another unit, as you will need help to transport both the mother and baby. Continue CPR until the baby breathes on its own or is pronounced dead by a physician. Do not give up! Many babies have survived and developed without brain damage if they have been given effective CPR, even after long periods without spontaneous breathing.

Keep the baby warm, not hot, at all times. The baby is not yet able to regulate its body temperature well and must be kept warm.

If the baby is obviously born dead, and is covered with blisters, has a foul smell, and the head is soft, then, and only then, should you not attempt CPR. If there is any doubt in your mind that the baby has a chance for survival, you should start resuscitation efforts.

## FIGURE 21-17

Umbilical cord preceding the baby

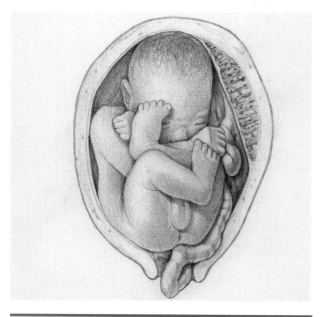

Reproduced with permission from *Mayo Clinic Complete Book of Pregnancy and Baby's First Year.* NY, NY, William Morrow and Co., 1994, © Mayo Foundation for Education and Research.

# ABNORMAL DELIVERIES

## PROLAPSED UMBILICAL CORD

On rare occasions, the umbilical cord may come out of the vagina before the baby. This is called a prolapsed umbilical cord (Figure 21-17). This situation is very dangerous, because the baby's head presses on the cord during birth. As a result, all circulation to the baby is cut off. A prolapsed umbilical cord is usually seen early in labor. Thus, you should inform medical control and provide transport. *Do not attempt to push the cord back into the vagina.* This condition must be treated in the hospital.

Your job at the scene is to keep the baby from pressing on the cord. Your first steps are to complete the initial assessment and obtain the history and baseline vital signs. Next, place the mother on a spine board with her head down, and her hips elevated on a pillow or folded sheet. This is Trendelenburg's position, which helps reduce the pressure on the baby in the vagina. Once the mother is in this position, carefully insert your sterile gloved hand into the vagina. Gently push the baby away from the umbilical cord, taking care to avoid the fontanels. Keep your hand in this position until the physician at the hospital tells you to remove it. Note that this situation and breech delivery are the only occasions where you should place your hand into the vagina. Wrap a sterile towel moistened with saline around the exposed cord. Give the mother high-flow oxygen and provide rapid transport.

## BREECH DELIVERY

Most babies are born head first. In rare cases, the buttocks come out first. This delivery is called a **breech presentation** (Figure 21-18). You will not know or be able

## FIGURE 21-18

A breech delivery

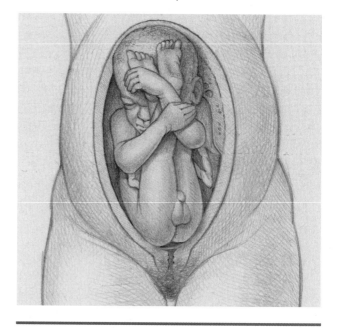

Reproduced with permission from *Mayo Clinic Complete Book of Pregnancy and Baby's First Year.* NY, NY, William Morrow and Co., 1994, © Mayo Foundation for Education and Research.

to tell ahead of time whether a breech presentation is occurring. You will know only when you see the buttocks, rather than the head, appear. With this presentation, the baby is at great risk for delivery trauma. Prolapsed cords are more common with breech deliveries as well. Breech deliveries are usually slow, so that there is time to get the mother to the hospital. If the mother does not deliver within 10 minutes of the buttocks presenting, provide rapid transport. However, if the buttocks have already passed through the vagina, delivery is underway. You should then follow the emergency procedures outlined below.

The preparations for a breech delivery are the same as for a head first delivery. Position the mother and unwrap the emergency delivery kit. Position yourself and your partner as you would for a head first delivery. Allow the buttocks and legs to deliver on their own. You can support them with your hand to prevent the baby from "popping out." The buttocks will usually come out easily. Let the legs dangle on either side of your arm as you support the trunk and chest as they are born. The head is almost always face down and should be allowed to deliver on its own. As the head is delivering, make sure to keep the baby's airway open. The best way to do this is to put your gloved finger into the mother's vagina to keep the walls of the vagina from pressing on the baby's airway.

***Never try to pull the baby's head out during a breech delivery.*** If the head is stuck in the vagina, you should support the baby's body with one hand and apply firm pressure to the uterus with your other hand. You may be able to feel the head. This maneuver often helps the head deliver on its own. If the head delivers on its own, you can continue the delivery as you would with a head first delivery. However, if the head does not deliver within 3 minutes, give the mother oxygen, place her in Trendelenburg's position, and provide rapid transport.

## FIGURE 21-19

Limb presentation

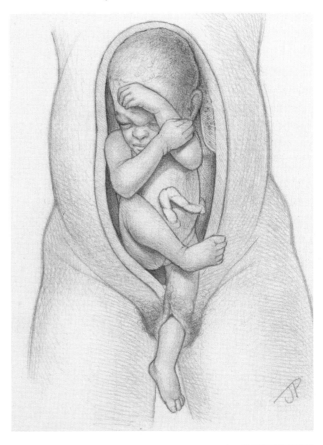

## LIMB PRESENTATION

On very rare occasions, you will see a single arm or leg or foot emerging from the vagina first, rather than the head. This is called a limb presentation (Figure 21-19). You cannot successfully deliver such a presentation in the field. These babies must be delivered in a hospital. Thus, if you are faced with a limb presentation, give the mother oxygen and provide rapid transport. Place the mother on her back with her head lower than her pelvis. If a limb is protruding from the vagina, cover it with a sterile towel. Never try to push it back into the vagina.

## MECONIUM STAINING

**Meconium** is the sterile fecal material that can be released from the baby's bowels before birth. When this occurs, the amniotic fluid will appear green or brownish-yellow. At times, the baby's skin will appear this color as well. Meconium staining usually indicates fetal distress before or during the labor. Aspiration of meconium can cause breathing problems. Thus, it is important to inform medical control of this finding. Make sure that you suction the mouth and oropharynx first—before you stimulate the baby. Suction and monitor the baby's airway carefully and provide prompt transport.

## MULTIPLE BIRTHS

Twins occur about once in every 80 births. Sometimes there is a family history of twins. The mother may suspect she is having twins because of an ultrasound she had earlier in the pregnancy, or because she has an unusually large abdomen.

Twins are usually smaller than single babies, and the delivery is usually not difficult. Twins should be suspected if the first baby is small, or if the mother's abdomen remains fairly large after the birth. If the mother is having twins, the second baby is usually born within 45 minutes after the first. About 10 minutes after the first birth, contractions will begin again, and the birth process will repeat itself.

### DELIVERING TWINS

You can usually deliver twins the same way you would a single birth. Clamp and cut the umbilical cord of the first baby as soon as it is born and before the second baby is delivered. The second baby may deliver before or after the first placenta. There may be only one placenta or there may be two. It is especially important to save the placenta when twins are born, as this will help hospital personnel determine whether the twins are identical or fraternal. Identical twins develop from one egg and will have one placenta with two umbilical cords attached. Fraternal twins develop from two eggs and will be born with two placentas and cords, one for each twin.

It is important to remember that if you only see one umbilical cord coming out of the first placenta, there is still another placenta to be delivered. On the other hand, if both cords are attached to one placenta, there will not be a second placenta, and the delivery is over. Record the time of birth and the Apgar score of each twin separately. Twins may be so small as to be premature; handle them very carefully and keep them warm. The Apgar score can be used as a guide in the same way you would use it for a single birth.

## PREMATURE INFANTS

The usual period for the development of a baby, called the gestation period, is 9 months or 40 weeks. A normal, single baby will weigh about 7 lb at birth. Any baby that delivers before 8 months gestation or weighs less than 5½ lb at birth is considered **premature.** However, in the field, it is often difficult to determine the exact gestation period, and you probably have no scale to weigh the baby. A premature baby is smaller and thinner, and its head is proportionately larger compared with the rest of its body than a full-term baby (Figure 21-20).

Premature babies need special care to survive. With such care, even babies as small as 1 lb have survived and developed into normal, healthy children. You should follow

## FIGURE 21-20

Footprints of full-term and premature infants

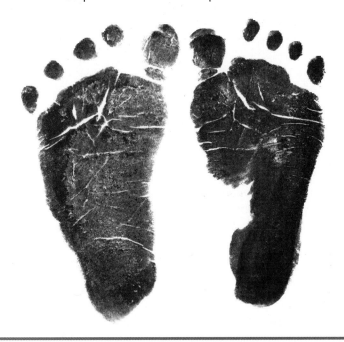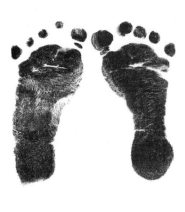

certain, specific procedures when you are handling a premature infant, as follows:

1. Premature babies often require resuscitation. Always resuscitate unless it is physically impossible due to extreme prematurity.

2. Keep the baby warm. Wrap it in a warm blanket as soon as it is born. Keep the face exposed, but keep the head covered. Keep the baby in a place where the temperature is between 90° and 95°F.

3. Keep the mouth and nose clear of mucus. Like all newborn babies, premature babies are nose breathers. Thus, their small nasal passages can be obstructed easily. Use the bulb syringe to suction the mouth and nostrils frequently. Handle the baby and all its parts very gently.

4. Give oxygen. Open the valve on your oxygen cylinder slowly to give a steady stream of oxygen (about 70 to 100 bubbles per minute through the water bottle that is attached to the oxygen tank). Do not direct the stream of oxygen directly into the baby's mouth. Rather, make a small tent over the baby's head using a blanket or a piece of aluminum foil, and then direct the oxygen into the tent. There is no danger in giving high concentrations of oxygen, if it is given over a short period of time.

5 Carefully observe the cut end of the cord attached to the baby and be sure that it is not bleeding. The loss of even a few drops of blood can be very serious.

6. Protect the baby from possible infection and contamination. Premature babies are very susceptible to infection. Do not breathe directly into the baby's face. Keep everyone else as far away from the baby as possible.

7. Inform medical control that you are transporting a premature baby and its mother. Bring a family member with you to the hospital.

## SURPRISE, SURPRISE!

You are stopped at a traffic light at a busy intersection when a man runs up to the ambulance, points to a small restaurant, and tells you to "Come quick! A lady is having a baby!" You hop out of the rig to check things out, while your partner contacts dispatch and pulls around the corner to park the rig. As you follow the man into the sandwich shop, you see a pregnant woman lying on the floor next to one of the booths. Even from the doorway, it's obvious that the baby's head is almost out. As you get closer, you note that the umbilical cord is wrapped around the baby's neck.

### For Discussion

1. Describe briefly the following conditions and the focus of prehospital care associated with each: prolapsed cord, breech birth, limb presentation, meconium staining, miscarriage.

2. Discuss the similarities and differences between placenta previa and placenta abruptio.

---

Some large medical centers have mobile infant carriers for the transportation of high-risk infants. If such a vehicle is available, the hospital personnel may want to send it rather than have you transport the baby in the ambulance. If such a vehicle is not available, you should transport the baby in a special carrier. The premature infant carrier has supplies that can be used for the immediate care of the premature infant as well as for its transport.

Fill the hot water bottles and pad them well so they do not come in direct contact with the baby's skin. Place them in the carrier so that one is on the bottom and on each side of where the baby will lie. Once you have wrapped the baby in a blanket and placed it inside the carrier, secure the carrier inside the vehicle. Keep the temperature of the vehicle at 90° to 95°F while the baby and mother are being transported to the hospital.

## GYNECOLOGIC EMERGENCIES

Occasionally major gynecologic problems will occur in females who are not pregnant, but who still require urgent medical care.

Excessive vaginal bleeding may be seen and may prompt a request for transport to the hospital. Injuries of the external female genitalia can include all types of soft tissue injuries. These genital parts have a rich nerve supply; injuries are, thus, very painful. Lacerations, abrasions, and avulsions should be treated with moist, sterile compresses, local pressure to control bleeding, and a diaper-type bandage to hold the dressings in place. You must, under no circumstances, pack or place dressings into the vagina. Leave foreign bodies in place after you stabilize them with bandages. Transport patients promptly to the emergency department. Contusions and other blunt injuries all require careful in-hospital evaluation.

While multiple potential causes exist, the EMT-B must treat these individuals as any other victim of blood loss, observing body substance isolation, ensuring maintenance of the airway, giving oxygen, documenting vital signs, and treating for shock, if necessary, while arranging for rapid transport.

Trauma to the external genitalia requires appropriate external dressings of any wounds, giving oxygen, carrying out ongoing patient assessment, and arranging transport. Never pack the vagina.

Instances of sexual assault and rape are all too common. Often you can do little beyond soothing and calming the patient and providing transportation to the emergency department. Do not examine the genitalia unless obvious bleeding requires the application of a dressing. Advise the patient not to wash, douche, urinate, or defecate until after a physician has had the opportunity to make an examination in the emergency department. Treat all other injuries according to appropriate procedures and note that they dictate the urgency of transport to the emergency department. You must obtain and record as clear a history of the incident as possible. Questioning and all necessary treatment must be handled quietly, as rapidly as possible, and away from onlookers. A calm professional manner is appropriate, with no display of personal curiosity.

You must be aware that the patient has the right to refuse assistance and to refuse to be taken to the emergency department. Such refusal sometimes occurs in cases of rape or sexual assault because the patient wishes to avoid publicity. It is not unusual for assistance to be refused after you arrive at the scene, even though help may originally have been requested. This choice, too, is the patient's prerogative. Referral to a rape counseling center can often be helpful in these circumstances.

Sexual assault requires that all the usual treatment principles be followed for victims of trauma. In addition, the following special steps should be included:

1. Body substance isolation is especially important in these instances.

2. Airway maintenance is always a major priority.

3. The SAMPLE focused assessment should be carried out in an objective and nonjudgmental fashion.

4. The crime scene should be protected as much as possible.

5. The genitalia should not be examined unless necessary because of profuse bleeding.

6. Same sex EMT-Bs should be used for care when available and whenever possible.

7. The patient should be discouraged from bathing, voiding, or cleaning any wounds until after transport and assessment at the hospital has been completed.

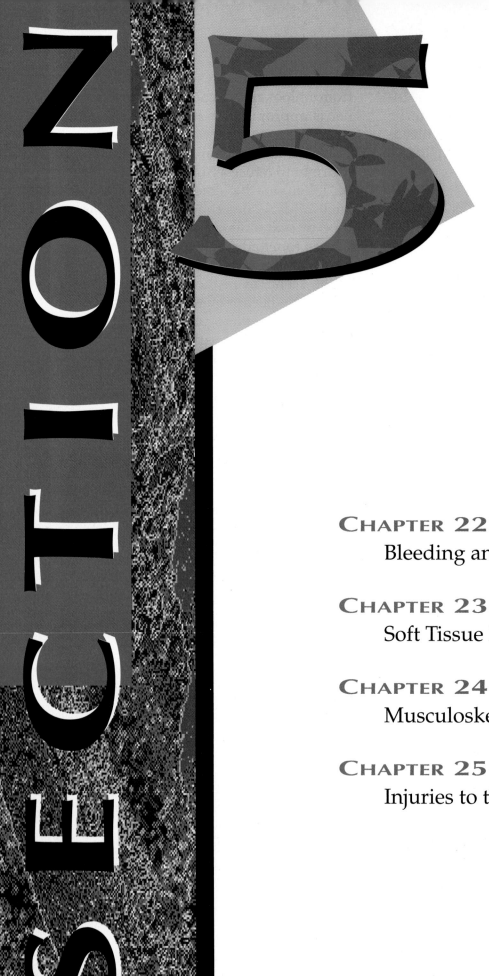

SECTION 5

# Trauma

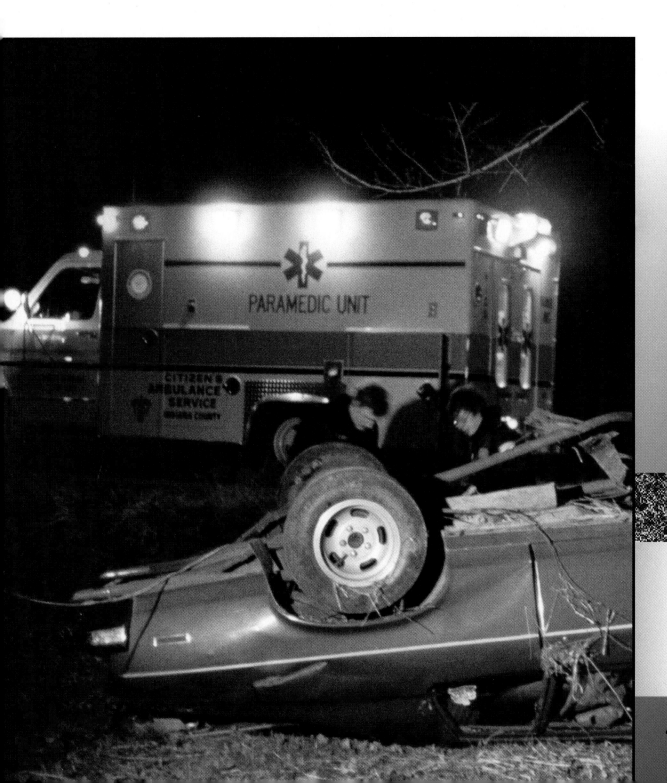

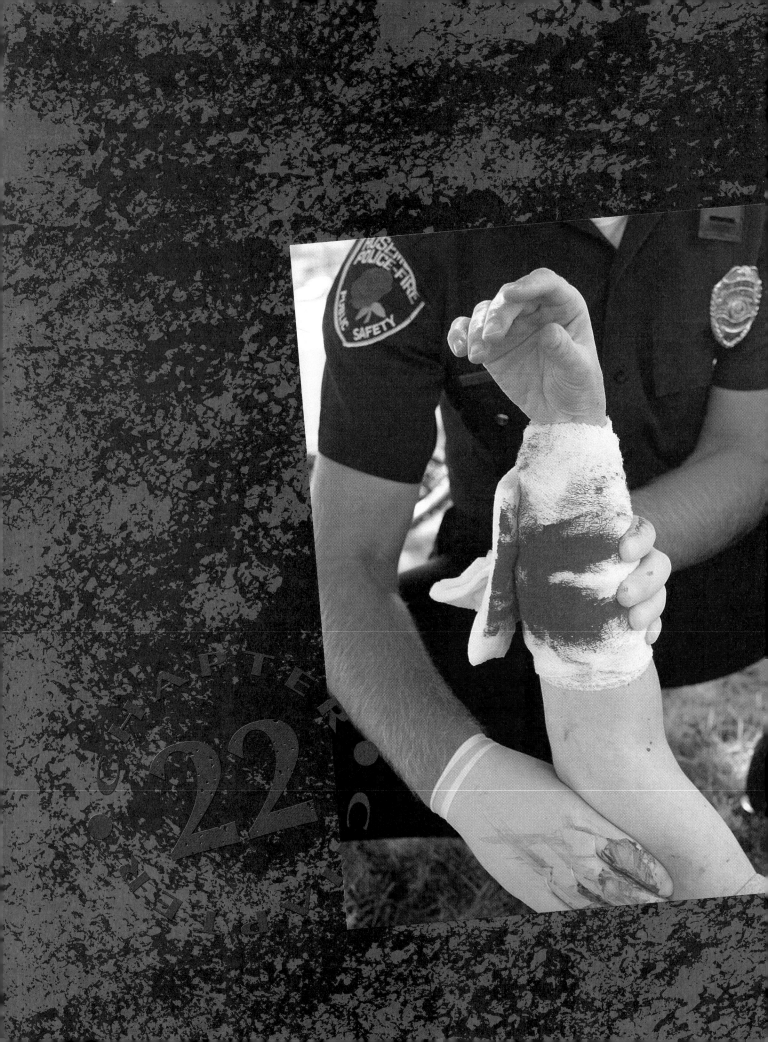

# CHAPTER 22

# Bleeding and Shock

After you have read this chapter, you should be able to:

- Describe the structure and function of the circulatory system.
- Differentiate among arterial, venous, and capillary bleeding.
- Describe the emergency medical care of external bleeding.
- Establish the relationship between body substance isolation and bleeding.
- Establish the relationship between airway management and trauma.
- Establish the relationship between the mechanism of injury and internal bleeding.
- Describe the signs of internal bleeding.
- List the steps in managing a patient who has signs or symptoms of internal bleeding.
- Discuss the signs and symptoms of shock.
- List the steps in managing a patient who has signs and symptoms of shock.

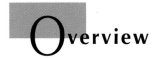

# Overview

Bleeding can be external and obvious, or internal and hidden. Either way, it is dangerous. Hemorrhage initially causes weakness and, if left uncontrolled, eventual shock and death. The most common cause of shock after trauma is bleeding. The purpose of this chapter is to help you understand how the cardiovascular system reacts to blood loss. After managing the airway, recognizing bleeding and how it affects the body are perhaps the most important skills you will learn. The first section of the chapter provides a brief review of the anatomy of the circulatory system. The second section describes the common signs and symptoms of external bleeding and how to provide emergency medical care. The third section explains internal bleeding—its signs and symptoms and how to provide emergency medical care.

Shock is a direct result of prolonged and inadequate tissue perfusion. As the body attempts to adjust to a lower blood volume, the cardiovascular system can fail. This chapter concludes with a discussion of shock, including specific steps for caring for a patient in shock.

# Key Terms

**Coagulation**   Formation of clots to plug openings in injured blood vessels and arrest blood flow.

**Epistaxis**   Nosebleed.

**Hemophilia**   Condition of lacking one or more of the blood's normal clotting factors.

**Hemorrhage**   Bleeding.

**Hypovolemic shock**   Condition in which low blood volume, due to massive internal or external bleeding, results in inadequate perfusion.

**Perfusion**   Circulation of blood within an organ or tissue in adequate amounts to meet the cells' current needs.

**Shock**   Condition in which the circulatory system fails to provide sufficient circulation so that every body part can perform its function. Also called hypoperfusion.

# ANATOMY REVIEW

The cardiovascular system circulates blood to all of the body's cells and tissues. It delivers oxygen and nutrients and carries away metabolic waste products. Certain parts of the body, such as the brain, spinal cord, and heart, require a constant flow of blood to live. The cells in these organs cannot tolerate a lack of blood for more than a few minutes. Any longer and the cells begin to die. Furthermore, without constant flow of blood, these tissues cannot generate new cells. Once their cells die, they are replaced with scar tissue. This can lead to a permanent loss of function or, if enough cells die, death. The cardiovascular system consists of two parts: a container and its contents. The "container" is the heart and blood vessels (tubes that reach every cell in the body). The second part of the cardiovascular system is the "contents," or the blood. Normally, there is just enough blood to fill the system entirely. In an average adult, this is 6 L.

## THE HEART

The heart is a hollow muscular organ about the size of a clenched fist. It is an involuntary muscle under the control of the autonomic nervous system. However, the heart has its own regulatory system. Thus, it can function even if the external nervous system shuts down.

The heart is always working. Because it works continuously, the heart has a number of special features that other muscles do not.

First, the heart can tolerate a serious interruption of its blood supply for only a very few seconds before the signs of a heart attack develop. Thus, its blood supply is as rich and well distributed as possible.

Second, the heart works as two paired pumps. A wall called the septum divides the heart down the middle into two sides.

Each side of the heart has an upper chamber (atrium) and a lower chamber (ventricle). Blood leaves each chamber of the heart through a one-way valve. These valves keep the blood moving in the proper direction by preventing a backflow.

The right side of the heart receives oxygen-poor (deoxygenated) blood from the veins of the body. Blood enters into the right atrium from the vena cava, then fills the right ventricle. After the right ventricle contracts, blood flows into the pulmonary artery and the pulmonary circulation.

The now oxygen-rich (oxygenated) blood returns to the left side of the heart from the lungs through the pulmonary veins. Blood enters the left atrium then passes into the left ventricle. This side of the heart is more muscular than the other because it must pump blood into the aorta and on to the arteries.

## BLOOD VESSELS

There are five types of blood vessels, as follows:

1. Arteries
2. Arterioles
3. Capillaries
4. Venules
5. Veins

Capillaries are small tubes, just the size of a red blood cell, that pass among all the cells in the body. Capillaries link the arterioles and the venules. Oxygen and nutrients easily pass from these tiny tubes into the cells. Waste and carbon dioxide move out of the cells and into the capillaries.

## PHYSIOLOGY AND PERFUSION

The heart is a muscular pump that circulates blood through the entire cardiovascular system. Normally, the heart pumps 6 L of blood per minute through an adult's system. Thus, every part of the system receives a regular supply of blood every minute.

**Perfusion** is the circulation of blood within an organ or tissue in adequate amounts to meet the cells' current needs. Blood enters an organ or tissue through the arteries and leaves it through the veins (Figure 22-1). To reach the veins, blood must first pass through the arterioles, connecting capillaries, and venules. While passing through the capillaries, the blood delivers nutrients and oxygen to the surrounding cells and picks up the wastes they have generated.

## FIGURE 22-1

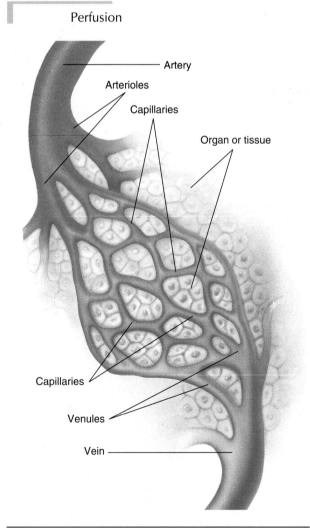

Perfusion

Artery

Arterioles

Capillaries

Organ or tissue

Capillaries

Venules

Vein

Blood must pass through the cardiovascular system at such a speed that circulation is maintained at the same time that each cell receives sufficient oxygen and nutrients and adequately rids itself of wastes.

Perfusion of the whole body keeps its cells alive and working. Certain tissues cannot live without a constant, high level of blood flow. The heart, central nervous system (brain and spinal cord), lungs, and kidneys all work continuously. Thus, they require a constant supply of blood.

Other parts of the body do not require a steady flow all the time. Certain tissues are used heavily, but they are used only from time to time. Muscles are a good example. They are at rest while you sleep and thus require a minimal blood supply. However, during exercise they need a very large blood supply. The gastrointestinal tract requires a high flow of blood after a meal. After digestion is completed, it can do quite well with a small fraction of that blood flow.

Thus, the cardiovascular system is dynamic—constantly adapting how it delivers blood, depending on the needs of each body part. The autonomic nervous system monitors the needs of the body moment to moment and adjusts the blood flow as needed. During emergencies, the autonomic nervous system automatically redirects blood away from other organs and to the heart, brain, lungs, and kidneys.

At times, the circulatory system fails to provide sufficient circulation so that every body part can perform its function. This condition is called hypoperfusion, or **shock.**

No part of the body can tolerate inadequate perfusion indefinitely. It is important for you to know which organs need adequate perfusion. In order, they are the heart, the central nervous system, the lungs, and the kidneys. The heart requires constant perfusion, or it will not function properly. The brain and spinal cord cannot go for more than 4 to 6 minutes without perfusion.

Any longer and the nerve cells will be permanently damaged. The kidneys will be permanently damaged after 45 minutes of inadequate perfusion. Skeletal muscles cannot tolerate more than 2 hours of inadequate perfusion. The gastrointestinal tract can exist with limited (but not absent) perfusion for several hours.

These times are based on a normal body temperature (98.6°F or 37.0°C). An organ or tissue is much more resistant to damage from hypoperfusion if it is considerably colder than normal.

It is important that you understand perfusion. Inadequate perfusion causes shock. It is just as important knowing which organs need constant perfusion and which can survive for longer periods without adequate perfusion.

# EXTERNAL BLEEDING

External bleeding is a visible hemorrhage. Examples include nosebleeds and bleeding from open wounds. As an EMT-B, you must understand how to control external bleeding.

*BSI always*

## EMT SAFETY

The risk of infection from a bleeding patient is the same as with any other routine, noncoughing patient. However, more than any other situation, a bleeding patient exposes you to potentially infectious body fluids. Thus, you must follow BSI techniques. Under BSI, you must consider blood or any other body fluid containing blood a potential risk. Wear gloves and eye protection in all situations. Wear a gown and mask if there is a risk for extensive blood splatter. Follow your local protocol. Avoid direct contact with body fluids, if possible. You should take great care if you have an open sore, cut, scratch, or ulcer. Also remember that frequent, thorough handwashing between patients and after every run is a simple, yet important protective measure.

## THE SIGNIFICANCE OF EXTERNAL BLEEDING

The body will not tolerate an acute blood loss of greater than 20% of blood volume. The typical adult (80 kg) has approximately 6 L of blood (7 mL/kg of body weight). This means that if a typical adult loses more than 1 L of blood (about 2 pt), significant changes in vital signs will occur. These changes include increasing heart rate and decreasing blood pressure. The same effect is seen in infants and children. However, because they have less blood volume, these same changes occur with lower amounts of blood loss. For example, a 1-year-old infant has a total blood volume of 800 mL. Significant symptoms of blood loss will occur after only 150 mL of blood loss.

How rapidly a person bleeds is related to the severity of bleeding. The average adult can comfortably donate a unit (500 mL) of blood over 15 to 20 minutes. Over this period of time, a normal, healthy individual can adapt well to the decrease in blood volume. However, if a similar loss occurs rapidly, hypovolemic shock may develop and the individual may even die. Under these circumstances, the body simply cannot compensate for the rapid blood loss.

In any situation, blood loss is an extremely serious problem. It demands your immediate attention as soon as you have cleared the airway and stabilized the breathing.

## CHARACTERISTICS OF BLEEDING

Injuries and some illnesses can disrupt blood vessels and cause bleeding. Characteristically, bleeding from an open artery

**FIGURE 22-2**

Types of bleeding

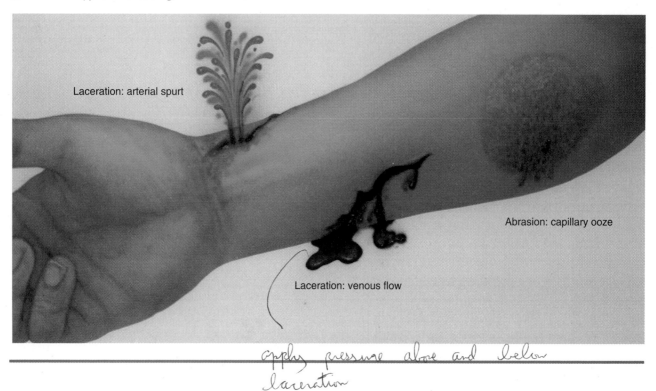

Laceration: arterial spurt

Abrasion: capillary ooze

Laceration: venous flow

*apply pressure above and below laceration*

is bright red and spurts in time with the pulse. The pressure that causes the blood to spurt also makes this type of bleeding difficult to control. As the amount of blood circulating in the body drops, so does the patient's blood pressure and, eventually, the arterial spurting.

Blood from an open vein is much darker and flows steadily. Because it is under less pressure, venous blood does not spurt and is more easily managed. Bleeding from damaged capillary vessels is dark red and oozes from a wound steadily but slowly. It may clot spontaneously (Figure 22-2).

Bleeding typically stops on its own after 6 to 10 minutes because the body has effective systems to stop bleeding. When we are cut, blood gushes from the open vessel. Soon afterward, the cut ends of the vessel begin to narrow. This reduces the amount of bleeding. Then a clot forms, plugging the

hole. This process is called **coagulation.** It is the mechanism that ultimately stops blood flow from injured vessels of every size. Bleeding will never stop if a clot does not form—unless the injured vessel is completely cut off from the entire blood supply. Direct contact with body tissues and their fluids is the common trigger that activates the blood's clotting factors. When exposed to these tissues and fluids, blood clots rapidly form to seal the injured portions of the damaged vessel.

Despite the efficiency of this system, it may fail in certain situations. A number of medications, including aspirin, interfere with normal clotting. With a severe injury, the damaged vessel may be so large that a clot cannot completely block the hole. Sometimes only part of the vessel wall is cut, preventing it from constricting. In these cases, bleeding will continue unless it is stopped by external means. Occasionally, blood loss occurs very rapidly. In these instances, the patient might die before the body's defenses, such as clotting, could help.

A very small portion of the population lacks one or more of the blood's clotting factors. This condition is called **hemophilia.** There are several forms of hemophilia. Most are hereditary. Some are severe. Almost all result in a significant increased capability to bleed. Sometimes, bleeding may occur on its own in hemophilia. Because the hemophiliac's blood does not clot, all injuries, no matter how trivial, are potentially serious. A patient with hemophilia should be transported immediately.

## CONTROLLING EXTERNAL BLEEDING

As you begin to care for a patient with obvious external bleeding, remember to follow BSI techniques. As with all patient care, make sure the patient's airway is open and oxygen provided, if necessary. You may then concentrate on controlling the bleeding. Six ways to control external bleeding are presented below. Practically speaking, the first three methods presented are commonly used. The other three methods are used less often.

The three most commonly used methods are as follows:

1. Direct local pressure
2. Splinting and elevation
3. Air splinting

The three less common methods are as follows:

4. Pneumatic antishock garments (PASG)
5. Proximal arterial pressure
6. Tourniquets

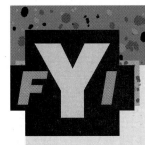

## How Climate Affects Pressurized Devices

Whenever the external temperature or air pressure changes, it will affect a pressurized device, like an air pressure splint or PASG. Thus, you must watch for changes in these devices whenever you transport a patient in a helicopter or through an area with marked temperature or pressure changes, such as a mountainous region.

In helicopters (and unpressurized airplanes), external pressure drops as you go up. In response, the air in a splint or PASG expands, and the device tightens.

Cold makes air within the device contract. Under these conditions, the splint or PASG will loosen. Similarly, if you apply a splint or PASG in a cold environment, you must adjust the pressure as you move the patient into a warm vehicle or room. Otherwise, the device will tighten as the air inside expands.

## FIGURE 22-3

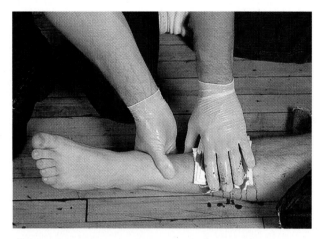

**A** Apply direct pressure with your gloved hand

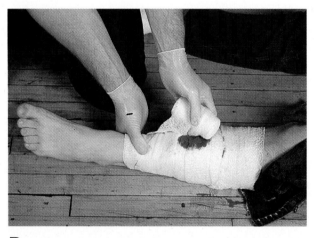

**B** Secure a pressure dressing with a roller bandage

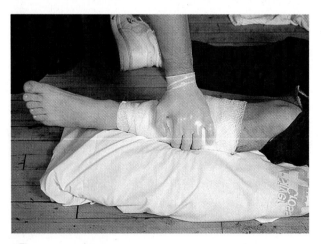

**C** Elevate the extremity and continue applying pressure

### Local Pressure and Elevation

Almost all instances of external bleeding can be controlled simply—by applying direct local pressure to the bleeding site. Pressure stops the flow of blood and permits normal coagulation to occur. This method is, by far, the most effective way to control local external bleeding.

You can apply direct pressure to the wound with your gloved finger or hand, but a pressure dressing is preferred (Figure 22-3a). Use 4" × 4" or 4" × 8" sterile gauze pads for small wounds and a sterile universal dressing for large wounds. If sterile gauze pads are not immediately available, use a clean handkerchief, sanitary napkin, clean cloth, or gloved hand to apply pressure.

Once you have controlled the bleeding, you can maintain the pressure by firmly wrapping a sterile, roller, self-adhering bandage around the entire wound. Then cover the entire sterile compressive dressing—above and below the wound—with the roller bandage, stretched sufficiently tight to control the bleeding (Figure 22-3b). Make sure that the bandage is not too tight, or it may decrease blood flow to the extremity.

Do not remove a dressing until a physician has evaluated the patient. If the bleeding continues after a dressing is in place, the dressing is probably not tight enough. In addition, you may have to pack large gaping wounds with sterile gauze pads. Apply additional manual pressure through the dressing. Then add additional gauze pads over the first dressing and secure them both with a second, tighter, roller bandage. Do not remove the original dressing and replace it with a clean dressing. Bleeding will almost always stop when the pressure of the dressing exceeds arterial pressure.

Elevating a bleeding extremity is also important. Elevation by as little as 6" often stops venous bleeding. Whenever possible,

TRAUMA

## FIGURE 22-4

A simple splint

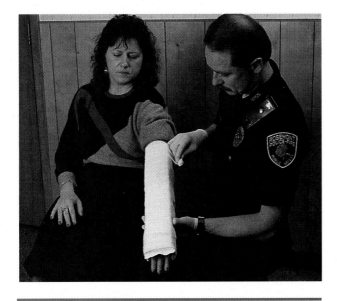

use both techniques—local pressure and elevation. In most cases, this will stop the bleeding (Figure 22-3c). However, if it does not, you still have several options.

Proximal compression, as described below, can be very effective when used in combination with direct pressure. If a wound continues to bleed after you have applied direct local pressure, try placing additional pressure over a proximal pulse point. This may help slow and eventually stop the bleeding.

### Splints

Much of the bleeding associated with broken bones occurs because the sharp ends of the bones cut muscles and other tissues. As long as a fracture remains unstabilized, the bone ends will move and continue to injure partially clotted vessels. Therefore, stabilizing a serious fracture is a high priority in the prompt control of bleeding. Often, a simple splint will quickly control bleeding associated with a fracture (Figure 22-4). Complete step-by-step instructions on the use of splints are presented in chapter 24, Musculoskeletal Care.

### Air Splints

Many ambulances carry air splints. Air splints can control the bleeding associated with severe soft tissue injuries, such as massive or complex lacerations, or fractures (Figure 22-5). An air splint acts like a pressure bandage. But it is applied to an entire extremity rather than to a small, local area. An air splint can effectively stabilize a fracture. You should monitor circulation in the distal extremity once an air splint has been applied. You may also use this type of splint on a patient who does not have a fracture, if you are just trying to control bleeding.

## FIGURE 22-5 *a pressure*

An air splint

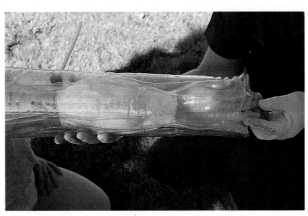

### Pneumatic Antishock Garments

Bleeding is often a severe or even fatal complication of injuries to the pelvis or the proximal femur. You may not even see the bleeding because the blood may collect behind the peritoneum and in the tissues around both hips. If a patient has injuries to the lower extremities, you can use a pneumatic antishock garment (PASG) to prevent or minimize hypovolemic shock.

A PASG may be effective in a few, very specific instances, such as the following:

- stabilizing fractures of the pelvis and proximal femurs
- controlling significant internal bleeding associated with fractures of the pelvis and proximal femurs
- controlling shock due to significant internal bleeding
- supporting the systolic blood pressure when it falls below 100 mm Hg following trauma (The source of bleeding may not be evident.)

The PASG is an effective device for stabilizing complicated pelvic and proximal femoral fractures. Ordinarily, it is not used to control obvious external bleeding. The device is normally used to treat shock as a result of internal bleeding. However, in rare instances, these fractures produce significant external bleeding. In these cases, the PASG helps compress the soft tissues.

A PASG works by compressing the abdomen and lower extremities, increasing peripheral resistance in the circulatory system.

## FIGURE 22-6

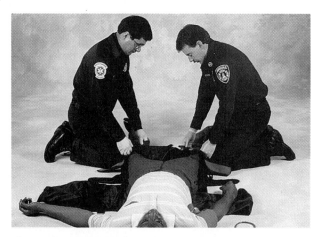

**A** Place the PASG under the patient

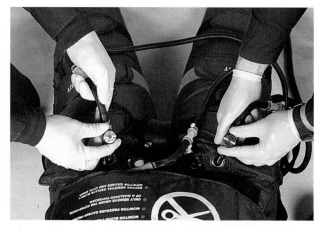

**B** Connect the inflation tubes to the leg compartment

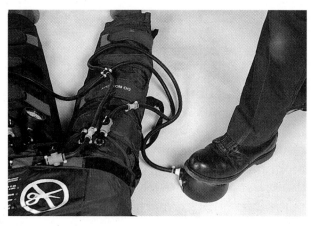

**C** Inflate the leg compartments

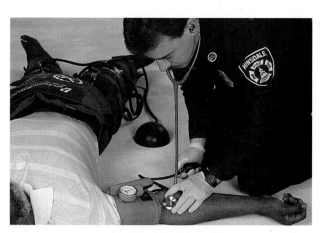

**D** Reassess the patient's vital signs

This increases the amount of blood available to the vital organs.

Do not use the PASG if any of the following conditions exist:

- pregnancy
- chronic pulmonary edema secondary to long-standing heart disease
- acute heart failure
- penetrating chest injuries
- groin injuries
- major head injuries
- relatively short transport time (less than 30 minutes)

In these situations, the PASG may needlessly worsen or complicate the patient's condition. In any case, do not keep a PASG inflated for more than 2 hours or the time needed to transport a patient to the hospital. Consult with medical control if you think prolonged use, or use in unusual circumstances, may be necessary.

In applying the PASG, you should carefully inflate the device in increments (Figure 22-6). As a general rule, gradually inflate the legs of the PASG before inflating the abdominal portion. Monitor the patient's blood pressure constantly.

Remember that the PASG's pressure gauges measure the air pressure in the device. They in no way reflect the patient's blood pressure. Thus, you should monitor and record the patient's blood pressure at least every 5 minutes before, during, and after application. Do not increase the garment's pressure any more than necessary. You should stop once the patient's systolic blood pressure exceeds 100 mm Hg. Avoid increasing the pressure around the lower extremities above 30 mm Hg. Higher pressures will damage tissue locally.

If the PASG has no pressure gauges, monitor the distal neurovascular status of the limbs. Make sure you can still detect pulses, sensation, and motion. The device has been effective if the patient's blood pressure increases and the vital signs stabilize.

*You should not remove a PASG in the field.* Rather, it should be gradually deflated in the hospital under careful supervision and only after appropriate IV solutions are given. Before turning over your patient, notify hospital personnel of the patient's blood pressure, the time you applied the PASG, and the results.

### Proximal Arterial Pressure

Sometimes when you cannot control the bleeding with direct pressure and elevation, or when pressure dressings are not available, you can use proximal arterial pressure. However, you must be thoroughly familiar with the location of the pulse points (Figure 22-7).

Proximal compression of a major artery rarely stops bleeding completely. This is because a wound usually draws blood from more than one major artery. However, this technique can help slow the loss of blood (Figure 22-8). Therefore, it is not the best way of controlling bleeding.

### Tourniquets

Tourniquets are effective for a very limited number of injuries. You should rarely need to use a tourniquet to control bleeding. Applying a tourniquet is considered a last resort, because it is rarely necessary and is generally not effective. In fact, most of the situations in which they might be effective do not produce much bleeding. Thus, a tourniquet often creates, rather than solves, problems. In addition, tourniquets are often improperly applied.

When applied properly, a tourniquet may save a patient's life. If you cannot control bleeding from an extremity's major vessel any other way, you may need to apply a tourniquet. Specifically, the tourniquet is useful if a patient is bleeding severely from a partial or complete amputation. Be sure to notify hospital personnel on your arrival that your patient has a tourniquet in place. Record this same information on the ambulance run report form.

FIGURE 22-8

Applying direct pressure to the brachial artery

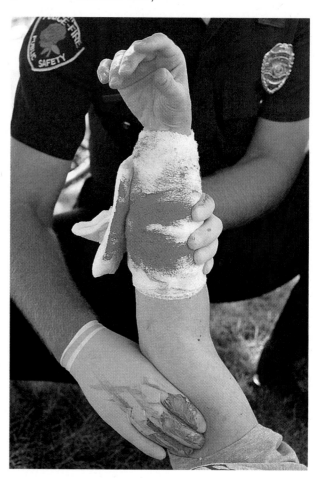

FIGURE 22-7

Arterial pressure points

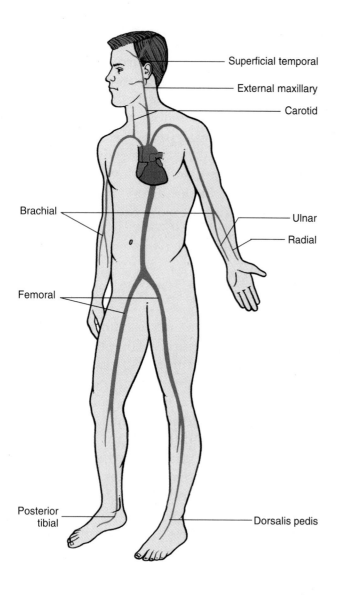

Superficial temporal

External maxillary

Carotid

Brachial

Ulnar

Radial

Femoral

Posterior tibial

Dorsalis pedis

## Applying a Tourniquet

1. Fold a triangular bandage until it is 4" wide and six to eight layers thick.

2. Wrap this long, 4" wide bandage around the extremity twice. Choose a point proximal to the bleeding but as distal on the extremity as possible (Figure 22-9a).

3. Tie one knot in the bandage. Place a stick or rod on top of the knot and tie the ends of the bandage over the stick in a square knot (Figure 22-9b).

4. Use the stick as a handle and twist it to tighten the tourniquet until the bleeding has stopped (Figure 22-9c). Once the

**FIGURE 22-9**

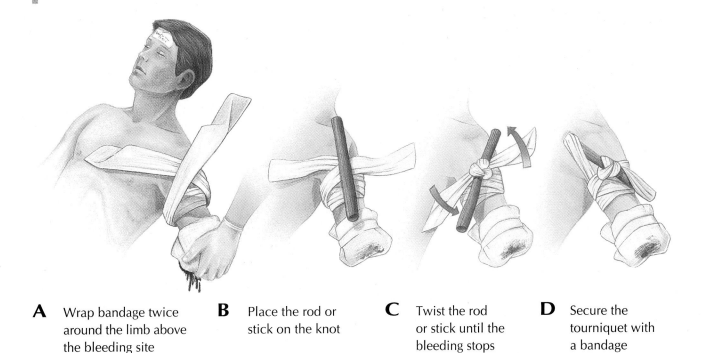

**A** Wrap bandage twice around the limb above the bleeding site

**B** Place the rod or stick on the knot

**C** Twist the rod or stick until the bleeding stops

**D** Secure the tourniquet with a bandage

bleeding has ceased, do not turn the stick any more. Secure it in place and make the wrapping neat and smooth (Figure 22-9d).

5. Write TK and the time you applied the tourniquet on a piece of adhesive tape. Securely fasten the tape to the patient's forehead. The phrase to use is "time applied." Indicate the correct hour and minute.

You can also use a blood pressure cuff as an effective tourniquet (Figure 22-10). Position the cuff proximal to the bleeding point. Inflate the cuff just enough to stop the bleeding. Leave the cuff inflated. If you use a blood pressure cuff, monitor the gauge continuously. You must be sure that the pressure is not gradually dropping. It may be necessary to clamp the tube with a hemostat leading from the cuff to the inflating bulb to prevent loss of pressure.

**FIGURE 22-10**

Use of a blood pressure cuff as a tourniquet

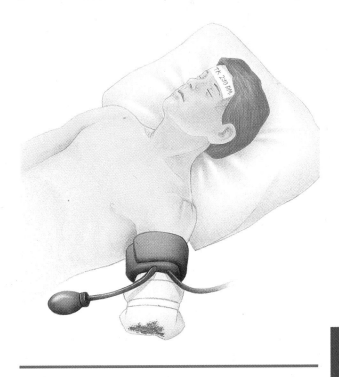

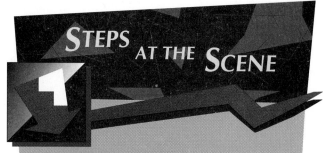
## APPLYING A TOURNIQUET

☐ Fold a triangular bandage until it is 4" wide and six to eight layers thick.

☐ Wrap this long, 4" wide bandage around the extremity twice. Choose a point proximal to the bleeding but as distal on the extremity as possible.

☐ Tie one knot in the bandage. Place a stick or rod on top of the knot and tie the ends of the bandage over the stick in a square knot.

☐ Use the stick as a handle and twist it to tighten the tourniquet until the bleeding has stopped. Once the bleeding has ceased, do not turn the stick any more. Secure it in place and make the wrapping neat and smooth.

☐ Write TK and the time you applied the tourniquet on a piece of adhesive tape. Securely fasten the tape to the patient's forehead. The phrase to use is "time applied." Indicate the correct hour and minute.

Whenever you apply a tourniquet, make sure you observe the following precautions:

1. Do not apply a tourniquet directly over any joint. Keep it as close to the injury as possible.

2. Use the widest bandage possible. Make sure that it is tightened securely.

3. Never use wire, rope, a belt, or any other narrow material. It could cut into the skin.

4. Use wide padding under the tourniquet, if possible. This will protect the tissues and helps with arterial compression.

5. Never cover a tourniquet with a bandage. Leave it open and in full view.

6. Do not loosen the tourniquet once it has been applied. Hospital personnel will loosen it once they are prepared to manage the bleeding.

## BLEEDING FROM THE NOSE, EARS, AND MOUTH

Several conditions can result in bleeding from the nose, ears, and/or mouth, including the following:

- skull fracture
- facial injuries, including those caused by a direct blow to the nose
- sinusitis, infections, nose drop use and abuse, dried or cracked nasal mucosa, or other abnormalities
- high blood pressure
- coagulation disorders
- digital trauma (nose picking)

**Epistaxis** (nosebleed) is a common emergency. Occasionally, a patient can lose enough blood to go into shock. The blood you see may be only a small part of the total blood loss. Much of the blood may pass down the throat into the stomach as the patient swallows. A person who swallows a large amount of blood may become nauseated and start vomiting. This can sometimes be confused with internal bleeding.

**FIGURE 22-11**

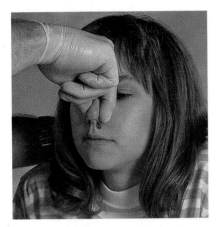

**A**  Pinch the nostrils together with gloved fingers

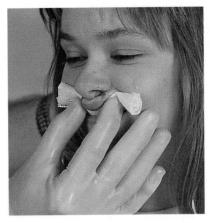

**B**  Place gauze under upper lip

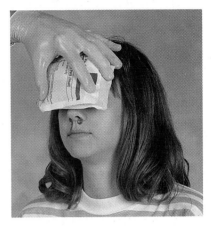

**C**  Place ice over the nose

Bleeding from the nose or ears following a head injury may indicate a skull fracture. In these instances, you should not attempt to stop the blood flow. First, such bleeding is difficult to control. Plus, applying excessive pressure to the injury may force the blood leaking through the ear or nose to collect within the head. This could increase the pressure on the brain and possibly cause permanent damage. If you suspect a skull fracture, collect the blood with a loose, dry sterile local dressing. Apply light compression by wrapping the dressing loosely around the head.

## EMERGENCY MEDICAL CARE

Caring for a patient with epistaxis involves the following steps:

1. Help the patient to sit, leaning forward, with the head tilted forward. This position stops the blood from trickling down the throat or being drawn into the lungs.

2. Apply direct pressure for at least 15 minutes by pinching the fleshy part of the nostrils together (Figure 22-11a).

3. Another option is to place a rolled 4" × 4" gauze bandage between the upper lip and the gum. Press the gum against the bandage with your gloved fingers. The patient can sometimes apply enough pressure by stretching the upper lip tightly against the rolled bandage and pushing it up into and against the nose (Figure 22-11b).

4. Keep the patient calm and quiet. This step is particularly important if the patient has high blood pressure or is anxious. Anxiety tends to increase blood pressure, which could worsen the nosebleed.

5. Apply ice over the nose (Figure 22-11c).

6. Spend enough time with the patient to completely control the bleeding, if this is the patient's only problem. Usually, 15 minutes is sufficient. Most often, failure to stop a nosebleed is due to the pressure being released too soon.

## WATCH YOUR STEP

It's a beautiful spring day. The rain that has been falling for the last 3 days finally lets up enough for Vern Fredericks, proprietor of Vern's Orchards, to get out and start trimming his trees. He's standing in his shorts and T-shirt on the very top step of a 12' stepladder. As he reaches to finish up the last of a trim job on an apple tree, he loses his footing and falls into the tree. A co-worker watches helplessly as Vern tumbles through the branches, finally crashing to the soft, muddy ground. He is still lying there when you arrive, complaining that his body "hurts." You ask him to be more specific. He says it's mostly his nose, neck, ribs, and right arm that hurt. He has multiple abrasions and minor cuts, and his right upper arm is swollen and very discolored. His nose is bleeding badly.

### For Discussion

1. Compare elements of urban trauma with rural trauma.
2. Describe the system approach to trauma management.

---

Most nosebleeds are the result of an injury of the mucous membrane covering the nasal septum. Thus, the procedure described above is often successful in stopping a nosebleed. Once the bleeding has been stopped, provide prompt transport. If you cannot control the bleeding or if the patient has a history of frequent nosebleeds, you should provide prompt transport to the hospital.

Some nosebleeds originate in the nasopharynx. Normal emergency methods cannot stop this type of nosebleed. Provide transport to any patient whose nosebleed does not respond to normal procedures to the hospital. Otherwise, hypovolemic shock might develop.

## INTERNAL BLEEDING

Internal bleeding can be very serious, especially because you may not be aware that it is happening. Severe internal bleeding may cause hypovolemic shock before you realize the extent of blood loss. Injured or damaged internal organs commonly result in extensive bleeding. However, you cannot see it. A person with a bleeding stomach ulcer may lose a large amount of blood very quickly. Similarly, a person who has a lacerated liver or spleen may lose a considerable amount of blood within the abdomen. Yet the patient has no outward signs of bleeding.

Broken bones may also result in serious internal blood loss. Broken ribs, in particular, may produce severe internal bleeding. Sometimes this bleeding extends into the chest cavity and the soft tissues of the chest wall. A broken femur can easily result in the loss of 1 L or more of blood into the soft tissues of the thigh. Often, the only signs of such bleeding are local swelling and bruising. These signs are due to the accumulation of blood around the ends of the broken bone.

Because internal bleeding is concealed, you should be particularly alert for it. Assess for signs and symptoms of internal bleeding, particularly if the mechanism of injury is severe.

## MECHANISM OF INJURY

Internal bleeding is possible whenever the mechanism of injury suggests that severe forces impacted the abdomen. These forces include rapid acceleration, deceleration, shearing, or compression. Internal bleeding commonly occurs as a result of falls, and automobile or motorcycle accidents. Likewise, any pedestrian who is hit by an automobile or motorcycle is at significant risk for internal bleeding.

As you assess a patient, look for signs of injury over the chest or abdomen. If the patient has contusions, abrasions, lacerations, or other signs of injury or deformity, you should suspect internal bleeding. You should always suspect internal bleeding in a patient who has a penetrating injury, such as a knife or gunshot wound. Provide rapid transport anytime you suspect internal bleeding.

## SIGNS AND SYMPTOMS

A common sign of internal bleeding is bruising around the abdomen. Bruising is also called contusion or ecchymosis. A mass of blood in the soft tissues beneath the skin is called a hematoma. Such discoloration indicates bleeding into the soft tissues and may be the result of either a minor or severe injury.

Bleeding, however slight, from any body opening is serious. It usually indicates internal bleeding that is not readily seen or controllable. Bleeding from the mouth, rectum (hematochezia), or blood in the urine (hematuria) may indicate serious internal injury or disease. Nonmenstrual vaginal bleeding is always significant.

Other signs and symptoms of internal bleeding include the following:

1. *Hematemesis.* This is vomited blood. It may be bright red or dark red. If the blood has been partially digested, it looks like coffee grounds vomitus.

2. *Melena.* This is dark, foul-smelling tarry stools that contain digested blood.

3. *Hemoptysis.* This is bright red blood that has been coughed up.

4. *Pain, tenderness, bruising, or swelling.* These signs and symptoms around an injury site could mean a closed fracture is bleeding.

5. *Broken ribs, bruises over the lower chest, or a tender, rigid, or distended abdomen.* These signs and symptoms could mean a lacerated spleen or liver. These patients may also complain of pain in the shoulder on the same side as the internal injury. A patient with a liver injury may have pain in the right shoulder. A patient with an injured spleen may have pain in the left shoulder. This is called referred pain. You should suspect internal abdominal bleeding in a patient with referred pain.

You should also look for the following late signs of hypovolemic shock (hypoperfusion), which could be the result of internal bleeding:

- tachycardia
- anxiety, restlessness, combativeness, or an altered level of consciousness

- weakness, faintness, or dizziness
- thirst
- nausea and vomiting
- weak, rapid (thready) pulse
- cold, moist (clammy) skin
- shallow, rapid breathing
- dull eyes
- slightly dilated pupils that are slow to respond to light
- decreasing blood pressure
- capillary refill in infants and children of more than 2 seconds

Patients with these signs and symptoms are at risk. Some may be in danger. They could continue to bleed. Even if the bleeding stops, it could begin again at any moment. Therefore, prompt transport is necessary.

## EMERGENCY MEDICAL CARE

Controlling internal bleeding depends on the source of the bleeding. There is nothing you can do in the field to control internal bleeding or bleeding from the major organs. Usually, such bleeding can be controlled only through surgery or with the help of complex equipment. If you suspect internal bleeding, given the mechanism of injury and the patient's signs and symptoms, provide immediate transport.

You can usually control bleeding into the extremities quite well. You may slow blood flow simply by splinting an injured extremity. In most cases, air pressure splints effectively control bleeding. You will rarely need to use a PASG. You should not use a tourniquet to control the bleeding from closed, internal, soft tissue injuries.

Caring for a patient with possible internal bleeding involves the following 10 steps:

1. Follow BSI techniques.
2. Maintain the airway, giving artificial ventilation and maintaining the cervical spine, if necessary.
3. Give the patient oxygen. As the blood volume drops, the body's tissues are deprived of oxygen.
4. Control all obvious external bleeding.
5. Treat obvious internal bleeding in an extremity by applying a splint or an air pressure splint.
6. Treat severe uncontrolled hypovolemic shock with a PASG, as described in the next section.
7. Monitor and record the vital signs at least every 10 minutes, especially pulse, respirations, and palpable systolic pressure.
8. Give the patient nothing (not even small sips of water) by mouth.
9. Elevate the patient's legs 6" to 12" to help the blood return to the vital organs. Keep the knees straight. Remember that the entire weight of the abdominal organs will fall on the diaphragm. The patient may be unable to breathe easily in this position and may require assisted ventilation.
10. Transport the patient as soon as possible.

## SHOCK

When trauma patients lose too much blood either externally or internally, they can go into **hypovolemic** (or hemorrhagic) **shock.** Like internal bleeding, shock cannot be seen. It is not a specific disease or injury. However, it is a dangerous condition that

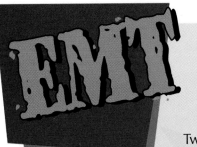

## NOT QUITE A TOUCHDOWN

Two young brothers are throwing a football in the house, despite the repeated warnings and scolding of their mother to "be careful." Moments later, one of the boys falls through the lower pane of a glass storm door as he tries to catch the football. As the glass shatters, it lacerates his arm in the area of his right wrist. On arrival, you find an anxious, but otherwise calm 9-year-old boy sitting in the kitchen in the care of his mother. She has a blood-soaked dish towel wrapped around the injury. You also note some blood splattered on the wall by the door, and several small puddles on the kitchen floor. A quick peek under the towel reveals very active bleeding. You also suspect that the wrist may be broken.

### For Discussion

1. Explain how capillary, venous, and arterial bleeding differ in appearance. Describe the proper care for each.

2. Describe proper BSI techniques when caring for a patient with severe external bleeding.

results in the inadequate flow of blood to the body's cells. Without adequate blood flow, organs and tissues do not receive the oxygen and nutrients they need. In addition, they do not rid themselves of the metabolic wastes they create. They begin to die. In an attempt to compensate, the body redirects blood flow from nonessential organs (skin, intestines, kidneys) to the essential organs (heart, lungs, brain). If the conditions causing shock are not promptly addressed, the patient will eventually die.

There are really only three ways shock can occur: 1) damage to the heart, 2) dilated blood vessels, and 3) inadequate blood volume in the circulatory system. First, the heart can be damaged by disease or injury. But no matter what the cause, a damaged heart does not pump blood properly. It does not generate enough energy to move blood through the system. Second, blood vessels can dilate so that the blood within them, even though it is of normal volume, is inadequate to fill the system. Thus, blood flow to the vital organs is inadequate. Third, a patient can bleed so much that the volume of blood within the system cannot provide adequate blood flow. Whatever the cause of shock, damage occurs because blood flow to organs and body tissues is inadequate (Figure 22-12). As soon as this perfusion stops or is impaired, tissues start to die. No matter what the cause, the end result is exactly the same. Inadequate perfusion affects the way our body works.

## FIGURE 22-12

Three causes of shock

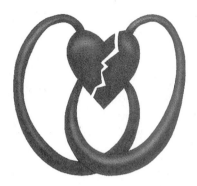

**1. Poor pump function**

Causes: Heart attack, trauma to heart

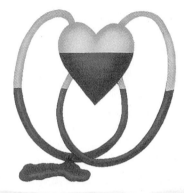

**2. Blood or fluid loss from blood vessels**

Causes: Trauma to vessels or tissues, fluid loss from GI tract (vomiting/diarrhea can also lower the fluid component of blood)

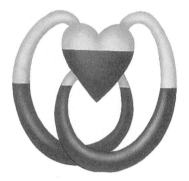

**3. Blood vessels dilate**

Causes: Infection, drug overdose (narcotic), spinal cord injury

---

## SIGNS AND SYMPTOMS

You must learn to recognize the signs and symptoms of shock based on your assessment. You should expect shock in many patient situations. For example, you would expect shock to accompany massive external or internal bleeding. You should also expect shock if a patient has any one of the following conditions:

- multiple severe fractures
- abdominal or chest injury
- spinal injury
- a severe infection
- a major heart attack
- anaphylaxis

You must quickly identify the signs and symptoms of early shock, begin treatment,

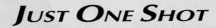

## JUST ONE SHOT

Dispatch sends you and your new partner down the road in the middle of a driving rain to a local convenience store for a "man down." En route, the call is upgraded to a "CPR in progress." On arrival, you find that the scene has just been secured as the gun-wielding patron is being hauled off in handcuffs by the county sheriff. You also find the patient lying on the floor behind the cash register. The patient is the 36-year-old cashier who was shot when an argument with a patron turned ugly. A quick look under the patient's shirt shows a single bullet wound in the center of the left side of the chest. The initial assessment shows that the patient has no pulse and is not breathing.

### For Discussion

1. Give at least two examples of how a trauma emergency can result in a respiratory emergency and vice versa.

2. Describe why a patient who goes into cardiac arrest as a result of trauma has such a poor chance of survival.

and provide immediate transport. The early stages of shock, while the body can still compensate for blood loss, is called compensated shock. The late stage of shock, when blood pressure is falling, is called decompensated shock.

The most common signs and symptoms of early (compensated) shock include the following:

- agitation, anxiety, restlessness, or an altered level of consciousness (the patient often experiences a feeling of impending doom)

- weak, rapid (thready) pulse

- pale, ashen, cool, moist (clammy) skin

- pallor, with cyanosis to the lips

- profuse sweating

- shallow, labored, or irregular breathing

- shortness of breath, especially if there is a chest injury

- nausea or vomiting

- capillary refill in infants and children of longer than 2 seconds

- marked thirst

The most common signs and symptoms of late (decompensated) shock include the following:

- gradual and steadily falling blood pressure (In general, assume an adult is developing shock if the systolic blood pressure is 90 mm Hg or lower.)

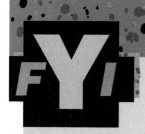

# The Complications of the PASG

The most common complication associated with using a PASG is severe hypovolemic shock. This usually occurs if the device is deflated too rapidly in the emergency department. This problem is not your direct concern because you would rarely participate in this aspect of the patient's care. You do, however, apply the device. Therefore, you should be aware of the problems that can arise from removing it.

Hospital personnel must be prepared to administer large volumes of IV fluid and blood to restore adequate blood volume before deflating the PASG. Otherwise, the patient may develop hypovolemic shock as the device is deflated.

Recently, there have been reports that the garment may exert excessive pressure if it remains inflated for a prolonged period. This can lead to the death of muscle tissues. The medical literature also reports the device is sometimes used inappropriately. Because of the potential for serious complications, you should only use the PASG for the specific situations outlined in this chapter.

Although several researchers have studied the benefits of using the PASG, they have so far failed to identify a positive effect on patient care. In general, it has not yet proven to be a lifesaver for patients that would otherwise be lost.

Despite this, there is general agreement that the PASG can stabilize major pelvic and femoral fractures. It can also provide some support for a low blood pressure when a patient is in hypovolemic shock. You must remember, however, that this support comes at a high cost:

- The pressures on the tissues in the lower extremities and abdomen can be lethal.

- The application of the device delays transport and more definitive care.

Just remember: the PASG is not an aid for controlling bleeding but a device to help manage shock. Serious problems have been identified with the use of this device. You should use it only when it is absolutely needed.

---

- poor urinary output
- dull eyes, dilated pupils
- weak or absent peripheral pulses

Remember that blood pressure may be the last measurable parameter to change. The body has several automatic mechanisms to compensate for initial blood loss and to help maintain blood pressure. By the time you detect a drop in blood pressure, shock is well developed. This is particularly true of infants and children, who can maintain their blood pressure until they have lost more than half their blood volume. By the time their blood pressure drops, infants and children are close to death.

You should vigorously treat any patient for shock as soon as you suspect that the condition exists. As with any type of patient care, you should begin by following BSI techniques and making sure the patient has an open airway. Give oxygen as needed. Make sure the patient can breathe well. Assist or control respirations as needed.

Lack of oxygen can rapidly lead to shock. Thus, you must carefully monitor the patient's breathing. Inadequate ventilation may be the primary cause of or a major factor in the development of shock. Establish and maintain an open airway and make sure that breathing is adequate. Give oxygen to all patients who are at risk for developing shock. A few assisted ventilations can increase the amount of oxygen in the patient's blood. In general, keep the patient in a supine position. Remember that some patients in shock after a severe heart attack or with a lung disease cannot breathe as well lying down. With such patients, place them in a position of comfort, either sitting up or in a semisitting position.

If the lower abdomen is tender, and you suspect a pelvic injury (but there is no evidence of chest injuries), apply and inflate a PASG—if approved by medical direction. You should apply (but not inflate) a PASG if the patient has any of the following:

- a critical injury
- a systolic blood pressure of less than 100 mg Hg
- a falling blood pressure
- a rising pulse rate

You can then inflate the garment rapidly should the patient's condition deteriorate and you have approval from medical direction.

Next, control all obvious external bleeding. Place sterile gauze compresses over the bleeding sites, then secure the compresses with circumferential pressure dressings. If there are no broken bones, elevate the lower extremities 6" to 12". This allows the blood in the legs to return to the heart more rapidly. It is a simple way to supply the heart with as much blood as possible after severe bleeding. It also helps stop venous bleeding in an extremity. If the legs are broken, splint the patient on a spine board, and then elevate the foot of the board.

Splint any bone or joint injuries. This minimizes pain, bleeding, and discomfort, all of which can aggravate shock. It also prevents the broken bone ends from further damaging adjacent soft tissue. In general, splinting also makes it easier to move the patient. Avoid rough or excessive handling.

To prevent the loss of body heat, place blankets under and over the patient. Be careful not to overload the patient with covers or attempt to warm the body too much. It is better for the patient to be slightly cool rather than too hot. Do not use any external heat sources, such as hot water bottles or heating pads. They may harm a patient in shock by causing vasodilation and decreasing blood pressure even more.

Do not give the patient anything to eat or drink. Specifically, you should not give anything by mouth, regardless of the patient's urgent requests. To alleviate the intense thirst that often accompanies shock, give the patient a moistened piece of gauze to chew or suck. Never give a patient in shock an alcoholic drink or other depressant. A stimulant, such as coffee, also has little value in treating shock.

Accurately record the patient's pulse, blood pressure, and other vital signs. Continue to monitor and record the vital signs throughout treatment and transport. Transport patients in shock promptly.

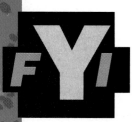

# Types of Shock

| Type of Shock | Causes | Signs/Symptoms | Treatment |
|---|---|---|---|
| Anaphylactic | Most severe form of allergic reaction | Can develop within seconds<br>Mild itching<br>Burning skin<br>Vascular dilation<br>Generalized edema<br>Profound coma<br>Rapid death | Supply respiratory support<br>Assist ventilations<br>Determine cause<br>Epinephrine<br>Transport promptly |
| Cardiogenic | Inadequate heart function<br>Disease of muscle tissue<br>Impaired electrical system<br>Disease or injury | Chest pains<br>Irregular pulse<br>Weak pulse<br>Low blood pressure<br>Cyanosis (lips, under nails)<br>Anxiety | Position comfortably<br>Administer oxygen<br>Assist ventilations<br>Transport promptly |
| Hypovolemic | Loss of blood or fluid | Rapid, weak pulse<br>Low blood pressure<br>Change in mental status<br>Cyanosis (lips, under nails)<br>Cool, clammy skin | Secure airway<br>Assist ventilations<br>Control external bleeding<br>Elevate legs<br>Prevent aspiration<br>PASG (if medical control approves)<br>Transport promptly |
| Metabolic | Excessive loss of fluid and electrolytes due to vomiting, urination, or diarrhea | Rapid, weak pulse<br>Low blood pressure<br>Change in mental status<br>Cyanosis (lips, under nails)<br>Cool, clammy skin | Secure airway<br>Assist ventilations<br>Determine illness<br>Transport promptly |

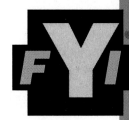

| Type of Shock | Causes | Signs/Symptoms | Treatment |
|---|---|---|---|
| Neurogenic | Damaged cervical spine, causing blood vessels to dilate widely | Bradycardia (slow pulse) Low blood pressure Signs of neck injury | Secure airway Assist ventilations Conserve body heat Maximize circulation PASG (if medical control approves) Transport promptly |
| Psychogenic (fainting) | Temporary, generalized vascular dilation Anxiety, news, sight of injury/blood, prospect of medical treatment, severe pain, illness, tiredness | Rapid pulse Normal or low blood pressure | Determine duration of unconsciousness Record initial vital signs and mental status If patient is confused or slow to regain consciousness, suspect head injury Transport promptly |
| Septic | Severe bacterial infections | Warm skin Tachycardia Low blood pressure | Transport promptly Administer oxygen en route Provide full ventilatory support Elevate legs Keep patient warm |

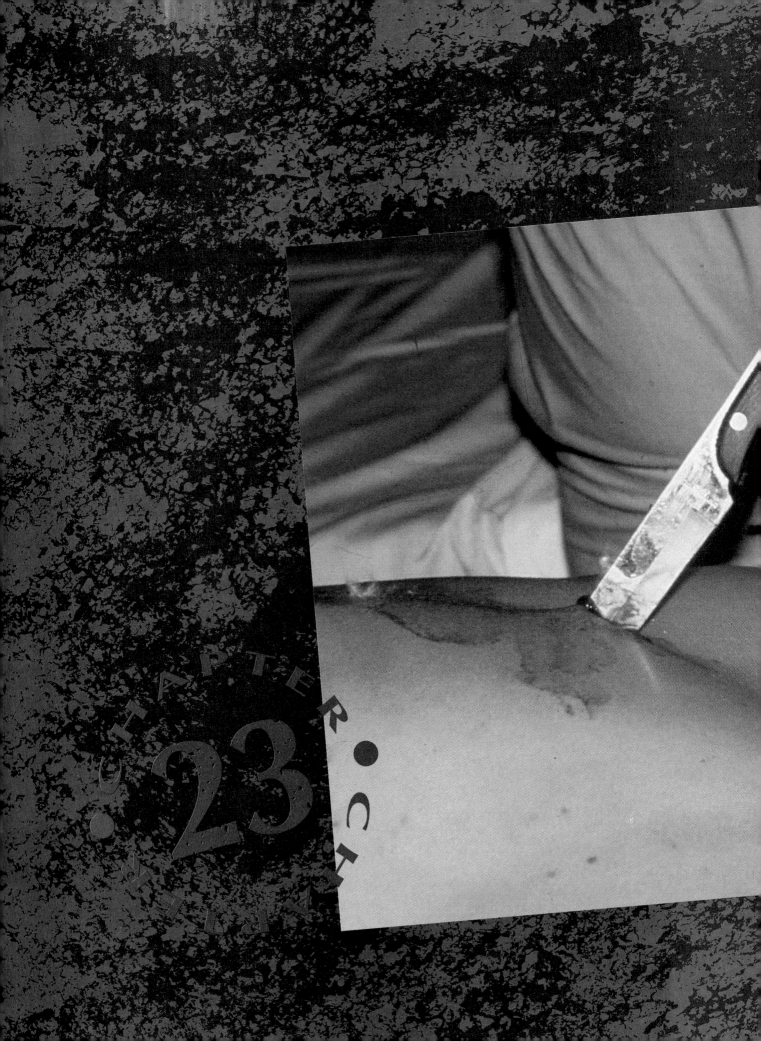

CHAPTER 23

# Soft Tissue Injuries

After you have read this chapter, you should be able to:

- Discuss the layers of the skin and its major functions.
- Establish the relationship between body substance isolation (BSI) and soft tissue injuries.
- Establish the relationship between airway management and the patient with chest injury, burns, or blunt or penetrating injuries.
- List the types of closed and open soft tissue injuries.
- Describe the emergency medical care of closed and open soft tissue injuries.
- Discuss the emergency medical care of a penetrating chest injury and an open wound to the abdomen.
- Differentiate between the care of open wounds to the chest and to the abdomen.
- Describe the emergency medical care of a patient with an impaled object.
- List the classifications of burns.
- Define a superficial burn, list its characteristics, and describe the emergency medical care.
- Define a partial-thickness burn, list its characteristics, and describe the emergency medical care.
- Define a full-thickness burn, list its characteristics, and describe the emergency medical care.
- Define the various types of electrical burns.
- Describe the emergency care for an electrical or chemical burn.
- List the functions of dressing and bandaging.
- Describe the purpose of a bandage.
- Describe the steps in applying a pressure dressing and the effects of improperly applied dressings, splints, and tourniquets.

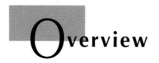

# Overview

Your skin is your first line of defense against external forces. And though it is relatively tough, your skin is still quite susceptible to injury. Injuries to soft tissues range from simple bruises and abrasions to serious lacerations and amputations. In all instances, you must control bleeding, prevent further contamination, and protect the wound from further damage. Therefore, you must know how to apply dressings and bandages to various parts of the body.

# Key Terms

**Abrasion**   Loss or damage of the superficial layer of skin after a body part rubs or scrapes across a rough or hard surface.

**Avulsion**   An injury in which a piece of skin is either torn completely loose or is hanging as a flap.

**Contamination**   The presence of infective organisms.

**Contusion**   A bruise.

**Dermis**   Inner layer of the skin containing hair follicles, sweat glands, nerve endings, and blood vessels.

**Ecchymosis**   Discoloration associated with a closed wound.

**Epidermis**   Outer layer of skin that acts as a watertight protective covering.

**Full-thickness burn**   All skin layers are burned; the subcutaneous layers, muscle, bone, or internal organs may also be burned. The area is dry, leathery, and may appear white, dark brown, or charred. Clotted blood vessels may be visible under the burned skin, or the subcutaneous fat may be visible.

**Hematoma**   Blood collected within the body's tissues or in a cavity, occasionally palpable as a discrete mass.

**Laceration**   A smooth or jagged open wound.

**Mucous membrane**   The lining of body cavities and passages that are in direct contact with the outside environment.

**Partial-thickness burn**   The epidermis and some portion of the dermis are burned. The subcutaneous tissue is not injured. Blisters form, and the skin is white to red, moist, and mottled.

**Superficial burn**   Only the epidermis is burned. The skin turns red but does not blister or actually burn through.

# THE SKIN

## ANATOMY REVIEW

The skin is the largest organ in the body. It varies in thickness, depending on age and its location. The skin of the very young and very old is thinner than the skin of a young adult. The skin covering your scalp, back, and the soles of your feet is quite thick, while the skin of your eyelids, lips, and ears is very thin. Thin skin is more easily damaged than thick skin.

The skin has two principal layers—the epidermis and the dermis. The **epidermis** is the tough, external layer. It forms a watertight covering for the body. The epidermis is itself composed of several layers. The cells on the surface layer of the epidermis are constantly worn away. They are replaced by cells pushed to the surface when new cells form in the germinal layer at the base of the epidermis. Deeper cells in the germinal layer contain pigment granules. Along with blood vessels in the dermis, these granules produce skin color (Figure 23-1).

The **dermis** is the inner layer of the skin. It lies below the germinal cells of the epidermis. The dermis contains the structures that give the skin its characteristic appearance—hair follicles, sweat glands, and sebaceous glands.

The sweat glands act to cool the body. They discharge sweat onto the surface of the skin through small pores, or ducts, that

## FIGURE 23-1

Layers of the skin

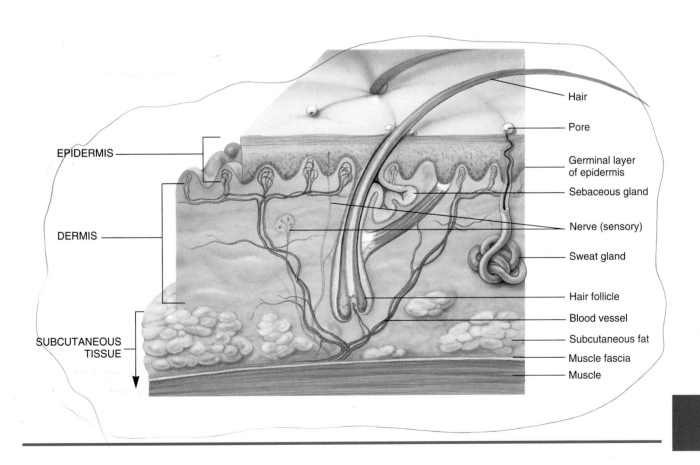

EPIDERMIS

DERMIS

SUBCUTANEOUS TISSUE

Hair

Pore

Germinal layer of epidermis

Sebaceous gland

Nerve (sensory)

Sweat gland

Hair follicle

Blood vessel

Subcutaneous fat

Muscle fascia

Muscle

pass through the epidermis. Sebaceous glands produce sebum, the oily material that waterproofs the skin and keeps it supple. Sebum travels to the skin's surface along the shaft of adjacent hair follicles.

Hair follicles are small organs that produce hair. There is one follicle for each hair. Each follicle is connected with a sebaceous gland and a tiny muscle. This muscle pulls the hair erect whenever you are cold or frightened.

Blood vessels in the dermis provide the skin with nutrients and oxygen. Small branches reach up to the germinal cells, but no blood vessels penetrate farther into the epidermis. There are also specialized nerve endings within the dermis.

The skin covers all external surfaces of the body. The various openings in our body, including the mouth, nose, anus, and vagina, are not covered by skin. Instead, these openings are lined with **mucous membranes.** These membranes are similar to skin. They, too, provide a protective barrier against bacterial invasion. But mucous membranes differ from skin because they secrete a watery substance that lubricates the openings. Thus, mucous membranes are moist, while skin is dry.

## FUNCTIONS OF THE SKIN

The skin serves many functions. It protects the body by keeping bacteria out and water in. The nerves in the skin report to the brain on the environment and on many sensations.

The skin is also the body's major organ for regulating temperature. In a cold environment, the blood vessels in the skin constrict. Thus, blood is diverted away from the skin. This decreases the amount of heat that is radiated from the body's surface. In hot environments, the vessels in the skin dilate. The skin becomes flushed or red, and heat radiates from the body's surface. Also, sweat glands secrete sweat. As the sweat

evaporates from the skin's surface, your body temperature drops—you begin to cool down.

Any break in the skin allows bacteria to enter. Infection, fluid loss, and loss of temperature control are also possible. Any one of these problems can cause serious illness and even death.

# SOFT TISSUE INJURIES

Because the soft tissues are exposed to the environment, they are often injured. There are three types of soft tissue injuries: closed injuries, open injuries, and burns. When soft tissue damage occurs beneath the skin or mucous membrane but the surface remains intact, this injury is called a "closed" injury. An injury is considered "open" when there is a break in the surface of the skin or the mucous membrane. This type of injury exposes deeper tissue to potential contamination. Burns occur when soft tissue receives more energy than it can absorb without injury. The sources of this energy could be thermal heat, frictional heat, toxic chemicals, electricity, or nuclear radiation.

## CLOSED INJURIES

Closed soft tissue injuries are characterized by a history of blunt trauma, pain at the site of injury, swelling beneath the skin, and discoloration. Such injuries can vary from mild to quite severe.

### Types of Closed Injuries

A **contusion** (bruise) results from blunt force striking the body. The epidermis remains intact, but cells within the dermis are damaged and small blood vessels are usually torn. The depth of the injury varies, depending on the amount of energy absorbed. As fluid and blood leak into the damaged area, the patient may have swelling and pain. The buildup of blood produces a characteristic discoloration. Usually black or blue, this discoloration is called **ecchymosis** (Figure 23-2).

A **hematoma** is a pool of blood that has collected within damaged tissue or in a cavity (Figure 23-3). It occurs whenever a large blood vessel is damaged and bleeds rapidly. It is usually associated with extensive tissue damage. A hematoma can result from a soft tissue injury, a fracture, or any injury to a large blood vessel. In severe cases, the hematoma may contain more than a liter of blood.

## FIGURE 23-2

A contusion

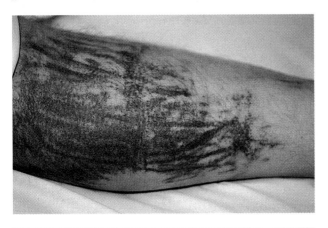

A crushing injury occurs when a great amount of force is applied to the body for a long period of time. The key with crushing injuries is the period of time in which the body is under the force. In addition to causing some direct soft tissue damage, continued compression of the soft tissues during the crushing will cut off their circulation. This will produce further tissue destruction.

## FIGURE 23-3

A hematoma

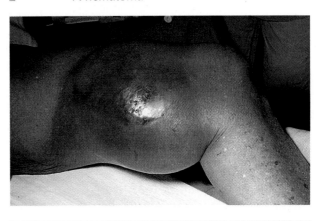

For example, a patient's legs are trapped under a collapsed pile of rocks. The tissues in the patient's legs will continue to be damaged until the compressing rocks are removed.

Another form of compression can result from the tissue damage itself. Whenever tissues are injured, swelling occurs. The cells that are injured leak watery fluid into the spaces between the cells. This results in swelling of the tissues. If swelling is excessive or occurs in a confined space such as the skull, the tissue pressure will increase to dangerous levels. The pressure of the fluid may become great enough to compress the tissue and cause further damage. This is especially true if the blood vessels become compressed, cutting off the blood flow to the tissue. Excessive swelling often follows injury of the brain, the spinal cord, and the extremities.

Severe closed injuries can also damage internal organs. The greater the amount of energy absorbed from the blunt force, the greater the risk of injury to deeper structures. Therefore, assess all patients with closed injuries for more serious hidden injuries. Remain alert for signs of shock or internal bleeding and begin treatment, if necessary.

## Emergency Medical Care

Small contusions require no special emergency medical care. More extensive closed injuries may involve significant swelling and bleeding beneath the skin. This could lead to hypovolemic shock. Before treating a closed injury, make sure to follow BSI techniques. Wash your hands thoroughly and wear gloves as you work with the patient.

Soft tissue injuries may look rather dramatic. However, you must make sure to focus on airway and breathing first. Always provide oxygen and maintain the airway in patients who need it. If the patient has difficulty breathing, you may have to assist ventilations.

You can control bleeding and swelling of a deep soft tissue injury by immediately applying ice and compression at the injury site. Ice or cold packs cause blood vessels to constrict, which slows the bleeding. Firm manual compression over the injury site compresses the blood vessels, which also slows bleeding.

Elevating the injured part just above the level of the patient's heart decreases swelling. Immobilizing a soft tissue injury or an injured extremity with a splint is another way to decrease bleeding. In addition, application of cold packs and splinting reduces pain. Therefore, you can treat a closed soft tissue injury with "ICES" (Ice, Compression, Elevation, and Splinting). You should also be alert for signs of developing shock.

Internal organs may be damaged or injured in patients with soft tissue injuries. This may result in internal bleeding. If the patient appears to be in shock, you should elevate the patient's legs, provide oxygen, and give IV fluids (if you are trained to do so and if allowed by medical control). Briefly, the signs and symptoms of shock include low blood pressure, high heart rate, and cool or clammy skin. Whenever a patient appears to be in shock, you must provide rapid transport to the hospital.

## OPEN INJURIES

Open injuries differ from closed injuries in that the protective layer of skin is damaged. This can produce more extensive bleeding. More important, however, a break in the protective skin layer means the wound is contaminated and may become infected. You must address these two problems in your treatment of open soft tissue wounds.

### Types of Open Injuries

There are four types of open soft tissue wounds: abrasions, lacerations, avulsions, and penetrating wounds.

An **abrasion** occurs when a friction rub damages the superficial layer of the skin. Blood may ooze from the injured capillaries in the dermis. An abrasion usually does not penetrate completely through the dermis. Known by a variety of names ("road rash," "road burn," "strawberry," and "mat burn"), abrasions can be extremely painful (Figure 23-4).

A **laceration** is a cut caused by a sharp object or a blunt force that tears the tissue. The depth of the injury can vary. A laceration may appear linear (regular) or stellate (irregular), and may occur along with other types of soft tissue injury. Lacerations may extend through the skin and subcutaneous tissue into the underlying muscles and adjacent nerves and blood vessels. Bleeding may be severe (Figure 23-5).

An **avulsion** is an injury that creates a flap of soft tissue, which is either completely unattached or hangs as a flap (Figure 23-6). Avulsed tissues ordinarily separate between the subcutaneous tissue and fascia. Usually there is significant bleeding. If the avulsed tissue is hanging from a small piece of skin, the circulation through the flap may be at risk. If an avulsion is complete, you should wrap the tissue in sterile gauze and bring it with you to the emergency department.

FIGURE 23-4

An abrasion

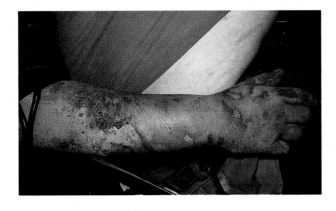

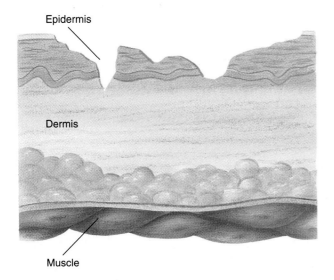

Epidermis

Dermis

Muscle

FIGURE 23-5

A laceration

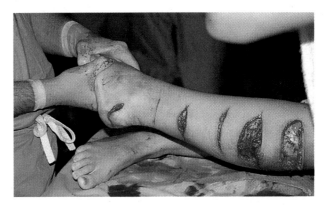

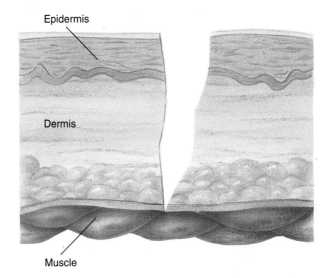

Epidermis

Dermis

Muscle

We usually think of amputations as involving the upper and lower extremities. But other body parts, such as the scalp, ear, nose, or lips, may also be totally avulsed, or amputated. You can easily control the bleeding from some amputations, such as the fingers. But, if an avulsion involves large areas of muscle mass, such as a thigh, there may be massive bleeding. In this situation, you need to treat the patient for hypovolemic shock.

A **penetrating wound** is an injury resulting from a sharp, pointed object, such as a knife, ice pick, splinter, or bullet. Such ob-

jects leave relatively small entrance wounds, so there may be little external bleeding (Figure 23-7). However, these objects can damage structures deep within the body. If the wound is in the chest or abdomen, the injury could cause rapid, fatal bleeding. Assessing the amount of damage a puncture wound has created is very difficult.

Stabbings and shootings often result in multiple penetrating injuries. It is essential that you assess these patients carefully to identify all wounds. Since a penetrating object can pass completely through the body, always look for both entrance and

## FIGURE 23-6

An avulsion

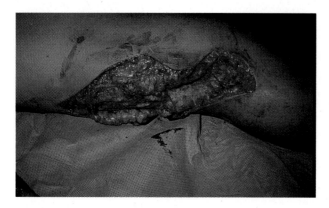

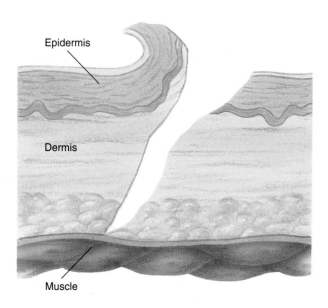

Epidermis

Dermis

Muscle

## FIGURE 23-7

A puncture wound

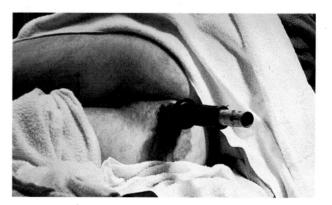

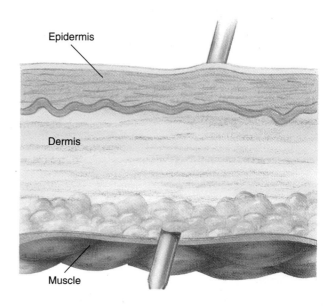

Epidermis

Dermis

Muscle

exit wounds. This is especially important with gunshot wounds. An entrance wound is usually smaller than an exit wound. A gun shot at close range will leave an entrance wound with powder burns around the edges (Figure 23-8). Because of its larger size, an exit wound may bleed excessively and yet be less apparent than an entrance wound.

Gunshot wounds have some unique characteristics that require special care. The amount of damage from a gunshot wound is directly related to the speed of the bullet. Thus, it is important to find out the type of

gun used in the shooting. This information can help the hospital personnel better care for the patient.

Often, the victim of a shooting will have multiple wounds. Assess the patient carefully to identify the number and locations of all bullet wounds. Sometimes the patient or bystanders can tell you how many rounds were fired. This information can be useful to hospital personnel.

Carefully document the circumstances surrounding any gunshot injury, the patient's condition, and the treatment given. Most shootings involve litigation at some

## FIGURE 23-8

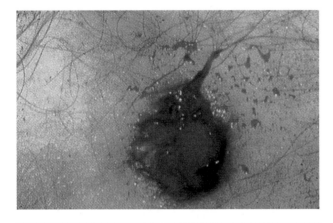

A close-range gunshot wound

future date. You may be called by the court to testify regarding conditions at the scene or any treatments you gave the patient. Only a carefully written record will be of any use to you in court.

Crushing injuries may cause extensive soft tissue damage. As with closed wounds caused by crushing, the internal organs may be damaged or bones may be broken. Although there may be minimal external bleeding, internal bleeding may be severe, even life threatening.

### Emergency Medical Care

Before you begin caring for a patient with an open wound, you should be sure to protect yourself by following BSI techniques. Wash your hands well and then put on gloves. Eye protection is essential to prevent contamination. Gowns provide additional protection, if necessary. Remember that before you can care for the wound, you must be sure the patient has an open airway and is given oxygen if necessary.

It is critical that you assess the severity of the wound. Remove any clothing covering the wound. Now you can complete your assessment and begin treatment.

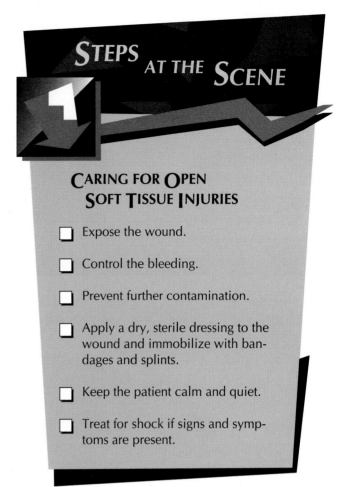

### STEPS AT THE SCENE

#### CARING FOR OPEN SOFT TISSUE INJURIES

- ☐ Expose the wound.
- ☐ Control the bleeding.
- ☐ Prevent further contamination.
- ☐ Apply a dry, sterile dressing to the wound and immobilize with bandages and splints.
- ☐ Keep the patient calm and quiet.
- ☐ Treat for shock if signs and symptoms are present.

The amount of bleeding with open wounds can be extensive and severe. Thus your first priority is to control the bleeding. To do this, apply a dry, sterile compression dressing over the entire wound. Apply pressure to the dressing with your gloved hand and then maintain this pressure by firmly applying a roller bandage to the injured part (Figure 23-9). If bleeding continues or recurs, leave the original dressing in place. Apply a second dressing on top of the first and secure it with another roller bandage. Once you have controlled the bleeding, keep the dressing in place with a splint.

All open wounds are contaminated and present a risk of infection. **Contamination** occurs as soon as the protective covering of the skin or mucous membrane is broken.

**FIGURE 23-9**

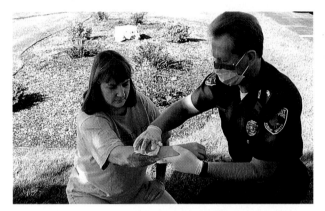

**A** Apply direct pressure with your gloved hand

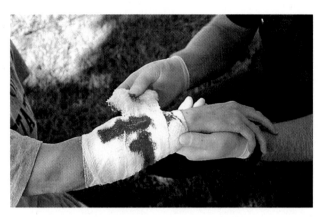

**B** Apply a compression dressing and secure with a roller bandage

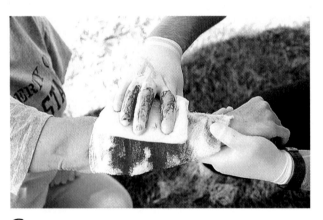

**C** Continue to apply pressure

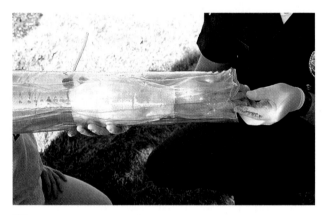

**D** Apply an air splint

You will prevent further contamination of an open wound when you apply the dry, sterile dressing. This keeps foreign material, such as hair, clothing, and dirt, out of the wound and decreases the risk of secondary infection. However, do not try to remove material from an open wound—no matter how dirty the wound is. Rubbing, brushing, or washing an open wound will only cause additional bleeding. Only hospital personnel should clean out an open wound.

Often, you can better control bleeding from open soft tissue wounds—whether or not they are associated with fractures—by splinting the extremity. Splinting can also help you keep the patient calm and quiet, as it often reduces pain. In addition, splinting keeps sterile dressings in place, minimizes damage to an already injured extremity, and makes moving the patient easier.

A patient who is bleeding significantly from an open wound can go into hypovolemic shock. You must be alert for this possibility and provide treatment, as needed.

### Chest Wounds

A penetrating wound to the chest may result in air entering the chest from the outside (pneumothorax). This type of wound may also cause blood to collect in the chest (hemothorax). Outside air may be sucked through the open wound as the patient inhales. Ordinarily the pressure inside the chest cavity is slightly less than that of the atmosphere. Inhalation further reduces this pressure. If there is an open wound in the chest wall, air will move through the wound just as easily as it moves through the nose and mouth during normal breathing. The air that enters through the wound remains in the pleural space, and the lung does not expand. When the patient exhales, air passes back through the wound. Such open wounds are called sucking chest wounds. With these wounds, each time the patient breathes there is a sucking sound at the wound caused by the passage of air. This reduces the lungs' ability to provide fresh oxygen to the blood.

As an initial emergency step, after providing oxygen to the patient, you must seal a sucking chest wound with an occlusive (airtight) dressing. The purpose of the occlusive dressing is to seal the wound and prevent air from passing through it. Several sterile materials, including aluminum foil, Vaseline gauze, or a folded universal dressing may be used to seal the wound. Use a large enough dressing so it is not pulled or sucked into the chest cavity. Tape three sides of the dressing to the chest wall. Leave one edge free to allow air to escape if pressure builds up in the chest.

Blood can also collect in the chest as a result of injury. This buildup of blood can result in difficulty breathing and/or shock. Emergency medical care should include giving the patient oxygen, elevating the patient's legs, and giving IV fluids (if you are trained to do so and if approved by medical control). Rapid transport is essential.

### Abdominal Wounds

An open wound in the abdominal cavity may expose internal organs (Figure 23-10). In some cases, the organs may even protrude through the wound (evisceration). Do not touch or move the exposed organs. Instead, cover the exposed organs with a sterile dressing moistened with sterile water or saline. Secure the dressing in place. If the patient's legs and knees are uninjured, flex them to relieve pressure on the abdomen. Rapid transport is essential with all abdominal wounds.

### FIGURE 23-10

An abdominal evisceration

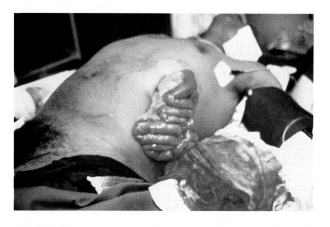

### Penetrating Wounds

Occasionally, a patient will have an object, such as a knife, a wood splinter, or a piece of glass impaled in the body (Figure 23-11a). *Do not attempt to move or remove the object, unless it is impaled through the cheek.* As with all open wounds, remove any clothing covering the injury. Control bleeding and use a bulky dressing to stabilize the object (Figure 23-11b). Remember,

## FIGURE 23-11

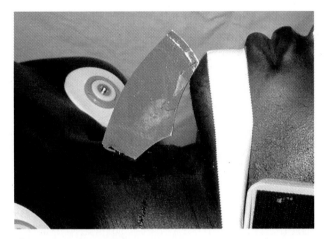

**A**    Glass impaled in the neck

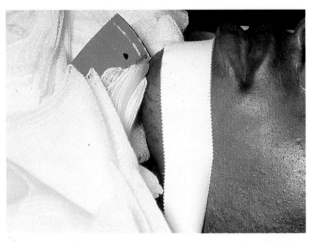

**B**    Apply a dressing over the wound

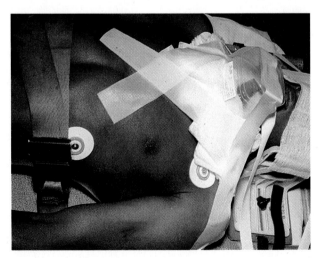

**C**    Secure the dressing with gauze and tape

do not remove the object. Moving the object may damage nerves, blood vessels, or muscles within the wound. Ordinarily, the patient needs surgery to remove the object. To prevent further injury, manually secure the object by incorporating it into the dressing (Figure 23-11c). The only exception to this rule is if the object is impaled in the cheek and obstructs breathing. In this situation, it is more important to restore the airway. If the object is very long, cut off (shorten) the exposed portion. This will make transport much easier. However, before cutting the object, secure it to minimize any motion, which could cause further internal damage and pain. Once the object is secured, and the bleeding is under control, provide prompt transport.

### Amputations

If a patient has experienced an amputation, it is now often possible to replace or reimplant the amputated part (Figure 23-12). However, correct prehospital care of the amputated part is vital for successful reattachment. With partial amputations, make sure you immobilize the part with bulky compression dressings and a splint.

## FIGURE 23-12

An amputated arm

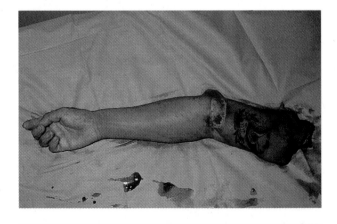

Do not sever any partial amputations. This may make it impossible to reimplant the part. With a complete amputation, make sure you wrap the part in a dry, sterile dressing and place it in a dry, plastic bag. Put the bag in a cool container. Do not soak the part in water or saline or allow it to freeze.

### Neck Injuries

An open neck injury could be life threatening. If the veins of the neck are open to the environment, they may suck in air. If enough air is "sucked" into a blood vessel, it can actually block the flow of blood in the lungs. The patient could go into cardiac arrest. This condition is called air embolism. To control bleeding and prevent the possibility of air embolism, cover the wound with an occlusive dressing. Apply manual pressure, but do not compress both carotid vessels at the same time. If you do, this may impair circulation to the brain. Secure a pressure dressing over the wound by wrapping roller gauze loosely around the neck and then firmly through the opposite axilla (Figure 23-13).

## FIGURE 23-13

Proper dressing of a neck wound

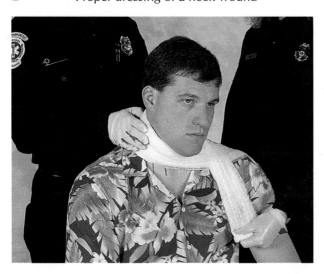

# BURNS

As an EMT-B, you will often provide care to patients who have been burned. Burns are a common cause of accidental death in the United States. Burns account for over 10,000 deaths a year. Most cases involve children under the age of 6. Burns are also among the most serious and painful of all injuries.

A patient is burned when the body, or a body part, receives more energy than it can absorb without injury. Potential sources of this energy include heat, toxic chemicals, and electricity. The proper emergency care of a burn may enhance a patient's survival and decrease the risk or duration of a long-term disability. While a burn may be the most obvious injury, you should always perform a complete assessment to determine if there are other serious injuries.

## BURN SEVERITY

It is important to try to estimate the seriousness of a burn injury. This information will help medical control direct you to the proper treatment facility. The following five factors will help you determine the severity of a burn:

1. Depth of the burn (superficial, partial thickness, or full thickness)
2. Extent of the burn
3. The involvement of critical areas
4. Pre-existing medical conditions or the presence of other injuries
5. The age of the patient

### Depth

Burns are first classified according to their depth (Figure 23-14). You must be able to identify the following three types of burns:

## FIGURE 23-14

Classification of burns

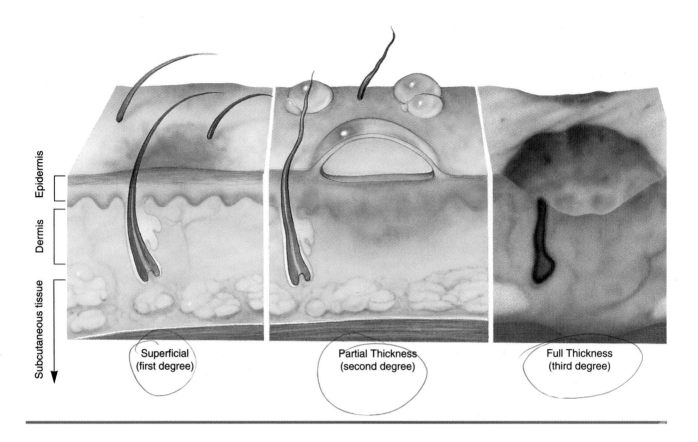

Superficial (first degree)

Partial Thickness (second degree)

Full Thickness (third degree)

1. Superficial (first-degree) burns
2. Partial-thickness (second-degree) burns
3. Full-thickness (third-degree) burns

Many burn centers prefer the more descriptive terminology of superficial, partial-thickness, and full-thickness burns over the traditional terms first-degree, second-degree, and third-degree burns. In this text, we will be using the descriptive terms.

**Superficial burns** involve only the top layer of skin, the epidermis (Figure 23-15). The skin turns red but does not blister or actually burn through. The burn site is painful. A sunburn is a good example of a superficial burn.

**Partial-thickness burns** involve the epidermis and some portion of the dermis (Figure 23-16). These burns do not destroy the entire thickness of the skin nor is the subcutaneous tissue injured. Typically, the skin is moist, mottled, and white to red. Blisters are common. Partial-thickness burns cause intense pain.

**Full-thickness burns** extend through all skin layers and may involve subcutaneous layers, muscle, bone, or internal organs (Figure 23-17). The burned area is dry and leathery and may appear white, dark brown, or even charred. Some full-thickness burns feel hard to the touch due to their leathery consistency. Clotted blood vessels may be visible under the burned skin, or

## FIGURE 23-15

Superficial burns

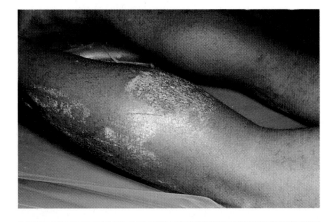

## FIGURE 23-16

Partial-thickness burns

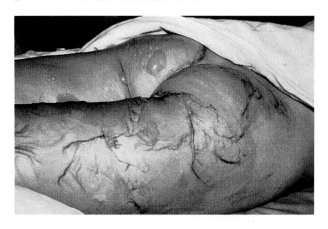

## FIGURE 23-17

Full-thickness burns

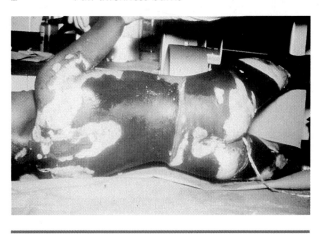

the subcutaneous fat may be visible. If the nerve endings have been destroyed, a severely burned area may have no feeling. However, the surrounding, less severely burned areas may be extremely painful.

Severe burns are typically a combination of superficial, partial-thickness, and full-thickness burns. It is unusual to have a purely full-thickness burn. Superficial burns heal well without scarring. Small partial-thickness burns also heal without scarring. However, deep partial-thickness burns and all full-thickness burns are best managed surgically.

It may be impossible to accurately estimate the depth of a particular burn. Even experienced burn surgeons underestimate or, more commonly, overestimate the extent of a particular burn.

### Extent

One quick way to estimate the surface area that has been burned is to compare it to the size of the patient's hand, which is roughly equal to 1% of the body's total surface area.

Another useful system is the Rule of Nines. The **Rule of Nines** is a system that divides the body into sections, each of which is approximately 9% of the body's total surface area (Figure 23-18). Remember that, for infants and small children, the head is relatively larger than in adults, and the legs are relatively smaller.

These two factors—depth and extent—are critical in assessing the severity of a burn. There are three other factors you should take into account, as follows:

1. Are any critical areas (face, upper airway, hands, genitalia) burned?

## FIGURE 23-18

Rule of Nines

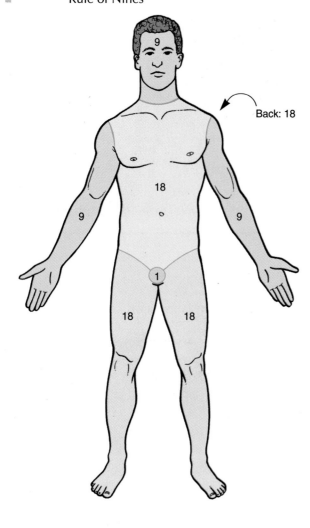

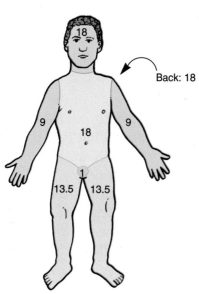

2. Are there any pre-existing conditions or other injuries?

3. Is the patient younger than 5 or older than 55?

If the answer to any of these questions is "Yes," you should upgrade the burn's classification (Table 23-1).

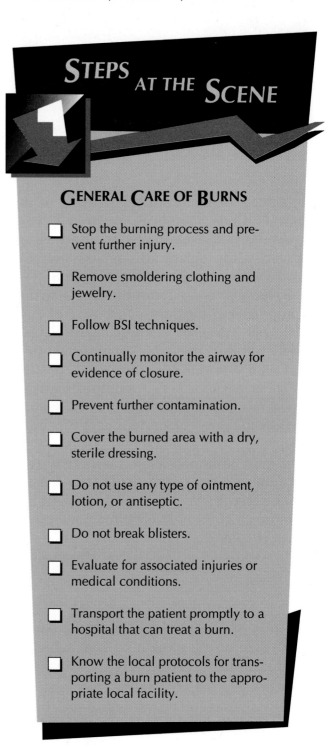

# STEPS AT THE SCENE

## GENERAL CARE OF BURNS

☐ Stop the burning process and prevent further injury.

☐ Remove smoldering clothing and jewelry.

☐ Follow BSI techniques.

☐ Continually monitor the airway for evidence of closure.

☐ Prevent further contamination.

☐ Cover the burned area with a dry, sterile dressing.

☐ Do not use any type of ointment, lotion, or antiseptic.

☐ Do not break blisters.

☐ Evaluate for associated injuries or medical conditions.

☐ Transport the patient promptly to a hospital that can treat a burn.

☐ Know the local protocols for transporting a burn patient to the appropriate local facility.

TABLE 23-1    CLASSIFICATION OF BURNS IN ADULTS

**Critical Burns**
- Full-thickness burns involving the hands, feet, face, upper airway, or genitalia
- Full-thickness burns covering more than 10% of the body's total surface area
- Partial-thickness burns covering more than 30% of the body's total surface area
- Burns associated with respiratory injury (smoke inhalation)
- Burns complicated by a painful, swollen, and deformed extremity
- Burns on patients younger than 5 or older than 55 that would be classified as "moderate" on young adults

**Moderate Burns**
- Full-thickness burns involving 2% to 10% of the body's total surface area (excluding hands, feet, face, genitalia, or upper airway)
- Partial-thickness burns covering 15% to 30% of the body's total surface area
- Superficial burns covering more than 50% of the body's total surface area

**Minor Burns**
- Full-thickness burns covering less than 2% of the body's total surface area
- Partial-thickness burns involving less than 15% of the body's total surface area
- Superficial burns covering less than 50% of the body's total surface area

## EMERGENCY MEDICAL CARE

### General Care of Burns

Your first responsibility when responding to a burn patient is to stop the burning process and prevent additional injury. Move the patient away from the burning area. If any clothing is on fire, wrap the patient in a blanket or use a dry chemical fire extinguisher to put out the flames. Remove any smoldering clothing and/or jewelry.

If the skin or clothing is hot, immerse the area in cool water or cover with a wet, cool dressing. This not only stops the burning, it also relieves pain. Always use clean dressings and clean or sterile water to minimize the risk of infection. However, do not keep a burned area under water for more than 10 minutes. If the burning stops before you arrive, do not immerse the affected part in water. Immersion increases the risk of infection.

Because a burn destroys the patient's protective skin layer, you must follow BSI techniques. Always wear gloves and eye protection when treating a burn patient.

More fire victims die from smoke inhalation than from skin burns. A patient with burns about the face or who has inhaled smoke or fumes may develop respiratory distress (Figure 23-19). Therefore, you must be sure to give the patient oxygen and provide prompt transport. Sometimes, respiratory problems do not develop immediately. A patient who appears to be breathing well at first may suddenly develop severe respiratory distress. Therefore, continually assess the airway for possible problems.

## FIGURE 23-19

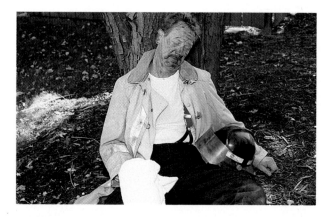

Patient with possible smoke inhalation and burns

An extensive burn can produce hypothermia (loss of body heat). Prevent further heat loss by covering the patient with warm blankets.

Rapidly estimate the burn's severity. Then cover the burned area with a dry dressing. Sterile gauze is best if the burned area is not too large. You may cover larger areas with a clean, white sheet. Most important, do not put anything else on the burned area. Use only a dry, sterile dressing or a clean, white sheet. Never use ointments, lotions, or antiseptics of any kind. In addition, do not intentionally break any blisters.

If the patient has a critical burn, give oxygen. Most burn patients have normal vital signs and can communicate at first. Always check for traumatic injuries or other medical conditions, which may be more immediately life threatening. Treat the patient for shock, if necessary.

It is important that you provide prompt transport for burn patients. If you are within 20 minutes of a hospital, do not delay transporting an adult victim by prolonged assessment and applying coverings to burns. With pediatric burn victims, it is best to "scoop and run" if transport time is less than 1 hour.

## PEDIATRIC CONSIDERATIONS

Burns to children are generally considered more serious than adult burns (Table 23-2). Infants and children have more surface area relative to total body mass than do adults. This means greater fluid and heat loss. In addition, children do not tolerate burns as well as adults. Plus, children are more likely to go into shock, develop hypothermia, and experience airway problems.

## TABLE 23-2    CLASSIFICATION OF BURNS IN INFANTS AND CHILDREN

**Critical Burns**
- Full-thickness or partial-thickness burns covering more than 20% of the body's total surface area
- Burns involving the hands, feet, face, airway, or genitalia

**Moderate Burns**
- Partial-thickness burns covering 10% to 20% of the body's total surface area

**Minor Burns**
- Partial-thickness burns covering less than 10% of the body's total surface area

You are listening on the scanner and hear law enforcement dispatched to an automobile accident out in the county. Moments later, you and your partner are dispatched to the same location. As you are pulling up, you see a small sports car smashed up against a concrete bridge abutment. There is extensive damage to the front end. The rescue team is already at work trying to free the unbelted driver who has gone down under the steering wheel. You climb through the shattered rear window to access the 17-year-old boy. From what you can see, he has two broken legs, and extensive soft tissue injuries. He is responsive to pain by withdrawing. He has no radial pulse, but has a fast, but weak carotid pulse at 138/min. He has a blood pressure of 98/62 mm Hg, respirations of 26/min, and pale, cool, clammy skin.

### For Discussion

1. Describe the philosophy and goals behind the Rapid Extrication technique.

2. Explain the concept of the Golden Hour. How does it impact survival of the trauma patient?

Many burns in infants and children result from child abuse. You should report suspected cases to the proper authorities. The classic burn resulting from deliberate immersion involves the hands and wrists as well as the feet, lower legs, and buttocks. Similarly, burns around the genitals and multiple cigarette burns should be viewed as possible abuse.

## CHEMICAL BURNS

A chemical burn can occur whenever a toxic substance contacts the body. Most chemical burns are caused by strong acids or strong alkalis. The eyes are particularly vulnerable to chemical burns. Sometimes the fumes of strong chemicals can cause burns, especially to the respiratory tract.

To prevent exposure to hazardous materials, you must wear gloves and eye protection whenever you are caring for a patient with a chemical burn. Be particularly careful not to get any chemical, dry or liquid, on yourself or on your uniform.

The emergency care of a chemical burn is basically the same as that for a thermal burn. To stop the burning process, remove any chemical from the patient. A dry chemical that is activated by contact with water may damage the skin more when it is wet than when it is dry. Therefore, always brush dry chemicals off the skin and clothing before flushing the patient with water (Figure 23-20). Remove the patient's clothing, including shoes, stockings, and gloves because there may be small amounts of chemicals in the creases.

FIGURE **23-21**

Flush chemical burns with water

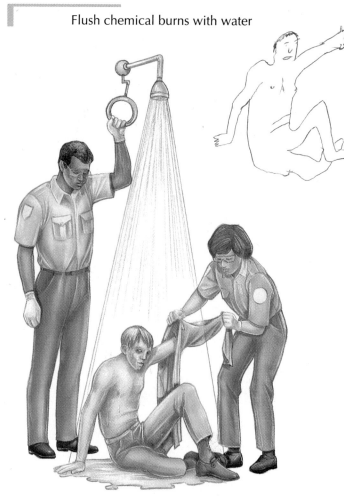

## FIGURE **23-20**

Brush dry chemicals off the patient before flushing with water

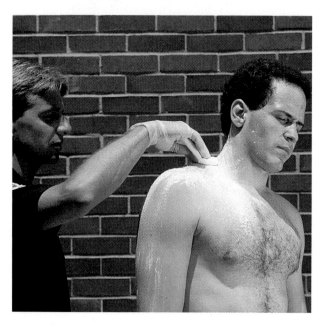

Immediately begin to flush the burned area with large amounts of water (Figure 23-21). Make sure you do not contaminate un-injured areas while flushing the burned area. Do not direct a forceful stream of water from a hose at the patient. The extreme water pressure may mechanically injure the burned skin. Continue flooding the area with gallons of water for 10 minutes after the patient says the burning pain has stopped. If it is the eye that is burned, hold the eyelid open while flooding with a gentle stream of water (Figure 23-22). Continue flushing the contaminated area while en route to the hospital.

## FIGURE **23-22**

Flush the eyes with water after a chemical burn

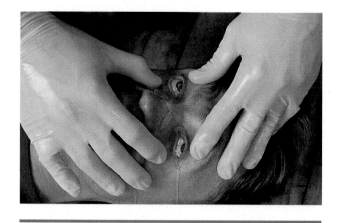

# EMT

## BEAT THE MACHINE

YOU ARE THE EMT

The new employee at the Triple Star Beef plant has been assigned to operate the beef jerky machine and is given a brief orientation as to the operation of the machine. Because he's working too slow and is behind quota, he decides to remove a safety guard so he can feed the beef in faster. Moments later he finds himself being pulled into a small auger on the top of his machine. A co-worker hears his screams, and hits the drive lever, shifting the machine into neutral. The co-worker then runs over to the phone and calls 9-1-1. On arrival, you find a 24-year-old man whose hand is entrapped, pulled into the machine up to the wrist. The machine is still running in neutral.

### For Discussion

1. Why would it be safer to manually remove the patient rather than reverse the machine mechanically?

2. How can assessment of the mechanism of injury be helpful with planning patient assessment as well as planning extrication?

## ELECTRICAL BURNS

Electrical burns may be the result of contact with high- or low-voltage electricity. Ordinary household current is powerful enough to cause severe burns. High-voltage burns may occur when utility workers make direct contact with power lines.

In order for electricity to flow, there must be a complete circuit between the electrical source and the ground. Any substance that prevents this circuit from being completed is called an "insulator." Rubber, for example, is an insulator. Any substance that allows a current to flow through it is called a "conductor." The human body, which is primarily water, is a good conductor. Electrical burns occur when the body, or a part of it, completes a circuit connecting a power source to the ground (Figure 23-23).

Your safety is of particular importance when you are called to the scene of an emergency involving electricity. You can be fatally injured from accidental contact with power lines.

If, upon your arrival, the patient is still in contact with the electrical source—or you are unsure—do not touch the patient. Touching someone in contact with a live power line will put you in the circuit and injure you as well. ***Never attempt to remove someone from an electrical source unless you are specially trained to do so.*** Likewise, you should never move a downed line unless

## FIGURE 23-23

The body forms a circuit for electricity to travel

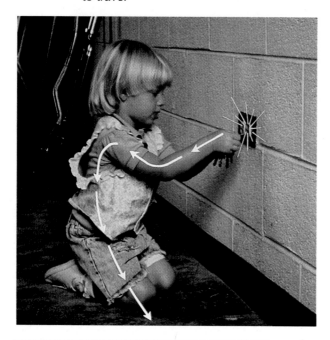

## FIGURE 23-24

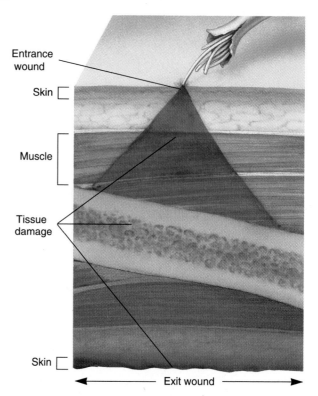

Entrance wound

Skin

Muscle

Tissue damage

Skin

Exit wound

**A** Tissue damage as a result of electrical burn

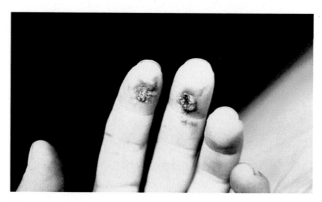

**B** Electrical burns often have entrance and exit wounds

you are absolutely certain it is not live—or you have the special training and equipment necessary to handle live power lines. Before approaching anyone who may still be in contact with a power line or an electrical appliance, make certain the power is turned off.

To cause injury, electricity must flow through the body. There is always a burn injury where the electricity entered the body (an entrance wound) and another where it exited (an exit wound). The entrance wound may be quite small, but the exit wound can be extensive and deep (Figure 23-24).

Two dangers are specifically associated with electrical burns. First, there may be a large amount of deep tissue injury. Electrical burns are always more severe than the external signs indicate. The patient may have only a small burn to the skin but have massive damage to the deeper tissues. Second, the patient may go into cardiac arrest from the electric shock.

If indicated, begin CPR. CPR may be a prolonged procedure in these cases. However, success rates are high when CPR is begun promptly and then sustained. If CPR is not indicated, give oxygen and monitor the patient closely for respiratory and cardiac arrest. Treat the soft tissue injuries by placing dry, sterile dressings on all burn wounds and splinting suspected fractures. Provide prompt transport of all patients with electrical burns. All electrical burns are potentially severe injuries that require further treatment in the hospital.

## DRESSING AND BANDAGING

All wounds require bandaging. In most instances, splints help control bleeding and provide firm support for the dressing. There are many different types of dressings and bandages. You should be familiar with the function and proper application of each. In general, dressings and bandages have three primary functions: 1) to control bleeding, 2) to protect the wound from further damage, and 3) to prevent further contamination and infection.

### STERILE DRESSINGS

All ambulances carry sterile dressings. Universal dressings, conventional 4" × 4" and 4" × 8" gauze pads, and assorted small adhesive-type dressings and soft self-adherent roller dressings will cover most wounds.

Measuring 9"× 36", the universal dressing is ideal for covering large open wounds (Figure 23-25). It also makes an efficient pad for rigid splints. Made of thick, absorbent material, these dressings are available in compact, commercially sterilized packages. The universal dressing material is also available in 20-yard rolls. Some EMS personnel cut this material into 3' lengths, which they package and sterilize themselves.

Gauze pads are appropriate for smaller wounds. Adhesive-type dressings are useful

for minor wounds. Occlusive dressings, made of Vaseline gauze, aluminum foil, or plastic, prevent air and liquids from entering (or exiting) the wound (Figure 23-26). They are used to cover sucking chest wounds and abdominal eviscerations.

## FIGURE 23-25

A universal dressing

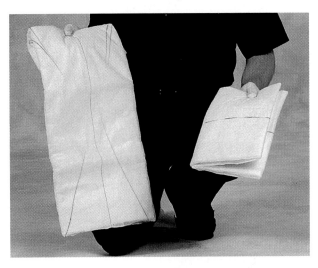

## FIGURE 23-26

An occlusive dressing

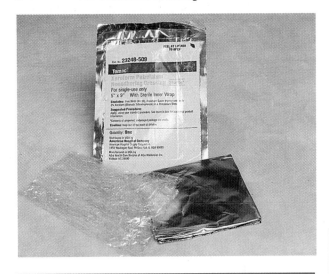

## BANDAGES

Dressings must remain in place during transport. You can use soft roller bandages, rolls of gauze, triangular bandages, or adhesive tape to secure dressings. The self-adherent, soft roller bandages are probably easiest to use (Figure 23-27). They are slightly elastic, which makes them easy to apply. The layers adhere somewhat to one another, and you can tuck the end of the roll into a deeper layer to secure it in place.

Adhesive tape holds small dressings in place and helps secure larger dressings. Some people, however, are allergic to adhesive tape. Use paper or plastic tape for these patients, if you have this information.

**FIGURE 23-27**

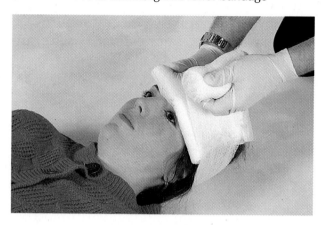

A self-adhering soft roller bandage

## FROM PAINT TO PAIN

A young first-time homeowner has just finished painting his garage and is now cleaning the paint brushes with gasoline. As he finishes cleaning each brush, he tosses them into the sink in the laundry room so he can rinse them out later with soap and water. Without warning, the hot water heater kicks on, and the gasoline fumes explode, momentarily engulfing the young man. The patient's wife calls 9-1-1 and then the fire department. As it turns out, she quickly extinguishes the fire, and there is no work for the fire department. You arrive to find her 27-year-old husband lying supine in the front yard in obvious distress. He is complaining of severe pain and has a dry cough. The anterior part of his chest, both arms, and his face are burned and blistered.

### For Discussion

1. Why are children at high risk when they are burned?

2. Discuss the similarities and the differences in the prehospital care given for chemical and electrical burns.

YOU ARE THE EMT

TRAUMA

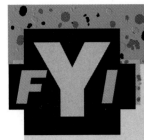

## Gas Inhalation

Poisonous gas can be just as dangerous as smoke. Fires produce two particularly dangerous gases: carbon monoxide and cyanide. There's a good chance that someone trapped in a burning building or room has inhaled carbon monoxide. This odorless and tasteless gas does not irritate the respiratory tract. Thus, a patient who has inhaled carbon monoxide does not always cough, bring up sputum, or even know that he or she has inhaled a toxin.

Cyanide gas is produced when plastics burn. It has a characteristic odor of burnt almonds. A patient may not recognize the odor, however, and may be unaware of the inhaled cyanide.

Both carbon monoxide and cyanide gases are poisons. They interfere with the red blood cells' ability to transport oxygen. If you suspect a patient has inhaled either gas, move the patient out of the burning area as rapidly as possible. Remember to protect yourself from inhaling poison gas by wearing the proper mask system.

Once the patient is in an open area, treat any burns and immediately administer 100% oxygen through a nonrebreathing mask. Transport the patient rapidly to the hospital.

Do not use elastic bandages to secure dressings. If the injury swells, the elastic bandage may become a tourniquet and cause further damage. Bandages should never interfere with a limb's circulation. Always check a limb distal to a bandage for signs of impaired circulation or loss of sensation. An improperly applied bandage can result in additional tissue damage or even the loss of a limb if it impairs circulation.

Air splints are useful in stabilizing broken extremities. They can be used with dressings to help control bleeding from soft tissue injuries.

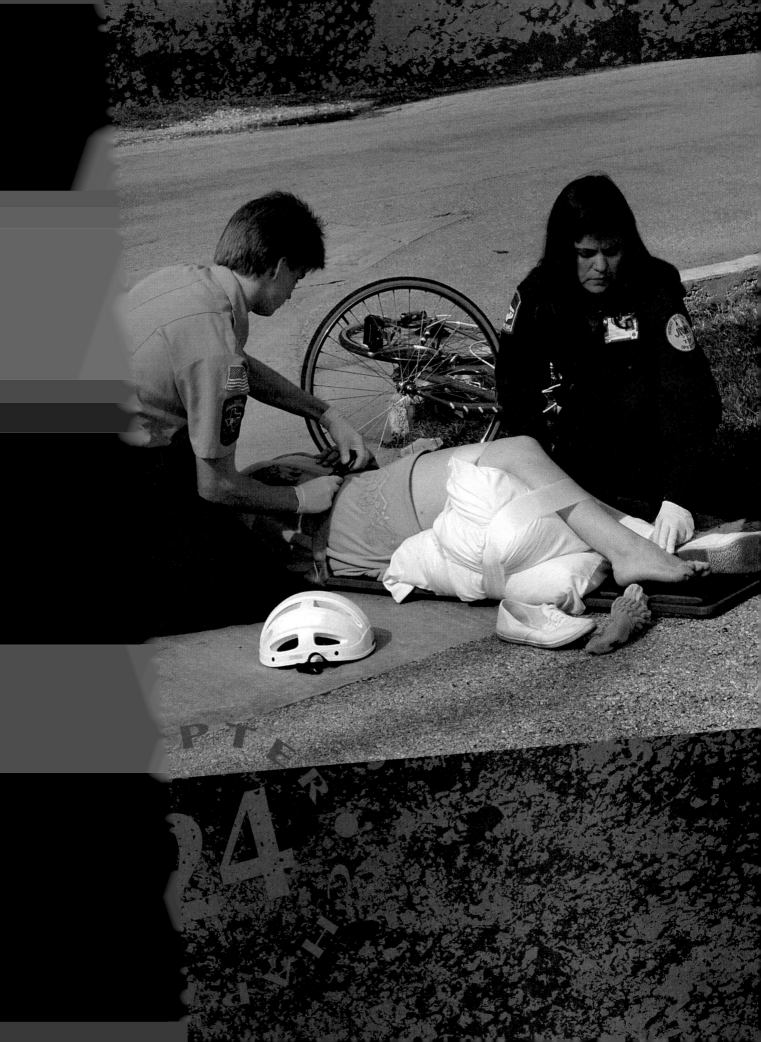

# Musculoskeletal Care

## Objectives

After you have read this chapter, you should be able to:

- Describe the function of the muscular and skeletal systems.
- List the major bones or bone groupings of the spinal column, the thorax, and the upper and lower extremities.
- Describe the difference between an open and a closed painful, swollen, deformed extremity (fracture).
- Explain the importance of splinting at the scene.
- List the general rules and complications of splinting.
- Describe the proper emergency medical care of a patient with a deformed extremity, particularly why immobilization is important.

## Overview

The form, upright posture, and movement of the human body are provided by the musculoskeletal system. The term musculoskeletal refers to the bones and voluntary muscles of the body. The musculoskeletal system also protects the vital internal organs of the body. While our bones and muscles are strong, they can be injured by external forces. More than our muscles and bones are at risk. Our tendons, joints, and ligaments may also be injured.

As an EMT-B, you must understand the basic anatomy of the musculoskeletal system. Although muscles are technically soft tissue, they are discussed here because of their close anatomic and functional relationship to the skeleton.

Musculoskeletal injuries are among the most common problems you will see as an EMT-B. You must check each patient for possible injury to bones or joints and be prepared to care for that injury properly. Your care of musculoskeletal injuries immediately relieves pain. It also decreases the possibility of shock (hypoperfusion) and further nerve or vessel injury. Proper care of these injuries also improves the patient's chances for a rapid recovery and early return to normal activity.

This chapter begins with a brief review of the musculoskeletal system. The sections that follow outline common injuries and the proper sequence for assessment of musculoskeletal injuries. Care of musculoskeletal injuries—specifically, methods of splinting and transporting—is discussed in detail.

## Key Terms

**Articular cartilage**   A thin layer of cartilage, covering the articular surface of bones in synovial joints.

**Closed fracture**   Any fracture in which the skin has not been broken by the bone ends, and there is no wound anywhere near the injury site.

**Displaced fracture**   Any injury that makes the limb appear in an unnatural position. Also called a deformity.

**Joint**   The place where two bones come in contact.

**Ligament**   A band of fibrous tissue that connects bones to bones. It supports and strengthens a joint.

**Musculoskeletal**   Pertaining to or composing the skeleton and the muscles, as the musculoskeletal system.

**Open fracture**   Any break in the bone in which the overlying skin has been damaged as well.

**Osteoporosis**   Reduction in the amount of bone mass, leading to fractures after minimal trauma.

**Point tenderness**   Tenderness sharply localized at the site of the injury found by gently palpating along the bone with the tip of one finger.

**Skeletal muscle**   Striated muscles that are attached to bones and usually cross at least one joint.

**Splint**   A rigid or flexible appliance used to keep in place and protect an injured part.

**Tendon**   A tough, rope-like cord of fibrous tissue that attaches a skeletal muscle to a bone.

**Traction**   The act of exerting a pulling force on a structure.

# ANATOMY REVIEW

## SKELETAL MUSCLE

The musculoskeletal system includes more than 600 muscles, most of which is skeletal muscle. Muscles are a form of tissue that helps the body to move. **Skeletal muscle** attaches to the bones and forms the major muscle mass of the body. Skeletal muscle is also called voluntary muscle because it is under direct voluntary control of the brain. We can make these muscles relax or contract at will. Each time we move, our skeletal muscles are relaxing and contracting. Usually, a specific movement is the result of several muscles contracting and relaxing at the same time.

All skeletal muscles are supplied with arteries, veins, and nerves. Blood from the arteries carries oxygen and nutrients to the muscle. The veins carry away the waste products, such as carbon dioxide, of muscular contraction. Muscles cannot function without an on-going supply of oxygen and nutrients and removal of waste products. Muscle cramps result when there is not enough oxygen or nutrients carried to the muscle. Cramps also occur when waste products build up and are not carried away.

Skeletal muscle is under the direct control of the central nervous system. Simply put, the brain commands the muscles, and the muscles respond. A message from the brain passes through a series of nerves to a specific part of the body. Once the brain makes the command, the message moves along specific nerves that pass directly from the brain to the spinal cord. The message is then passed off to other nerves, much like a baton in a relay race. The muscle contracts or relaxes once the message arrives. However, if the control center, the brain, is injured or damaged in some way, the messages will not travel along the network of nerves. Thus, the voluntary control of the muscle is lost, and the muscle becomes paralyzed.

Most skeletal muscles are attached directly to bone by tough, rope-like cords of fibrous tissue called **tendons.** Tendons continue the fascia that covers all skeletal muscles. Fascia is much like the skin of a sausage in that it covers the muscle tissue. At either end of the muscle, the fascia extends beyond the muscle to attach to a bone. This combination of muscle and tissue crosses over a joint and is responsible for the movement of that joint. The proximal point of attachment of the musculotendinous unit is its origin, and the distal bony attachment is called the insertion of the muscle (Figure 24-1). When a muscle contracts, a line of force is created between the origin and the insertion, which pulls the points of origin and insertion closer together. This motion occurs at the joint between the two bones.

## FIGURE 24-1

Points of tendon origin and insertion

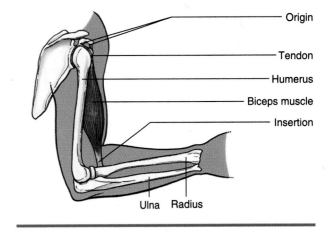

Origin
Tendon
Humerus
Biceps muscle
Insertion
Ulna   Radius

## THE SKELETON

The skeleton gives us our recognizable human form and protects our vital internal organs. The brain lies within the skull. The heart, lungs, and great vessels are protected by the thorax. Much of the liver and spleen is protected by the lower ribs. The spinal cord is contained within and protected by a bony spinal canal formed by the vertebrae.

The approximately 206 bones of the skeleton provide a framework for the attachment of muscles (Figure 24-2). The skeleton is also designed to allow motion of the body. Bones come in contact with one another at joints where, with the help of muscles, we are able to bend and move.

The major functions of the skeleton are to:

- give us form
- allow us to move
- protect our vital internal organs
- produce red blood cells
- serve as a reservoir for calcium, phosphorus, and other important body chemicals

In the center of bones is a substance called bone marrow. Bone marrow produces our red blood cells. Red blood cells have a short life span—about 120 days. Thus, our bone marrow is making new red blood cells all the time to make sure that our bodies get the oxygen and nourishment they need and to remove waste from our bodies.

Bone is living tissue as are muscle, skin, and other tissues. Bones receive oxygen and nutrients from a constant supply of blood. Bone also has an extensive nerve supply. Thus, when a bone is broken, we experience severe pain due to irritation of the nerves. Significant bleeding also occurs due to damage to the bone's blood vessels.

## FIGURE 24-2

The skeleton

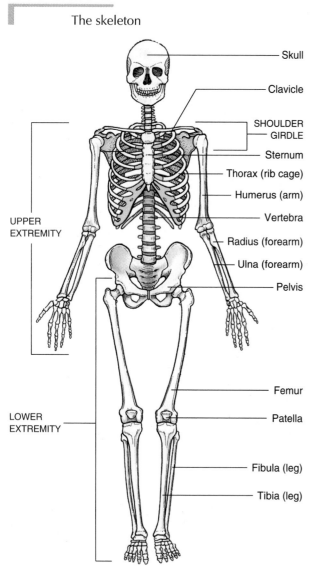

Skull

Clavicle

SHOULDER GIRDLE

Sternum

Thorax (rib cage)

Humerus (arm)

Vertebra

Radius (forearm)

Ulna (forearm)

Pelvis

UPPER EXTREMITY

Femur

Patella

LOWER EXTREMITY

Fibula (leg)

Tibia (leg)

### Joints

Wherever two bones come in contact, a **joint** is formed. The joint consists of the ends of the bones that make up the joint and the surrounding, connecting, and supporting tissue (Figure 24-3). Most joints are named by combining the names of the two bones that form that joint. For example, the sternoclavicular joint is the joint between the sternum and the clavicle.

Most joints allow motion—for example, the knee, hip, or elbow. Some bones fuse with one another at joints to create a solid, immobile, bony structure. For instance, the skull is composed of several bones that fuse as we grow. An infant, whose skull bones are not yet fused, has soft spots between the bones. The fontanels close as the bones fuse when the child's skull is finished growing.

**FIGURE 24-3**

The knee joint

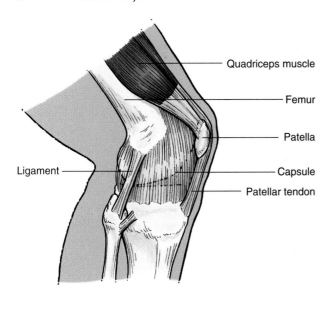

In joints that move, the ends of bones are covered with a smooth, shiny surface called **articular cartilage.** The bone ends of a joint are held together by a fibrous tissue joint capsule. At certain points around the joint, the capsule is lax and thin so that movement can occur. In other areas, it is quite thick and resists stretching or bending. These bands of thick, tough capsule are called **ligaments.**

How freely a joint can move is determined by the extent to which the ligaments hold the bone ends together. It is also determined by the shape and form of the bone ends themselves. The hip joint is a ball-and-socket joint that allows rotation as well as bending. The finger joints and the knee are hinge joints. Their motion is restricted to one plane. They can only flex (bend) and extend (straighten). Rotation is not possible because of the shape of the joint surfaces and the strong restraining ligaments on both sides of the joint. Thus, although the amount of motion varies from joint to joint, all joints have a definite limit beyond which

they cannot move. When a joint is forced beyond this limit, damage to some structure must occur: either the bones that form the joint will break, or the supporting capsule and ligaments will be disrupted.

## COMMON MUSCULOSKELETAL INJURIES

### CAUSES OF INJURY

Because musculoskeletal injuries occur so often, you must be able to evaluate them properly. Injury to the bones and joints is often associated with injury to the surrounding soft tissue, especially nearby nerves and blood vessels. Other areas of the body, even those some distance from the deformity, may be injured as well. Therefore, you must always first perform an initial assessment before you focus on an obviously deformed arm or leg. Remember that the purpose of the initial assessment is to identify life-threatening conditions.

#### Mechanisms of Injury

Significant force is usually required to cause a painful, swollen, deformed extremity (fracture). The force may be applied to the limb in several ways. Direct blows, indirect forces, twisting forces, or high-energy injury all may cause significant musculoskeletal injury (Figure 24-4). A direct blow is a common cause of deformity. The deformity from a direct blow occurs at the point of impact. For example, the patella (kneecap) may be injured when it strikes the dashboard in an automobile accident.

Indirect forces can also result in injury and deformity. In such instances, the force is applied to one part of the limb. The site of

## FIGURE 24-4

Mechanisms of injury

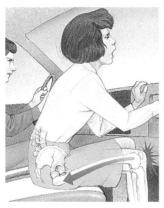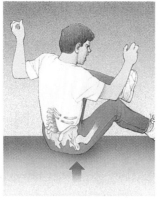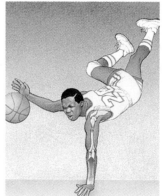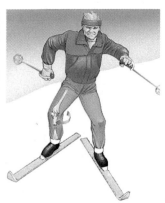

injury is some distance away from the point of impact, usually above it. The best example of this is the wide range of injuries that occur when a person falls and lands on an outstretched hand. The patient may injure the bones of the wrist, or forearm, the humerus, or even the clavicle. In fact, this is the most common mechanism of deformity of the clavicle.

Twisting forces can also result in injury, particularly injury to the leg. Such a force is a common cause of tibial deformity as well as knee and ankle ligament injuries. With this mechanism of injury, the foot is usually fixed to a point on the ground as the person falls. Skiing injuries often happen this way. A ski becomes caught and the skier falls, applying a twisting force to the lower extremity.

High-energy injury—as in automobile accidents, falls from heights, gunshot wounds, and injuries from other extreme forces—results in severe damage to the skeleton. Also damaged are the surrounding soft tissues and the vital internal organs. More than one bone in a limb may be injured and multiple injuries commonly occur following high-energy trauma.

Not all deformities result from violent force. For example, bone tumors weaken the bone so that only a slight force will cause it to break. Another common bone disease, osteoporosis, weakens the bones. Weakened bone is very prone to deformity, even with minimal force. Osteoporosis is common in elderly patients, particularly postmenopausal women. Minor falls, simple twisting injuries, or even muscle contraction can cause injury and deformity in people who have osteoporosis.

## BONE INJURY

As you assess a patient with a possible broken bone, or any extremity injury, you must check for any breaks in the overlying skin and soft tissue. Just as with soft tissue injuries, broken bones or fractures are classified as open or closed.

### Types of Injury

An **open fracture** is any break in the bone in which the overlying skin has been damaged as well (Figure 24-5). Laceration (tearing) of the skin often occurs when sharp bone ends break through it. A direct blow can also tear the skin at the time of the injury. Wounds may vary in size—from a small puncture wound to a gaping hole with much exposed bone and soft tissue. The bone may or may not be visible in the wound. No matter how little or how much damage to the skin, any broken bone in which the skin has been damaged is considered an open, contaminated fracture. A closed fracture is one in which the skin has not been broken by the bone ends, and there is no wound anywhere near the injury site.

## FIGURE 24-5

Open fracture of the tibia

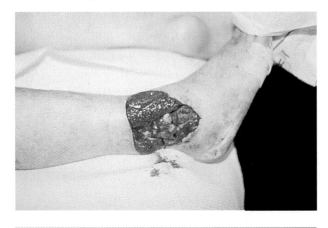

Open fractures to long bones and joints are much more serious than closed fractures for two reasons. First, greater blood loss occurs with open fractures. Second, and more important, the bone is contaminated by being exposed to the outside environment. As a result, the injury site may become infected. An infected bone sometimes causes serious life-long problems for the patient. For these reasons, all injuries, including possible fractures, should be described to

hospital personnel as either open or closed. Proper treatment can then be started immediately upon arrival at the hospital.

Fractures are also described by the degree of displacement of the bone fragments. A **displaced fracture** makes the limb appear in an unnatural position. This is called a deformity. The deformity is slight if the displacement is minimal. It may be extreme with gross (whole scale) displacement of the bone fragments. You will likely see many different types of limb deformities. Angulation at the injury site and rotation of the limb below the injury site are common types of displacement. A limb may appear shorter if the bone fragments are displaced and their ends overlap (Figure 24-6).

## FIGURE 24-6

X ray of a displaced fracture of the ankle

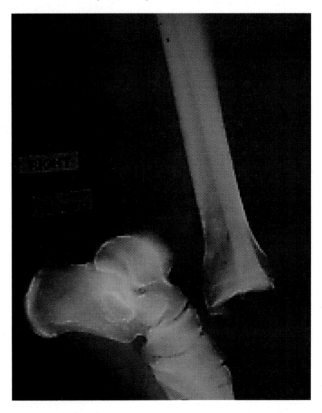

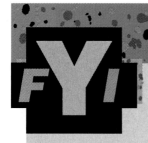

# Inside Our Bones

Bone is a living tissue. Just like muscle, skin and other tissues, our bones receive oxygen and nutrients from a constant supply of blood. They also have an extensive nerve supply. Thus a patient experiences severe pain and significant bleeding when he breaks a bone.

**Bone marrow,** a specialized tissue in the middle of every bone, produces red blood cells. Because these cells have a short life span (about 120 days), our bone marrow is making new red blood cells all the time.

At birth, our bones are not fully developed. Although the skeleton must be rigid and stiff to give a body shape, bones must also grow and change as we grow. Unless some abnormality exists, our bones stop growing when we reach our late teens.

Until then, bones are relatively flexible. This is why juvenile bones are often uninjured in accidents that would break an adult bone. However, because kids are so active, injuries still occur frequently.

Throughout your life, your body requires phosphorus and calcium to make your bones hard and strong. Phosphorus is a critical component of bone tissue. Calcium assures your skeletal muscles will contract normally.

As humans age, bones gradually weaken as they lose calcium. This condition, called **osteoporosis,** is particularly common in women and is especially severe after menopause. Thus elderly people, particularly post-menopausal women, are more susceptible to bone injury. Even trivial injuries may produce significant injury and deformity in patients with osteoporosis.

Bone is different than other tissues in your body; it heals by forming more of itself. Other tissues form scar tissue. But scar tissue is not strong enough to replace bone. So, your bones heal quite differently than any other tissue.

## Signs and Symptoms

You should suspect a bone or joint injury in any trauma patient who complains of musculoskeletal pain. Identifying possible fractures is relatively easy if bone ends are protruding through the skin, or a limb is grossly deformed. Many fractures and other bone injuries—particularly those in which there is no deformity—are less obvious. You must know the following eight signs and symptoms of bone and joint injury. All eight do not need to be present for you to suspect a possible fracture. You should suspect a possible fracture if a patient has just one of the following signs:

1. *Deformity.* The limb may lie in an unnatural position—shortened, angulated, or rotated where no joint exists. If you are not sure whether a deformity exists, use the opposite limb as a mirror image to compare. Always compare the injured

limb with the uninjured opposite limb when you check for deformity (Figure 24-7).

## FIGURE 24-7

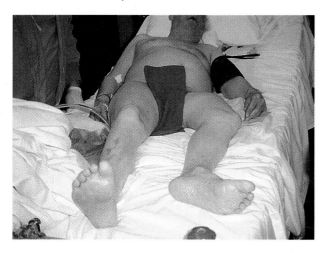

Compare the injured limb with the uninjured limb

2. *Pain and tenderness.* Tenderness is usually sharply localized at the site of the injury. You can find a painful spot by gently feeling along the bone with the tip of one finger. This sign, called **point tenderness,** is the most reliable indication of an underlying injury (Figure 24-8). Remember to use a gloved hand if there are any open wounds.

3. *Guarding (inability to use the extremity).* A patient who has a possible fracture usually guards the injured part and will refuse to use it because motion causes increased pain. It is the patient's way of "splinting" the injured limb to minimize motion and pain (Figure 24-9). Although the inability to use a limb is a reliable sign of a significant injury, the reverse is not true. The ability to use an extremity does not mean that the patient does not have a possible fracture. Occasionally,

nondisplaced fractures are not very painful. In fact, some patients may use an injured limb. This often happens with multiple fractures, where one area is very painful and masks the pain of the other injuries.

4. *Swelling and bruising.* Fractures are almost always associated with swelling and bruising (discoloration) of the surrounding soft tissues. These signs are

## FIGURE 24-8

Point tenderness

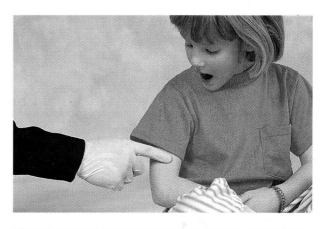

## FIGURE 24-9

Guarding

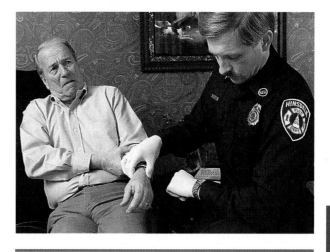

also present following almost any injury and are not specific for bone or joint injuries. However, rapid swelling that occurs immediately after an injury usually indicates bleeding from the injury site into the soft tissues. Swelling may be severe enough to mask deformity of a limb produced by the injury. Generalized swelling of the limb may occur several hours later.

5. *Exposed fragments.* In open fractures, bone ends may protrude through the skin or be seen in the depths of the wound itself. Both are obvious signs of open fracture.

6. *Crepitus (grating).* A grating or grinding sensation called crepitus can be felt and sometimes even heard when the raw bone ends rub together.

7. *False motion.* Motion at a point in the limb where it usually does not occur is a positive indication of fracture.

8. *Loss of distal pulses.* Loss of pulses in the distal extremity signals a circulation problem.

Crepitus and false motion only appear when a limb is moved or manipulated. Because these injuries are extremely painful, you should not move or manipulate the limb to elicit these signs. Simply looking at the limb with the clothing removed will allow you to see any deformity, swelling, bruising, or exposed bone fragments. Watch the patient for guarding and loss of function. Finally, palpation with one finger over the injured bone will elicit point tenderness. Any one of these signs is sufficient grounds to assume the patient has a possible fracture or joint injury.

### Joint Injuries

With displacement of a joint, injury to the supporting ligaments and capsule is so severe that the joint surfaces are completely separated from one another. The bone ends lock in the displaced position, making any attempt to move the joint difficult as well as painful. The joints most commonly injured in this way are the small joints of the fingers, the shoulder, the elbow, the hip, and the ankle.

You may see the following six signs and symptoms when a joint is displaced:

1. Marked deformity
2. Swelling in the area of the joint
3. Pain that becomes worse with any attempt at movement
4. Almost complete loss of normal motion (a "locked" joint)
5. Tenderness on palpation
6. Loss of pulses distal to the injured site

# EXAMINATION OF MUSCULOSKELETAL INJURIES

The following are three essential steps in caring for a patient who has musculoskeletal injuries:

1. Perform a general assessment.
2. Examine the injured part.
3. Evaluate the distal neurologic function.

## GENERAL ASSESSMENT

You should always perform an initial assessment of the patient before you focus attention on an injured limb. Multiple injuries often occur, so your first steps at any scene are to assess and stabilize the patient's overall condition. Bleeding from an extremity should be controlled as part of the primary stabilization. Further treatment of the extremities should begin only after the patient's vital functions are fully stabilized.

When the patient is critically injured and the vital functions cannot be stabilized in the field, rapid transport to a trauma center is necessary. In this situation, extensive assessment and splinting of limb injuries in the field wastes valuable time. Instead, you should secure a critically injured patient to a long spine board. This will rapidly immobilize the spine, pelvis, and extremities. You should then provide rapid transport to the hospital.

## EXAMINING INJURED EXTREMITIES

If the patient does not have life-threatening injuries and you have stabilized the patient's overall condition, you can then begin evaluating injured limbs. During the detailed physical exam, you should inspect and palpate the limbs to identify possible injuries. First, look at the injured limb and compare it with the opposite, uninjured side. Remember to follow BSI techniques. Gently and carefully remove the patient's clothing and look for any open injury, deformity, swelling, and/or discoloration (bruising). Next, gently palpate the extremities and the spine to identify any areas of point tenderness. Remember that point tenderness is the best indicator of an underlying bone or joint injury.

In most instances, inspection and palpation will help you to identify a significant limb injury. It is not important to distinguish or classify types of injuries. In most instances, your assessment will be reported as an "injury to the limb." *As an EMT-B, you will treat all limb injuries in the same manner.* Therefore, it is not important that you try to classify a specific injury among the various types of extremity injuries.

If the patient has no signs of injury following inspection and palpation, ask the patient to move each limb carefully. With any significant injury, movement of an injured part will be painful. The patient can usually identify the point that is most painful. If even the slightest movement produces pain, you should immediately direct the patient to stop moving. You should not attempt to move the painful limb either. Also remember that the patient should not be directed to move if he or she has any neck or back pain. In these instances, even the slightest movement may cause permanent damage to the spinal cord.

## EVALUATING NEUROLOGIC FUNCTION

Once you have identified an injury to a limb, you must periodically assess distal neurologic function. Many important blood vessels and nerves lie close to the bone, especially around the major joints. Therefore, any injury or deformity may have associated vessel or nerve injury. You must assess neurologic function during the detailed physical exam, and then repeat this assessment every 15 minutes until the patient arrives at the hospital.

You must also recheck neurologic function after any manipulation of the limb, such as splinting. Reassessment after a splint is applied is most important. Movement of the limb during splinting may cause a bone fragment to press against or pierce an important nerve or blood vessel. A pulseless limb will die if circulation is not restored. Therefore, you must give priority to such patients.

You should complete the following four steps in the neurologic examination and record the results for each injured limb:

1. *Pulse.* Palpate the pulse distal to the point of injury. Palpate the radial pulse in the upper extremity and the posterior tibial pulse in the lower extremity (Figure 24-10).

## FIGURE 24-10

## FIGURE 24-11

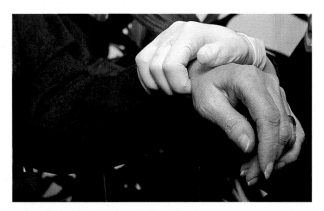

**A**   Palpation of the radial pulse

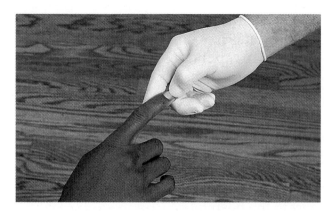

**A**   Press the fingernail until it blanches

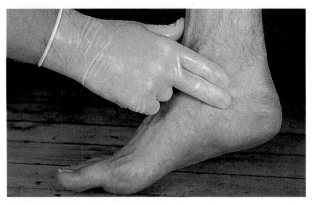

**B**   Palpation of the posterior tibial pulse

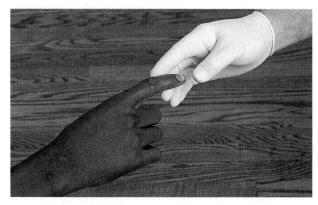

**B**   Release the fingernail and look for rapid return of pink color

2. *Capillary refill.* Note and record skin color, looking for signs of paleness or cyanosis. The capillary bed is best seen in the finger or toe underneath the nail. Applying firm pressure on the tip of the nail will cause the nail bed to blanch (turn white). On release of the pressure, the nail bed should return to its normal pink color in the time it takes to say "capillary filling." If the nail bed does not turn pink in this 2-second interval, it is considered delayed and indicates impaired circulation. Capillary refill should be pink and brisk (Figure 24-11).

3. *Sensation.* Check sensation to light touch in two places in the hand: on the pulp of the index finger and the little finger. In the foot, check the pulp of the big toe and laterally on the dorsum of the foot. The patient's ability to sense light touch in the fingers or toes distal to the injury site is a good indication that the nerve supply remains intact.

4. *Motor function.* Evaluate muscular activity when the injury is above the patient's hand or foot. Do not perform this test if the injury involves the hand or foot itself, as it will cause pain. Ask the patient to

open and close the fist for an upper extremity injury and wiggle the toes or move the foot up and down for a lower extremity injury. Sometimes, attempting to move will produce pain at the injury site. If pain occurs, stop this part of the examination.

Taken together, these examination findings are often referred to as CMS (circulation, motor, and sensory functions). Thus, a patient with good pulses, capillary refill, motor response, and sensation is said to have "good CMS" on examination.

Performing some parts of the CMS evaluation will not be possible if the patient is unconscious, because many of the steps require patient cooperation. With an unconscious patient, first perform an initial assessment and stabilize the vital functions, if necessary. You should then examine the extremities. Any limb deformity, swelling, discoloration, or false motion should be considered evidence of a limb injury and treated as such. You can monitor the distal pulses and capillary refill in an unconscious patient. However, assessing sensation and motor function cannot be done without patient cooperation. Remember, you must always assume that any unconscious, injured patient has a spinal injury that will require spinal immobilization.

## EMERGENCY MEDICAL CARE

### GENERAL PRINCIPLES

Your first steps in caring for any patient are to perform an initial assessment and stabilize the patient's ABCD. Once you have done so, you can focus on specific injuries.

You should completely cover all open wounds with a dry, sterile dressing and apply local pressure to control bleeding. Remember to follow BSI techniques when blood or other body fluids are present. Once you apply a sterile compression dressing, an open fracture is handled in the same way as a closed fracture.

Your next step is to apply the appropriate splint and elevate the extremity. Cold packs may be applied to the area, if needed, to reduce swelling. Avoid placing cold packs directly on the skin or other exposed tissues. Placing a cold pack on top of an air splint or other thick, insulating material will not help reduce swelling.

Once an injured limb is adequately splinted, you should prepare the patient for transport. The exact position of the patient will vary somewhat, depending on the type of injury. With most isolated upper extremity injuries, the patient will be most comfortable in a semiseated position rather than lying flat. However, either position is acceptable. With lower extremity injuries, the patient should lie supine, with the limb elevated about 6" to minimize swelling. In all cases, the injured limb should be positioned

## FIGURE 24-12

Transport the injured limb above the level of the heart

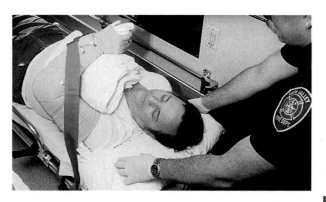

slightly above the level of the heart (Figure 24-12). The injured limb should never be allowed to flop about or dangle off the edge of the backboard.

You must inform hospital personnel about all wounds that have been dressed and splinted.

## PRINCIPLES OF SPLINTING

All extremity injuries should be splinted before a patient is moved, unless the patient's life is in immediate danger. A splint is a rigid or flexible appliance used to keep in place and protect an injured part. However, your first step, no matter what type of splint you are using, is to follow BSI techniques before you cover any open wounds. Also before you apply any type of splint, you should assess the distal neurologic function in the injured limb. Splinting is important because it reduces pain and it prevents motion of the following:

- bone fragments
- injured joints
- damaged soft tissues

Loose, broken bone fragments in a closed fracture can damage nerves, blood vessels, and muscles. *One of the main reasons for splinting is to prevent a closed fracture from becoming an open fracture.* Splinting also helps make patient transfer and transport easier for you and less painful for the patient. Because splinting has so many advantages, all extremity injuries should be splinted before a patient is transported.

Splinting will also prevent the following:

- further damage of muscles, peripheral nerves, and blood vessels from broken bone ends
- laceration of the skin by broken bone ends
- impaired circulation distal to the site of injury

- excessive bleeding due to tissue damage caused by bone ends at the injury site
- paralysis of extremities due to a damaged spine

A splint can be made from any material. It is simply a device to prevent movement of the injured part. However, you should have an adequate supply of standard commercial splints in your unit. Only occasionally should you have to improvise.

### General Principles of Splinting

1. In most instances, remove clothing from the area of any suspected fracture or joint injury. This allows you to look for open wounds, deformity, swelling, and bruising.

2. Note and record the patient's pulse, capillary refill, sensation, and movement in the area below the site of injury before and after the splint is applied. Continue to monitor the neurologic status until the patient reaches the hospital.

3. Cover all wounds with a dry, sterile dressing before applying a splint. Make sure to follow BSI techniques. Inform hospital personnel of any open wounds.

4. Do not move the patient before splinting extremity injuries, unless the patient's life or your life is in immediate danger.

5. Immobilize the joint above and the joint below the injury site in a suspected fracture of the shaft of any bone.

6. Immobilize the bone above and the bone below the injury site in a suspected injury of a joint.

7. Pad all rigid splints to prevent local pressure.

8. As you apply a splint, use your hands to minimize movement of the limb and to support the injury site until the limb is completely splinted.

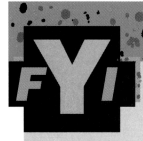

## Sprains

When a joint is twisted or stretched beyond its normal range of motion, the supporting capsule and ligaments are stretched or torn. Because it is an injury to a joint, this injury should be considered to be a partial separation. The bone ends are not completely displaced from one another by the force of injury, so they can fall back into alignment when the force is released. Therefore, the severe deformity seen with a separated joint is not present.

Joint injuries vary in severity from a slight injury to severe disruption of the supporting ligaments and capsule. A severe sprain often causes as much damage to the supporting ligaments and the joint capsule as does a complete dislocation. Although injuries most often occur in the knee and ankle, any joint may be involved.

The following are signs of soft tissue injury to joints:

- Tenderness. Point tenderness can be elicited over the injured ligaments.

- Swelling and ecchymosis. A sprain usually tears blood vessels, producing swelling and ecchymosis at the point of ligament injury.
- Inability to use the extremity. Because of the pain of injury, the patient often cannot move or use the limb normally.

It should be noted that the signs of joint injuries are the same as some of those for a fracture. At times it is impossible to differentiate between a nondisplaced fracture and a joint injury. The point to remember is that although an injury may appear to be a joint injury, a fracture may be present as well.

In evaluating musculoskeletal injuries, the topic of sprains should be mentioned. A strain, unlike a sprain, causes no ligament or joint damage. A strain is a stretching or tearing of a muscle. The muscle fibers are partially pulled apart, producing pain and occasional swelling and ecchymosis of the local soft tissues.

9. Align a severely deformed limb with the shaft of a long bone above it. Use constant, gentle manual traction so that the limb can be placed into a splint. This is particularly important if the distal part of the extremity is cyanotic or lacks a pulse.

10. Splint the limb in the position in which you found it if you encounter resistance to limb alignment when you apply traction.

11. Immobilize all suspected spinal injuries in a neutral in-line position.

12. If the patient has signs of shock, align the limb in normal anatomic position and transport.

13. *When in doubt, splint.*

# KITE RESCUE GONE BAD

A father is teaching his young daughter how to fly a kite when a sudden gust of wind blows it into a tree. Not wanting to write off the kite, Dad gets a ladder and heads up the tree. About 15' up, his right foot slides off a rung and his leg slides through. As he turns and falls, he pulls the ladder and himself to the ground. The little girl runs home crying, and her mother calls 9-1-1. On arrival, you find a 25-year-old man still tangled in the ladder, complaining of pain in his right leg and shoulder. His skin is slightly cool and moist. A bone end protrudes through his shorts.

## For Discussion

1. Describe the rationale behind splinting extremities.

2. What problems occur when a closed injury becomes an open injury?

## General Principles of Traction

Traction is the most effective way to re-align a fracture of the shaft of a long bone so that the limb can be splinted more effectively. **Traction** is the action of drawing or pulling on an object. Excessive traction can be very harmful to an injured limb. However, when applied correctly, traction stabilizes loose bone fragments and improves the overall alignment of the limb. You should not attempt to reduce a fracture or force all the bone fragments back into alignment. This is the physician's responsibility. In the field, the goals of traction are as follows:

- to stabilize deformed bone fragments to prevent excessive movement

- to align the limb enough so that it can be placed in a splint

The amount of pull needed to stabilize the bone fragments and to adequately align the limb varies, but it rarely exceeds 15 lb. Therefore, you should use the least amount of force necessary to align the limb. Grasp the patient's foot or hand firmly as you apply traction. Once you begin pulling, do not release the traction until the limb is fully splinted. To minimize the patient's discomfort, make sure your partner supports the injured limb under the fracture site.

When applying traction, the direction of pull is always along the long axis of the limb. Imagine the normal position of the limb if it was not injured. Next, pull along the line of that normal position. The injured limb will come to rest in this position as you apply gentle traction (Figure 24-13). The patient may have discomfort as you grasp the foot or hand and/or as you begin

## FIGURE 24-13

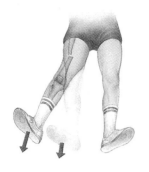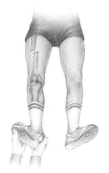

Applying gentle traction

to pull. However, this discomfort quickly subsides, and you may then apply further gentle traction. If the patient strongly resists, or if it causes more pain, you must stop immediately. In these instances, you must splint the limb in the position in which you found it.

## TYPES OF SPLINTS

Many different materials can be used as splints. Even when no splinting materials are available, the arm can be bound to the chest and an injured leg can be splinted to the uninjured leg for temporary stability. Splints can be made from materials such as pillows, rolled up magazines or newspapers, or even a T-shirt. However, you will use three basic types of splints, as follows: 1) rigid splints, 2) formable splints, and 3) traction splints.

### Rigid Splints

Rigid (nonformable) splints are made of firm material to prevent motion at the injury site. These splints can be applied to the sides, front, and/or back of an injured limb. Common examples include padded board

splints, molded plastic and metal splints, padded wire ladder splints, and folded cardboard splints (Figure 24-14).

## FIGURE 24-14

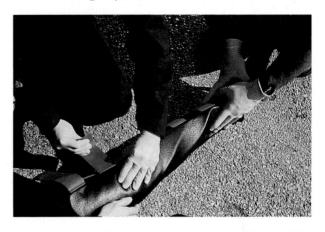

Rigid splint

In some instances, a patient will have a severe limb deformity or will have pain as you apply gentle traction to the shaft of a long bone. When this occurs, or if you feel resistance as you apply gentle traction, you should splint the limb in the position of deformity. In this situation, apply padded board splints to each side of the limb and secure the splints with soft roller bandages (Figure 24-15).

## FIGURE 24-15

Padded board splint to the elbow

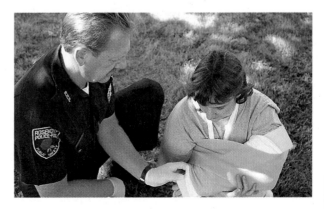

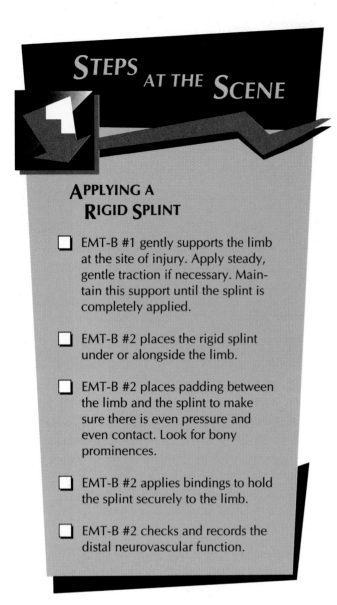

## APPLYING A RIGID SPLINT

- ☐ EMT-B #1 gently supports the limb at the site of injury. Apply steady, gentle traction if necessary. Maintain this support until the splint is completely applied.

- ☐ EMT-B #2 places the rigid splint under or alongside the limb.

- ☐ EMT-B #2 places padding between the limb and the splint to make sure there is even pressure and even contact. Look for bony prominences.

- ☐ EMT-B #2 applies bindings to hold the splint securely to the limb.

- ☐ EMT-B #2 checks and records the distal neurovascular function.

### Pneumatic Splints

Pneumatic splints are formable or soft splints, such as air and vacuum splints. These splints are available in a variety of sizes and shapes. They may or may not have a zipper that runs the length of the splint. The most commonly used splint is the precontoured, inflatable, clear plastic air splint. Air splints are comfortable, provide uniform contact, and apply firm pressure to a bleeding wound. This type of splint is used to immobilize injuries below the elbow or below the knee only.

Air splints do have some disadvantages, particularly in cold weather areas. The zipper can stick, clog with dirt, or freeze. With extreme temperature changes, the air pressure in the splint will vary, decreasing in cold air and increasing in warm air. Changes in pressure will also occur with changes in altitude. This is sometimes a problem with helicopter transport of patients.

The way to apply an air splint depends on whether it has a zipper. Your first step, no matter what type of splint you are using, is to follow BSI techniques to cover all wounds with a dry, sterile dressing. If the splint has a zipper, hold the injured limb slightly off the ground applying gentle traction. Support the limb under the site of injury. Place the open, deflated splint around the limb, zip it up, and inflate it by mouth—never with a pump.

Vacuum splints are another type of formable splint. They can be easily shaped, like an air splint, to fit around a deformed limb (Figure 24-16). Suction is then applied to a valve in the splint to remove the air from inside. When all the air is out and the valve is sealed, the vacuum splint becomes rigid. Thus, the limb is immobilized in a splint that conforms to the shape of the deformity.

The pneumatic antishock garment (PASG) is also a type of formable splint used to immobilize pelvic injuries. Other soft splints such as pillow splints, SAM splints, and a sling and swathe are described in the Atlas of Common Musculoskeletal Injuries at the end of this chapter.

### Applying an Air Splint

If you use a nonzippered or partially zippered type of air splint, two EMT-Bs should follow these steps:

1. EMT-B #1 places his or her arm through the splint. Once the hand is extended beyond the splint, grasp the hand or foot of the patient's injured limb (Figure 24-17a).

## FIGURE 24-16

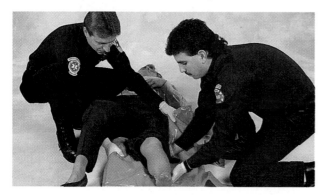

**A** Place the vacuum splint around the extremity

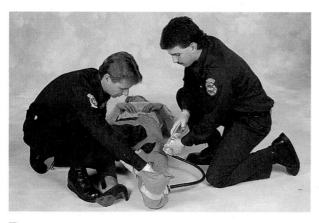

**B** Remove air from the splint

2. EMT-B #2 supports the patient's injured limb until splinting is complete.

3. EMT-B #1 applies gentle traction to the hand or foot while sliding the splint onto the injured limb (Figure 24-17b). Make sure to include the hand or foot of the injured limb in the splint.

4. EMT-B #2 inflates the splint by mouth (Figure 24-17c).

5. EMT-B #1 tests the air pressure after the splint is applied. With proper inflation, you should be just able to press the walls of the splint together with a firm pinch between the thumb and index finger near the edge of the splint (Figure 24-17d).

## FIGURE 24-17

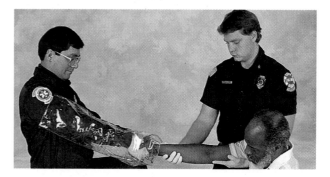

**A** Place the patient's limb in a splint

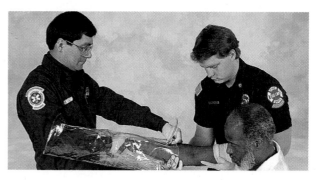

**B** Maintain traction while applying an air splint

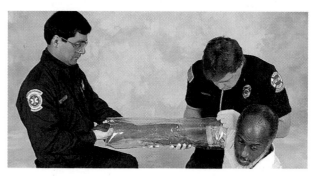

**C** Inflate the splint by mouth

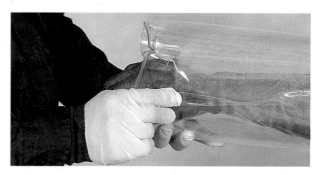

**D** Test the air pressure after a splint is applied

6. EMT-B #1 checks and records the distal neurologic function after the splint is applied. Monitor distal neurologic function periodically until the patient reaches the hospital.

## Traction Splints

Traction splints are used primarily for fractures of the shaft of the femur. Traction splints should not be used for the following conditions:

- injuries of the upper extremity
- injuries close to or involving the knee
- injuries of the hip
- injuries of the pelvis
- partial amputations or avulsions with bone separation

Several types of bipolar traction splints for the lower extremity are available. Each brand has its own unique method of application. Therefore, you must be thoroughly familiar with and have practiced applying the several types of traction splints. One of the most commonly used splints is the Hare traction splint. Another commonly used traction splint is the Sager splint. Its method of application is presented in the Atlas of Common Musculoskeletal Injuries at the end of the chapter.

When traction is applied to the foot through the ankle hitch, a force is exerted by the upper end of the splint against the ischial tuberosity of the patient's pelvis. This force is called countertraction. The Hare traction splint must be seated well on the ischial tuberosity for effective countertraction.

Two well-trained EMT-Bs are needed to properly apply a Hare traction splint. *It is impossible for one person to properly apply this splint.* You and your partner must thoroughly understand how this splint is applied. You should practice the steps until the sequence and necessary teamwork

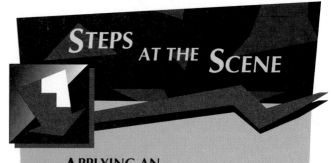

**STEPS AT THE SCENE**

1

### APPLYING AN AIR SPLINT

☐ EMT-B #1 places his or her arm through the splint. Once the hand is extended beyond the splint, grasp the hand or foot of the patient's injured limb.

☐ EMT-B #2 supports the patient's injured limb until splinting is complete.

☐ EMT-B #1 applies gentle traction to the hand or foot while sliding the splint onto the injured limb. Make sure to include the hand or foot of the injured limb in the splint.

☐ EMT-B #2 inflates the splint by mouth.

☐ EMT-B #1 tests the air pressure after the splint is applied. With proper inflation, you should be just able to press the walls of the splint together with a firm pinch between the thumb and index finger near the edge of the splint.

☐ EMT-B #1 checks and records the distal neurovascular function after the splint is applied. Monitor distal neurovascular function periodically until the patient reaches the hospital.

become routine. Your first step, no matter what type of splint you are using, is to follow BSI techniques to cover all wounds with a dry, sterile dressing.

## Applying a Bipolar Traction Splint

1. Assess and record the distal pulse, motor function, and sensation distal to the site of injury. Cut open the patient's trouser leg or otherwise expose the injured lower extremity so that you can see the limb as you splint it.

2. Place the splint beside the patient's uninjured leg and adjust it to the proper length (with the ring at the ischial tuberosity and the splint extending 12" beyond the foot) (Figure 24-18a). Open and adjust the four Velcro support straps. These should be positioned at the midthigh, above the knee, below the knee, and above the ankle.

3. EMT-B #1 gently supports and stabilizes the injured limb so that it will not move.

4. EMT-B #2 fastens the proper sized ankle hitch about the patient's ankle and foot (Figure 24-18b). Customarily, the shoe is removed from the patient's foot.

5. EMT-B #1 supports the leg at the site of the injury (Figure 24-18c).

6. EMT-B #2 applies gentle longitudinal traction to the ankle hitch and foot. Apply only enough traction to align the limb so that it will fit into the splint. Do not attempt to align the deformed fragments anatomically.

7. EMT-B #1 slides the splint into position under the patient's injured limb (Figure 24-18d). Make sure that the ring is seated well on the ischial tuberosity. Pad the groin and gently apply the ischial strap (Figure 24-18e).

**FIGURE 24-18**

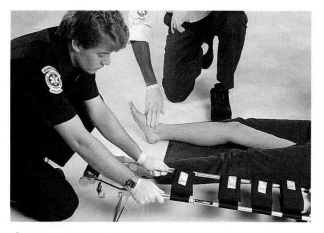

**A**   Place the traction splint alongside the injured limb

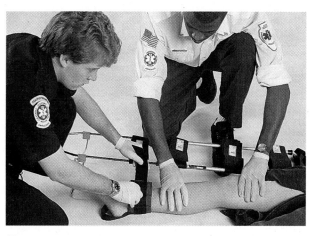

**B**   Fasten the ankle hitch

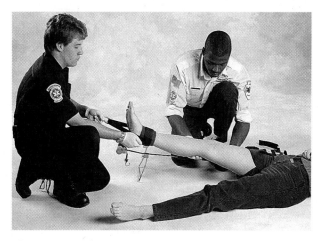

**C**   Support the limb at the site of injury

8. EMT-B #1 connects the loops of the ankle hitch to the end of the splint as the traction is maintained (Figure 24-18f). Apply gentle traction to the connecting strap between the ankle hitch and the splint, just strongly enough to maintain limb alignment. This splint comes with a ratchet mechanism to tighten the strap. This mechanism can generate an excessive amount of force, which can overstretch the limb and injure the patient.

9. Once proper traction has been applied, EMT-B #1 fastens the support straps so that the limb is held securely in the splint (Figure 24-18g).

10. Check all the support straps to make sure they are secure.

11. Reassess and record the distal pulse, motor function, and sensation distal to the site of injury.

12. Secure the patient's torso on a long spine board to immobilize the hip. Then secure the splint to the spine board to prevent movement en route to the hospital (Figure 24-18h).

A bipolar traction splint immobilizes the limb by producing countertraction on the ischium and in the groin. Therefore, make sure you pad these areas well—especially to avoid placing excessive pressure on the external genitalia. Use commercial padded ankle hitches rather than pieces of rope, cord, or tape. Such improvised hitches are painful and can impair circulation in the foot.

## HAZARDS OF SPLINT USE

All splints must be applied properly. There are several hazards associated with improper splinting, as follows:

- compression of nerves, tissues, and blood vessels
- delay in transport of a patient with a life-threatening injury

**FIGURE 24-18** *continued*

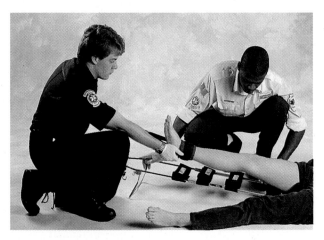

**D**  Slide the splint under the limb while applying traction

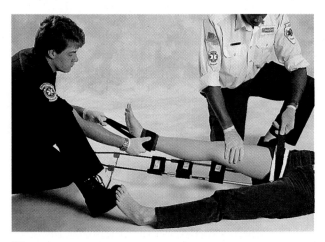

**E**  Pad the groin and fasten the ischial strap

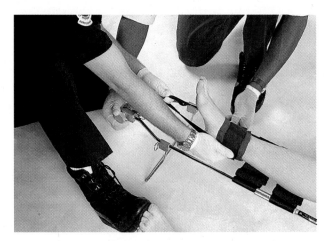

**F**  Loop the ankle hitch to the end of the splint

## *HARD AS A ROCK*

It's been a long Saturday at the state park, and with sunset not too far away, the party is still going strong. The beer has been flowing freely all day, so when one teenager dares another to jump the creek, he immediately accepts the challenge. Unfortunately, he comes up short on his landing and crashes into a large, slick boulder. As his feet go out from under him, he slams his upper arm and shoulder into the rock before splashing into the creek. One of the party-goers runs to the ranger station and calls EMS. On arrival, you find a 19-year-old man with slurred speech who is complaining of pain in the ankle and shoulder. You can see the end of his tibia bulging through his sock. Aside from that, and the saucer-sized abrasion on his shoulder, he appears to be in remarkably good shape.

### For Discussion

1. What mechanism of injury can produce neurologic injury in association with a broken extremity?

2. Why is communication with the patient an essential part of traction splinting?

**FIGURE 24-18** *continued*

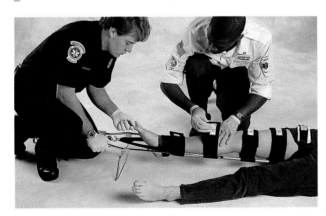

**G** Fasten the support straps

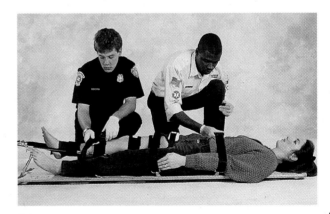

**H** Place the patient on a long spine board

- impaired distal circulation from applying a splint too tight
- aggravation of the bone or joint injury
- conversion of a closed fracture to an open fracture

## TRANSPORTATION

Very few, if any, patients with musculo-skeletal injuries need extremely rapid transport. Once dressed and splinted, the limb is stable. The patient can then be transported in an orderly fashion. With the pulseless limb, a sense of urgency develops. This patient must be transported with a higher priority. If the hospital is only a few minutes away, reckless speeding will make little or no difference to the patient's eventual outcome. However, if the hospital is an hour or more away, a patient with a pulseless limb should be transported by helicopter or rapid ground transportation. In every instance in which a patient has impaired circulation to the distal limb, you should inform medical control. The proper steps can be taken once the patient arrives at the hospital.

# Atlas of
# Common Musculoskeletal Injuries

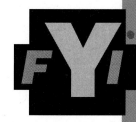

## THE SHOULDER

### Clavicle

The clavicle (collar bone) is one of the most commonly injured bones in the body. Clavicle injuries most commonly occur in children, usually from a fall on an outstretched hand. These injuries also occur with crushing injuries of the chest. Patients with a deformity of the clavicle will have pain in the shoulder girdle (Figure 24-19). They will also usually hold the injured arm against the chest, supporting the elbow or

forearm with their opposite hand. This "splints" the site of injury.

A young child will often complain of pain all along the arm and will usually refuse to use the arm. These complaints sometimes make it difficult to pinpoint the exact site of injury. Generally, there is swelling and point tenderness over the clavicle. Sometimes, the skin will look "tented" over deformed bone fragments. This is because the clavicle lies just beneath the skin. The clavicle lies directly over the major arteries, veins, and nerves that supply the upper extremity. As such, deformities of the clavicle may damage these important neurovascular structures.

### Scapula

Injuries of the scapula (shoulder blade) are less common, because this bone is well protected by many large muscles. These injuries almost always occur as a result of a violent blow to the back, directly over the scapula. Patients limit use of the arm because of pain at the injury site.

The force required to break the scapula is so great, a patient may have broken ribs or other chest injuries. These may result in respiratory problems. Thus, the patient may have breathing problems and must be monitored carefully. Administer oxygen and provide rapid transport if the patient shows signs of severe respiratory distress. Other signs and symptoms of injury to the scapula include abrasions, contusions, swelling, and tenderness about the scapula (Figure 24-20).

---

## FIGURE 24-19

A clavicle injury

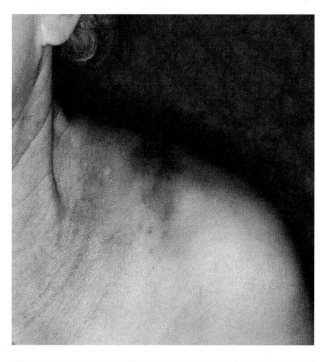

---

## FIGURE 24-20

A scapula injury

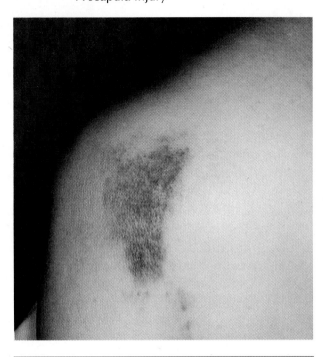

## FIGURE 24-21

An A/C separation

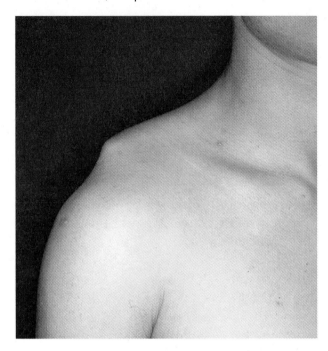

### Acromioclavicular (A/C) Joint Separation

The joint between the outer end of the clavicle and the acromion process of the scapula is called the acromioclavicular (A/C) joint. This joint is often injured, especially in football players. The injury is commonly called a shoulder separation or an A/C separation. Deformity occurs when the patient falls and lands on the point of the shoulder. The impact drives the scapula away from the outer end of the clavicle. Pain, including point tenderness over the joint, is common. The appearance is classic—prominence of the distal end of the clavicle (Figure 24-21).

### The Shoulder Joint

The shoulder joint is where the humeral head and the glenohumeral joint meet. This joint is the most commonly displaced large joint in the body. Almost always, the humeral head displaces anteriorly, coming to lie in front of the scapula. This anterior displacement is caused by forceful abduction and external rotation of the arm. The patient will often hold the displaced arm with the opposite hand to "splint" it. As you look at a patient from the front, you will see that the injured shoulder does not have the normal rounded contour of the opposite uninjured shoulder. Instead, the injured shoulder is squared off—flattened laterally (Figure 24-22). The humeral head protrudes anteriorly, lying underneath the pectoralis muscle on the anterior chest wall. There is often numbness in the upper extremity because the head of the humerus is pressing on the major nerves in the axilla (armpit).

### Treatment of Shoulder Injuries

Injuries of the clavicle and scapula and A/C separations can be splinted effectively

**FIGURE 24-22**

Dislocation of the shoulder joint

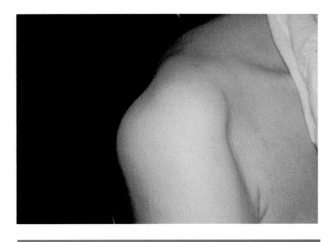

**FIGURE 24-23**

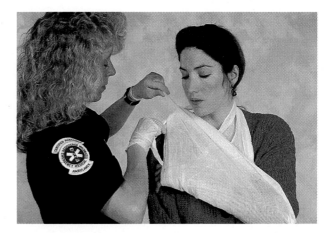

**A**  Apply the sling with the knot to one side of the neck

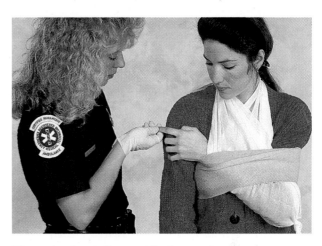

**B**  Check capillary refill after applying a sling and swathe

with a sling and swathe. The sling supports the weight of the upper extremity and relieves the pull of gravity on the injury site. To be effective, a triangular sling must apply gentle upward support to the olecranon process of the ulna. The knot of the sling should be tied to one side of the patient's neck so that it does not press uncomfortably on the cervical spine (Figure 24-23).

However, a sling alone does not fully immobilize the shoulder region. A swathe must be added to bind the arm to the chest for adequate immobilization. The swathe should be tight enough to secure the limb to the chest and prevent it from swinging freely. The swathe should not be so tight that it compresses the chest, affecting the patient's breathing. The hand should remain exposed so that you can assess neurovascular function at regular intervals after you have applied the splint.

Immobilizing a displaced shoulder is difficult, because the patient will hold the arm in a fixed position away from the chest. Any attempt to move the arm toward the chest will produce pain. Therefore, you must splint the joint in the position that is most comfortable for the patient. First,

gently place a pillow or rolled blanket between the arm and the chest to fill up the space between them (Figure 24-24). Once the arm is stabilized against the pillow, you can flex the elbow to 90° without causing additional pain. Next, apply a sling to the forearm and wrist to support its weight. Secure the arm in the sling to the pillow and chest with a swathe. Transport the patient in a sitting or semi-seated position.

**FIGURE 24-24**

Use of a pillow splint provides additional support

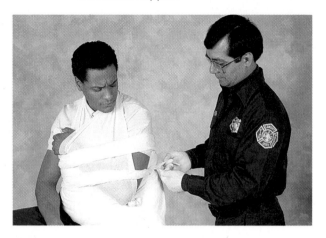

**FIGURE 24-25**

X ray of fractured humerus

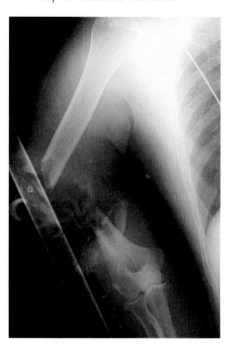

## THE UPPER EXTREMITY

### Humerus

Two regions of the humerus are prone to injury: 1) the proximal shaft near the shoulder joint, and 2) the midshaft. In the elderly, the proximal shaft is often injured as a result of a fall. In younger adults, injury near the midshaft is more common, usually as a result of violent trauma.

Injury to the proximal shaft causes mild to moderate deformity. Note that deformity is often hidden by swelling and by the large muscles that surround the upper part of the arm. With displacement of the midshaft, there is usually gross angulation at the deformity site and visible instability of the bone fragments (Figure 24-25).

Occasionally, the radial nerve is lacerated, compressed, or trapped at the site of a midshaft deformity (Figure 24-26). When this nerve is injured, the patient cannot extend (dorsiflex) the wrist or fingers. The patient may also complain of numbness on the dorsum (top) of the hand. This weakness produces a characteristic "wristdrop" appearance of the arm.

**FIGURE 24-26**

Compression of the radial nerve from fracture

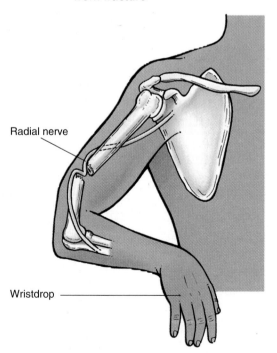

Radial nerve

Wristdrop

A sling and swathe or a shoulder immobilizer is effective for displacement of the proximal shaft and all minimally displaced deformities of the humeral shaft. Use the chest as a splint and secure the injured arm to the chest, as you would with injuries about the shoulder. You can place a short padded board splint on the lateral side of the arm under the sling and swathe to provide additional lateral support.

With a severely angulated injury of the humeral shaft, you should apply traction to realign the bone fragments before splinting them. Support the site of the deformity with one hand and with the other hand grasp the two humeral condyles just above the elbow. Pulling gently in line with the normal axis of the limb will align the arm (Figure 24-27). You can then splint the arm more effectively. Once you achieve gross alignment of the

**FIGURE 24-27**

Applying traction to the humeral condyles

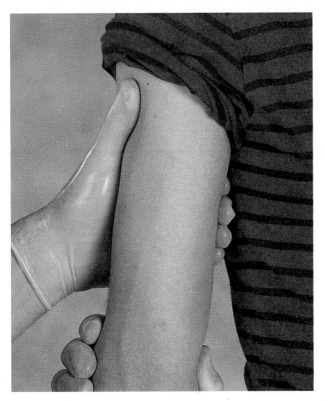

limb, apply a sling and swathe, along with a padded board splint on the lateral side of the arm. If the patient has significant pain or resists gentle traction, splint the arm in the position in which you found it. Use a padded wire ladder splint or a padded board splint and pillows to support the injured limb.

### Elbow

All elbow injuries should be considered serious and treated with extreme care. Inappropriate care can result in injury to the nearby nerves and blood vessels. Therefore, avoid excessive movement of the joint as you assess and immobilize the limb. Careful, periodic assessments of distal neurovascular function are also necessary.

Displacement of the distal end of the humerus often occurs in children. Frequently, this deformity is caused by a significant rotation of the bone fragments. This injury exposes the surfaces of the bones to the nearby vessels and nerves, which often damages these structures (Figure 24-28). Swelling occurs rapidly and may be severe.

**FIGURE 24-28**

Nerve and vessel injury due to distal humeral fracture

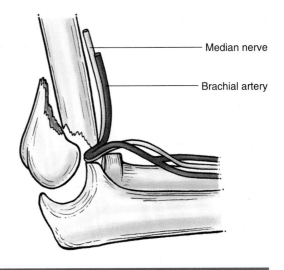

Median nerve

Brachial artery

Separation of the elbow usually occurs in teenagers and young adults as a result of an athletic injury. With this injury, the ulna and radius are most commonly displaced posteriorly. This makes the olecranon process of the ulna much more prominent (Figure 24-29). The joint is locked with the forearm moderately flexed on the arm. Any attempt to move the elbow is very painful. As with all injuries in this region, swelling is common, as is the potential for significant vessel or nerve injury. Deformity of the olecranon process of the ulna is usually the result of a direct blow. Therefore, you will likely see abrasions or lacerations at the injury site.

padded board splints, applied to each side of the limb and secured with soft roller bandages, to provide adequate stability. The splints should extend from the shoulder joint to the wrist joint. This will immobilize the entire bone above and below the injured joint. A padded wire ladder splint or a SAM splint can also be molded to the shape of the limb to splint it in the position in which you found it (Figure 24-30). You can add a wrist sling to support the weight of the arm and further support the limb with a pillow, if necessary.

**FIGURE 24-30**

Use of a molded splint for elbow immobilization

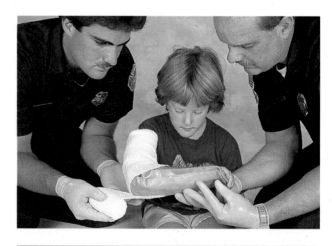

**FIGURE 24-29**

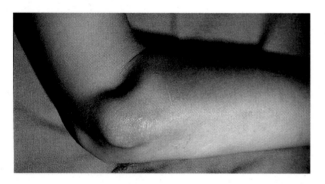

**A**   Elbow dislocation

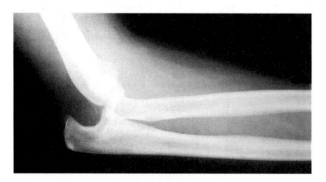

**B**   X ray of an elbow dislocation

If the patient has strong pulses and good capillary refill, splint an elbow injury in the position in which you found it. Use two

If the patient's hand is cold, pale, or has a weak or absent pulse and poor capillary refill, the vessels have likely been injured. These signs suggest serious injury, and medical control should be notified immediately. A physician should advise you about further care of this injury until the patient arrives at the hospital. If the patient is within 10 to 15 minutes of the hospital, splint the limb in the position in which you found it and provide prompt transport. If the hospital is farther away than 10 to 15 minutes, then medical control may direct you to try to realign the limb. This will improve circulation to the hand. If the pulseless limb is significantly deformed at the elbow, apply gentle manual traction in line with the long axis of the limb. This maneuver may restore the pulse. Do not try to move the limb excessively, as this will only injure or damage the blood vessels more.

If you restore the pulse with gentle manual traction, splint the limb in the position that allows the strongest pulse. If no pulse returns after one try to realign the limb, splint it in the position most comfortable for the patient. Provide prompt transport for all patients with impaired distal circulation.

## Radius and Ulna

Injuries to the shaft of the radius and the ulna (forearm) are especially common in children, but occur routinely in persons of all ages. If a patient falls on an outstretched hand, both bones usually break at the same time (Figure 24-31). An isolated deformity of the shaft of the ulna may occur as the result of a direct blow.

Injuries to the distal radius are common in the elderly, especially those who have osteoporosis. If a patient falls on an outstretched hand, the injured wrist may appear curved, much like the curve of a dinner fork. This injury is commonly called a "silver fork deformity" because of its striking appearance (Figure 24-32).

You can use a variety of splints to immobilize these injuries. Padded board, air,

**FIGURE 24-31**

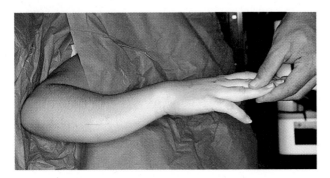

**A**   Displaced fracture of the forearm

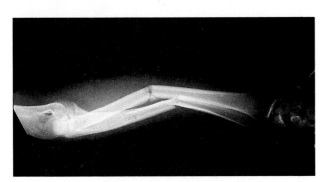

**B**   X ray of a fracture of the forearm

**FIGURE 24-32**

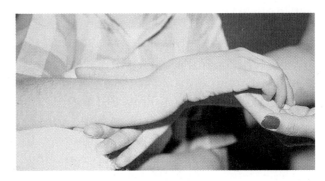

**A**   Fracture of the distal radius

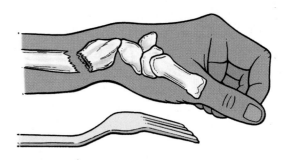

**B**   Silver fork deformity

vacuum, or pillow splints are all effective. To immobilize deformities of the shaft of radius and ulna, you must include the elbow joint. Splinting the elbow joint is not needed with injuries near the wrist. However, the patient will be more comfortable if a sling or supporting pillow is added.

### Wrist and Hand

All injuries to the wrist and hand can be potentially serious, because they often include injury to the underlying nerves, tendons, or blood vessels. The very intricate function of the fingers and hand is so important that any injury may result in permanent deformity and disability. Therefore, prompt, proper treatment of these injuries is critical. All injuries to the hand must be evaluated promptly by a physician. Even simple lacerations should be treated quickly and carefully (Figure 24-33). Deformed finger joints should not be "popped back" into place (Figure 24-34). Any amputated parts should be brought with the patient to the hospital.

You should splint all hand and wrist injuries with a bulky hand dressing. First, cover all wounds with a dry, sterile dressing. Make sure you follow BSI techniques. Next, gently form the injured hand into the position of function. In this position, the wrist is slightly dorsiflexed, and all finger joints are flexed moderately (Figure 24-35). One way to visualize this position is to think about the position in which you would most comfortably hold a baseball. After you have positioned the patient's hand, place a soft roller bandage into the palm of the hand. Apply a padded board splint to the palmar side of the hand and wrist. Secure the splint with a soft roller bandage down the length of the splint. Prop the splinted hand and wrist on a pillow or on the patient's chest during transport to the hospital.

**FIGURE 24-33**

Laceration of the thumb

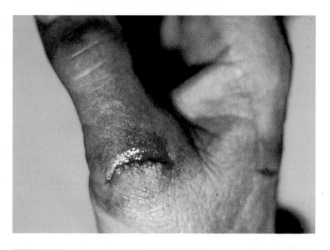

**FIGURE 24-34**

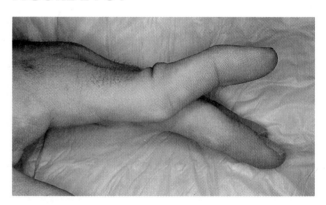

**A**   Dislocation of the finger joint

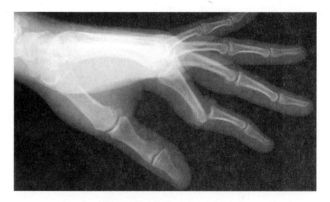

**B**   X ray of a dislocated finger joint

**FIGURE 24-35**

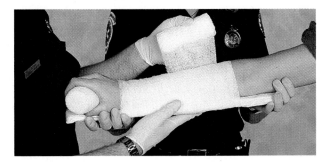

**A**    Place the hand in the position of function

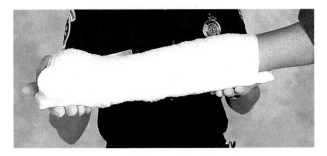

**B**    Wrap the hand and arm with gauze

**FIGURE 24-36**

A common mechanism of injury

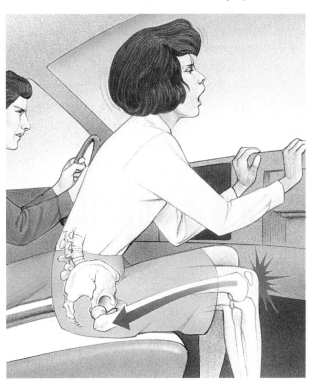

## THE PELVIS

Closed injuries to the pelvis commonly result when the pelvis is crushed, such as after a fall from a height or a direct crushing blow. Indirect forces can also result in injury. For example, the knee can strike the dashboard in a car accident. The impact of the force travels along the femur, driving the femoral head into the pelvis (Figure 24-36). However, pelvic injuries are not always caused by violent trauma. A simple fall can result in a pelvis injury, especially among the elderly who have osteoporosis.

Severe blood loss can occur with injuries of the pelvis. Large blood vessels lie next to the pelvis and are easily torn or lacerated at the time of the injury. A large amount of blood can drain from these lacerated vessels into the retroperitoneal space, an area in the abdomen that can hold several liters of blood. This space contains the kidneys, stomach, the spleen, and the intestines. As a result, hypovolemic shock may develop and the patient could die from blood loss. Therefore, you must carefully monitor the patient for signs of shock. If signs of shock develop, you must begin treatment immediately, even if there is only minimal swelling or other external signs of bleeding. Remember that the extent of blood loss in a closed injury may not be apparent because blood drains into the retroperitoneal space.

Open injuries of the pelvis are quite rare, because the pelvis is surrounded by heavy muscles. Occasionally, bone fragments will lacerate the rectum or vagina and create an open injury. According to the principles of Prehospital Trauma Life Support (PTLS), a critically injured patient with a pelvis injury should be transported immediately to the hospital.

Any patient who has been in a high-velocity accident will likely have a pelvis injury. Frequently, the patient will have pain in the pelvic region or the lower abdomen. Because the area is covered by heavy muscles and other soft tissues, deformity or swelling in the pelvic region is difficult to see. The most reliable sign of pelvis injury is tenderness on firm compression and palpation. If this sign is absent, the patient could still have a pelvic fracture (the absence of a sign does not exclude the possibility of injury). You can assess for tenderness by applying firm compression on the two iliac crests. First, place the palms of your hands over the lateral aspect of each iliac crest and apply firm inward pressure on the pelvic ring (Figure 24-37a). Then, with the patient lying supine, place your palms over the anterior aspect of each iliac crest and apply firm downward pressure (Figure 24-37b). Next, place your palms over the symphysis pubis and apply firm compression. This will also elicit tenderness if there is injury to the anterior portion of the pelvic ring (Figure 24-37c).

The bladder is especially prone to injury following a deformity of the pelvis. Pelvic bone fragments may lacerate the bladder, or the force of impact may cause the bladder to rupture. With an injury to the bladder or the urethra, the patient will have lower abdominal tenderness. The patient may also have hematuria (blood in the urine) or a bloody discharge from the urethral opening. Thus, important structures such as blood vessels, the bladder, the vagina, and the rectum are susceptible to injury once the pelvic ring has been broken.

## Treatment of Pelvis Injuries

Your first step in caring for a patient with a possible pelvis injury is to perform an initial assessment. You must also monitor vital signs closely due to the potential for hypovolemic shock. If the patient's condition is stable, you can immobilize isolated deformities of the pelvis by securing the patient on a long spine board. Place a pneumatic antishock garment (PASG) on the spine board before you transfer the patient onto the board (Figure 24-38). During transport, elevate the foot of the board 6" to 12". If the patient is in shock or has signs of hypovolemic shock, supplement the immobilization by inflating the PASG. The PASG provides adequate immobilization of the

**FIGURE 24-37**

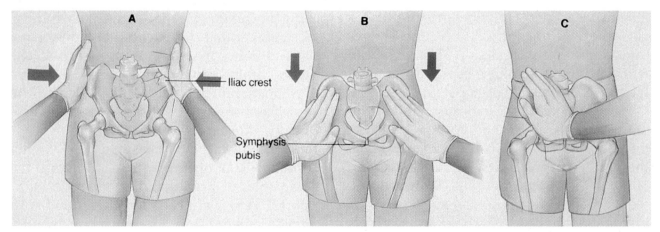

**A** Compress the pelvis from the side    **B** Compress the pelvis from the front    **C** Compress the symphysis pubis

**FIGURE 24-38**

Place the PASG on the spine board before log rolling the patient

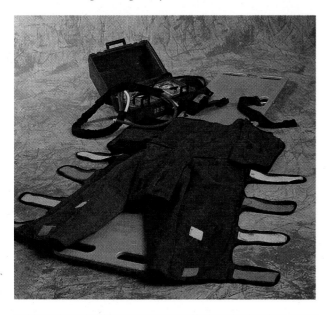

injury and decreases the severity of the hypovolemic shock. Once the PASG is applied and inflated, you must carefully follow all the rules governing its use, particularly the method of deflation and removal. For these patients, rapid transport is essential.

## THE HIP JOINT

The hip joint is a stable ball-and-socket joint that displaces only after significant injury. The femoral head almost always displaces posteriorly, coming to lie in the muscles of the buttock. The femoral head very rarely displaces anteriorly. When this happens, the legs are suddenly and forcefully spread wide apart. Posterior displacement most commonly occurs as a result of an automobile accident. Often, the knee meets with a direct force, such as the dashboard, and the entire femur is driven posteriorly, separating the joint. Thus, you should look carefully for contusions, lacerations, or obvious deformity in any patient involved in a car accident.

Injury to the sciatic nerve commonly occurs with this type of hip injury. Located directly behind the hip joint, the sciatic nerve is the most important nerve in the lower extremity. It controls the activity of some of the muscles in the thigh, all the muscles below the knee, and all sensation in the leg and foot.

When the head of the femur is forced out of the acetabulum (hip socket), it damages the sciatic nerve by pressing on it or stretching it (Figure 24-39). Partial or complete paralysis of this nerve can result from posterior displacement of the hip. Paralysis of the sciatic nerve will decrease sensation in the leg and foot and weaken the foot muscles—particularly the muscles that raise the toes or the foot. This muscular weakness is commonly called a "foot drop."

The appearance of a posterior displacement is classic. The patient lies with the knee drawn up toward the chest and the thigh rotated inward and adducted across the midline of the body (Figure 24-40). The

**FIGURE 24-39**

Posterior dislocation of the hip

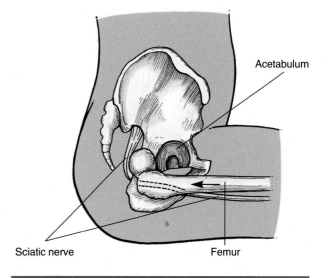

**FIGURE 24-40**

Position of the limbs in posterior dislocation of the hip

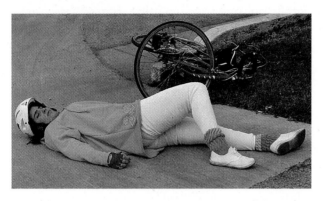

**FIGURE 24-41**

Splinting a posterior dislocation of the hip

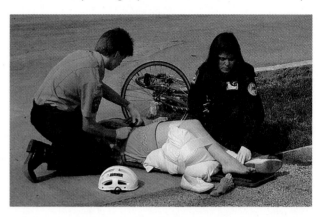

flexed thigh on the injured side lies across the midline of the body over the top of the thigh of the uninjured, normal leg. With the rare anterior displacement, the limb lies in the opposite position—extended straight out, rotated outward, and pointing away from the midline of the body.

With these injuries, the patient will have severe hip pain. Any attempt to move the joint will be met with great resistance. Palpation of the lateral and posterior aspects of the hip region will elicit tenderness. Careful examination of sensation and motor function in the lower extremity may identify a sciatic nerve injury.

### Treatment of Hip Joint Injuries

As with any other injured joint, you should make no attempt to reduce the displaced hip in the field. Splint the injury in the position in which you found it. Place the patient supine on a long spine board. Support the limb with pillows and rolled blankets, particularly under the flexed knee. Then secure the entire limb to the spine board with long straps. Stabilize the limb well enough to the spine board to eliminate all motion in the hip region (Figure 24-41).

## THE FEMUR

### Proximal Femur

Injuries of the proximal (upper end) femur, also called "hip fractures," occur in two distinct groups of patients—the elderly and young adults. Injuries of the hip most commonly occur in the elderly (particularly women) with osteoporosis. Because of the brittleness of the osteoporotic bone, a simple fall could result in injury. On rare occasions, injury of the proximal femur occurs in younger adults as a result of severe trauma. All patients with hip injuries may lose significant amounts of blood. Therefore, you should watch for signs of shock and monitor vital signs carefully.

A deformed proximal femur has a characteristic appearance. The patient lies with the injured leg externally rotated, and the leg appears shorter than the opposite, uninjured limb (Figure 24-42). Most patients are unable to walk or move the leg due to pain. Usually the pain is in the hip region or along the inner aspect of the thigh. Apply gentle manual pressure to the greater trochanter to elicit tenderness if you believe a patient has an injury of the proximal femur (Figure 24-43). Occasionally, the patient will have knee pain. In fact, an elderly patient

**FIGURE 24-42**

Position of the limbs in a displaced right hip fracture

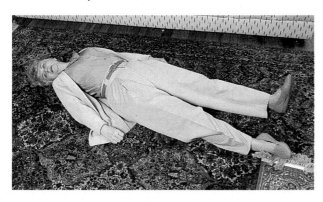

**FIGURE 24-43**

Palpation of the greater trochanter

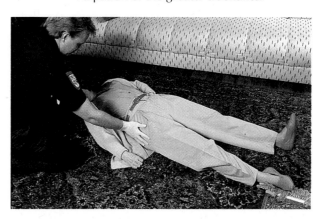

with this type of injury will often complain of knee pain. Because this injury is so common, any elderly patient who complains of hip or knee pain after a fall should be splinted and transported.

### Treatment of Proximal Femur Injuries

The way you splint this injury is based on the age of the patient and the severity of the deformity. In young adults, injuries of the proximal femur that result from violent trauma are best immobilized with a traction splint or a PASG and a spine board. The traction splint is applied in the same way as for femoral shaft deformities. Remember to protect the injured area around the hip from excessive pressure from the ring of a Hare traction splint. In a patient with serious or multiple injuries, apply and inflate a PASG on top of a long spine board. This combination will effectively immobilize the pelvis and hip region. The PASG will also help control hemorrhage in the region.

In an elderly patient with an isolated hip injury, traction is not necessary to adequately immobilize the limb. In this instance, place the patient on a long spine board using pillows or rolled blankets to support the injured limb in the deformed

**FIGURE 24-44**

Securing the patient with a hip fracture to a spine board

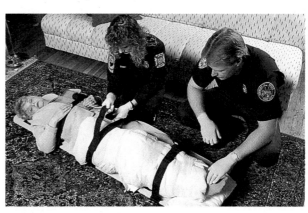

position. Secure the injured limb to the stretcher with long straps or cravats (Figure 24-44).

### Femoral Shaft

Injuries of the femur can occur in any part of the shaft, from the hip to just above the knee joint. After any injury, the large muscles of the thigh begin to spasm to "splint" the unstable limb. This muscle spasm often results in significant deformity, with severe angulation or rotation at the injury site. The limb usually shortens significantly as well. Injuries of the femoral shaft are often open, and bone fragments may protrude through the skin.

There is always significant blood loss with injuries of the femoral shaft—as much as 50 to 1,000 mL of blood. With open injuries, the amount of blood loss may be even greater. Therefore, you should closely watch for signs of hypovolemic shock. Use extra care in handling these patients, because any extra movement or manipulation will increase the amount of blood loss.

Because of the severe deformity that occurs with these injuries, bone fragments may also penetrate or press on important nerves and vessels. This may result in serious damage to these structures. Therefore, you must periodically assess distal neurovascular function in patients with these injuries.

### Treatment of Femoral Shaft Injuries

Because these injuries often include wounds, you must first inspect the thigh to identify any open wounds. Be sure to follow BSI techniques as you inspect the thigh. Cover any wounds with a dry, sterile compression dressing. If the area below the injury shows signs of impaired circulation (pale, cold, or pulseless), apply gentle traction in line with the long axis of the limb. Gradually turn the lower extremity from the deformed position to restore overall alignment. Turning the limb to a more normal position often restores or improves circulation to the foot. The patient likely has a serious vascular (blood vessel) injury if circulation does not return or improve after you have applied traction and realigned the limb. Monitor the patient's vital signs closely and watch for signs of hypovolemic shock. Be prepared to provide prompt transport.

A femoral shaft injury is best immobilized with a traction splint. The Sager traction splint is often used for this type of injury. It is lightweight, applies a measurable amount of traction, and can be used with a PASG. Unlike the Hare traction splint, a Sager splint can be applied by one person, if necessary. But as with the Hare traction splint, you and your partner must practice applying this splint. You should practice the steps until the sequence becomes routine.

#### APPLYING A SAGER TRACTION SPLINT

1. Before applying the splint, adjust the thigh strap so that it will lie anteriorly when secured in place (Figure 24-45a).

2. Estimate the proper length for the splint by placing it next to the injured limb. Make sure that the wheel is at the level of the heel (Figure 24-45b).

3. Arrange the ankle pads to fit the patient's ankle.

4. Place the splint along the inner aspect of the limb and slide the thigh strap around the upper thigh. Make sure that the perineal cushion is snug against the groin and the ischial tuberosity. Tighten the thigh strap snugly (Figure 24-45c).

5. Secure the ankle harness tightly around the patient's ankle just above the malleoli (Figure 24-45d).

6. Snugly pull the cable ring up against the bottom of the foot.

7. Pull out the inner shaft of the splint to apply traction of approximately 10% of body weight to a maximum of 15 lb (Figure 24-45e).

8. Secure the limb to the splint using elasticized cravats (Figure 24-45f).

9. Secure the patient to a long spine board (Figure 24-45g).

**FIGURE 24-45**

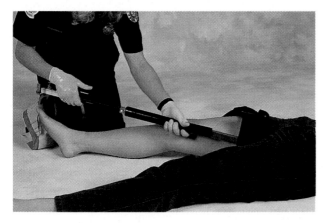

**A** Adjust the thigh strap

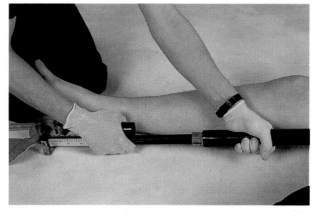

**B** Estimate the proper length of a splint by placing it next to the injured limb

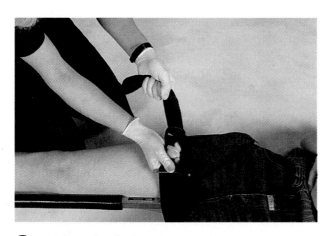

**C** Tighten the thigh strap

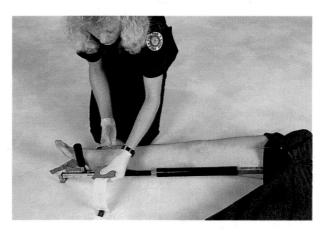

**D** Secure the ankle harness

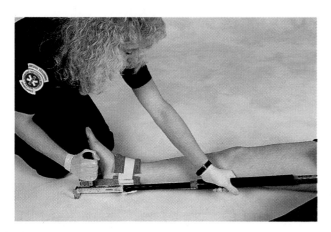

**E** Apply traction to the splint

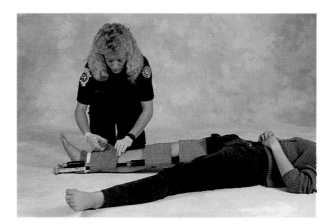

**F** Secure the limb to the splint

**FIGURE 24-45** *continued*

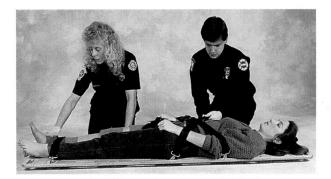

**G** Secure the patient to a long spine board

# THE KNEE

### The Knee Ligaments

Injuries to the knee ligaments range in severity from mild stretching to complete disruption of one or more of the stabilizing ligaments. These injuries occur when the knee abnormally bends or twists, as is common in sports injuries. Patients with knee ligament injuries often complain of joint pain and usually cannot use the extremity normally. The knee will be swollen and occasionally bruised. Point tenderness is also common in the area of the ligament injury.

### Treatment of Knee Ligament Injuries

Splint all suspected knee ligament injuries with a splint that extends from the hip joint to the foot. The splint must immobilize the bone above the injured joint (the femur) and the bone below (the tibia). You may use any of the following splints:

- a padded rigid long-leg splint
- two padded board splints applied to the medial and lateral aspects of the limb
- a long spine board
- a pillow splint
- binding the injured limb to the opposite uninjured limb

The patient is usually able to straighten the knee so that you can apply the splint. If the patient resists or complains of pain when you attempt to straighten the knee, splint it in the flexed position. Make sure you monitor distal neurovascular function until the patient reaches the hospital.

### The Knee Joint

Complete disruption of the ligaments supporting the knee may result in separation of the joint. When this happens, the proximal end of the tibia completely displaces from its articulation with the lower end of the femur, usually producing a significant deformity. Although substantial ligament damage always occurs with this type of injury, the immediate seriousness is not related to the ligament damage but to injury to the popliteal artery. Often, the popliteal artery is lacerated or compressed by the displaced tibia (Figure 24-46). When this severe injury of the knee is suspected because of gross deformity, severe pain, and an inability to move the joint, you must always check the distal circulation carefully before taking any other step. If the distal pulses are absent, notify medical control immediately because further steps in field stabilization must be directed by medical control.

**FIGURE 24-46**

Injury to the popliteal artery behind the knee

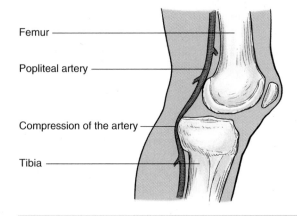

Femur

Popliteal artery

Compression of the artery

Tibia

On rare occasions, medical control may request that you realign a deformed, pulseless limb in order to restore distal circulation. You should only make one attempt to realign the limb and thus reduce compression of the popliteal artery. Gently straighten the limb by applying gentle longitudinal traction in the axis of the limb. Monitor the posterior tibial pulse during the application of traction to determine whether the pulse returns. Splint the limb in the position in which the strongest pulse is felt. If traction significantly increases the patient's pain, make no further attempts to realign the limb. Once you apply manual traction, maintain it until the limb is fully splinted; otherwise, the limb will return to its deformed position.

If you are unable to restore the distal pulse, splint the limb in the position most comfortable for the patient; then transport the patient promptly to the hospital. Medical control should be notified of the status of the distal pulse so that arrangements can be made in advance to receive the patient.

### The Patella

Displacement of the patella (dislocated kneecap) usually occurs in teenagers and young adults as a result of a sports injury. Some patients will have repeated dislocations, even after only minor twisting of the knee. Usually the patella displaces to the lateral side, and the knee is held in a partially flexed position. This injury produces a significant deformity (Figure 24-47).

### Treatment of Patella Injuries

The knee should be splinted in the position in which it is found, usually with the knee flexed to a moderate degree. Apply padded board splints to the medial and lateral aspects of the joint, extending from the hip to the ankle. When combined with pillows, this splinting technique will provide adequate immobilization.

**FIGURE 24-47**

A displaced patella

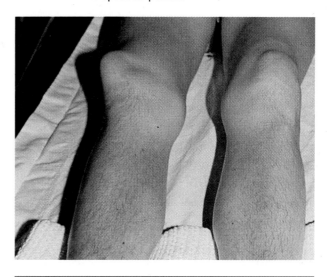

Occasionally, as the splint is being applied, the patella will return to its normal position on its own. When this occurs, immobilize the limb in a padded long-leg splint, as you would for a knee ligament injury. If the patella returns to its normal position, you must still transport the patient and report your findings.

## THE LEG

### The Tibia and Fibula

Injuries of the tibia or the fibula may occur at any place between the knee joint and the ankle joint. Usually both bones are injured at the same time. Because the tibia is located under the skin, open injuries of this bone are quite common. These injuries may result in severe deformity, with significant angulation or rotation (Figure 24-48).

### Treatment of Tibia and Fibula Injuries

You should immobilize injuries of the tibia and fibula with a padded, rigid long-leg splint or an air splint that extends from the foot to the upper thigh. You can also use

**FIGURE 24-48**

Open fracture of the tibia

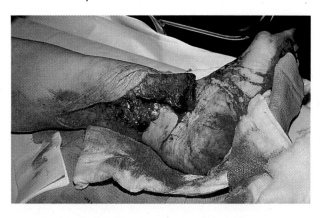

a traction splint. However, constant traction is not usually necessary with isolated tibial injuries. When both the tibia and femur have been injured, a traction splint will provide adequate immobilization for both bones.

As with most other injuries of the shaft of long bones, you apply gentle in-line traction before applying the splint. You must first apply traction to restore adequate alignment of the limb so that a standard splint can be applied. It is not necessary to replace the deformed fragments in their anatomic position.

Injuries to the blood vessels are also common with injuries of the tibia and fibula. These vascular injuries are often due to the extreme deformity following injury. Realigning the limb will often restore the blood supply to the foot. If realignment of the limb does not restore adequate circulation, you should provide prompt transport. You should also advise medical control of the patient's condition while you are en route.

## THE ANKLE AND FOOT

### The Ankle

It is difficult to distinguish serious ankle injuries from simple ones. Therefore, any ankle injury characterized by pain, swelling, localized tenderness, or the inability to

bear weight must be evaluated by a physician (Figure 24-49). The most common mechanism of injury is twisting, which stretches or tears the supporting ligaments. A more extensive twisting force may result in deformity of one or both malleoli. With displacement of the ankle, both malleoli are usually involved.

### Treatment of Ankle Injuries

You should treat all ankle injuries in the same way. Dress all open wounds, assess distal neurovascular function, apply gentle in-line traction to the heel if necessary, and apply a splint. You may use a padded rigid splint, an air splint, or a pillow splint for ankle injuries. Make sure you splint the entire foot and leg up to the knee joint.

### The Foot

Injuries of the foot can result in the deformity of the tarsals, metatarsals, or phalanges. Toe injuries are especially common.

Of the tarsal bones, the calcaneus is injured most often. Injuries of the calcaneus usually occur when the patient falls or jumps from a height and lands directly on the heel(s). The force of injury compresses the calcaneus, resulting in immediate swelling and bruising about the heel.

**FIGURE 24-49**

A swollen ankle

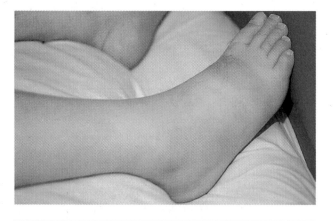

If the force of impact is great enough, as from a fall from a roof or tree, additional injuries may occur as well. Frequently, the force of the trauma is transmitted up the legs to the spine, resulting in an injury of the lumbar spine (Figure 24-50). For any patient who complains of heel pain after falling from a height, you should splint the foot and transport the patient on a long spine board to immobilize any possible spinal injury.

Injuries of the foot are often quite swollen, but they rarely result in significant deformity (Figure 24-51). Vascular injuries are not common. As with injuries of the hand, lacerations on the ankle and foot may damage important underlying nerves and tendons. Puncture wounds of the foot are common and may cause serious infection if not treated early. All of these injuries must be evaluated and treated by a physician.

**FIGURE 24-50**

Energy transmitted up the lower extremity

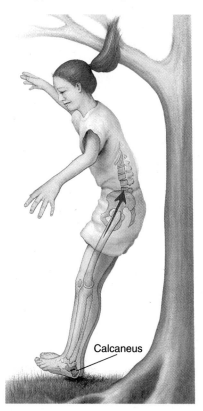

Calcaneus

**FIGURE 24-51**

A swollen foot

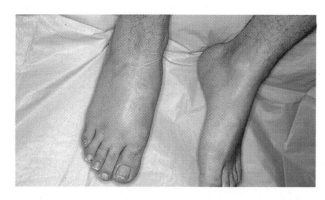

### Treatment of Foot Injuries

You should use a rigid padded board splint, an air splint, or a pillow splint for foot injuries. The splint must immobilize the ankle joint as well as the foot (Figure 24-52). The toes should remain exposed so that you can assess for distal neurovascular function. Slightly elevate the foot after splinting to minimize swelling. When the patient is lying on a stretcher, prop the foot up about 6". Transport the patient in a supine position so that the limb can be elevated. The foot and leg should never be allowed to dangle off the stretcher on the floor or ground.

**FIGURE 24-52**

Pillow splint

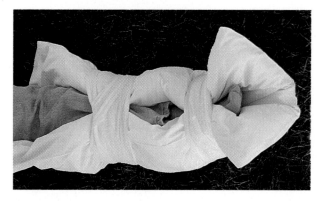

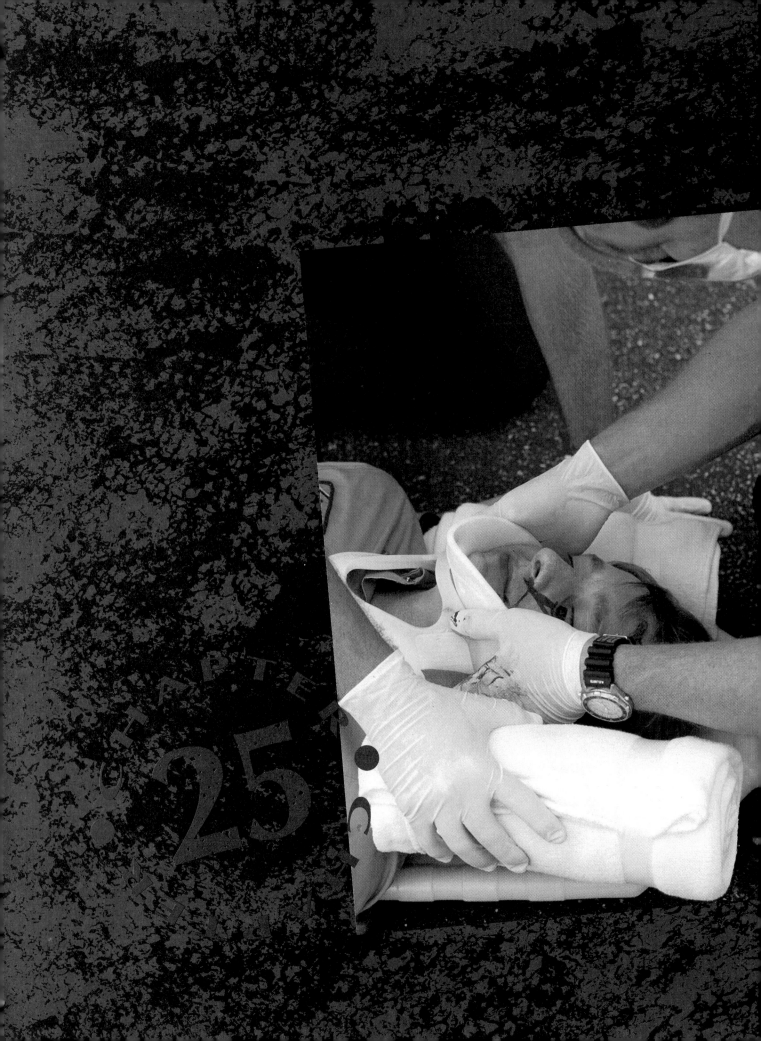

# Injuries to the Head and Spine

## Objectives

After you have read this chapter, you should be able to:

- List the components and functions of the nervous system and discuss how the structure of the skeletal system relates to the nervous system.
- Relate mechanisms of injury to potential head and spinal injuries.
- State the signs and symptoms of a potential spinal injury and describe how to determine if a responsive patient has such an injury.
- Describe the implications of improperly caring for potential spinal injuries.
- Relate the airway emergency medical care techniques to the patient with suspected head or spinal injuries.
- Describe when and how to immobilize a patient and stabilize the cervical spine, using a cervical spine immobilization collar and a short or long spine board.
- Describe how to size a cervical spine immobilization collar.
- List the indications for Rapid Extrication.
- Describe how to log roll a patient with a suspected spinal injury.
- Identify different types of helmets and describe the unique characteristics of sports helmets.
- Discuss when and how to remove a helmet, including stabilizing the patient's head in or out of a helmet.

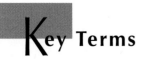

# Overview

The nervous system is a complex network of nerve cells that enables all parts of the body to function. It includes the brain, the spinal cord, and several billion nerve fibers that carry information to and from all parts of the body. Because the nervous system is so vital, it is well protected. The brain lies within the skull, and the spinal cord is inside the bony spinal canal. Despite this protection, serious impacts and blows can damage the nervous system. To accurately assess injuries to the nervous system, you must understand its anatomy and how it functions.

This chapter first briefly reviews the anatomy and function of the central and peripheral nervous systems and of the skeletal system. You will then explore the treatment of specific head and spinal injuries. Extrication of patients with potential spinal injuries is also discussed.

# Key Terms

**Autonomic (or involuntary) nervous system** The part of the nervous system that regulates functions, such as digestion and sweating, that are not controlled by conscious will.

**Brain stem** The part of the central nervous system that controls virtually all the functions that are absolutely necessary for life, including the cardiac and respiratory systems.

**Central nervous system (CNS)** The brain and spinal cord.

**Cerebellum** The part of the brain that coordinates body movements.

**Cerebral edema** Swelling of the brain.

**Cerebrum** The largest part of the brain, containing about 75% of the brain's total volume.

**Connecting nerves** Nerves that connect the motor and sensory nerves.

**Distraction** When the spine is pulled along its length.

**Eyes forward position** Position in which head is gently lifted until the patient's eyes are looking straight ahead and the head and torso are in line.

**Four-person logroll** Procedure for moving a patient from the ground to a long spine board. Recommended if you suspect a spinal injury.

**Intervertebral disk** Cushion that lies between the vertebrae.

**Involuntary activity** Those actions we do not control.

**Meninges** Three distinct layers of tissue that surround and protect the brain and the spinal cord within the skull and the spinal canal.

**Motor nerves** Nerves that carry information from the CNS to the muscles.

**Peripheral nervous system** 31 pairs of spinal nerves and 12 pairs of cranial nerves in the form of long fibers that link the nuclei and cell bodies of the CNS to the body's various organs.

**Sensory nerves** Nerves that carry information from the body to the CNS and transmit senses, such as touch, taste, heat, cold, or pain.

**Somatic (or voluntary) nervous system** The part of the nervous system that regulates our voluntary activities, such as walking, talking, and writing.

**Voluntary activity** Those actions we consciously perform in which sensory input determines the specific muscular activity.

# THE NERVOUS SYSTEM

## ANATOMY REVIEW

The nervous system is divided into two anatomic parts: the central nervous system (CNS) and the peripheral nervous system. The **central nervous system** is the part of the nervous system covered and protected by bones—the brain and spinal cord. While the nuclei and cell bodies of most nerve cells are within the CNS, long fibers link these cells to the body's various organs through openings in the bony coverings. These "cables" of nerve fibers make up the **peripheral nervous system.**

The major types of peripheral nerves are sensory, motor, and connecting nerves. The **sensory nerves** carry information from the body to the CNS; the **motor nerves** carry information from the CNS to the muscles. **Connecting nerves** connect the sensory and motor nerves.

### Central Nervous System

The central nervous system is composed of the brain and spinal cord. The brain is the organ that controls the body. It is the center of consciousness. It is divided into three major areas: the cerebrum, the cerebellum, and the brain stem.

The largest part of the brain, the **cerebrum,** contains about 75% of the brain's total volume. The cerebrum controls a wide variety of activities. Underneath the cerebral tissue lies the **cerebellum,** which coordinates body movements. The most primitive part of the CNS, the **brain stem,** controls virtually all the functions that are absolutely necessary for life, including the cardiac and respiratory systems. Deep within the cranium, the brain stem is the best-protected part of the CNS.

The spinal cord, the other major portion of the CNS, is mostly made of fibers that extend from the brain's nerve cells. The spinal cord carries messages between the brain and body.

## Protective Coverings

The cells of the brain and spinal cord are soft and easily injured. Once damaged, these cells cannot be regenerated or reproduced. Therefore, the entire CNS is contained within a protective framework. The thick, bony structures of the skull and spinal canal withstand injury very well.

The skull is covered by the "scalp," a thick vascular layer of skin. Underneath this skin is a layer of muscle fascia. The spinal canal is also surrounded by a thick layer of skin and muscles.

The CNS is further protected by the **meninges**—three layers of tissue that suspend the brain and the spinal cord within the skull and the spinal canal. The three layers are distinct. The outer layer, the dura mater, is a tough, fibrous layer that closely resembles leather. This layer forms a sac to contain the CNS. The peripheral nerves exit through small openings.

The inner two layers of the meninges, called the arachnoid and the pia mater, are much thinner than the dura mater. The blood vessels that nourish the brain and spinal cord are in these layers. Cerebrospinal fluid is produced by and fills the spaces between the arachnoid and the pia mater. The brain and spinal cord essentially float in this fluid. Cerebrospinal fluid is an excellent shock absorber, which buffers the CNS from injury.

If an injury penetrates all of these protective layers (the skin, muscle fascia, skull, and dura mater), you may see leaking cerebrospinal fluid. Most often you will see such leaks from the nose and the ears. Cerebrospinal fluid is clear and watery. If a patient with a head injury has a "runny nose" or watery fluid draining from the ear or an open skull fracture, you should assume the fluid is cerebrospinal fluid.

All of these protective layers isolate the CNS and protect it from injury. However, these same protective tissues can lead to serious problems in closed head injuries. Severe injury may cause the vessels under the dura mater to bleed. The subdural hematoma that develops increases the pressure inside the skull and compresses softer brain tissue. Only prompt surgery can avert permanent brain damage.

## Peripheral Nervous System

The peripheral nervous system has two anatomic parts: 31 pairs of spinal nerves and 12 pairs of cranial nerves.

The 31 pairs of spinal nerves conduct sensory impulses from the skin and other organs to the spinal cord. They also conduct motor impulses from the spinal cord to the muscles. Because the arms and legs have so many muscles, the spinal nerves serving the extremities are arranged in complex networks. The brachial plexus controls the arms and the lumbosacral plexus controls the legs.

Cranial nerves are the 12 pairs of peripheral nerves that pass through holes in the skull and transmit sensations directly to the brain. For the most part, they perform special functions in the head and face. These special functions include sight, smell, taste, hearing, and facial expressions.

There are three types of peripheral nerves: sensory nerves, motor nerves, and connecting nerves. The specialized nerve endings of each sensory nerve can perceive one and only one type of sensation. These nerves send their messages to the brain via the spinal cord. Each muscle has its own motor nerve. Connecting nerves are found only in the brain and spinal cord. These cells have short fibers that connect sensory nerves with motor nerves, allowing them to exchange messages.

## HOW THE NERVOUS SYSTEM WORKS

The nervous system controls virtually all of our body's activities, including those we can control and those we cannot. There are three types of nervous system activity: reflex, voluntary, and involuntary.

The connecting nerves in the spinal cord actually "connect" the sensory and motor nerves of the limbs, forming a reflex arc. If a sensory nerve in this arc detects an irritating stimulus (such as heat), it will bypass the brain and send a message directly to the motor nerve (Figure 25-1).

**Voluntary activities** are those actions we consciously perform. For example, we reach across the table for a salt shaker or to pass a dish. Sensory input determines the specific muscular activity. **Involuntary activities** are those actions we do not control. Many of our body's functions occur independently of thought, or involuntarily. In most instances, we breathe without consciously thinking about inhaling and exhaling.

## FIGURE 25-1

The reflex arc

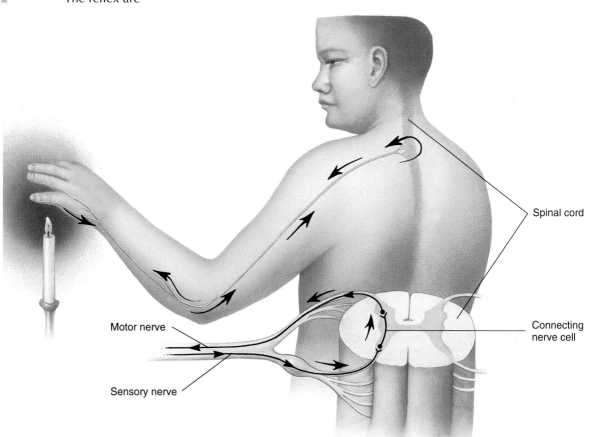

Spinal cord

Connecting nerve cell

Motor nerve

Sensory nerve

## SOMATIC NERVOUS SYSTEM

The part of the nervous system that regulates our voluntary activities, such as walking, talking, and writing, is called the **somatic (or voluntary) nervous system.** The somatic nervous system controls almost all coordinated muscular activities. The mechanism is straightforward. The brain interprets the sensory information it receives from the peripheral nerves. It then responds by sending signals to the voluntary muscles.

## AUTONOMIC NERVOUS SYSTEM

The body functions that occur without conscious effort are controlled by the **autonomic (or involuntary) nervous system.** The autonomic nervous system is a much more primitive system. It controls the functions of many of the body's vital organs. The brain has no voluntary control over this activity.

The autonomic nervous system is composed of two parts: the sympathetic nervous system and the parasympathetic nervous system. The sympathetic nervous system reacts to stress with the "fight or flight" response whenever it is confronted with a threatening situation. The parasympathetic nervous system has the opposite effect on the body. These two divisions of the autonomic nervous system tend to balance each other so basic body functions remain stable and effective.

# SKELETAL SYSTEM

## ANATOMY REVIEW

The skull has two layers of bone that protect the brain. It is divided into two large structures: the cranium and the face. The lower jaw (mandible) is the only movable facial bone. The temporomandibular joint attaches to the cranium just in front of each ear. A complete discussion of the skeletal system is presented in chapter 4, The Human Body.

The spinal column is the body's central supporting structure. It is divided into five sections (listed from the top down):

- cervical (neck)                          7 vertebrae
- thoracic or dorsal              12 vertebrae
  (upper part of the back)
- lumbar                                     5 vertebrae
  (lower part of the back)
- sacral (part of the pelvis)   5 vertebrae
- coccygeal                               4 vertebrae
  (coccyx or tailbone)

Each of the spine's 33 bones is called a vertebra. The front part of each vertebra consists of a round, solid block of bone. This is called the "body." The back part of each vertebra forms a bony arch. This series of arches from one vertebra to the next forms a tunnel that runs the length of the spine. It is called the "spinal canal." The spinal canal encases and protects the spinal cord.

The vertebrae are connected by ligaments. A cushion, called the **intervertebral disk,** lies in between them. These ligaments and disks allow the spine some motion, enabling the trunk to bend forward and back. However, they also limit motion so the spinal cord is not injured. When the spine is injured or fractured, the spinal cord and its nerves are left unprotected. Therefore, until the spine is stabilized, you must keep it aligned as best you can to prevent further injury to the spinal cord.

The spinal column itself is virtually surrounded by muscles. However, you can palpate the posterior spinous process of each vertebra. This process lies just under the skin in the midline of the back. The most prominent and most easily palpable spinous process is at the seventh cervical vertebra at the base of the neck (Figure 25-2).

## FIGURE 25-2

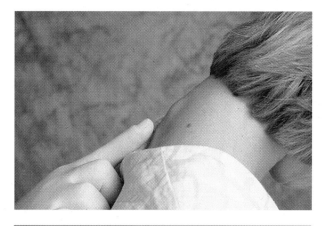

The spinous process of C7

Because of its extreme range of motion for head function, the cervical spine is commonly injured in automobile accidents. The lumbar spine is also vulnerable to injury. Injury often occurs as a result of motion at the junction of the lumbar and sacral spine.

## SPINAL INJURIES

The cervical, thoracic, and lumbar portions of the spine can be injured in a variety of ways. Compression injuries can occur as a result of a fall, regardless of whether the patient landed on his feet, his coccyx, or on the top of his head (as occurs in diving accidents). Motor vehicle accidents or other types of trauma can excessively flex, extend, or rotate the spine. Any one of these unnatural motions, as well as excessive lateral bending, can result in fractures or neurologic deficit.

Any time the spine is **distracted,** or pulled along its length, you can expect to find serious injuries to the spine. For example, hangings typically fracture the vertebrae high up in the cervical spine.

## MECHANISMS OF INJURY

You should always suspect a possible spinal injury any time you encounter one of the following mechanisms of injury:

- motor vehicle collisions
- pedestrian-motor vehicle collisions
- falls
- blunt trauma
- penetrating trauma to the head, neck, or torso
- motorcycle collisions
- hangings
- diving accidents
- unconscious trauma victims

Motor vehicle collisions and pedestrian-motor vehicle collisions can easily lead to spinal injuries. You should assume that anyone who has fallen or had blunt trauma to the body has a possible spinal cord injury, until proven otherwise. Certainly, any type of penetrating trauma to the head, neck, or torso can injure the spinal cord. Likewise, anyone involved in a motorcycle crash, a hanging, or diving accident can have a spinal cord injury. *You should always assume that any unconscious trauma victim has a spinal cord injury.* If you fail to "protect the spine" or follow "spinal precautions" in these instances, the patient may have permanent numbness, paralysis, and/or other neurologic problems.

## ASSESSMENT OF SPINAL INJURIES

### SIGNS AND SYMPTOMS

As you assess a patient, look carefully for signs or symptoms of a spinal injury. Remember that the ability to walk, move the extremities, or feel sensation does not necessarily rule out a spinal cord injury. Nor does an absence of pain. Do not ask patients with possible spinal injuries to move as a test for pain. In fact, you should remind them to be still as you ask questions.

However, pain or tenderness when you palpate the spinal area is certainly a warning sign that a spinal injury may exist. Patients with spinal injuries may complain of pain along the spinal column or in their extremities. This may be a constant or intermittent pain. A spinal cord injury may also produce pain independent of movement or palpation.

At times, you will feel an obvious deformity as you palpate the spine. Another sign of spinal injury is soft tissue injuries in the spinal region. If there is a soft tissue injury of the head and neck, a cervical spine injury is certainly a possibility (Figure 25-3). Obvious injury to the shoulders, back, or abdomen may indicate injury to the thoracic or lumbar spine. Injuries of the lower extremities may indicate a problem with the lumbar spine or sacrum.

## FIGURE 25-4

Paralysis from L1 (left) and
C5-6 (right) injury

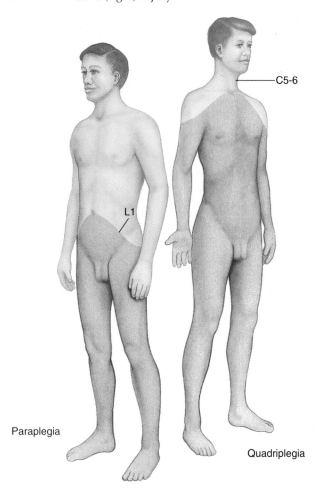

Paraplegia

Quadriplegia

Any complaint of numbness, weakness, or tingling in the extremities is another warning sign. Patients with severe injury may lose sensation or experience paralysis below the suspected injury, or even be incontinent (Figure 25-4).

## ASSESSING RESPONSIVE PATIENTS

As with all patients, begin with an initial assessment, focusing on ABCD. When assessing for possible spinal injuries in responsive patients, make sure you ask pertinent questions about the mechanism of injury and

## FIGURE 25-3

Soft tissue injury to the face

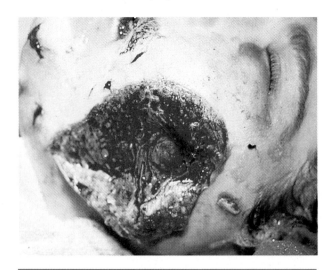

their symptoms. Begin by asking the following five questions:

1. Does your neck or back hurt?
2. What happened?
3. Where does it hurt?
4. Can you move your hands and feet?
5. Can you feel me touching your fingers? Your toes?

As part of your focused assessment, inspect the spinal area for contusions, deformities, lacerations, punctures, penetration injuries, and swelling. Palpate for tenderness or deformity. Make sure that you do not move the patient or any body parts excessively. Finally, assess the strength of each extremity. Check the strength of the patient's hand grasp. To check the lower extremities, ask the patient to gently push his or her feet against your hands.

## ASSESSING UNRESPONSIVE PATIENTS

As with all patients, begin with an initial assessment, focusing on ABCD. With unresponsive patients, you should try to identify the mechanism of injury. First responders, family members, or bystanders may have information relevant to the mechanism of injury. They may also know when the patient lost consciousness or the patient's previous level of consciousness. As part of your focused assessment, inspect the spinal area for contusions, deformities, lacerations, punctures, penetrations, and swelling. Palpate for tenderness or deformity.

## COMPLICATIONS

Complications that occur secondary to spinal cord injuries are serious. They may be life threatening or may result in lifelong disability. Respiratory failure can occur

from direct injury to the brain stem. This is usually fatal. Injury to the spinal cord usually causes paralysis. The damage to the spinal cord may be complete, resulting in no function below the level of injury. A patient will have some function if the damage is not complete. This complication results in lifelong disability. Thus, as you care for and transport patients with possible spinal cord injuries, you must take care to avoid any movement that could further injure the spine. All patients with injuries must be treated as if they have a spinal injury, until proven otherwise. This is the safest approach to caring for these patients.

## EMERGENCY MEDICAL CARE

Emergency medical care of a patient with a possible spinal injury begins, as does all patient care, with your protection. Follow BSI techniques any time you may be exposed to blood or other body fluids. Next, you must maintain the airway in the proper position, assess respirations, and give oxygen.

### RESTORING THE AIRWAY

Improper handling of a spinal injury can leave a patient permanently paralyzed. However, this possibility should not prevent you from opening the patient's airway. Just remember: Patients die if they cannot breathe.

If a patient with a spinal injury has an airway obstruction, you should perform the trauma jaw-thrust or trauma chin-lift maneuver to open the airway (Figures 25-5 to 25-6). Do *not* use the head-tilt/chin-lift maneuver. It extends the neck and may further damage the cervical spine. If the patient is unconscious, you can lift or pull the tongue forward so you do not have to move the neck. Once the airway is open, hold the head still, in a neutral, in-line position, until it can be fully immobilized.

After you open the airway, consider inserting an oropharyngeal airway, but make sure to monitor the airway closely. Make sure a suctioning unit is available because you will often need to clear blood, saliva, or vomitus from the airway. Give oxygen to any patient who is having trouble breathing.

If you cannot open the airway, realign the neck. Firmly grasp the patient's head with both hands. Next, pull the head gently and firmly away from the trunk and turn it to the front, bringing the eyes forward. Maintain the head in this in-line position while you repeat the trauma jaw-thrust maneuver. You can also maintain this in-line position as your partner performs the trauma chin-lift maneuver.

## MANUAL IMMOBILIZATION

Once the airway is secure, you must stabilize the head and trunk so bone fragments do not damage the spinal cord. Otherwise, continued motion—even as little as 1 mm—can significantly injure the spinal cord.

Begin manual in-line immobilization by holding the head firmly with both hands, as described above. Whenever possible, kneel behind the patient and place each hand around the base of the skull. Support the lower jaw with your index and long fingers. Support the occiput with your thumbs and palms. Gently lift the head until the patient's eyes are looking straight ahead and the head and torso are in line. This is called the **eyes forward position.** Align the nose with the navel. Never twist, flex, or extend the head or neck excessively. Moving the head to this neutral in-line position makes immobilization easier.

Once you have placed the head in a neutral, in-line position, you must manually maintain the position as you establish the airway and ventilate the patient. Do not remove your hands from the patient's head until the patient is properly secured to a backboard and the head immobilized. The patient must remain immobilized until he or she is examined at the hospital.

Once the patient's head and neck are immobilized, assess the pulse, motor functions, and sensation in all extremities. Then assess the cervical spine area. As you continue to support the head manually, your partner should place a rigid spinal immobilization collar (cervical collar) around the neck to provide some stability. Make sure the collar is the proper size. If you do not have a properly sized collar, you can place

## FIGURE 25-5

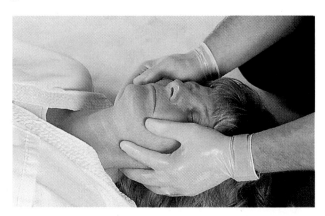

**A**  Stabilize the neck in a neutral, in-line position

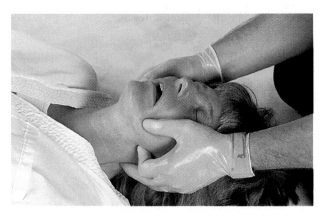

**B**  Push the angle of the lower jaw forward

a rolled towel around the head and tape it to the spine board as you immobilize the patient on the board. Remember that an improperly fitting collar will do more harm than good. The cervical collar provides some support, but it does not replace manual support. Thus, it is important to maintain manual support until the patient is fully secured to a backboard.

### Exceptions to Manual Immobilization

In certain situations, you should not force the head into a neutral, in-line position. Do not move the head if any of the following causes the patient to complain of pain:

- muscle spasms in the neck
- increased pain
- numbness, tingling, or weakness
- compromised airway or ventilations

In these situations, immobilize the patient in the position in which you found him or her.

# PREPARATION FOR TRANSPORT

## SUPINE PATIENTS

A patient who is supine can be effectively immobilized by securing him or her to a long spine board. The ideal procedure for moving a patient from the ground to a long spine board is the **four-person logroll.** This procedure is recommended if you suspect a cervical spine injury. For a patient with no suspected spinal injury, you may choose to slide the patient onto a spine board, use one of many lifts described earlier in this text, or use a scoop stretcher. The patient's condition, the scene, and the available resources will dictate the method you choose. You may recruit bystanders to assist with the logroll, if necessary, but make sure you instruct them fully before moving the patient.

## FIGURE 25-6

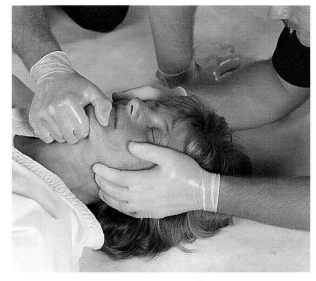

**A**  Stabilize the neck in a neutral, in-line position

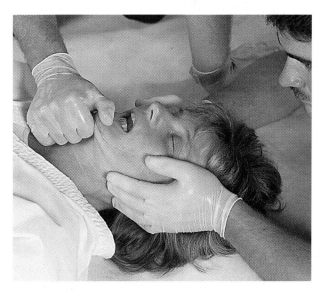

**B**  Lift the chin forward to open the airway

## Four-Person Logroll

You should kneel by the patient's head to maintain manual in-line immobilization. In this position, you will direct the team during the logroll (Figure 25-7a). Your job is to ensure that the head, torso, and pelvis move as a unit. Your team members control the movement of the body. Next, make sure that the spine board is near the patient so that you may slide it under the patient's back. Also, make sure a cervical collar is in place before you begin the logroll (Figure 25-7b).

The team moving the body should place their hands on the far side of the patient (Figure 25-7c). This will increase their leverage. Members of the team moving the body should use their body weight and their shoulder and back muscles to ensure a smooth, coordinated pull. The team should then concentrate their pull on the heavier portions of the patient's body.

At your command, the team should roll the patient onto the spine board (Figure 25-7d). Avoid rotating the head, shoulders, or pelvis while transferring the patient.

Place foam padding or a blanket roll around the head to support it in the in-line position (Figure 25-7e). Pads may also be placed in the space between the patient's torso and the spine board. However, if you place pads under the torso, be careful to avoid excessive patient movement.

Once the patient is centered on the long spine board, secure the upper torso to the

## STEPS AT THE SCENE

### PERFORMING THE FOUR-PERSON LOGROLL

- ☐ EMT-B #1 kneels at the head and maintains manual in-line immobilization to the cervical spine and provides direction for the logroll.

- ☐ EMT-B #2 applies a cervical collar while EMT-B #1 maintains manual in-line immobilization.

- ☐ EMT-B #2 positions his hands on the upper arm and upper thigh, on the far side of the patient.

- ☐ EMT-B #3 positions his hands on the far side of the torso and the far knee.

- ☐ EMT-B #4 positions his hands on the far side of the pelvis and on top of the ankles.

- ☐ EMT-B #1 directs the team to log roll the patient.

- ☐ Position the spine board as close to the patient as possible.

- ☐ Assess the patient's back for bleeding or obvious signs of injury.

- ☐ Slowly and gently roll the patient onto the spine board.

- ☐ Secure the head and neck to the spine board with foam blocks or a blanket roll. Secure the torso and legs to the spine board.

- ☐ Place straps over the patient's forehead.

# FIGURE 25-7

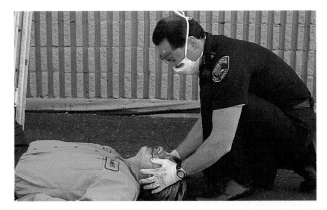

**A** EMT-B #1 maintains in-line immobilization and directs the logroll

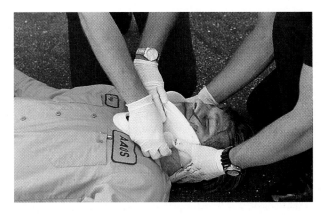

**B** Apply a cervical collar

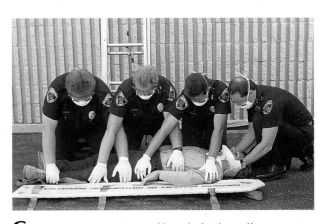

**C** Proper positioning of hands for logroll

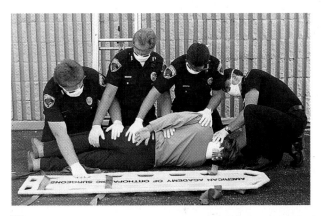

**D** Log roll the patient onto a spine board

board with long straps (Figure 25-7f). Secure the pelvis with a strap over the iliac crests or with groin loops (Figure 25-7g).

Once the patient is adequately padded, secure the patient's head to the board with two straps (Figure 25-7h). One strap passes over the forehead and the second goes over the pads and cervical collar. Straps should never be placed around the chin, in the event that an airway problem develops. Secure the legs to the board with straps that pass above and below the knees (Figure 25-7i). Place the arms securely under a second strap passing across the lower torso so they do not move during transport. Alternatively, you can loosely tie

the patient's wrists together with a cravat or soft, rolled bandage (Figure 25-7j). Reassess the patient's pulses, motor function, and sensation periodically to make sure that the straps are not too tight.

## SITTING PATIENTS

You may find a patient with a possible spinal injury in a sitting position, such as after an automobile accident. In this instance, you need a different approach to immobilization. Use a short spine board or other short spinal extraction device to immobilize the cervical

**FIGURE 25-7** *continued*

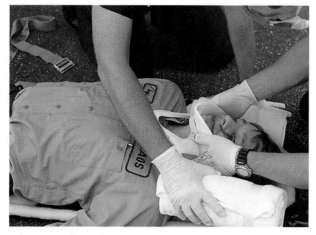

**E** Place rolled towels around the head to maintain the in-line position

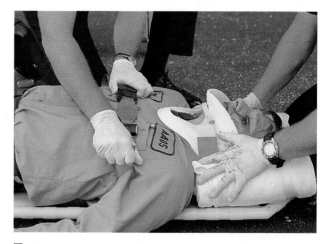

**F** Secure the upper torso to the spine board

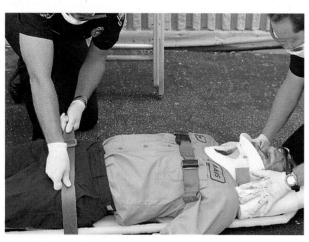

**G** Secure the pelvic area to the spine board

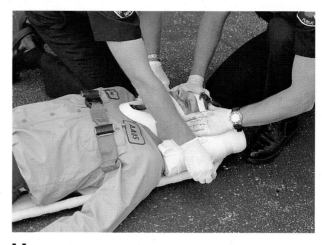

**H** Secure the head to the spine board

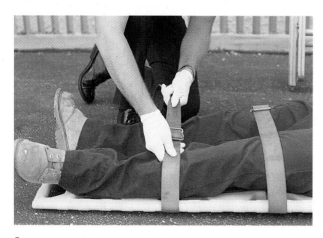

**I** Secure the lower extremities to the spine board

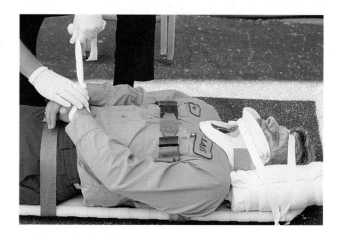

**J** Secure the hands with the cravat

and thoracic spines. However, at times you may have to remove the patient quickly, without taking the time to secure the patient to the short spine board. This may occur in the following situations:

- when the situation is dangerous to you or the patient

- when you need to gain immediate access to other patients

- when the patient's injuries warrant urgent removal

In these cases, your team should lower the patient directly onto a long spine board as you provide manual in-line immobilization.

As with the supine patient, you must first stabilize the head and maintain manual in-line immobilization until the patient is secured to a long spine board. Next, secure the airway and apply the cervical collar (Figure 25-8a). Once you have completed this sequence, wedge the short board between the patient's upper back and the seat (Figure 25-8b). Open the board's side flaps and position them around the patient's torso and snug to the armpits (Figure 25-8c). Make any adjustments necessary without excessive movement of the patient.

Once the board is properly positioned, secure the upper torso straps. Next, secure the midtorso straps (Figure 25-8d). Position and fasten both groin loops (Figure 25-8e). Then, check all torso straps to make sure they are secure. You should next pad any space between the patient's head and the board. Secure the forehead strap and then fasten the lower head strap around the cervical collar (Figure 25-8f).

Your next step is to secure the patient to a long spine board. Place the long board next to the patient's buttocks, perpendicular to the trunk (Figure 25-9a). Then turn the patient until he or she is parallel to the long board. Slowly lower the patient onto the board (Figure 25-9b). Lift the patient (without rotating him or her) and slip the long board under the short board. You can now secure the short and long boards together (Figure 25-9c). Once the patient has been secured to the long spine board, reassess the pulses, motor function, and sensation in all four extremities. Note your findings and prepare to transport the patient.

Remember that, if the patient is critically injured or the situation is dangerous, you should perform the Rapid Extrication technique as described in chapter 6, Lifting and Moving Patients.

## STANDING PATIENTS

You may arrive at a scene in which you find a patient standing or wandering around after an accident or injury. You must immobilize the patient if you suspect there may be underlying head, neck, or spinal injuries. In this situation, you must quickly apply a cervical collar and then instruct the patient to remain still. Once you have applied the cervical collar, you should begin to immobilize the patient to a long spine board. This will require three EMT-Bs. First, position the board upright directly behind the patient. EMT-B #1 and EMT-B #2 should stand on either side of the patient, with EMT-B #3 directly in front of the patient. EMT-Bs #1 and #2 should grasp the spine board with the hand closest to the patient (Figure 25-10a). With the other hand, EMT-Bs #1 and #2 should secure the patient's head (Figure 25-10b). Once this position is secure, EMT-Bs #1 and #2 should place the leg closest to the patient behind the board. EMT-B #3 secures the board and the patient to prevent the patient from sliding off the board (Figure 25-10c). EMT-Bs #1 and #2 then lower the board to the ground (Figure 25-10d). Once the board is on the ground, you should assess the patient's vital signs and proceed with assessment.

**FIGURE 25-8**

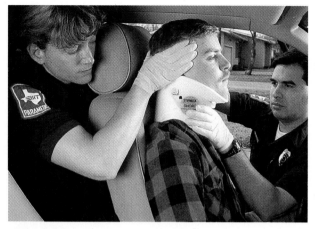

**A** Stabilize the neck in a neutral, in-line position and apply a cervical collar

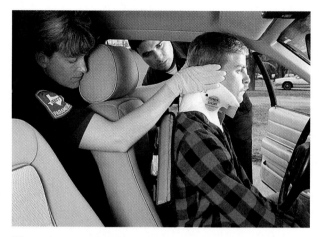

**B** Insert a short spine board between the upper back and the seat

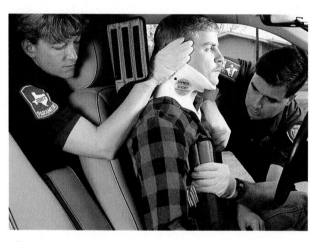

**C** Position side flaps around the patient's torso

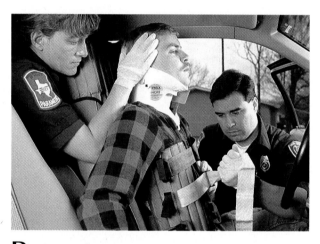

**D** Secure the torso straps

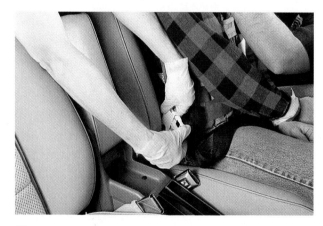

**E** Secure the groin loops

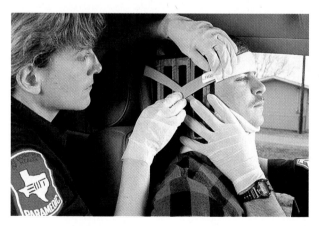

**F** Secure the forehead strap and the lower head strap

**FIGURE 25-9**

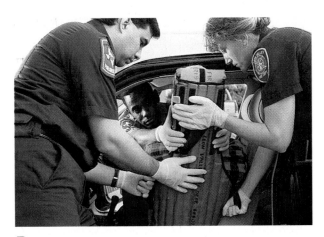

**A** Wedge a long spine board next to the buttocks, perpendicular to the trunk

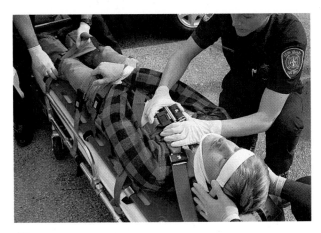

**B** Turn the patient parallel to the spine board and slowly lower the patient

**C** Secure the short spine board to the long spine board

# COMMON HEAD INJURIES

## *BRAIN INJURIES*

### Intracranial Bleeding

If a blood vessel inside the brain or in the meninges is cut, intracranial bleeding (hematoma) will develop. The brain almost completely fills the skull. There is very little room for anything else. Thus, bleeding from a lacerated or torn vessel compresses the brain tissue, resulting in a loss of brain function.

There are three kinds of intracranial hematomas, as follows (Figure 25-11):

1. Epidural, which occurs outside the dura mater but under the skull
2. Subdural, which occurs beneath the dura mater but outside the brain
3. Intracerebral, which occurs within the brain tissue itself

An epidural hematoma develops rapidly, while a subdural hematoma develops very slowly over several days. When the bleeding occurs rapidly, the patient's neurologic status may deteriorate within minutes. If not treated promptly, an expanding hematoma will cause progressive loss of brain function and, eventually, death.

An expanding hematoma inside the skull often requires prompt surgical treatment. Assume that any patient whose neurologic signs deteriorate rapidly following a head injury has an intracranial hematoma. It is important to quickly evaluate such patients. Give the patient oxygen, continue to monitor the airway, elevate the head of the stretcher, and provide immediate transport.

### Cerebral Edema

**Cerebral edema**, or swelling of the brain, is one of the most common and serious complications of any head injury. Like any other tissue, the brain swells when it has been

**FIGURE 25-10**

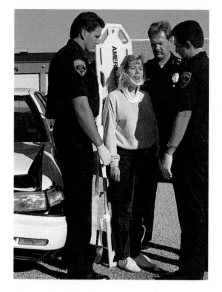

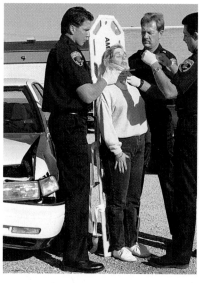

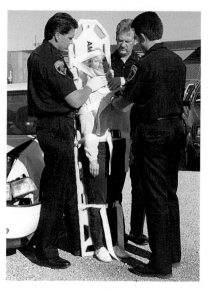

**A**    Position the spine board behind the patient

**B**    Secure the head to the spine board

**C**    Secure the torso and extremities to the spine board

injured. Swelling in the skull, however, compresses the brain tissue, which results in a loss of brain function.

Cerebral edema becomes worse if there are low oxygen levels in the blood. Thus, you must make sure that the airway is open and that adequate ventilations and high-flow oxygen are given. This is especially true if the patient is unconscious. Do not wait for cyanosis or other obvious signs of hypoxia to develop. Many patients need oxygen and ventilatory support before cyanosis appears. You should give high-flow oxygen to any patient with a head injury.

### Other Brain Injuries

Brain injuries are not always a result of trauma. Certain medical conditions, such as blood clots or hemorrhaging, can also cause brain injuries. Nontraumatic injuries can still produce significant bleeding or swelling in the brain. Problems with the blood vessels, high blood pressure, or any number of other causes may cause spontaneous bleeding in the brain. As a result, the patient's level of consciousness will be affected. The signs and symptoms of nontraumatic injuries are the same as those of traumatic brain injuries. However, there is no obvious mechanism of injury or any evidence of trauma.

### SKULL INJURIES

All head injuries are potentially serious. If improperly treated, head injuries that seem minor initially may become life threatening. Severe scalp lacerations or skull fractures that seem serious may not injure the brain or produce long-term problems. Thus, you should not rely on simple appearance. You should suspect a skull injury if the patient has any of the following:

- scalp laceration or contusion
- severe mechanism of injury (trauma)
- visible skull deformities

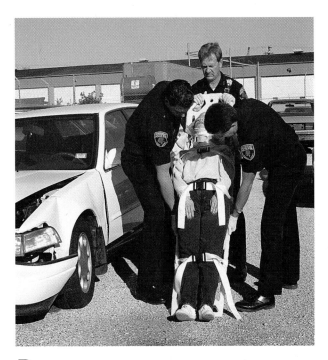

**D**  Lower the spine board to the ground

## FIGURE 25-11

Types of intracranial hematomas

- bruising and discoloration around the eyes (raccoon eyes)
- bruising and discoloration behind the ear over the mastoid process (Battle's sign)
- cerebrospinal fluid leaking from a scalp wound, the nose, or the ear
- failure of the pupils to respond to light
- unequal pupil size
- loss of sensation and/or motor function

### Scalp Lacerations

Scalp lacerations can be minor, or they can be very serious (Figure 25-12). Because both the face and scalp have unusually rich blood supplies, even small lacerations can quickly lead to significant blood losses. Occasionally, this blood loss may be severe enough to cause hypovolemic shock, particularly in children. In patients with multiple injuries, bleeding from scalp or facial lacerations contributes to hypovolemia. In addition, scalp lacerations are usually the result of direct blows to the head. Thus,

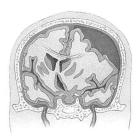

A.  Subdural

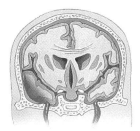

B.  Intracerebral

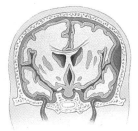

C.  Epidural

## FIGURE 25-12

A scalp laceration

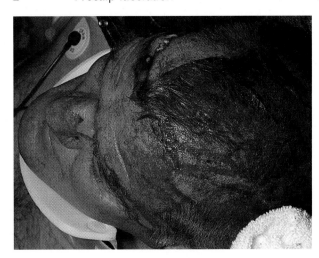

# FIGURE 25-13

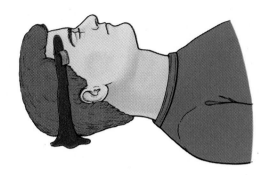

**A**  A flap-type scalp laceration

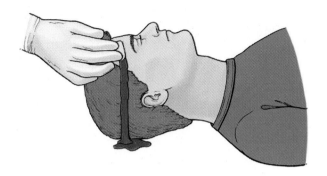

**B**  Fold the flap back down onto the skin bed

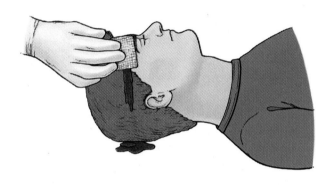

**C**  Apply firm pressure with a dry, sterile dressing

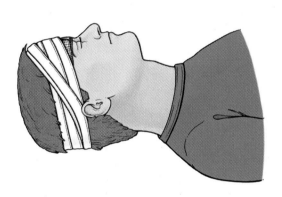

**D**  Secure the dressing with a soft roller bandage

these injuries often indicate other, deeper, more serious injuries.

You can almost always control bleeding from a scalp laceration by applying direct pressure over the wound. Remember to follow BSI techniques. Use a dry, sterile dressing. Fold any skin flaps torn from the skin back down onto the bed before applying pressure. In some instances, you will have to apply firm compression for several minutes to control the bleeding. If you suspect a skull injury, do not apply excessive pressure to the open wound. Otherwise, you may increase intracranial pressure or push bone fragments into the brain.

If the dressing becomes soaked, do not remove it. Rather, place a second dressing over the original. Continue applying manual pressure until the bleeding is controlled. Once the bleeding is under control, secure the compression dressing in place with a soft, self-adhering roller bandage (Figure 25-13).

## Closed Injuries

Closed head injuries are usually associated with trauma. A closed head injury is an injury in which the brain has been injured, but the skin has not been broken. In addition, there is no obvious bleeding. When assessing a patient with a possible closed head injury, consider the mechanism of injury. Did the patient fall? Was he or she in an automobile accident? Was the patient an assault victim? Look for scalp lacerations and hematomas or skull deformities. Sometimes, the skull may appear as if it has been pushed into the brain.

Certainly, closed head injuries can lead to neurologic deficit. Decreased level of consciousness is the most reliable sign of this type of injury. Monitor the patient for changes in level of consciousness, including signs of confusion, disorientation, or deteriorating mental status. Is the patient unresponsive or repeating questions? Is the patient experiencing any seizures? Next, assess for decreased movement and/or numbness and tingling in the extremities. Also assess the vital signs carefully. People with head injuries may have irregular respirations, depending on which region of the brain is affected. Nausea and vomiting are also common.

As you perform your focused assessment, look for blood or fluid leaking from the ears, nose, or mouth. Blood or fluid leaking (cerebrospinal fluid or CSF) from these areas may indicate an injury to the base of the skull. Discoloration around the eyes, known as "raccoon eyes," is another indication of a CSF leak and possible injury at the base of the skull. Bruising or discoloration behind the ear over the mastoid process is known as Battle's sign (Figure 25-14).

You may also evaluate the patient's pupils, especially if the patient has a decreased level of consciousness. Often, unequal pupil size after a head injury signals a serious problem. Developing blood clots may be pressing on the third cranial nerve, causing one pupil to dilate.

## FIGURE 25-14

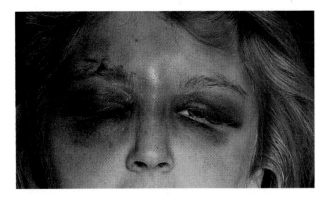

**A**  Raccoon eyes

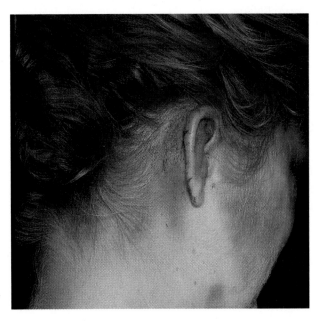

**B**  Battle's sign

### Open Injuries

As with closed head injuries, open head injuries may be present if there are scalp contusions, lacerations, or hematomas. Obvious skull deformities are another sign of this type of injury. A penetrating injury is an open head injury. Remember, do not remove any impaled objects. Open and closed head injuries have essentially the same signs and symptoms, including seizure activity, and nausea and vomiting.

You should also suspect an open head injury if you detect a soft or depressed area of the skull. There may be bleeding and exposed brain tissue if there is an open wound. Once again, blood or CSF leaking from the ears, nose, or mouth suggests a head injury. Bruising around the eyes or behind the ears can be present with an open head injury. Do not probe open scalp lacerations with your gloved finger. This may cause bone fragments to be pushed into the brain.

## EMERGENCY MEDICAL CARE

Your care of a patient with a possible head injury begins with ABCD—regardless of the severity of the head injury. Be sure to follow BSI techniques.

### RESTORING THE AIRWAY

If a patient with a head injury has an airway obstruction, you should perform the trauma jaw-thrust or trauma chin-lift maneuver to open the airway. Once the airway is open, maintain the head in a neutral, in-line position, until it can be fully immobilized with a cervical collar. Remove any foreign bodies, secretions, or vomitus from the airway. Make sure a suctioning unit is available because you will often need to clear blood, saliva, or vomitus from the airway. Give oxygen to any patient who is having trouble breathing.

Once you have cleared the airway, you need to provide adequate ventilation. Monitor the patient's respirations. If the part of the brain that controls respirations has been damaged, the patient's breathing may be ineffective. Chest injuries or paralysis of some or all respiratory muscles due to a spinal injury may also affect breathing.

By giving the patient high-flow oxygen, you help reduce hypoxia and possible cerebral edema. An injured brain is even less tolerant of hypoxia than a healthy brain. More than any other part of the body, the brain requires a constant, rich supply of oxygen. Without it, severe brain damage or death may occur in minutes.

### MANUAL IMMOBILIZATION

Once you have established an airway and given the patient oxygen, you must immobilize the patient and perform your initial assessment. Any patient with a head injury should be immobilized as if he or she has a spinal injury as well. As described above, provide manual, in-line immobilization as you open the airway and apply a cervical collar. Next, secure the patient to a long spine board. Elevate the head of the spinal immobilization device about 6" (Figure 25-15). Keep a suctioning unit available to clear any buildup of fluids in the airway.

### FIGURE 25-15

Elevate the head of the stretcher to transport a patient with a head injury

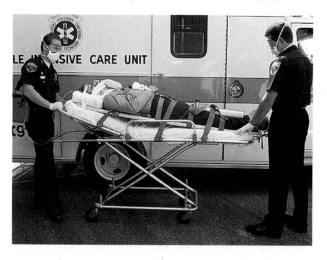

## ASSESSING THE PATIENT

You should now continue your initial assessment. Plan on completing your complete detailed physical exam en route. Determining whether a patient with a head injury also has a spinal injury is often very difficult, even with a conscious patient. The patient may not report any pain along the spine, and there may be no loss of neurologic function. The patient may not feel any pain along the spine due to shock or more painful injuries elsewhere. Thus, your care of a patient with a head injury should include immobilizing the spine. Identifying a spinal injury in an unconscious patient is even more difficult. Moving an injured cervical spine may cause permanent, irreversible damage. With an unconscious patient, you should make spinal immobilization part of your routine care.

As you continue to treat the patient, closely monitor the airway, respirations, pulse, and level of consciousness. Patients with head injuries may also experience seizures. Control external bleeding of soft tissue injuries with direct pressure. Remember, do not apply pressure to an open or depressed skull injury. This pressure may damage the brain further.

If the patient has a medical condition or nontraumatic injury along with the head injury, place him or her on the left side. Be sure to maintain the head in the in-line neutral position, with the cervical collar in place. This position will prevent aspiration if the patient happens to vomit. Thus, you should have a suctioning unit available. Provide immediate transport for these patients.

## IMMOBILIZATION DEVICES

### CERVICAL COLLARS

Rigid cervical immobilization devices, or cervical collars, provide preliminary, partial support. A cervical collar should be applied to every patient who has a possible spinal injury, based on mechanism of injury, history, or signs and symptoms. Although cervical collars are used routinely in spinal immobilization, they do not fully immobilize the cervical spine. Therefore, you must maintain manual support until the patient is completely secured to a spinal immobilization device, such as a long or a short spine board.

To be effective, a rigid cervical collar must be the correct size for the patient. It should rest on the shoulder girdle and provide firm support under both sides of the mandible. It must not obstruct the airway or ventilation efforts in any way. If you do not have the correct size, use a rolled towel and tape it to the spine board around the patient's head and provide continuous manual support (Figure 25-16). If the cervi-

## FIGURE 25-16

Use a rolled towel as a cervical collar if a properly fitting collar is not available

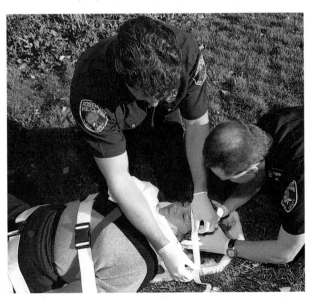

cal collar fits properly, either you or your partner should apply the collar while the other provides continuous manual in-line support of the head.

## SHORT SPINE BOARDS

There are several types of short board immobilization devices. The most common are the vest-type device and the rigid short board (Figure 25-17). These devices are designed to stabilize and immobilize the head, neck, and torso. They are used to immobilize noncritical patients who are found in a sitting position and have possible spinal injuries.

## FIGURE 25-17

Types of short spine boards

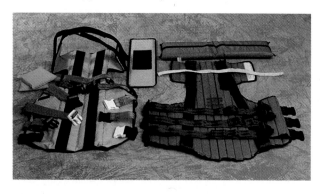

As described earlier in this chapter, the first step in securing a patient to a short spine board or device is to provide manual, in-line support of the cervical spine. Then assess the pulses, motor function, and sensation in all extremities. Next, assess the cervical area and apply an appropriately sized cervical collar.

Position the device behind the patient and secure it to the patient's torso. Evaluate how well the torso and groin are secured and make adjustments, as necessary. Avoid excessive movement of the patient. Next, evaluate the position of the patient's head.

Pad behind the head, as needed, to maintain neutral, in-line immobilization.

Next, secure the patient's head to the device. You can now release manual support of the head. Rotate or lift the patient to the long spine board. At this point, you must reassess the pulses, motor function, and sensation in all four extremities. Reassessment is important to determine if this change in position has affected the patient's vital signs or neurologic status. Finally, you should immobilize the patient to the long spine board.

## LONG SPINE BOARDS

There are several types of long board immobilization devices (Figure 25-18). These devices provide full body spinal immobilization. Long spine boards are used to immobilize patients found in any position—standing, sitting, or supine. They are sometimes used in conjunction with short spine boards.

## FIGURE 25-18

Types of long spine boards

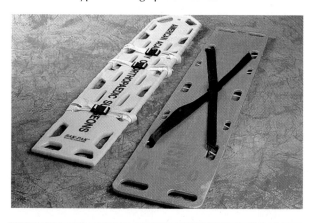

Securing a patient to a long spine board was described in detail earlier in this chapter. Briefly, you should begin by providing manual, in-line support of the head. Next, assess pulses, motor function, and sensation in all extremities. After assessing the cervical area, apply an appropriately sized cervical collar.

Now position the device. Log roll the patient onto the device. As you maintain in-line support, your partner should kneel by the patient's head and direct the other two EMT-Bs as you roll the patient. Your partner's job is to make sure that the head, torso, and pelvis move as a unit.

As the patient's back comes into view, quickly assess its condition if you did not do so during initial assessment. One EMT-B should position the device under the pa-

tient. Then, at your partner's command, roll the patient onto the board.

If there are voids between the patient's head and torso and the board, fill them with pads. In an adult, these voids are usually under the head and torso. In a child, place padding under the shoulders to the toes to establish a neutral position.

Next, secure the torso to the device by applying straps across the chest and pelvis. Adjust these straps as needed. Next, secure the patient's head to the board. Secure the legs, above and below the knees, to the board last. At this point, reassess pulses, motor function, and sensation in all extremities. When the patient is properly secured, you can safely lift the board or turn it on its side, if necessary (Figure 25-19).

## FIGURE 25-19

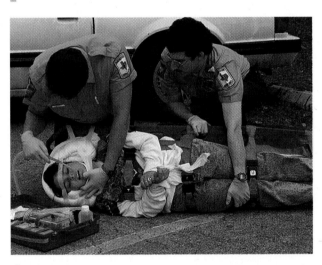

**A**   Properly secured patient turned to the side

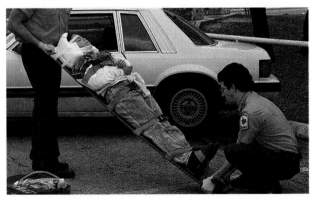

**B**   Properly secured patient lifted vertically

## SPECIAL CONSIDERATIONS

### RAPID EXTRICATION TECHNIQUE

Rapid extrication may be necessary in any number of situations. The scene may be dangerous to you and/or the patient. It may be necessary if the patient's condition is unstable or if you must reach a more seriously injured patient. Base your decision on time constraints and the patient's condition, not on your personal preference. The steps of the Rapid Extrication technique are discussed in detail in chapter 6, Lifting and Moving Patients.

### HELMET REMOVAL

As you plan your care of a patient wearing a helmet, ask yourself the following questions:

- Is the patient's airway clear?
- Is the patient breathing adequately?

## ROLLOVER ROULETTE

While returning to quarters after a call, you notice a car in the oncoming lane moving erratically. Without warning, the driver loses control of the car and veers off the road. The car rolls over at least twice on the way down the embankment. As you attempt to turn around, your partner notifies dispatch of the accident and requests a tow truck and another ambulance. You find the car upside down. The 31-year-old woman driving the car was not wearing a seat belt. You find her lying on the inside of the roof. She is alert only to name, belligerent in responding to your questions, and has the distinct smell of alcohol. She is moving all four extremities and doesn't even want you to take her vital signs. You finally convince her she's been in a serious accident. She says you can treat her. She has a blood pressure of 110/64 mm Hg, a pulse of 104/min, and respirations of 16/min. She says she's been at a party since 5 pm, where she was drinking tequila shooters. It's currently 1 am.

### For Discussion

1. What are the implications of improper care of a potential spinal injury?

2. What makes a rollover accident potentially fatal—especially for unbelted occupants?

---

- Can you maintain the airway and assist ventilations if the helmet remains in place?

- How well does the helmet fit?

- Can the patient move within the helmet?

- Can the patient's spine be immobilized in a neutral position with the helmet on?

A helmet that fits well prevents the patient's head from moving. If the patient's helmet fits well, leave it on. Leave the helmet in place if it does not interfere with assessing and treating airway or ventilation problems. You should also leave the helmet on if there is any chance that removing it will further injure the patient. Finally, leave the helmet on if you can properly immobilize the spine.

You should remove a helmet if it makes assessing or managing airway problems difficult. A poorly fitting helmet that allows excessive head movement must be removed. A helmet that prevents you from

## FIGURE 25-20

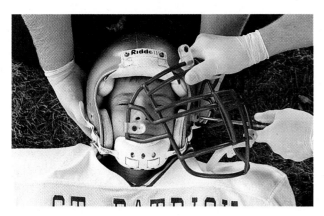

**A**    Stabilize the neck in a neutral, in-line position

**B**    Remove the face guard to access the airway

## FIGURE 25-21

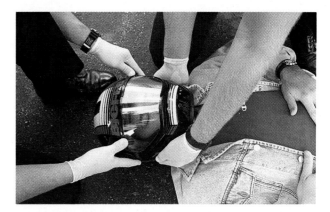

**A**    Stabilize the neck in a neutral in-line position

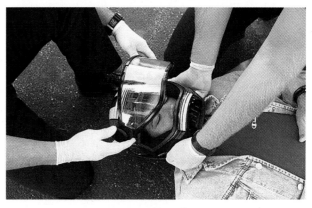

**B**    Remove the face shield to access the airway

properly immobilizing the spine should also be removed. You must always remove a helmet if the patient is in cardiac arrest.

### Types of Helmets

How you remove a helmet depends on the type of helmet the patient is wearing. Sports helmets are typically open in the front. They may or may not include an attached face mask. The mask can be removed without affecting the helmet position or function. This is done by simply removing or cutting the straps that hold the mask to the helmet. As such, sports helmets allow easy access to the airway (Figure 25-20). Motorcycle helmets often have a shield covering the face. This shield can be unbuckled to allow access to the airway (Figure 25-21). Some motorcycle helmets have face shields that cannot be removed. In these situations, the helmet will have to be removed to access the patient's airway.

### Removing a Helmet

You and your partner should first consult with medical control, if possible, about your decision to remove the patient's helmet. Begin by kneeling down at the patient's

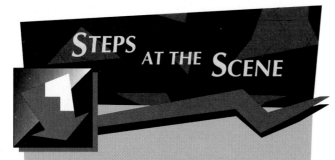

## STEPS AT THE SCENE

### REMOVING A HELMET

☐ Remove the patient's eyeglasses, if he or she is wearing them.

☐ EMT-B #1 should place his or her hands on each side of the helmet and his or her fingers on the mandible. This stabilizes the helmet.

☐ EMT-B #2 loosens the strap on the helmet.

☐ EMT-B #2 places one hand on the lower jaw at the angle of the jaw and the other hand behind the head at the occipital region.

☐ EMT-B #1 pulls the sides of the helmet apart and gently slips the helmet halfway off the head. Remember to stop pulling when the helmet is halfway off the head.

☐ EMT-B #2 slides the hand supporting the occipital region toward the top of the patient's head. This prevents the head from falling back after the helmet is completely removed.

☐ EMT-B #1 removes the helmet and begins immobilizing the cervical spine.

head. Your partner should kneel on one side of the patient, at the shoulder area. First, open the face shield, such as on a motorcycle helmet, and assess the patient's airway and breathing. Remove any eyeglasses, if the patient is wearing them.

Next, you must stabilize the helmet by placing your hands on either side of the helmet. Your fingers should be on the patient's lower jaw to prevent movement of the head. Once your hands are in position, your partner can loosen the face strap (Figure 25-22a).

Once the strap is loosened, your partner should place one hand on the lower jaw at the angle of the jaw. The other hand should be placed behind the head at the occipital region (Figure 25-22b). Once your partner's hands are in position, you may pull the sides of the helmet away from the patient's head. Gently slip the helmet halfway off the patient's head. Be sure to stop pulling once the helmet is pulled to the halfway point (Figure 25-22c). Your partner then slides his or her hand from the occiput to the back of the head. This will prevent the head from snapping back once the helmet is completely removed (Figure 25-22d). With your partner's hand in place, you may then remove the helmet and immobilize the cervical spine (Figure 25-22e). You may then apply the cervical collar and secure the patient to the spine board.

Remember that during helmet removal, one EMT-B is always providing in-line support as the other EMT-B moves. You and your partner should not move at the same time. Remember also that in many instances, removing a patient's helmet is not necessary. This is the case in the following situations:

- if you can access the airway

- if the head is snug inside the helmet so that the helmet can be secured to an immobilization device.

FIGURE 25-22

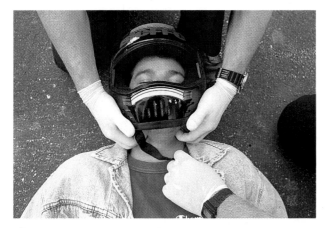

**A** EMT-B #1 maintains the neck in a neutral, in-line position, as EMT-B #2 removes the chin strap

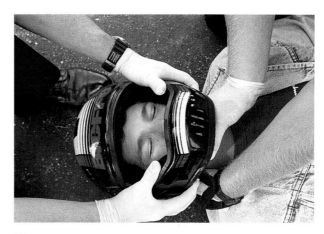

**B** EMT-B #1 grasps the helmet, as EMT-B #2 supports the occiput

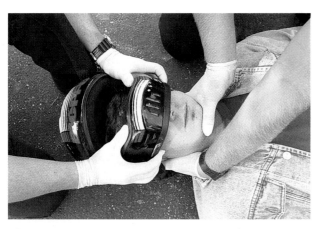

**C** EMT-B #1 slips the helmet halfway off the head

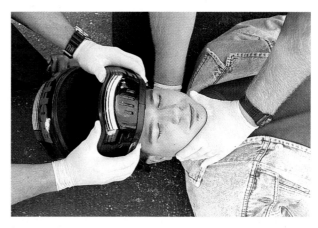

**D** EMT-B #1 removes the helmet, as EMT-B #2 now supports the back of the head

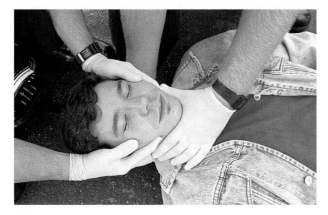

**E** Maintain the neck in a neutral, in-line position until the cervical collar is applied

With large helmets or small patients, you may need to pad under the shoulders. This will prevent flexion of the neck.

## PEDIATRIC CONSIDERATIONS

You are likely to find infants and children involved in automobile accidents still in their car seats. Your best course of action is to immobilize the child in the car seat, if

## FIGURE 25-23

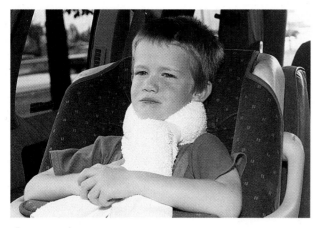

**A** Use a rolled towel as a cervical collar to immobilize a child in a car seat

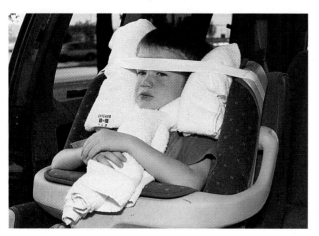

**B** Pad the sides of the car seat to prevent lateral movement

possible. Whenever you apply a cervical collar, make sure it is properly sized. If a properly fitting collar is not available, use a rolled towel and tape it to the car seat (Figure 25-23a). An improperly fitting collar does more harm than good. Apply a properly fitting cervical collar and pad the sides of the car seat, if necessary, to prevent lateral movement (Figure 25-23b). Place additional padding in any spaces between the patient and the car seat. If the child is not in a car seat or was removed before your ar-

rival, use an appropriately sized immobilization device.

Remember that small children may require additional padding to maintain the in-line neutral position. Children are not small adults. They have smaller airways, so padding is important to maintain the airway. Pad under the shoulders to the toes, as needed, to avoid excessive neck flexion (Figure 25-24a). In addition, place blanket rolls between the child and the sides of an adult- sized board to prevent the child from slipping to one side or the other (Figure 25-24b). Appropriately sized spine boards are available for children.

## FIGURE 25-24

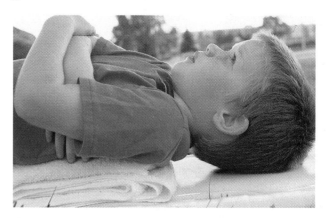

**A** Pad between the child's shoulders and the spine board

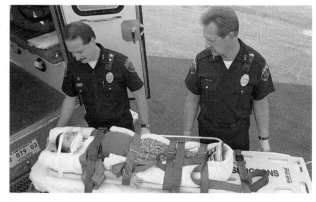

**B** Place blanket rolls between the child and the sides of an adult spine board

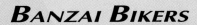

## *BANZAI BIKERS*

Taunts turn to trouble, as two young men step from the bar and decide to test just exactly who has the "baddest ride." They hop on their new motorcycles and head to the interstate's frontage road to have a little run for the money. On cue from a mutual friend, they take off and run side by side for a quarter mile until one loses control and swerves off the road. As his bike crashes into the ditch, he is launched through the air, crashing into some small birch trees. You find a 21-year-old man, wearing a T-shirt, sandals, and no helmet. He is responsive only to pain when you move his arms and legs. He has a blood pressure of 168/92 mm Hg, a pulse of 64/min, and irregular respirations of 28/min. His pupils are unequal. The left is fixed and dilated. His left femur is severely angulated, and he has multiple abrasions on his arms, legs, shoulders, and hands.

### For Discussion

1. Discuss the importance of airway management to a patient with a suspected cervical spine injury.

2. Describe the importance of your assessment of the mechanism of injury as it relates to injuries of the cervical spine and spinal cord.

# CHAPTER 26
Infants and Children

# Infants and Children

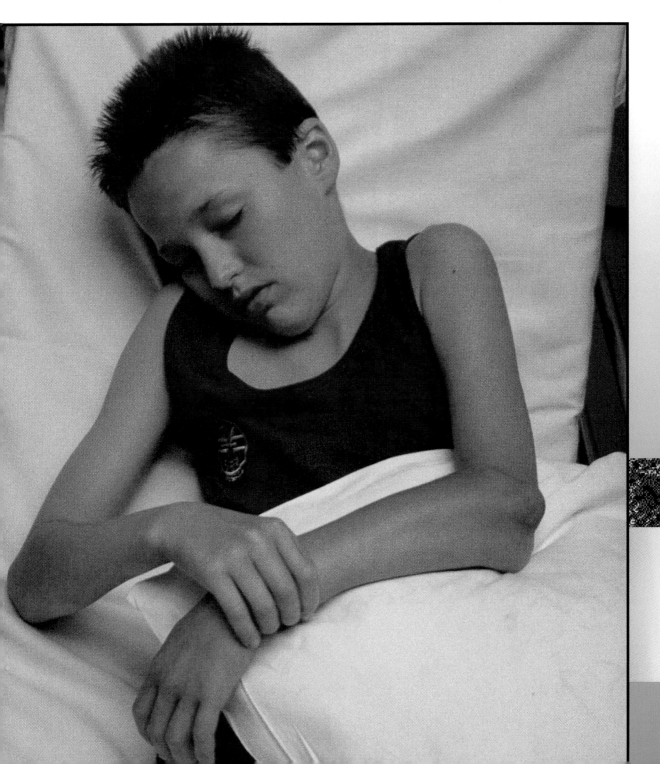

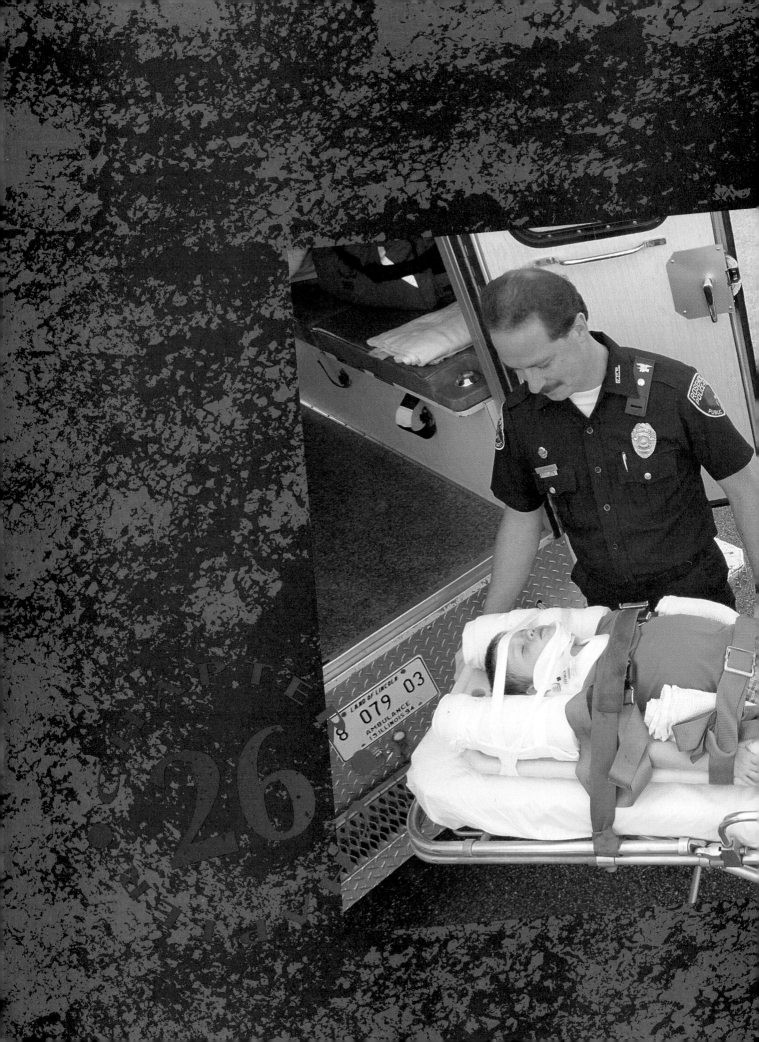

# Infants and Children

## Objectives

After you have read this chapter, you should be able to:

- Identify the developmental considerations for infants; toddlers; preschool, school-age, and adolescent children.
- Describe differences in the anatomy and physiology of infants, children, and adults.
- Differentiate the response of the ill or injured infant or child from that of an adult.
- Indicate various causes of respiratory emergencies.
- Differentiate between respiratory distress and respiratory failure and summarize the emergency medical care strategies for both.
- List the steps in the management of foreign body airway obstruction.
- Identify the signs and symptoms of shock (hypoperfusion) in infants and children.
- Describe the methods of determining end organ perfusion in infants and children.
- State the usual cause of cardiac arrest in infants and children.
- List the common causes of seizures in infants and children and describe how to manage them.
- Differentiate between the injury patterns in adults, infants, and children.
- Discuss the field management of the infant and child trauma patient.
- Summarize the indicators of possible child abuse and neglect.
- Describe the medicolegal responsibilities in suspected child abuse.
- Recognize the need for debriefing following a difficult transport of an infant or child.

# 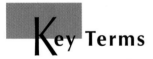Overview

As an EMT-B, some of the most difficult emergencies you will handle involve injured, ill, or physically or sexually abused infants and children. At the same time, perhaps no part of the job is as rewarding. Saving an infant's life or rescuing a child from permanent, disabling injury means giving back the promise of years of life and happiness.

It is important for you to understand that children differ from adults in more than just body size and build. Several conditions, particularly certain infections, occur more often in children. However, trauma is the leading cause of death in children over the age of 1 year. Although the basic principles of caring for children are similar to those for adults, certain differences do exist.

The chapter begins with a description of pediatrics and various developmental stages. Next, the chapter addresses the initial approach to pediatric assessment. You will then learn about a number of specific emergencies involving infants and children. These include fever, abdominal pain, poisoning, drowning, infectious diseases, and sudden infant death syndrome (SIDS). The chapter also discusses physical abuse, neglect, and sexual abuse. It concludes by explaining that you must deal with the emotions of the patient's family as well as your own.

# Key Terms

**Child abuse**   Any improper or excessive action that injures or harms a child or infant.

**Dehydration**   Loss of water from the tissues of the body.

**Meningitis**   An inflammation of the meningeal coverings of the brain and spinal cord caused by either a virus or a bacterium.

**Neonate**   A newborn infant.

**Pediatrics**   Medical practice devoted to the care of children up to age 18.

**Sudden infant death syndrome (SIDS)**   Death from unknown cause occurring during sleep in an otherwise healthy infant. Also called "crib death."

# THE PEDIATRIC PATIENT

Children have many unique health problems. Similarly, many problems common in adults do not occur in children. Thus, there is a separate medical practice devoted to the care of the young called **pediatrics.**

Handling a sick or injured child can be extremely challenging. It is almost always a trying experience to care for a seriously ill or injured child. Not everyone is comfortable caring for children. In most situations, handling an infant or child means you must manage the parents as well. Thus, it is vital that you are calm and professional when you care for a child. Hard as it is, you must keep your personal feelings in check as you work with infants, children, and their families.

Despite these challenges, you have an opportunity to make a real difference in the lives of these children and their families.

## DEVELOPMENTAL CONCERNS

Traditionally, pediatrics pertains to children up to age 15. Recently, however, the upper age limit has been extended to the age of 18 years. This is when many children move away from home. Within this span of 18 years, a child experiences major changes. Therefore, the following developmental stages have been created by pediatricians. Each stage has typical behavior patterns and specific medical problems (Figure 26-1).

## FIGURE 26-1

Developmental stages of infants and children

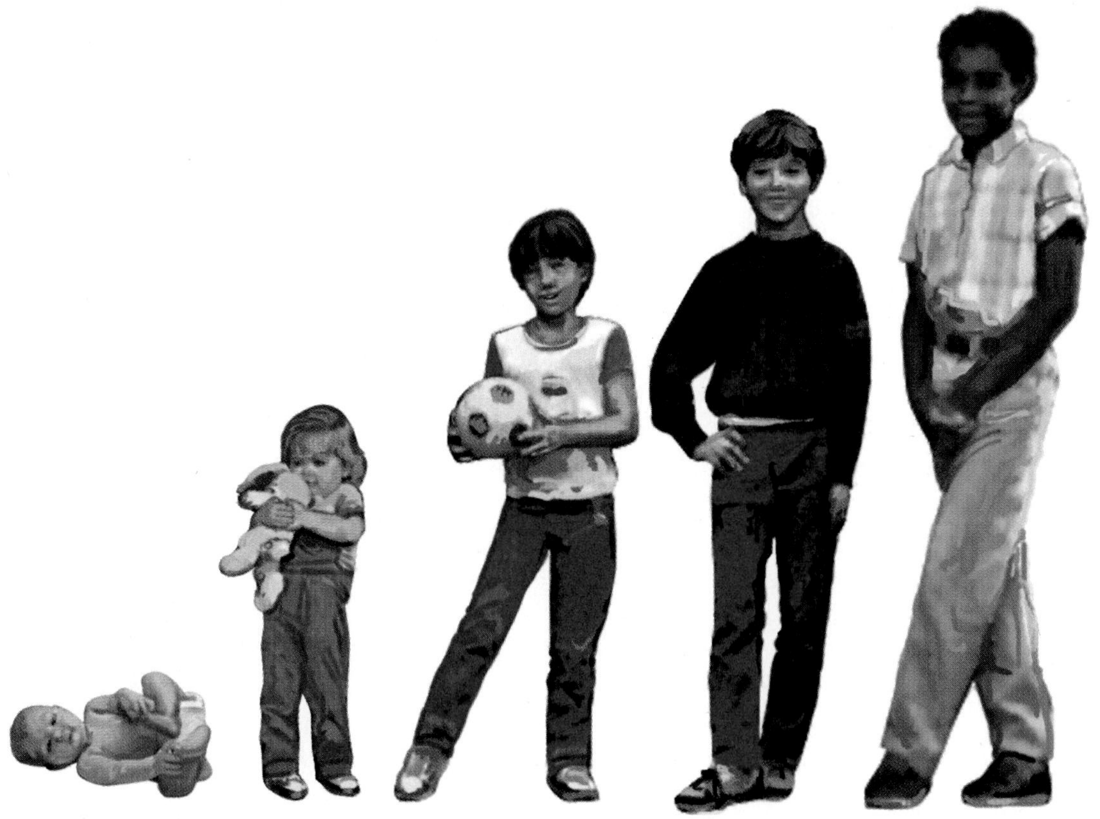

Infant     Toddler     Preschool Child     School-Age Child     Adolescent

## Infants

From birth until the age of 1 year, a child is regarded as an infant. However, in the first 30 days following birth, an infant is sometimes referred to as a newborn or **neonate.**

During infancy, the major causes of death are problems related to birth. This includes premature birth and birth defects.

Infants are not usually frightened of strangers. However, they do not like to be separated from their parents or caregivers.

You need to keep infants warm. Make sure your hands and stethoscope are warm before touching an infant. Assess an infant's breathing as you approach, before you touch the child. You can determine the rate by watching the chest rise and fall. Infants will resist an oxygen mask being placed over their face. Before approaching the infant, also note the skin color and level of activity. Begin your assessment by examining the heart and lungs first. Examine the head last.

## Toddlers

Children between the ages of 1 and 3 years are considered toddlers. During this stage, children are very active. They are developing physical skills but do not understand the concept of danger and possible injury. Toddlers often find a way around gates and other devices designed to ensure their safety. As a result, injuries are the leading cause of death among toddlers.

Toddlers know what they dislike or do not wish to do, and they will make sure you know, too. Toddlers do not like being touched, especially by strangers. Nor do they like being separated from their parents. Also, they do not want to remove their clothing. Thus, your assessment will be more successful if you uncover one area at a time or remove a single piece of clothing. Replace the clothing before moving on to another area.

Toddlers are afraid of needles. They will also resist an oxygen mask being placed over their faces because they fear being held down and suffocated.

Typically, toddlers are afraid, especially if they are in pain or bleeding. As a result, take great care to examine them gently and carefully. Examine the body before examining the head. Throughout the process, tell the toddler that you are there to help. It is particularly important to reassure a toddler that he or she has not been hurt or is sick as punishment for being bad.

## Preschool Children

Children between the ages of 3 and 6 years are considered preschoolers. Although they are larger and more active than toddlers, preschool children are very similar to toddlers. Preschoolers can be particularly shy and fearful of strangers. They will resist separation from their parents and are increasingly modest. Thus, you should replace clothes you have removed during assessment as soon as possible.

Like infants and toddlers, preschool children fear that an oxygen mask will suffocate them. In most emergency situations, they are also afraid of pain, bleeding, and permanent injury. Plus, they still worry that an injury or illness is a punishment for being bad. In addition, their active imaginations may invent strange, elaborate, and, at times, frightening ideas about what is occurring and what is about to happen. You may not be able to reassure them, but you should try.

## School-Age Children

School-age children are between the ages of 6 and 12 years. These children are more developed and mobile than younger children. As a result, they are more likely to be victims of trauma, particularly injuries from car accidents. They are also commonly involved in bicycle-car or pedestrian-car accidents. They are more likely to have sports injuries than younger children.

School-age children are better able to understand an emergency and are often easier to deal with than younger children. Nonetheless, they remain quite modest, especially around strangers. They fear pain, blood, and permanent injury. They also worry that permanent injury will make them look strange or different to their friends.

### Adolescents

Children between the ages of 12 and 18 years are considered adolescents. A number of problems are unique to this age group. However, this group also experiences several injuries and illnesses common to adults. Unfortunately, major adolescent health issues include some very adult problems, including the following:

- trauma, especially automobile accidents
- drug use and overdose
- alcohol abuse
- gunshot wounds and other injuries due to violence
- complications related to pregnancy

Adolescents can act in a variety of ways during an emergency, depending on how well they understand what is happening. Adolescents who have had a traumatic injury are often most concerned with permanent injury and/or how they will look as a result. Adolescents may be extremely modest, a behavior that may be affected if they have been using drugs or alcohol.

It is important for you to treat adolescents as if they were adults. Many adolescents are sensitive about being treated like children (Table 26-1).

## ANATOMY AND PHYSIOLOGY

The basic difference in caring for a child compared with an adult is that a child is smaller in size. However, you should remember that a child is not a small adult. For more detailed information on specific anatomic differences, review chapter 4, The Human Body.

A patient's size affects which basic airway techniques you should use. For children older than 8 years, adult techniques are effective. For patients younger than 8 years, you must modify your techniques. For example, you need to position a young child's airway differently than an adult's to avoid hyperextending the neck. This distinction is a guideline, not a rigid rule. If the patient is a small 9- or 10-year-old, manage that individual as a child. Specific CPR techniques for infants, children, and adults are presented in appendix A, BLS Review.

**TABLE 26-1**     **EXAMINATION TIPS**

| Age Group | Examination Tip |
| --- | --- |
| Infants | Make sure your hands are warm! Start exam with the heart and lungs. |
| Toddlers | Do not remove all their clothing at once. Uncover them area by area, then recover. |
| Preschoolers | Reassure them they have not been bad. |
| School-Age | Respect their modesty. |
| Adolescents | Make sure you treat them as adults. |

As you review the CPR techniques for infants and children, it is important to remember that a child's tongue is large relative to the jaw and airway. Thus, it can easily obstruct the airway of an unconscious child. In addition, the air passages in a child's respiratory system are smaller than those in an adult's. Therefore, secretions or swelling can easily block these passages.

Remember that infants are nose breathers and cannot breathe easily from their mouths. Therefore, suctioning the nose can significantly improve an infant's breathing.

Children usually compensate well for breathing problems for a short period of time. They do so by using their accessory muscles and by breathing faster. However, this is only a short-term solution. Their breathing muscles tire as they become more tired from the extra work of breathing. Thus, they can develop serious breathing problems rather quickly. You must be alert for changes in a child's breathing and ready to intervene.

Respiratory emergencies are very common in infants and children. These are covered later in this chapter. To review airway management in children, see chapter 8, Airway and Ventilation, as well as appendix A, BLS Review.

## ASSESSING INFANTS AND CHILDREN

As you approach a child for the first time, quickly gather a general impression of overall appearance. At the same time, ask the parents about the patient's history. You can begin to evaluate the ABCD from a distance. For example, assess the child's overall level of consciousness. Is the child awake, alert, crying, groggy, minimally responsive, or unconscious?

Assess the child's breathing. Does the child have to work hard to breathe? Is there nasal flaring, stridor, crowing, or noisy res-

pirations? Is the child grunting as he or she breathes? You can assess the respiratory rate from a distance or while you are at the child's side. Remember, a lack of oxygen will agitate a child. A build-up of carbon dioxide will reduce responsiveness.

Note the child's color. Is the skin pale, pink, mottled, or cyanotic? Listen for the quality of the cry or speech. Watch how the child interacts with his or her surroundings, especially with parents. Is the child playing and moving around, making eye contact? Or is the patient inattentive? Also evaluate the emotional state, overall body tone, and position. What is the child's response to you?

If you are a careful observer, you can gather a lot of information very quickly as you approach the scene.

Once you are at the child's side, assess the breath sounds. Is there any stridor or wheezing that you did not hear as you approached the child? Assess circulation at the brachial or femoral pulse. Also, check the peripheral pulses and capillary refill. In children older than 3 years, obtain a blood pressure reading. Be sure to use a cuff that is appropriately sized for small children (Figure 26-2).

## FIGURE 26-2

Adult and pediatric blood pressure cuffs

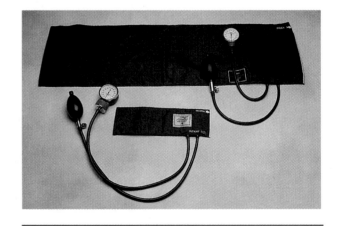

As you begin the detailed physical exam, start at the trunk and end at the head. Listen to the chest and examine the abdomen before moving to the head. Remember that the age of the child has a great impact on how well the child will cooperate with you. Young children will often cry or become agitated if you begin by examining the head. Thus, your exam of the heart or breath sounds becomes much more difficult.

# COMMON MEDICAL CONDITIONS

## AIRWAY OBSTRUCTION

An airway obstruction caused by swallowing a foreign body is an especially common problem in young children. This is especially true in small children who are crawling and exploring their environment. Sometimes the foreign body, such as a peanut, part of a hot dog, or small toy, is aspirated into a lung. If it is, it can only be removed under anesthesia at the hospital.

### Partial Airway Obstruction

With a partial, or incomplete, obstruction, the patient will still be able to breathe, although with some difficulty. You will usually find the patient conscious, alert, and sitting. If you hear stridor, crowing, or noisy respirations, there may be a partial obstruction. Also look for muscle retractions. Retractions are seen when the muscles of the chest and neck work extra hard as the child breathes. Because they are still getting some air, these patients will have healthy, pink skin and good capillary refill.

Children in respiratory distress will usually be in a position that helps them to breathe easier. Let them stay in that position as long as the partial airway obstruction does not become a complete one. Help younger children to sit up. They should not lie down. Try to have them sit on a parent's lap.

In addition, try not to agitate a child with a partial airway obstruction. Limit your initial assessment to ABCD. Do not attempt to assess the child's blood pressure.

Remove the foreign body only if it is clearly visible in the mouth and can be easily removed. If the object appears lodged in the upper airway or cannot be easily seen or dislodged with a finger, do not try to remove it if the child can still breathe. Improper manipulation of a foreign body can turn a partial obstruction into a complete one. The only other time you should try to dislodge a partial obstruction is if the patient is cyanotic after receiving 100% oxygen.

Administer high-flow oxygen by gently placing an oxygen mask over the child's mouth and nose. Remember that children are often afraid of having anything covering their mouths or faces. Therefore, you should explain what the mask is and how it will help them breathe. Hold the mask a short distance away if the child is too upset to tolerate it close to the face (Figure 26-3).

## FIGURE 26-3

Hold the oxygen mask slightly away from the child's face

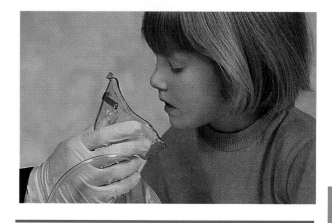

You should provide prompt transport for a child with a partial obstruction. Allow the parent to ride in the ambulance during transport.

### Complete Airway Obstruction

You should suspect a complete airway obstruction if the patient's chest does not rise and fall with your initial rescue breaths. Other common signs include decreased level of consciousness, cyanosis, and/or an inability to cry or speak. An infant with a complete obstruction may appear blue.

You should attempt to dislodge the foreign body if it is completely blocking the airway and the patient is unconscious or unresponsive. A foreign body that is completely blocking the airway can only be dislodged by applying energy to it. Thus, you should perform the abdominal thrust maneuver, modified to accommodate the patient's small size (Figure 26-4). However, if the patient is younger than 1 year, you should use back blows accompanied by chest thrusts. Once the airway is cleared, provide assisted ventilations with a BVM

### FIGURE 26-4

Modified abdominal thrust maneuver on a child

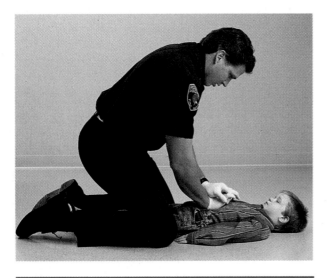

device and then transport. If you do not clear the airway, provide rapid transport.

## OTHER RESPIRATORY EMERGENCIES

It is important to recognize the differences between upper airway obstructions, such as those described above, and lower airway disease. Upper airway obstructions are characterized by stridor on inhalation. Lower airway disease produces wheezing and increased respiratory effort on exhalation. Lower airway disease is characterized by rapid respirations without stridor. Infants and children are particularly susceptible to several infectious diseases, such as croup and epiglottitis, that do not typically affect adults. See the FYI on Croup and Epiglottitis in this chapter for more information.

### Signs of Respiratory Problems

**Early distress**  Signs of early respiratory distress include audible wheezing, grunting, stridor, nasal flaring, intercostal, supraclavicular or subcostal retractions, or the use of accessory muscles.

**Severe distress**  A patient with respirations of more than 60 breaths/min is in severe respiratory distress or respiratory failure. In addition to the signs of early respiratory distress, a patient in severe distress may exhibit any of the following:

- cyanosis
- drooling
- decreased muscle tone
- an altered level of consciousness

Poor peripheral perfusion will change the patient's skin color and pulse. Capillary refill may also be affected. A child or infant in severe respiratory distress may use the abdominal or neck muscles to assist breathing. The use of accessory muscles is particularly pronounced.

**Respiratory arrest**    A child with respirations fewer than 10 breaths/min is in respiratory arrest. This patient is typically unconscious and unresponsive. Look for limp muscle tone in addition to the signs listed above. The heart rate has usually slowed to less than 80 beats/min, and distal pulses may be weak or absent.

It is important to assess the severity of a child's respiratory problems. Based on the severity, you can decide how to continue with treatment. For patients in early respiratory distress, give oxygen and transport. If the patient still shows sign of cyanosis, you will need to assist ventilations. Other indications for assisted ventilations include a decreased level of consciousness, poor muscle tone, and severe respiratory distress. For patients in full respiratory arrest, you must provide full ventilatory support with a BVM device. You may need to perform CPR, depending on the situation.

## SEIZURES

Seizures are relatively common among children. And, while they are rarely life threatening, they can cause great anxiety for parents and bystanders. This is especially true when the child has never had a seizure before. Although prolonged seizures are possible, most episodes are relatively brief, usually 15 seconds or less. A child may lose bowel or bladder control during a seizure. This can add to the confusion and embarrassment that follows a seizure.

Seizures are commonly caused by high fever in children who have underlying viral or bacterial infections. However, they can also be the result of specific infections involving the brain or central nervous system. Poisoning, trauma, and inadequate oxygen are all possible causes. Sometimes, seizures are the first sign of hypoglycemia in a diabetic child. Occasionally, children develop seizures for unknown reasons.

As you assess a child, it is important to determine if the seizure was caused by trauma, as this requires a different treatment. However, head injuries are usually quite obvious. Thus, it is usually easy to distinguish between seizures caused by trauma and those due to medical conditions.

Regardless of the cause, the emergency medical care for a seizure is the same. Your first priority is to make sure the patient's airway is open. If you do not suspect a possible spinal injury, place the child on his or her side. Have a suctioning unit ready. If the patient is cyanotic, open the airway and then assist ventilations.

You should transport a child who has had a seizure, even if the episode has ended. Brief seizures are not harmful in and of themselves, but there may be a more dangerous underlying condition. Make sure you obtain a history of the episode from the parents, if possible, so that you can record and report it to hospital personnel.

## ALTERED LEVEL OF CONSCIOUSNESS

As you assess patients, you are collecting information on signs and symptoms. Then, with the help of medical control, you can make treatment decisions based on your findings. Sometimes, the cause of a specific problem is not immediately clear. This is particularly true of a child with an altered level of consciousness.

A child's mental status may change for a variety of reasons, including the following:

- hypoglycemia due to diabetes
- poisoning
- infection
- insufficient oxygen
- head injury

It is also possible that the child is recovering from a seizure episode. You cannot rule out this possibility simply because no one witnessed or recognized the seizure.

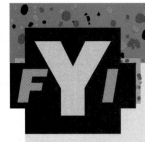

## Croup and Epiglottitis

Croup and epiglottitis swell airway tissues in children. Thus, both can lead to airway obstruction. Croup is a viral illness that causes acute swelling of the lining of the larynx, below its opening. Epiglottitis is a bacterial infection that produces severe swelling of the epiglottis, the flap of tissue that protects the opening to the larynx.

Children with either of these illnesses are likely to have a fever and have increasing difficulty breathing. Generally, patients will have a barking, brassy cough and hoarseness. You may also see progressive and excessive muscular effort with breathing.

Never put a tongue blade, finger, or artificial airway into the mouth of a child who has croup or epiglottitis. Doing so may cause the larynx to spasm or cause a complete airway obstruction. Oral or nasal airways should not be inserted because they are designed to support a flaccid tongue—not bypass a swollen epiglottis. With croup, the obstruction is far below the reach of an airway adjunct. Likewise, delivering back blows and chest thrusts, as you would with a foreign body obstruction, will obviously be of no help.

Instead, place the patient in a position that helps him or her to breathe easier. Warm, moist oxygen is the treatment of choice for epiglottitis, while cool mist is best for croup. Gently suction the mouth to remove any secretions. Transport the child as quickly as possible. Allow the parents to travel with the patient during transport.

Both croup and epiglottitis are very frightening illnesses to both the child and parents. Take time to reassure everyone. It is important to calm the parents to avoid excessively agitating the child, which will only aggravate the breathing problem.

---

The postseizure, or postictal, period is characterized by confusion, slurred speech, and an almost drunken appearance.

As with seizures, it is important to confirm or rule out trauma as a cause of an altered level of consciousness. Again, this should be relatively easy to do.

Your first step in caring for a child with an altered level of consciousness is to make sure the airway is open. Be prepared to assist ventilations or suction, if necessary.

You should provide transport so that the child can be examined by a physician at the hospital.

## POISONING

Many common household items are poisonous, and children are curious. They think brightly colored bottles or cans must contain something good to eat or drink. Sometimes, a child can swallow a large amount of a

## ALMOST A HOLIDAY OF HARM

It's a beautiful sunny 4th of July. Your day has been remarkably quiet so far. The peace comes to an end when dispatch sends you to a park for a "child hit by a car." On arrival, you find a 4-year-old child in her mother's arms. She has obviously been crying even though she's quiet now. She just looks scared. Her mother tells you the child chased a softball into the street. A car skidded about 20' before hitting the child, knocking her down. The mother also tells you the girl did not lose consciousness. Other than minor abrasions, you can only tell that the child appears to be breathing about 30 to 40 times a minute.

### For Discussion

1. Discuss the problems unique to immobilizing a child's spine.
2. Describe how children compensate for injuries.

substance before a parent or caregiver realizes the potential danger. Thus, poisonings are a common reason you are called to treat an infant or a child. If you are called to a possible poisoning, try to gather as much information about the poison as possible. Bring the container with you to the hospital. See chapter 18, Allergies and Poisoning, for more information.

If a child is responsive upon your arrival, inform medical control about the situation. You will need to discuss the possibility of giving activated charcoal. Then provide prompt transport. Continue to monitor the child for any changes in level of consciousness.

If the child is unconscious, first make sure the airway is open and be prepared to assist ventilations. Provide immediate transport. While en route, make sure the patient has not sustained any trauma, which could be the reason for the change in level of consciousness.

### FEVER

Children respond to many illnesses by developing a high fever very rapidly. Temperatures of 103°F (39.4°C) and higher are common in children and the reason for many ambulance calls. It is important to transport a child with a high fever so a physician can identify and treat the underlying cause.

In general, you should not try to obtain a rectal temperature in small children or in-

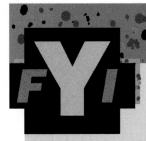

## Abdominal Pain

The most serious cause of abdominal pain in childhood is appendicitis. Although you can see it in a child of any age, appendicitis usually occurs between the ages of 10 and 25. An older child may give a history of progressive abdominal pain.

Appendicitis is characterized by crampy pain. Generally, the pain starts over the umbilicus and moves to the right lower quadrant of the abdomen in a matter of hours. After that, the pain becomes steady and severe. A child with appendicitis is usually nauseated, irritable or fussy, and has no appetite. Occasionally, the child will vomit. Low-grade fever is also common.

If a child is having abdominal pain, your best course of action is to transport the child to the hospital. Pinpointing the exact cause of abdominal pain, particularly in young children, is difficult at best. You should never attempt to determine the cause of abdominal pain in any patient.

fants in the field. The rectum is small, and the thermometer can easily damage the tissues. High fever is usually obvious. The child is flushed, crying, and feels warm to the touch. In older children, you should take an oral or rectal temperature using the appropriate type of thermometer.

Remember that fever is not a disease. Rather, it is a sign that there is an underlying problem, usually an infectious one. Most fevers are not serious in children and do not cause permanent brain injury. One exception is meningitis. **Meningitis** is a viral or bacterial infection of the membranes covering the brain and spinal cord. This is an extremely serious disease but usually not very contagious.

Children with meningitis are hot and obviously sick. Headache and a stiff neck are common. The child may have had a sore throat or upper respiratory problem before the fever developed. Provide rapid transport for children who have these signs and symptoms. Be alert for seizures en route to the hospital.

The most dangerous fevers in children are those caused by heat-related emergencies, especially heatstroke. In the treatment of serious heat-related emergencies, you should provide the same care for children as you do for adults. Body temperature must be reduced as quickly as possible. A child who has hot, dry skin after being in the sun, in an extremely warm, poorly ventilated room, or in a closed, parked car has a serious condition. If you cannot transport the child, or if prolonged transport is needed, you must cool the child at the scene. Undress the child to the underwear and then place him or her in a tub of cool water. Provide transport as soon as possible. Monitor the child carefully. Because the surface area of a child is large with respect to the child's volume, the body temperature may change rapidly.

About 5% of children under age 5 who have fevers above 100.4°F (38°C) will experience febrile convulsions. These seizures usually last less than 15 minutes and are rarely dangerous. Thus, they require no special treatment beyond airway maintenance.

Occasionally, a high fever may trigger a prolonged seizure in a child who has epilepsy. Treatment includes airway maintenance and prompt transport. When a child who is having a seizure becomes cyanotic, you must attempt to open the airway. *Remember, never place your fingers in the mouth, because the child may bite.* In addition, do not attempt to pry the jaws open. This will usually do more harm than good. Gentle extension of the neck will open the airway partially. If the patient's teeth are clenched, make sure the nasal passages are clear so that the patient can breathe. Make sure you give the patient oxygen.

Following an epileptic seizure, a child will have an altered level of consciousness and slow respirations. You should maintain the airway, continue to administer oxygen, and provide prompt transport.

## DEHYDRATION

**Dehydration,** or the loss of body fluids, is a common problem in infants and children. It is often associated with abdominal pain. Diarrhea or vomiting can quickly cause dehydration in infants and children. Sometimes diarrhea resulting from the flu can last for days. Dehydrated children may be lethargic. Their skin and mucous membranes are often dry. Dehydration may cause shock in infants and children. Therefore, prompt transport is necessary.

## CONTAGIOUS DISEASES

Occasionally, you must transport a child who has a common infectious childhood disease. These diseases are usually easy to spot. Measles (rubeola), German measles (rubella), and chicken pox produce characteristic rashes. Mumps causes swelling and tenderness of the glands directly in front of the ears.

Inform medical control that you are transporting a child with a contagious disease. If the child has a fever and rash, you should wear a mask. Remember, however, that these diseases are rarely a threat to you. You have probably already had the disease or been immunized against it. Careful handwashing as well as a thorough cleaning of exposed surfaces and equipment in the vehicle will usually protect you.

## SHOCK

Shock is rarely the result of a heart condition in infants and children. Rather, it can be the result of meningitis, a blood infection, dehydration due to vomiting, or an abdominal injury. Most often, shock in children and infants results from blood loss or dehydration.

A child tolerates far less blood loss than an adult. Common signs of shock in an infant or child include the following:

- rapid heartbeat
- delayed capillary refill
- pale, cool, clammy skin
- weak or absent peripheral pulses
- altered level of consciousness

Determine if the child's fluid levels have dropped. Is the patient producing tears as he or she cries? Is the child's urine output decreased? Has the number of wet diapers decreased? These, too, are signs of developing shock.

A late indicator of shock is a low systolic blood pressure. The minimum pressure is equal to 80 mm Hg plus twice the child's age. Thus, the patient's condition is extremely serious if the blood pressure reading is one of the following:

- less than 50 mm Hg in a child under 5 years
- less than 60 mm Hg in a child between 5 and 12 years
- less than 70 mm Hg in a teenager or young adult

Caring for a child in shock includes making sure the airway is open, giving oxygen, and preparing to assist ventilations, if necessary. Protect the cervical spine, manage any bleeding, and splint fractures if the patient has traumatic injuries. Elevate the legs, and keep the patient warm. Remember to handle the patient gently.

Often, children in shock will ask for water. Do not give anything by mouth, especially if the child has had a traumatic injury. If the child needs an emergency operation, the stomach should be completely empty. Remember to say no in a kind way.

Once you have completed the important treatments described above, you must begin transport. You can complete your detailed physical exam en route.

## NEAR DROWNING

A child's drowning or near drowning requires rapid response and prompt, appropriate treatment. Providing artificial ventilation is your top priority. However, you must also carefully consider the possibility of associated trauma. Diving accidents often lead to serious head or neck injuries as well as drowning. You should also be alert to the possibility of hypothermia. The possibility of alcohol or drug use in adolescents may complicate your treatment.

When you respond to a drowning or near-drowning incident, you should assess for possible spinal injury, begin ventilation, and provide oxygen. Children can sometimes completely recover from these incidents, even after prolonged periods of immersion. Reports indicate that children can recover even after lengthy periods of full CPR during rescue and transport. Always protect the child's airway and be prepared to suction, if necessary.

Prompt transport is critical after a near-drowning incident. A child may appear to fully recover from a near-drowning incident. However, you must transport the child for examination by a physician, as respiratory problems can develop.

## SUDDEN INFANT DEATH SYNDROME (SIDS)

Approximately 10,000 infants die each year in the United States from **sudden infant death syndrome (SIDS).** The exact causes of SIDS are unknown, although it is rarely due to child abuse. SIDS usually strikes otherwise healthy babies between 2 and 6 months old. Most times, the infant is discovered in the early morning. Because the infant dies during sleep, this syndrome is also called "crib death."

When you respond to a possible SIDS situation, be prepared to deal with the emotional needs of the parents. The parents will likely be in agony from shock, remorse, and imagined guilt. It is important for you to spend some time and effort comforting them. At the same time, however, you need to make every effort to revive the baby—even if a long period of time has passed since the infant's death. Begin BLS measures before transport and en route to the hospital. Continue your resuscitation efforts until a physician pronounces the infant dead.

Whenever you respond to a SIDS call, do not expect a good outcome, but try for one anyway. In the meantime, avoid making any comments that might suggest the parents are to blame for the infant's death.

# TRAUMATIC INJURIES

Traumatic injuries are the leading cause of death among infants and children. Blunt injuries are the most common life-threatening injuries. The number one killer of America's children today is the automobile. Children are injured as pedestrians, on bicycles, on motorcycles, or as passengers.

Occasionally, a serious injury results from a sports or recreational activity. Unfortunately, you will also be called to incidents in which children have been shot or are victims of child abuse.

The pattern of injuries seen in children can differ from that in adults. One reason is that the size of a child's head, in relation to his or her body, is larger than that of an adult. A child's neck muscles are weaker and less able to protect the head from sudden, violent stress and loads. Thus, head and neck injuries are a particular concern in children. A second reason is that the amount of circulating blood in children is less than that in an adult. Therefore, children cannot tolerate as much blood loss as an adult without going into shock.

A third reason is that a child's skeleton is more flexible and elastic than an adult's skeleton. This alters the pattern of fractures in children. Thus, a child may have serious injuries due to blunt trauma of the chest, abdomen, and pelvis without fractures. Similar blunt trauma would result in fractures in adults. Remember that even though the pattern of injury may differ from that of an adult, you provide the same care. First, you must focus on ABCD, then immobilize the cervical spine, control bleeding, and splint musculoskeletal injuries (Figure 26-5).

## HEAD, NECK, AND SPINAL INJURIES

Injuries of the head, neck, and spine in infants and children are usually due to automobile accidents, falls, or diving mishaps. Any unconscious child who has been involved in an accident should be treated as if he or she has a neck injury, as well as other internal injuries. If the child is showing signs of shock, you should consider the possibility of other internal injuries. Other common signs include nausea and vomiting.

Your care of a child with a possible spinal injury should be the same as that of an adult. The single most important step is to make sure that the patient's airway is open. The tongue often falls back into the throat of an unconscious child with a head injury, blocking the airway. This can lead to hypoxia. Therefore, you must perform the jaw-thrust maneuver to open the airway.

You are likely to find infants and children involved in automobile accidents still in their car seats. Your best course of action is to immobilize the child in the car seat, if possible. Whenever you apply a cervical collar, make sure it is properly sized. If a properly fitting collar is not available, use a rolled towel and tape it to the car seat. An improperly fitting collar does more harm than good. Apply a properly fitting cervical collar and pad the sides of the car seat to prevent lateral movement. Place additional padding in any spaces between the patient and the car seat (Figure 26-6).

If the child is not in a car seat or was removed before your arrival, use an appropriately sized immobilization device. Remember that children are not small adults. They have smaller airways. As such, you

# FIGURE 26-5

Differences in traumatic injury patterns in adults and children

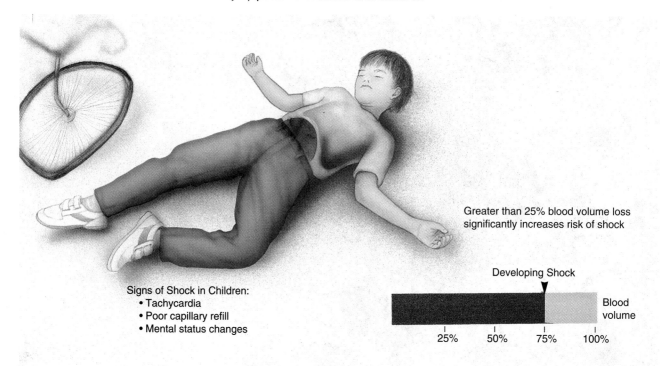

Greater than 25% blood volume loss significantly increases risk of shock

Signs of Shock in Children:
• Tachycardia
• Poor capillary refill
• Mental status changes

Developing Shock

Blood volume

25%    50%    75%    100%

Signs of Shock in Adults:
• Tachycardia
• Hypotension
• Mental status changes

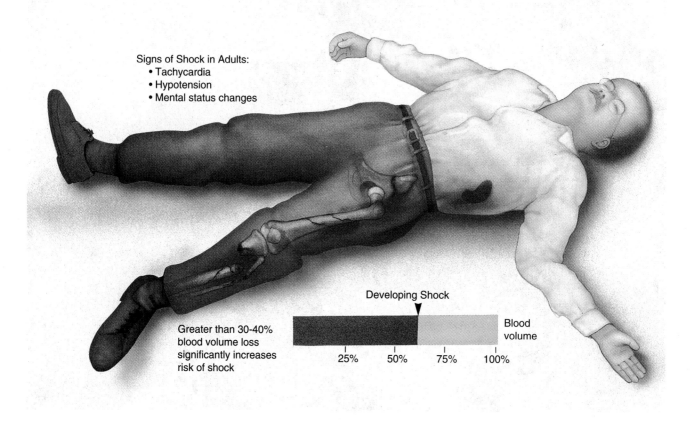

Greater than 30-40% blood volume loss significantly increases risk of shock

Developing Shock

Blood volume

25%    50%    75%    100%

## FIGURE 26-6

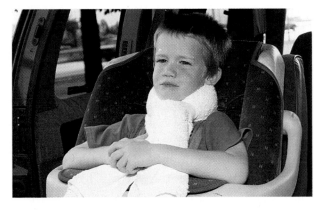

**A** Use a rolled towel as a cervical collar to immobilize a child in a car seat

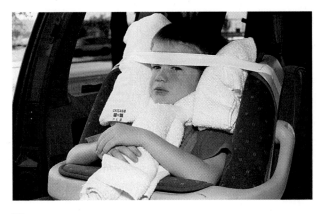

**B** Pad the sides of the car seat to prevent lateral movement

place padding as needed to maintain the head in a neutral position. You may need to fill space from the shoulders to the toes.

Avoid using sandbags to immobilize a child with a suspected spinal injury. The weight of the sandbags may cause further injury if you need to turn the spine board in the event the child vomits.

Avoid the urge to pick up and cradle an injured child unless there is an overriding need to move quickly, such as a fire or other environmental threat. Transport chil-dren with head injuries with the head slightly elevated and supported on the spine board.

During transport, carefully monitor the patient's ABCD. Assess the patient's breath-ing often, carefully watching for any sign that the patient has stopped breathing (apnea). This commonly occurs in infants and children. Monitor the patient's level of consciousness every 5 minutes. This is one of your most important duties after resusci-tation and care of injuries. From the time you first see the patient until you deliver the patient to the hospital, you should con-tinually assess the patient's level of con-sciousness. Report and record any changes. A patient with a head injury may be alert one minute and comatose only a few min-utes later. If this occurs, the patient is likely to need an urgent, lifesaving operation.

## CHEST AND ABDOMINAL INJURIES

Penetrating abdominal or chest injuries are not common in children. However, when they do occur, you should provide the same care as you would for adults. Blunt injuries from falls or automobile accidents are far more common.

Children have very soft, pliable ribs. Therefore, blunt injuries to the chest can lead to serious internal injuries—even though there are few external signs. There could be serious injuries to the heart or the lungs. Thus, you should provide immediate trans-port for all children with chest injuries. Pre-hospital care is identical to that for adults.

Children experience blunt trauma to the abdomen more often than do adults. In fact, this is often a site of hidden injury. You will be called to care for a seriously injured child with multiple trauma from time to time. When you do, keep in mind the possibility of a serious abdominal injury. While there are no external signs of abdominal injury, it is possible that the child has a ruptured liver, spleen, or kidney. Blunt injury may cause abdominal pain and lead to shock. Bruising, distention, and tenderness are common signs of blunt trauma. Be alert for these signs—even if there is no obvious external blood loss.

If air enters the stomach, it can distend the abdomen. This, in turn, can interfere with your efforts to provide artificial ventilation.

Provide prompt transport to patients with injuries of the chest and abdomen. Monitor vital signs carefully and watch for vomiting and signs of shock.

## EXTREMITY INJURIES

In general, extremity injuries are not life threatening. However, the prompt control of bleeding is especially important in children. Cover open soft tissue wounds with dry, sterile compression dressings. Open fractures tend to bleed considerably. You can almost always control this bleeding with local pressure.

In those rare circumstances when you must use a tourniquet to control bleeding, follow the same rules that apply to adults, as described in chapter 23, Soft Tissue Injuries.

### THINGS THAT GO WHEEZE IN THE NIGHT

It's a hot, humid summer night. The air conditioning in your ambulance has been working off and on since early afternoon. You and your partner are complaining about the air when you are called to a home where a child is having "breathing difficulty." On arrival, you find a 5-year-old girl sitting up, but slightly hunched forward. Her mother says her daughter was recently diagnosed with asthma. They tried her inhaler once, but it provided little relief. Afraid to try it again, the mother paged the family doctor twice. Since the doctor has not called, she called 9-1-1. The mother also reports that her daughter had the flu 3 days ago and has been running a fever since then.

#### For Discussion

1. Describe some of the feelings the mother may experience regarding her child's illness. What is the best way to deal with them?

2. Explain the differences between respiratory distress and respiratory failure.

INFANTS AND CHILDREN

If you use a blood pressure cuff as a tourniquet on a child, inflate the cuff to 100 mm Hg. This pressure will usually control the bleeding.

Splint injuries to a child's extremities in the same way you would splint an adult's extremities. Use an appropriately sized splint. Before you position a splint or align an injured extremity, assess the patient's distal pulse, capillary refill, sensation, and motor function. Continue to monitor the neurovascular status until you reach the hospital.

## OTHER COMMON TRAUMATIC INJURIES

### Severe Bleeding and Use of a PASG

Typically, a PASG is used in patients with signs of severe hypoperfusion or cases of pelvic instability. However, the use of a PASG is somewhat controversial, especially for children. You should always check with medical control about using a PASG on a child.

Regardless of the protocols, you should never use a PASG if it does not fit. Do not place small children or infants in one leg of the trouser. Likewise, do not inflate the abdominal compartment. Otherwise, the PASG might limit the patient's ability to move his or her chest. This, in turn, would affect the patient's ability to breathe.

### Burns

Burns are a critical problem, especially in children. Infants and children have a larger body surface area relative to total body mass than do adults. This increases their risk of life-threatening burns. In general, any time a child's clothing has caught fire, you are dealing with a serious burn problem. Usually, you will find full-thickness burns.

It is important to cover burn patients with dry bandages, clean white sheets, or sterile dressings, preferably nonstick dressings. Early in the process, you should attempt to identify patients who should be treated at a burn center. Rapid transport is indicated for burn patients. Begin aggressive fluid resuscitation as soon as possible, as this greatly improves the outcome for burn patients. For detailed information on treatment of burns, see chapter 23, Soft Tissue Injuries.

## CHILD ABUSE AND NEGLECT

Child abuse is considered any improper or excessive action that injures or harms a child or infant. The deliberate, intentional injury—whether physical or emotional—of a child is not rare in our society today. The exact incidence of child abuse is unknown. However, what is known is that child abuse is a far greater problem than was once suspected. Child abuse is found at all socioeconomic levels and can occur in any family. Child abuse is a progressive situation. In other words, a child may be continually abused with increasing severity until he or she ends up dead.

The most serious abuse results in injury to the central nervous system. "Shaken baby syndrome" is a common form of abuse in infants. With this syndrome, you will not see direct blows or fractures about the head. Severe injury and possible brain damage occurs from the forceful shaking of the body. Injuries include bleeding within the head and damage to the cervical spine.

### RECOGNIZING CHILD ABUSE

As an EMT-B, you must be aware of the condition to recognize the problem. You are most likely to spot the signs of physical, rather than emotional, abuse or neglect. In many cases, you and your partner will be called to the scene to care for a child who has had an "accidental" injury. You should be suspicious if you and/or your ambulance service have made repeated calls to the same address. Another clue is if the person who called gives a history that does not appear to fit the child's injury. Characteristically, an abused child has many injuries, all at different stages of healing. Fresh burns are another possible sign. An abused child may appear withdrawn, fearful, or hostile. You should be particularly concerned if the child refuses to discuss how the injury occurred.

Occasionally, the parent or caretaker reveals a history of several "accidents" in the past. Be alert for conflicting stories or a marked lack of concern from the parents or caregiver. Remember, the abuser may be a parent, relative, caregiver, or friend of the family. Sometimes, the abuser is an acquaintance of a single parent.

When you suspect child abuse, do not attempt to make a diagnosis or accuse the suspected abusers. This only delays transport and treatment. However, maintaining a professional approach in these instances is not easy. An obvious case of child abuse will arouse strong emotions and challenge your ability to think and act clearly. But you must remain calm. Carefully record the history you are given and promptly transport the child, even if the injuries are relatively trivial. Often a child who is a suspected victim of abuse will be admitted to the hospital for protection. This is often the case, even though the child's injuries are not severe enough to warrant hospitalization.

### Handling Possible Child Abuse

Remember that you cannot transport a child to the hospital without the parent's consent. Sometimes, you can persuade a parent to allow transport if you say the

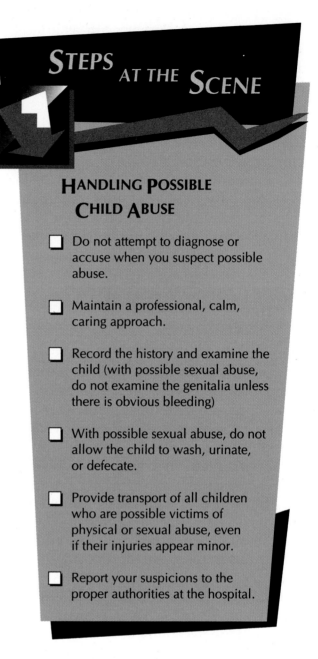

## STEPS AT THE SCENE

### HANDLING POSSIBLE CHILD ABUSE

- [ ] Do not attempt to diagnose or accuse when you suspect possible abuse.

- [ ] Maintain a professional, calm, caring approach.

- [ ] Record the history and examine the child (with possible sexual abuse, do not examine the genitalia unless there is obvious bleeding)

- [ ] With possible sexual abuse, do not allow the child to wash, urinate, or defecate.

- [ ] Provide transport of all children who are possible victims of physical or sexual abuse, even if their injuries appear minor.

- [ ] Report your suspicions to the proper authorities at the hospital.

child may need special X rays or tests. If the parent still refuses and you are concerned about the child's well-being, consult law enforcement.

## REPORTING CHILD ABUSE

Most states have laws that require health care providers to report cases of suspected child abuse to various social service or law enforcement agencies. There may be local regulations as well. Learn the regulations in your area. When you suspect child abuse, make sure to report it to the physician at the hospital. Be careful in how you report your observations. Your goal is to report what you saw and heard, not what you think.

The ultimate determination of child abuse is made by the courts, often after a long, complicated legal process. Your job, along with all other health care professionals, is to identify suspicious instances of child abuse so that the process can begin.

## SEXUAL ABUSE

Sexual abuse can happen to infants, young children, and adolescents, to both boys and girls. Most victims of rape are over 10 years of age. However, younger children are sometimes victims as well. This is often the result of long-standing abuse by a relative.

You should not examine a young child's genitalia unless there is obvious bleeding, or there is an injury that must be treated. Limit your exam to determining what type of dressing the injury requires. Sometimes, a sexually abused child is also beaten. Treat any bruises or fractures appropriately.

If you suspect that a child is a victim of sexual abuse, do not allow the child to wash, urinate, or defecate before a physician completes an exam. While this is difficult, it is important to preserve evidence. If the molested child is a girl, make sure a female EMT-B or police officer remains with the child unless finding one will delay transport.

It is important to maintain a professional composure throughout your time with a sexually abused child. Assume a concerned, caring approach. Shield the patient from onlookers and curious passersby.

Obtain as much history as possible from the child and any witnesses. The child may be hysterical or unwilling to say anything at all, especially if the abuser is a relative or family friend. You are in the best position to obtain the most accurate first-hand information concerning the incident. Thus, you should record any information carefully and completely on the run report.

Transport all children who are victims of sexual assault. You should carry the local phone numbers of agencies in your area that specialize in addressing these problems. Sexual abuse of children is a crime. Make sure you cooperate with law enforcement officials in their investigations.

## NEGLECT

Child abuse can also occur when a parent or caregiver does not provide basic care to a child. For example, providing food, clothing, and shelter is considered basic care. Not providing for these basic needs is considered neglect. Also, abandoning children without care or supervision for a long period of time is considered neglect.

## CHILDREN WITH SPECIAL NEEDS

Occasionally, you may be called repeatedly to treat children with chronic illnesses or special needs. These situations include the following:

- children who were born prematurely and have associated lung disease problems
- small children or infants with congenital heart disease
- children with neurologic disease (occasionally due to hypoxia at the time of birth, as with cerebral palsy)
- children with chronic disease or whose functions have been altered since birth

## TRACHEOSTOMY TUBES

Many of these children live at home but are dependent on technology to survive. For example, some children rely on various types of tracheostomy tubes to breathe. These tubes can be dislodged or become obstructed. Other complications include bleeding around the tracheostomy site, air leakage, and infection.

Whenever you respond to a child experiencing a problem with a tracheostomy tube, you should maintain an open airway. Be ready to suction the tube, if necessary. Place the child or infant in a position of comfort and provide prompt transport.

## ARTIFICIAL VENTILATORS

You may also be called on to care for a child who is dependent on some type of artificial ventilator. Usually, parents or home attendants know how to operate these devices. Your care should focus on making sure the child's airway is open. Give supplemental oxygen with artificial ventilation and provide rapid transport.

## CENTRAL IV LINES

Other children have IVs for the long-term administration of nutrition or medication. These IVs are often central lines placed through the arm or beneath the collar bone. In these locations, the line can feed directly into the circulation system near the heart. Occasionally, these lines can crack and leak. Sometimes a clot will block the line. Other potential complications include infection and bleeding. If a child with an IV in place is bleeding from the site, apply direct pressure over the site with your gloved hand. You should then provide transport.

## GASTROSTOMY TUBES

Some children with chronic illnesses cannot swallow or ingest solids or liquids normally. Therefore, they cannot be fed by mouth. These patients may be sent home with a gastrostomy tube, used for gastric feeding. Gastrostomy tubes come in a variety of shapes.

Because these patients cannot handle substances or secretions normally, you should be alert for potential respiratory problems. When treating a child or infant with a gastrostomy tube, make sure the airway is open. Have a suctioning unit available. If the patient is diabetic, monitor the patient for changes in the level of consciousness. Without food, an infant or child with diabetes can become hypoglycemic quickly. Giving these patients oxygen is usually appropriate.

Transport these patients either sitting or lying down on the right side with the head elevated. This reduces the chance that the patient will aspirate any material into the lungs.

## SHUNTS

Occasionally, you will be called to a scene in which a child has a central nervous system shunt. This device, used to treat a condition called hydrocephalus, diverts excess cerebral spinal fluid from the brain to the abdomen. You will find a reservoir on the side of the skull. Problems with a shunt may produce changes in level of consciousness or ventilation difficulties. Because these patients can stop breathing, it is important to make sure they are adequately ventilated. Make sure the airway is open, and then provide transport. Physicians can then determine the exact nature of the problem.

## FAMILY MATTERS

It is important to remember that with all children, especially those with chronic illnesses, you have not just one patient to treat but several. Family members, especially the primary caregiver, are also often in need of help or support when medical emergencies or problems develop. A calm parent usually helps contribute to a calm child. An agitated parent usually means that the child will act the same way. Make sure you are calm, efficient, professional, and sensitive as you deal with children and their families.

## TRANSPORTING INFANTS AND CHILDREN

Before you transport a sick or injured child, you should be aware of special transport considerations for infants and children. Infants and small children are very susceptible to temperature changes. They lose body heat rapidly and must always be transported wrapped in blankets. Very young and sick children are also extremely susceptible to infection. You should thus avoid breathing or coughing directly on a small or sick child. Isolate an infant or child from bacterial contamination, particularly from your own nose, mouth, and hands.

Newborns should be transported in special incubators. If an incubator is not available, wrap a newborn in blankets. Be sure to keep the newborn's face uncovered and make sure the ambulance is warm. Many large medical centers maintain specially equipped vehicles for transporting infants and small children. You should know the location and availability of these vehicles.

## EMS RESPONSE TO PEDIATRIC EMERGENCIES

After care and transport of a sick or injured child, you may experience a wide range of powerful emotions. These emotions result from the call itself, or from your previous experience (or inexperience) caring for infants and children. You may feel anxious if you have not had much experience dealing with infants and children. You may also think of your own children, or the children of a loved one.

As a result, you must be prepared to care for children. Practice with children and pediatric equipment is necessary. Children are not simply "small adults." However, many of the skills and principles you use to care for adults can be applied to children. You simply must remember that there are differences in anatomy and emotions.

After difficult incidents involving children, debriefing is helpful in working through the stress and trauma. It is also a means to help you in the future if you are faced with similar situations. The ability to seek out help following difficult episodes is a sign of maturity and confidence.

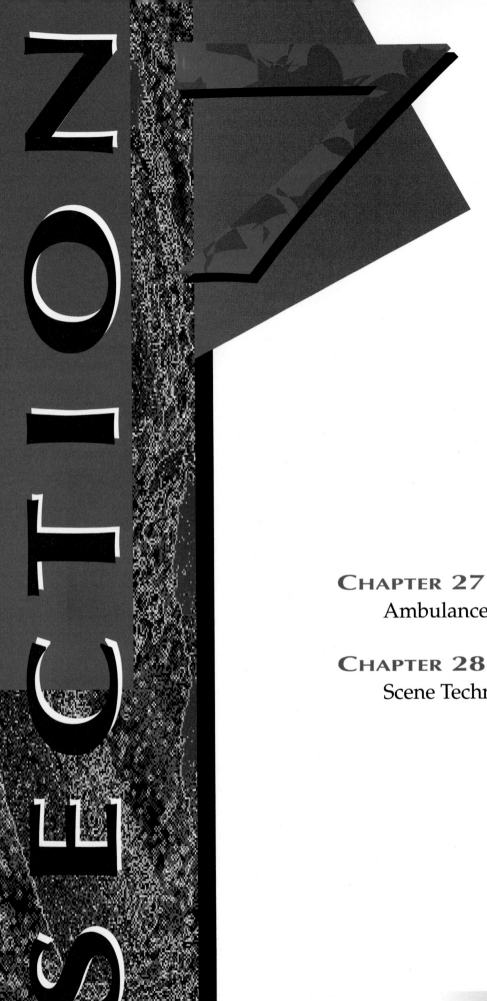

SECTION 7

# Operations

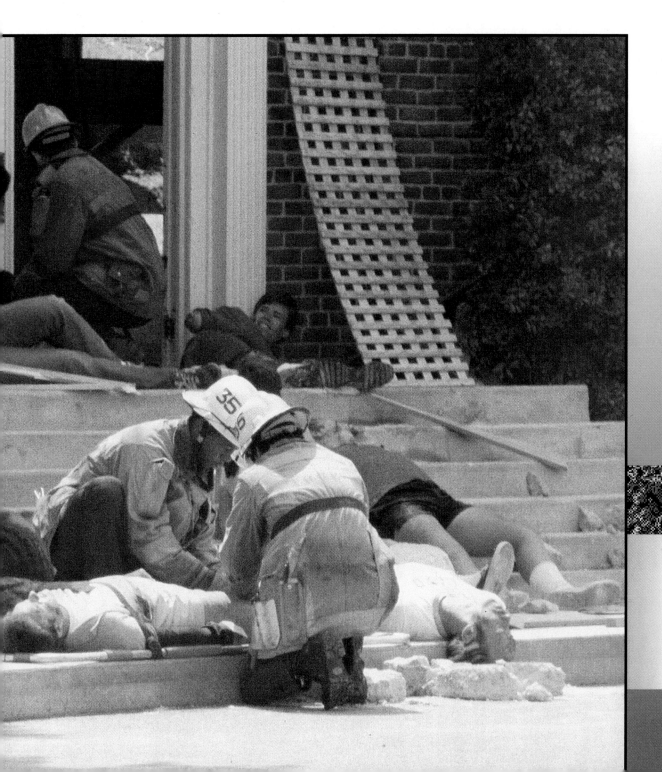

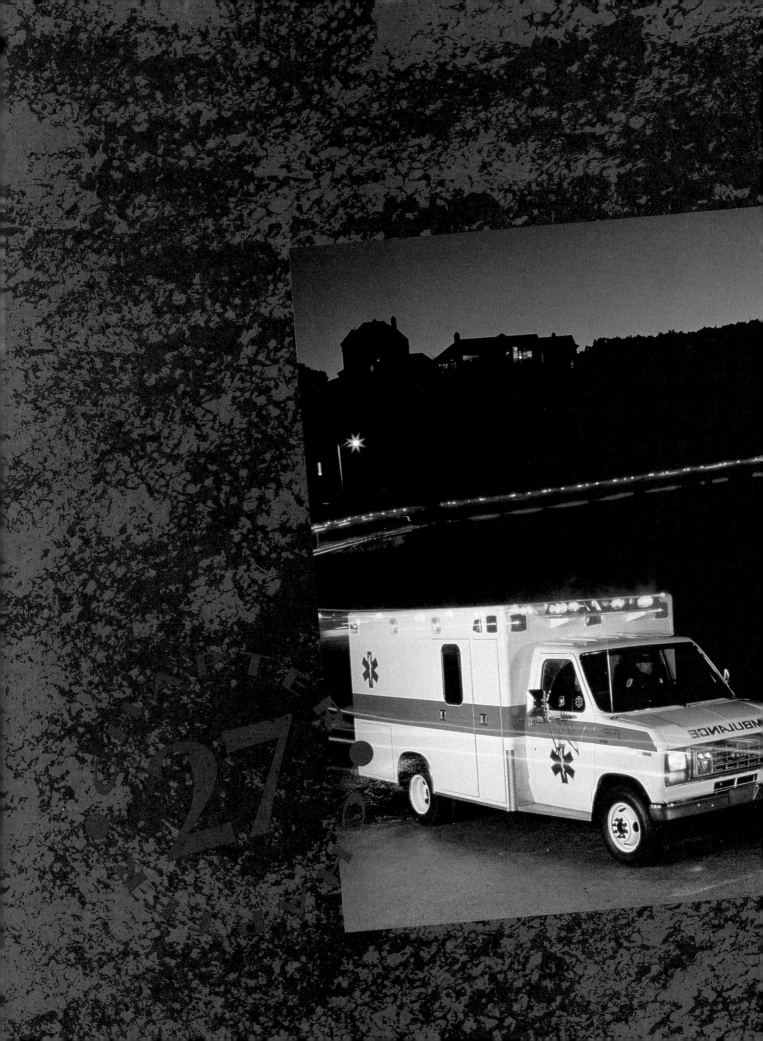

# Ambulance Operations

After you have read this chapter, you should be able to:

- Discuss the medical and nonmedical equipment needed to respond to a call.
- List the phases of an ambulance call.
- Describe the general provisions of state laws relating to the operation of an ambulance and any special privileges in any or all of the following categories: speed, warning lights, sirens, right-of-way, parking, turning.
- List contributing factors to unsafe driving conditions.
- Describe the consideration that should be given to requests for escorts, following an escort vehicle, and intersections.
- Discuss "Due Regard for Safety of All Others" while operating an emergency vehicle.
- Discuss essential information in order to respond to a call.
- Discuss various situations that may affect response to a call.
- Differentiate between the various methods of moving a patient to the ambulance based upon injury or illness.
- Apply the components of the essential patient information in a written report.
- Summarize the importance of preparing the unit for the next call.

- Identify what is essential for completion of a call.
- Distinguish among the terms cleaning, disinfection, high-level disinfection, and sterilization.
- Describe how to clean or disinfect items following patient care.

# Overview

An **ambulance** is a vehicle used for treating and transporting patients who need emergency medical care from the scene to the hospital. The first motor-driven ambulance was introduced in 1906. For many decades after that, a hearse was most often used as an ambulance because it was the only vehicle that could transport a person laying down. Few supplies were carried, and there was little space for an attendant in the back with the patient.

The hearse-ambulance has gone the way of its horse-drawn predecessor. Better-equipped and better-designed emergency vehicles have become available. Ambulances are currently designed in accordance with government regulations, such as KKK specifications and ASTM standards. These regulations are based on suggestions from the ambulance industry and the EMS personnel who use them. One of the most significant developments in ambulance design has been the greater width, length, and height of the patient compartment.

Many patients have said that the most frightening part of being suddenly ill or injured is the ambulance ride to the hospital. The terrifying effect of a bumpy fast swaying ride with a blaring siren is not very reassuring to an already upset patient. Although sometimes this kind of a ride is truly lifesaving, excessive speed is usually unnecessary. It rarely decreases the amount of time it takes to get to the hospital. What is necessary is that the patient be transported to a hospital safely in the shortest practical time. This takes common sense and defensive driving techniques. Speed should never be used to cover up a lack of these qualities. Only about 20% of all ambulance calls are for true emergencies. Unnecessary speed for nonurgent calls is not only foolish—it can be fatal.

This chapter focuses on the techniques and judgment that you will need to learn in order to drive an ambulance. The chapter discusses emergency vehicle control and emergency vehicle operation—both important factors in safe driving. The chapter describes the qualifications needed to drive an ambulance. Also discussed are how to equip an ambulance, parking considerations, the effects of bad weather on driving, and common hazards when driving an ambulance. The chapter concludes with a brief discussion of air medical operations.

## Key Terms

**Ambulance**    Vehicle used for treating and transporting patients who need emergency medical care from the scene to a hospital.

**CPR board**    Device that provides a firm surface under the patient's torso so that you can give effective chest compressions.

**Hydroplaning**    Condition in which the tires of a vehicle may be lifted off the road surface as water "piles up" under it. As a result, the tires are not in direct contact with the road surface. The vehicle then feels as if it is floating on the road surface.

**Jump kit**    A lightweight, durable, waterproof portable kit containing items used in the initial care of the patient.

# PHASES OF AN AMBULANCE CALL

## PREPARING FOR THE CALL

One important element in preparing for the call is the availability and readiness of equipment and supplies. Items that are missing or that do not work are of little use to you or the patient.

Equipment and supplies should be placed in the unit according to their relative importance and frequency of use. Give priority to items needed to care for life-threatening conditions. These include equipment for airway care, artificial ventilation, and oxygen delivery. Place these items within easy reach, at the head of the primary litter. Place items for cardiac care, control of external bleeding, and monitoring blood pressure at the side of the litter.

Your equipment and supplies should be durable and as standardized as possible. This is important so that you can exchange equipment between units or between your unit and the emergency department. Exchange is an important consideration for any ambulance service, as it decreases the time that you and your unit must stay at the hospital.

Storage cabinets and kits should open easily, but must be fastened securely to keep them from opening en route. The fronts of cabinets and drawers can be made of transparent materials so that you can identify equipment and supplies rapidly (Figure 27-1).

## MEDICAL EQUIPMENT

As an EMT-B, you have access to a large variety of equipment and supplies—far too many to describe in a detailed list here. The sections below group many of these items into categories for easier understanding.

## FIGURE 27-1

Transparent fronts of cabinets

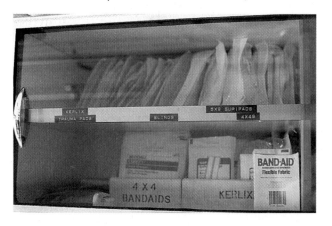

### Basic Supplies

All units should carry the following basic supplies:

- at least 2 pillows and pillowcases
- at least 2 spare sheets
- 4 blankets
- 4 towels
- 6 disposable emesis bags or basins
- 2 boxes of disposable tissue
- 1 bedpan (optional)
- 2 urinals (one male, one female; optional)
- 3 thermometers (one oral, one rectal, one hypothermia)
- 3 blood pressure cuffs (pediatric, adult, large adult)
- 1 stethoscope
- 1 pair trauma shears
- 1 package of disposable drinking cups
- 1 unbreakable container of water
- 1 package of wet wipes
- 4 chemical cold packs
- 4 L of sterile irrigation fluid
- 2 restraining devices

- 1 package of plastic bags for waste or severed parts
- latex disposable gloves (various sizes)
- 1 sharps container (minimum)
- 1 set of hearing protectors
- 2 infection control kits (goggles, masks, and waterproof gowns)

In addition, equipment for dealing with specific problems or conditions should be available.

## Airway Management

You must have on hand oropharyngeal airways for adults, children, and infants. Nasal airways for adults and children should also be available. If your service is authorized by your medical director to perform advanced airway procedures, you should have the proper equipment on hand in the unit, as well as in the jump kit that is carried to the patient.

## Ventilation

Portable artificial ventilation devices that operate independently of an oxygen supply must be provided. These include pocket masks and BVM devices. BVM devices capable of oxygen enrichment should also be carried on the unit. When attached to an oxygen supply, with the oxygen reservoir in place, the BVM device should be able to supply almost 100% oxygen. The device must be easy to clean and decontaminate. The nonrebreathing valve on the mask must permit inhalation of oxygen during both artificial ventilation and spontaneous respirations.

You should make sure you carry masks in a variety of sizes, from infant to adult. Make sure these masks are transparent. This will help you to monitor the patient's respirations, and any changes in respirations or vomiting, easily and rapidly.

## Suctioning Unit

You should have both portable and "on-board" installed suctioning units (Figure 27-2). These units must be powerful enough to provide an airflow of 30 L/min at the end of the tube and a vacuum of 300 mm Hg when the tube is clamped. The suctioning force must be adjustable for use on infants and children. The units should include large-bore, nonkinking suction tubing with a semirigid pharyngeal tip. Additional semirigid tips should be available. The "on-board" unit should include a suction yoke, an unbreakable collection bottle, water for rinsing the suction tips, and suction tubing.

## FIGURE 27-2

On-board suctioning unit

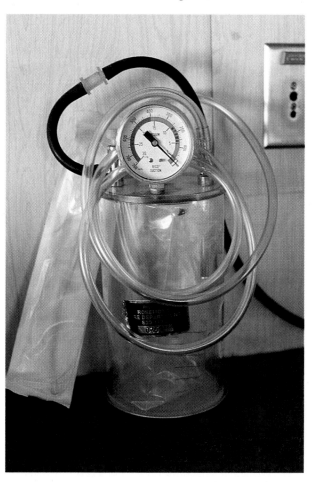

This equipment should be easily accessible to you when you are sitting at the head of the litter. The tubing must reach the patient's airway, regardless of the patient's position. All components of the suctioning unit must be made of material that is easily cleaned and decontaminated.

### Oxygen Delivery

Your unit must be equipped with at least two oxygen supply units—one portable unit and one on-board, installed unit. The portable unit should have a capacity of 300 L of oxygen. It should also be equipped with a yoke, pressure gauge, flowmeter, oxygen supply tubing, nonrebreathing mask, and nasal cannula. This unit must be able to deliver oxygen at a rate between 2 and 15 L/min. At least one extra portable 300-L cylinder should be kept on the ambulance. The portable unit should be located near a door for easy use outside the ambulance. Many services equip the backup cylinder with its own yoke, gauge, regulator, and tubing so that it can be used for a second patient, when needed.

The on-board oxygen unit should have a capacity of 3,000 L of oxygen (Figure 27-3). It should also be equipped with visible

flowmeters that are accessible to you if you are at the head of the litter. This unit must be able to deliver oxygen at a rate of between 2 and 15 L/min. The flowmeters must be so located that the oxygen supply tubing can reach a patient's face if he or she is on the stretcher or on the squad bench.

### CPR Equipment

A **CPR board** provides a firm surface under the patient's torso so that you can give effective chest compressions (Figure 27-4). It also establishes an appropriate degree of head tilt. If you do not have a special CPR board, you can place a long spine board under the patient on the litter. A tightly rolled sheet placed on the board will raise the patient's shoulders 3" to 4" above the level of the board. This will also keep the patient's head in a position of maximum backward tilt, with the shoulders and chest in a straight position without manual

**FIGURE 27-4**

CPR board

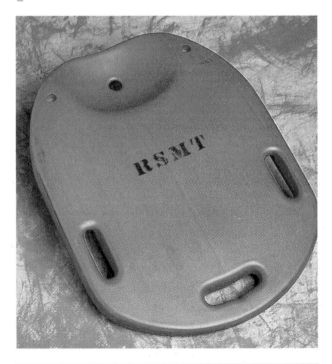

**FIGURE 27-3**

On-board oxygen delivery unit

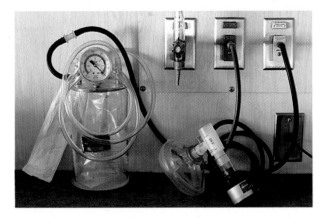

support. However, if you suspect a spinal injury, do not use this roll to hyperextend the neck.

Mechanical devices are also available. These operate on compressed gas and deliver chest compressions and ventilations.

## Basic Wound Care Supplies

Supplies for dressing open wounds include the following:

- large safety pins
- adhesive tape in several widths
- self-adhering, soft roller bandages, 4" × 5 yd
- self-adhering, soft roller bandages, 2" × 5 yd
- sterile dressings, gauze, 4" × 4"
- sterile dressings, ABD or laparotomy pads, usually 6" × 9" or 8" × 10"
- sterile universal trauma dressings, usually 10" × 36", folded into 9" × 10" packages
- sterile, nonporous, nonadherent dressings (aluminum foil sterilized in original package)

## Splinting Supplies

Supplies for splinting fractures and dislocations include the following:

- 1 adult-sized traction splint
- 1 child-sized traction splint
- a variety of arm and leg splints, such as inflatable, vacuum, cardboard, plastic, wire-ladder, or padded board (The number and types of splints should be determined by your medical director.)
- a variety of triangular bandages and roller bandages
- a short spine board
- a long spine board

- a variety of sizes of cervical collars
- 1 pneumatic antishock garment (PASG)

## Childbirth Supplies

You must carry a sterile emergency delivery pack, including the following supplies:

- 1 pair surgical scissors
- 3 hemostats or special cord clamps
- umbilical tape or sterilized cord
- small rubber bulb syringe
- 5 towels
- 1 dozen 2" × 10" gauze sponges
- 3 or 4 pairs of sterile gloves
- 1 baby blanket
- sanitary napkins
- plastic bag

## Medications

Activated charcoal in premeasured doses, as well as drinkable water and cups, should be carried on your unit. You should also have tubes of oral glucose on hand. Oxygen, as described above, should also be carried on the unit. Make sure that you have the telephone number and radio frequency of the local poison control center with you on the unit. One good place for this number is on the back of your clipboard.

You should also carry supplies for irrigating the skin and eyes. You may also need to carry a snakebite kit or other regional equipment, depending on your area and local protocol.

## Automated External Defibrillator

Automated defibrillation equipment, as permitted by the local medical director, should be carried on your unit.

## FIGURE 27-5

A typical jump kit

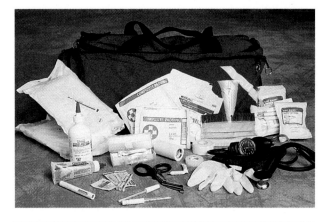

### The Jump Kit

Your unit should be equipped with a portable jump kit that you can carry to the patient. The **jump kit** must be light, durable, waterproof, quick to open, and easy to secure (Figure 27-5). Think of the jump kit as the "5-minute kit"—anything you might need in the first 5 minutes with the patient, except the oxygen bottle, defibrillator, and possibly the portable suctioning unit. A jump kit typically contains the following items in addition to the items carried on the ambulance:

- latex gloves
- triangular bandages
- trauma shears
- adhesive tape in various widths
- universal trauma dressings
- self-adhering soft roller bandages, 4" × 5 yd and 2" × 5 yd
- oropharyngeal airways in adult, child, and infant sizes*
- BVM device with masks for adults, children, and infants*
- blood pressure cuff

* These might be carried in a separate airway kit, along with the portable oxygen cylinder.

- stethoscope
- penlight
- sterile dressings, gauze, 4" × 4"
- sterile dressings, (ABD or laparotomy pads) 6" × 9" or 8" × 10"
- thermometer
- Band-Aid adhesive strips
- oral glucose
- activated charcoal

### Patient Transfer

Each unit should have a primary wheeled ambulance stretcher, as well as a folding litter and a collapsible chair device, or stair chair. The collapsible and folding litters may be combined as one unit. Litters must be easy to move, store, clean, and disinfect. The folding litter should keep the patient elevated above the floor when in the flat, extended position.

## NONMEDICAL EQUIPMENT

### Personal Safety Equipment

You should carry personal protective equipment so that you can work safely in a limited variety of hazardous or contaminated situations. You will not be equipped to face all HazMat and other exposure situations that you may encounter. These situations are the job of specially trained HazMat technicians and response teams. Rather, this equipment should protect you from being exposed to blood and other body fluids. It will also allow you to work for brief periods on the periphery of situations such as a structural fire or an explosion. Examples of such equipment might include the following:

- face shields
- gowns, shoe covers, and caps for protection from blood splatter or other potentially infectious materials

- turnout gear
- helmets with face shields or safety goggles

## MAPS AND DIRECTORIES

You should carry complete street and area maps, as well as preplanned directions to various locations, such as local hospitals, in the driver's compartment of the unit.

It is important to learn and be familiar with the various roads in your town or city. Knowing a variety of routes will enable you to plan alternate ways to reach a destination. In fact, switching to alternate routes will often save more time than driving faster. Knowing ways around frequently opened bridges or blocked railroad crossings is especially important.

## PERSONNEL

Obviously, an ambulance without EMTs does no good. As an absolute minimum, every ambulance must be staffed with at least one EMT-B in the patient compartment whenever a patient is being transported. Some services may operate with a non-EMT driver and a single EMT-B in the patient compartment. However, it is strongly recommended that at least two EMT-Bs be on every ambulance whenever a patient is being transported.

## DAILY INSPECTIONS

You and your team should inspect both the unit and equipment daily to ensure that everything is in proper working condition. An inspection of the vehicle should include checking each of the following:

- fuel levels
- oil levels
- transmission fluid levels
- engine cooling system and fluid levels
- battery(ies)
- brake fluid
- engine belts
- wheels and tires (including the spare, if any) for inflation pressure and unusual or uneven wear
- all interior and exterior lights
- windshield wipers and fluid
- horn
- siren
- air conditioners and heaters
- ventilating system
- doors for proper opening, closing, latching, and locking
- communications systems, vehicle and portable
- all windows and mirrors for cleanliness and position

Check all medical equipment and supplies at least daily, including all of the oxygen supplies, the jump kit, splints, dressings and bandages, backboards and other immobilization equipment, emergency delivery kit, and all other supplies. Equipment should be checked for proper function, while supplies are assessed for adequate quantity and cleanliness. All battery-operated equipment, including the defibrillator, should be operated and checked each day. The batteries should be rotated according to an established schedule.

## SAFETY PRECAUTIONS

A final part of the preparation phase is reviewing safety precautions. These safety precautions should be followed on every call. Check to make sure that safety devices, such as seat belts, are in proper working condition.

## DISPATCH

A readily accessible, 24-hour dispatch service must be available for your EMS service. Dispatch may be operated by the EMS service itself, or it may be a shared service that provides coverage for law enforcement, fire, and EMS. The dispatch center might serve only one jurisdiction, such as a single city or town. It might also be an area or regional center that serves several communities or an entire county.

The dispatch center should be staffed by trained personnel who are familiar with both the geography of the service area and the capabilities and characteristics of the agencies they are dispatching. For every emergency request, the dispatcher should gather and record the following information:

- the nature of the call
- the name, present location, and call-back telephone number of the person calling
- the location of the patient
- the number of patients and some idea of the severity of their conditions
- any other special problems or pertinent information concerning hazards or weather conditions

## RESPONSE PHASE

As you and your partner prepare to leave for the scene, make sure you fasten your seat belts and shoulder harnesses before you move the unit. At this point, you should inform dispatch that your unit is responding. You also need to confirm the nature and location of the call. This is also an excellent time to ask about any other available information about the location. For example, you might learn that the patient is on the third floor or that the best door to use is around the side of the house, and so on.

### CHARACTERISTICS OF THE DRIVER

In many ways, the en route or response phase of the call is the most dangerous for you. Collisions between automobiles and emergency vehicles account for most job-related injuries for EMS personnel. Thus, diligence and caution are important characteristics for safe driving. In addition, the driver must be physically and mentally fit, able to perform under stress. A positive attitude about your ability and tolerance of other drivers are also helpful characteristics. In many states you must successfully complete an approved emergency vehicle operations course before you are allowed to drive the unit on emergency calls.

One basic requirement is that the driver be physically fit. Many accidents occur as a result of physical impairment of the driver. Therefore, you should not be the driver if you are taking medications such as cold remedies, analgesics, or tranquilizers that may induce sleep or slow reaction times. And of course, you should never drive or provide medical care after drinking alcohol.

Another requirement is that the driver be emotionally fit. Emotions should not be taken lightly. In fact, personalities often change once an individual gets behind a steering wheel. Emotional stability is closely related to the ability to operate under stress. You must be capable of acting properly under the stresses of emergency conditions. In addition to knowing exactly what to do, you must be able to do it under trying conditions.

The driver must also be aware of the important responsibilities of emergency driving and develop the proper attitude. Although your unit is usually granted right-of-way privileges, state laws are very clear about the responsibility of the driver of an emergency vehicle. You must never get behind the wheel thinking you can do whatever you wish. Being able to drive to your destination without interruption, as granted in right-of-way privileges, and being able to move from one lane into the opposite lane are valuable, time-saving privileges that must never be abused.

## SAFE VEHICLE OPERATIONS

Safe driving is a very important part of the emergency care of sick and injured patients. Transport to the hospital is one of the tools that you use in caring for patients. Efficient, safe transport is just as important as many other treatment measures that you will use.

Operating an ambulance is a great responsibility. To do so, you must use good judgment and knowledge you have gained through training and experience. Only in extreme life-and-death emergencies is speed an important factor. *In most instances, if the patient is properly assessed and stabilized at the scene, speed during transport is unnecessary, undesirable, and dangerous.* The driver should never travel at a speed that is not safe.

There is an old adage that applies very well to emergency driving: Practice makes perfect. You can practice anytime, any place, and in any vehicle. No one is such a good driver that he or she would not benefit from practice.

Remember that you must always drive defensively. Never rely on what another motorist will do, unless you receive a clear visual signal from that motorist. Even then, be prepared to take defensive action in case of miscommunication, panic, or careless driving.

### Safe Driving Practices

The first rule in the safe driving of an emergency vehicle is that *speed does not save lives.* In most instances, on a multi-lane highway, keep the unit in the extreme left-hand (fast) lane. Using this lane allows other motorists to move over in a normal, pull to the right manner and causes the least possible disturbance to other traffic. The second rule is that the driver and all passengers must wear seat belts and shoulder harnesses at all times. Other EMT-Bs should wear them en route to the scene and when they are not performing direct patient care. Seat belts and shoulder harnesses are the most important items of safety equipment on every ambulance.

Learn how your vehicle works with regard to acceleration, cornering, swaying, and stopping. For example, disc booster brakes improve braking efficiency, but they increase sway. You must also know exactly what the vehicle will do and how it will respond to steering, braking, and acceleration under various conditions.

Getting the feel for the proper brake pressure comes with experience and practice driving your vehicle. Each vehicle has a different braking action and feel. For example, the brakes on types I and III vehicles have a heavier feel than do the brakes of a type II vehicle. Certain heavy vehicles use air brakes. These have yet another feel. Become familiar with each vehicle you drive, and be sure you understand its braking characteristics and the best down-shifting technique for that vehicle.

### Weather and Road Conditions

You should be constantly alert to changing weather, road, and driving conditions.

Warnings of ice or hazardous conditions must be taken seriously. Whether en route to an emergency or returning to the hospital, you must modify your speed according to road conditions. Although you should follow specified routes for most runs, you should have alternate routes available if needed. During a major disaster, it is especially important that all public safety and emergency services be coordinated with all vehicles following assigned routes. If you encounter unexpected traffic congestion, notify the dispatcher. That way other emergency vehicles can be informed about the congestion and delays and select alternate routes.

Even the most careful drivers will occasionally run into unexpected situations that may require special driving skills. Driving at a speed appropriate for the weather and road conditions will decrease the need to use these techniques.

**Hydroplaning**   On a wet road, a tire usually displaces the water on the road surface and stays in direct contact with the road. However, as a vehicle's speed increases above 30 mph, the tire may be lifted off the road surface as water "piles up" under it. At this speed, there is not enough time for the driver to slow down quickly and force the water out from under the tire. As a result, the tires are not in direct contact with the road surface. The vehicle then feels as if it is floating on the road surface. This is known as **hydroplaning** (Figure 27-6). If you are traveling at higher speeds on wet roadways, the front wheels of your vehicle may be riding on a sheet of water. This gives you little or no control over the vehicle. If hydroplaning occurs, you should gradually slow down, without jamming on the brakes.

**Water on the Roadway**   If at all possible, avoid driving through large pools of water. If it cannot be avoided, make sure you slow down and turn on the windshield wipers. After driving out of the pool, you should lightly tap the brakes several times until they are dry. Wet brakes will slow the vehicle and pull it to one side or the other.

**Decreased Visibility**   In areas where there is fog, smog, snow, or heavy rain, common sense dictates that you slow down after giving sufficient warning to following vehicles. At night, use only low headlight beams for maximum visibility without reflection. You should use headlights during the day to increase your visibility to other drivers. Also watch carefully for stopped or slow-moving cars.

**Ice and Slippery Surfaces**   A light mist on an oily, dusty road can be just as slippery as a patch of ice. Good all-weather tires and an appropriate speed can help decrease traction problems significantly. You should consider studded snow tires (where permitted by law) if you are in an area that often has snowy or icy conditions. You should be especially wary of bridges and overpasses when temperatures are close to freezing. These road surfaces will freeze much faster than surrounding road surfaces, because they lack the warming effect of the underlying ground.

**FIGURE 27-6**

Hydroplaning

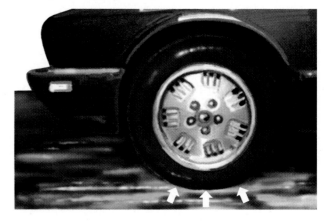

## LAWS AND REGULATIONS

While regulations regarding vehicle operations vary from state to state and city to city, some general similarities exist. While every state grants the driver of an emergency vehicle certain limited privileges, this in no way lessens or eliminates the driver's liability in the event of a collision. In fact, in most cases the driver is presumed to be guilty if a collision occurs while the unit is operating with warning lights and siren. Motor vehicle accidents are the single largest source of legal actions against EMS personnel and services.

You must follow three basic universal principles to legally and appropriately use the warning lights and siren, as follows:

1. The unit must be engaged in a true emergency response to your best knowledge.

2. Both audible and visual warning devices must be used simultaneously.

3. The unit must be operated with due regard for the safety of all others using the roadway.

Exemptions from usual vehicle operations are commonly granted to emergency vehicles that are on a valid emergency call. Again, you must be on a valid emergency call and your warning lights and siren must be turned on. These exemptions may include any one of the following:

- parking or standing in an otherwise illegal location
- proceeding through a red traffic light or stop sign
- driving faster than the posted speed limit
- driving against the flow of traffic on a one-way street, or making an otherwise prohibited turn
- traveling left of center to make an otherwise illegal pass

Remember that these regulations and exemptions vary by state and local jurisdiction. Therefore, you should check your local statutes for regulations and exemptions in your area.

In almost no case is an emergency vehicle exempted from passing a school bus that has stopped to load or unload children and that is displaying its flashing red lights or extended "stop arm." If you approach a school bus that has its lights flashing, you should stop before reaching the school bus and wait for the bus driver to secure the children, close the bus door, and turn off the warning lights. Only then can you carefully proceed past the stopped school bus.

### Use of Lights and Siren

The siren is probably the most overused piece of equipment on an ambulance. In general, the siren does not help you as you drive the ambulance. It does not really help other motorists in closed cars. Motorists driving at the speed limit with the windows up, and the radio on and/or the air conditioner or heater set on high cannot hear the siren until the ambulance is only a short distance away. If the radio is particularly loud, the other driver may not hear the siren at all.

If you do have to use the siren, be sure to warn the patient before you turn it on. If you must use the siren, do not speed up simply because the siren is on. Always travel at a speed that will enable you to stop safely at all times. This is especially important if other motorists do not give you the right-of-way. Never assume that warning lights and sirens will allow you to pass through a congested area. Always assume that other drivers will have their car windows rolled up, their radios playing, conversation going on, and the heater or air conditioner fan going at high speed. They will not be looking for an ambulance and will not hear the siren, even if it is only a short distance away.

The ambulance's headlights are sometimes equipped with a high-beam flasher unit. These are the most visible, effective warning devices for clearing traffic in front of the ambulance.

## Guidelines for Safe Ambulance Driving

1. Select the shortest and normally least congested route to the scene at the time of dispatch.

2. Avoid routes with heavy traffic congestion. Know alternate routes to each hospital during rush hours.

3. Avoid one-way streets, as they may become clogged by the sound of your siren. Do not go against the flow of traffic on a one-way street.

4. Watch carefully for bystanders as you approach the scene. Curiosity seekers rarely move out of the way.

5. Park the unit in a safe place once you arrive at the scene. If you park facing into traffic, turn off your headlights as they may blind on-coming traffic. Keep your warning lights on to alert oncoming motorists.

6. Drive within the speed limit en route with a patient, except for the rare extreme emergency.

7. Go with the flow of traffic.

8. Use the siren as little as possible en route.

9. Always drive defensively.

10. Always maintain a safe following distance. Use the "4-second rule." Stay at

## EMT

### FIRST DAY ON THE JOB

YOU ARE THE EMT

All your hard work has paid off. You've finally completed the EMT-B course, passed the state test, and have been certified! In addition, you've been hired as an EMT-B with a local private ambulance service. You put on your new uniform, hit the bathroom mirror for a quick once over, and it's off to work. You report to the shift supervisor, who introduces you to your new partner. Your partner will be doing your orientation. You say your "Hellos" and then start to check out your ambulance.

### For Discussion

1. Name the parts of the ambulance that require cleaning, those that need disinfecting, and those that need sterilizing.

2. Describe a variety of methods for moving a patient to the ambulance, based on injury or illness.

least 4 seconds behind another vehicle in the same lane.

11. Try to maintain an open space in the lane next to you as an escape route if the vehicle in front of you should stop suddenly.

12. Use your siren if you turn on the emergency lights, except when you are on a freeway.

### Right-of-Way Privileges

Right-of-way privileges granted to an ambulance vary from state to state. Some states allow you to proceed through a red light or stop sign after you stop and make sure that it is safe to go on. Other states allow you to proceed through a controlled intersection "with due regard" using flashing lights and siren. This means that you may proceed only if you consider the safety of all persons using the highway. Failure to use due regard may result in a liability claim against your service. It may also result in punitive damages against you if you are found at fault.

Thus, you must be familiar with the local right-of-way laws. Exercise these privileges only when it is absolutely necessary for the patient's well-being. The truth is, very few emergencies require extremely rapid transport.

### Reviewing Dispatch Information

In addition to safely operating the unit while en route, you and your team should prepare to assess and care for the patient. Review dispatch information regarding the nature of the call and the location of the patient. Each team member should be assigned specific initial duties, such as what type of equipment or stretcher to carry to the scene.

## PARKING CONSIDERATIONS

It is important that you park your unit in a position that will allow efficient traffic con-

### FIGURE 27-7

Park uphill/upwind of the scene if hazardous materials are present

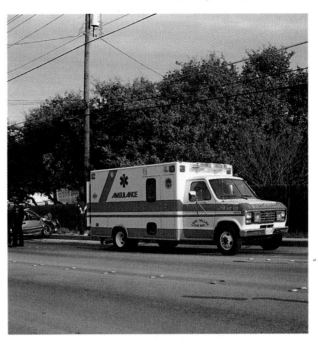

trol and flow around the accident scene. You should not park alongside the scene, as it may block the movement of other emergency vehicles. Rather, you should park about 100' past the scene on the same side of the road. It is best to park uphill and/or upwind of the scene if smoke or hazardous materials are present (Figure 27-7). If you must park on the backside of a hill or curve, leave your warning lights or devices on. This is also true when parking at night.

Make sure as you size up the scene that you park well away from any potential collapsing structures, fires, explosive hazards, or downed wires. Be sure to set the parking brake and leave the vehicle warning lights on. If your unit is parked facing on-coming traffic, turn off the headlights unless they are needed to illuminate the scene.

Given the safety guidelines above, you should still try to park your unit as close to the scene as possible to facilitate emergency medical care. As you approach the scene, quickly survey the area and select the best place to park to unload equipment and to load patients. If necessary, you can temporarily move the unit into a position to block traffic so that patients can be moved quickly and safely. If you must do this, try to do it as quickly as possible so that traffic is not blocked any longer than is absolutely necessary.

While traffic flow should continue with as little interruption as possible, patient care is the priority. Your first responsibility at the scene is to care for the patients. Only when all patients have been treated and the situation is under control should you be concerned with restoring the flow of traffic. If law enforcement is delayed in arriving at the scene, you may be required to take action.

## USE OF ESCORTS

The use of a police escort is an extremely dangerous practice. When other motorists hear a siren and see a police car passing, they may assume that the police car was the only emergency vehicle. As a result, they may not see you coming and collide with your unit. The only time that an escort is justified is when you are operating in unfamiliar territory and truly need a guide more than an escort. In such cases, neither vehicle should use any warning lights or sirens. If you are being guided by a police car, make sure you follow it at a safe distance.

You should never assume that motorists and the public will do the "right thing" when an emergency vehicle is in the area or is approaching from the rear. In most states, motorists must pull their vehicles to the right side of the road and stop upon the approach of an emergency vehicle with its warning lights and siren turned on. However, you should be ready for other motorists to do anything. This includes coming

to a screeching stop right in front of your unit. If you do not have your unit under control, a serious accident could occur.

## INTERSECTION HAZARDS

Intersection accidents are the most common and usually the most serious type of collision in which ambulances are involved. Thus, you must be alert and careful when approaching an intersection. If you are on an urgent call and cannot wait for traffic lights to change, you should still come to a momentary stop at the light. Once you have stopped, look around for other motorists before you proceed into the intersection.

Another serious hazard is when other motorists "time the traffic lights." This occurs when a motorist arrives at the intersection knowing that the traffic light is about to change and expects to go through. The theory is that by timing the lights, the motorist can avoid stopping. If you arrive at the intersection at the same time, a serious accident can occur. Even if the green light is in your favor, but about to change, a motorist "timing the lights" may drive through the intersection anyway.

A third common intersection hazard occurs when the driver of one emergency vehicle follows another emergency vehicle through an intersection without assessing the situation carefully. A motorist who has yielded the right-of-way to the first vehicle may proceed into the intersection, not expecting a second emergency vehicle to be close behind. Therefore, when following another emergency vehicle, you must exercise extreme caution. Use a siren tone different from that of the first vehicle. This may signal other motorists that a second unit is approaching.

Driving through an intersection when vision is obstructed, without stopping to make sure that the passage is clear, is like driving blindfolded. You may collide with another vehicle or strike a pedestrian, creating another emergency situation.

## ARRIVAL PHASE

Once you reach the scene, you should inform dispatch that you have arrived. You should also report any unexpected situations, such as the need for backup units, a heavy rescue unit, or a HazMat team.

Your scene size-up should include evaluating the need for BSI techniques, assessing for safety hazards, and determining the mechanism of injury in trauma patients or the nature of the illness on medical calls. Make sure you follow BSI techniques before you touch the patient. The type of personal protective equipment you wear depends on the type of problem or what the type of care is you expect to give.

Part of your size-up should include an assessment of where to park the unit. As stated earlier, make sure you park in a safe place and that it is safe to approach the patient. If there are dangerous hazards at the scene, you, your team, and the patient should be moved from the scene immediately before you begin caring for the patient.

In determining the mechanism of injury or the nature of the patient's illness, you must evaluate the need to stabilize the spine. If you are at the scene of a mass-casualty incident, or other incident in which there are many patients, quickly estimate the number of patients. Inform dispatch that backup units are needed at the scene. Once dispatch has been informed, you should begin the triage process to identify and then care for the most seriously sick or injured patient(s).

## CALL NUMBER ONE!

It finally happens! You've been sitting around for the last 3 hours, and your pager goes off. You are requested to respond to a car-truck collision out by the truck stop next to the interstate. Once you and your partner are seat belted in, you head out the door and put the rig in service.

### For Discussion

1. Describe at least four unsafe driving conditions and what you can do to remedy them.

2. What is the importance of being familiar with local directions, construction projects, etc.?

**YOU ARE THE EMT**

## TRANSFER TO THE AMBULANCE

In virtually every case, you should provide lifesaving care right where you find the patient—before moving him or her to the ambulance. When lifesaving care has been given, you may then begin less critical measures such as bandaging and splinting. The patient should then be packaged for transport and secured to a device such as a backboard, scoop litter, or the wheeled ambulance stretcher. You should then move to the ambulance and properly lift the patient into the patient compartment.

No matter how careful the driver may be, riding to the hospital while laying on your back on a stretcher can be an uncomfortable and even hazardous experience. The patient should be secured to the ambulance stretcher with at least three straps across the body (Figure 27-8). Make sure to use deceleration or stopping straps to secure the patient to the stretcher. These straps pass over the shoulders and prevent the patient from continuing to move forward should the ambulance (and stretcher) abruptly slow down or stop.

## FIGURE 27-8

Secure the patient to the stretcher with three straps

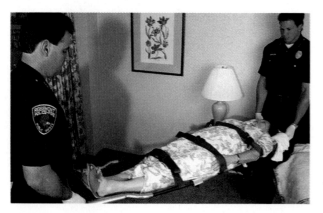

## TRANSPORT TO THE HOSPITAL

Inform dispatch when you are ready to leave the scene with the patient. Report the number of patients you have and the name of the receiving hospital. Even though you have assessed and treated the patient at the scene, you should monitor the patient en route. These on-going assessments signal changes in the patient's vital signs and overall condition. At this time, you should also contact the receiving hospital. Inform medical control about your patient(s) and the nature of the problem(s). Depending on how many EMT-Bs are available and how much care the patient needs, you may also want to begin working on your written report en route.

Finally, and most importantly, do not abandon the patient! It can be very easy to become engrossed in paperwork and on-going assessments. Do not ignore the patient's fears and emotions. This is a good time to reassure the patient. You are there to help and take care of the patient.

## DELIVERY AND POSTRUN PHASES

Inform dispatch once you arrive at the hospital. The transfer of the patient to the receiving hospital takes several forms. The first and most obvious is the physical transfer of the patient from your stretcher to the bed. Second, you must present a complete verbal report at the bedside to the nurse or physician who is taking over the care of the patient. Third, you must complete a detailed written report and then leave a copy with an appropriate staff member.

While at the receiving hospital, you may be able to restock any items that were used during the run, such as oxygen masks or dressings and bandages. Remember, though, that your priority is transfer of the patient and patient information to the hospital staff. Restocking your unit comes second.

Once you leave the hospital, inform dispatch whether or not you are in service and where you are going. You should clean and disinfect the unit and any equipment used as soon as you reach your station, if you did not do so before leaving the hospital. Restock any supplies that you were unable to obtain at the hospital.

At the station, refuel the unit, as needed, and complete and file any additional written reports. Check the oil level if you refuel. Once again, inform dispatch of your status, location, and availability. After each trip, clean and decontaminate the inside of the ambulance, according to state and local regulations. Blood, vomitus, and other substances must be scrubbed from the floors, walls, and ceilings. Clean the outside of the unit as needed. Replace or repair broken or damaged equipment without delay.

## AIR MEDICAL OPERATIONS

There are two basic types of air ambulances: fixed-wing and helicopters (rotary wing) (Figure 27-9). Fixed-wing aircraft are generally used for interhospital patient transfers over distances greater than 100 miles. For shorter distances, rotary-wing aircraft are more efficient. Specially trained medical flight crews accompany these flights. Your involvement with fixed-wing aircraft transfers will probably be limited to providing ground transport for the patient and medical flight crew between the hospital and the airport.

Rotary-wing aircraft have become an important tool in providing emergency medical care. In many areas, it is an everyday occurrence to see a medical helicopter land at an accident scene and transport the victims to a trauma facility. Medical helicopters speed the delivery of appropriate lifesaving care to a patient, as well as speed the delivery of the patient to a lifesaving treatment facility. In order to use them safely and effectively, you should be familiar with the capabilities, protocols, and methods for accessing helicopters in your area. Training for EMT-Bs in ground operations and safety when working in and around rotary-wing aircraft is readily available from the helicopter services.

### FIGURE 27-9

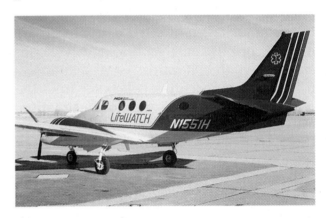

**A**   A fixed-wing aircraft

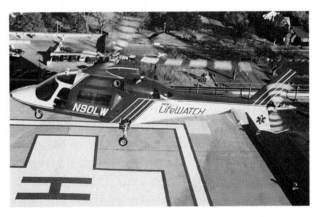

**B**   An air medical helicopter

## SAFETY PRECAUTIONS

The types of helicopters used for medical operations vary, but the dangers are the same. Helicopter safety is nothing more than good common sense, along with a constant awareness of the need for personal safety. If you are familiar with the way helicopters work and if you follow the instructions of the pilots, you should minimize any dangers involved. The most important rule is to stay a safe distance from the aircraft or helicopter whenever it is on the ground and "hot" (the rotors are spinning). The tips of the rotor blades are traveling near the speed of sound.

When accompanying a flight crew member, either to go on the mission or to help load a patient, you must follow the directions of the flight crew *exactly.* You should never try to open any aircraft door or move equipment unless a flight crew member tells you to. When directed to approach the aircraft, use extreme caution and pay constant attention to hazards.

Never approach the helicopter from the rear, even if it is not a "hot load" situation. The approach area is between nine and three o'clock as the pilot faces forward (Figure 27-10). The approach area has been strictly defined because of the hazard of the tail rotor. In addition, the pilot may need to swing the tail boom to a different direction for takeoff.

The tail rotor is a spinning blade that is almost impossible to see because of its extreme speed. Thus, it is important for you to stay away from the tail rotor. If you must move from one side of the helicopter to the other, go around the front of the aircraft. Never duck under the body, the tail boom, or the rear section of the helicopter. The pilot cannot see in these areas. When enough personnel are available, someone should stand toward the rear of the aircraft, outside the arc of the rotor blades, to warn bystanders and others away.

## FIGURE 27-10

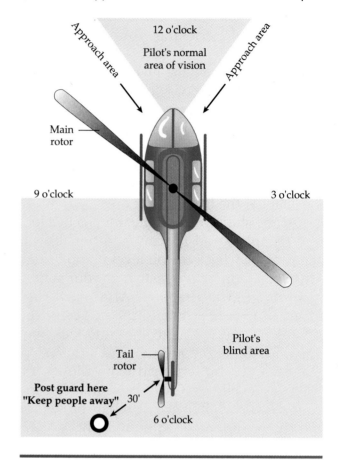

Approach routes for air medical helicopter

Another area of concern when approaching a helicopter is the height of the main rotor blade. Due to the flexibility of the blade, it may dip as low as 4' off the ground (Figure 27-11). When you approach the aircraft, walk in a crouched position until you reach the helicopter. Wind gusts can influence the blade height without warning. Therefore, protect equipment as you carry it under the blades. Air turbulence created by the rotor blades can blow off hats and loose equipment. These, in turn, can become a danger to the aircraft and personnel in the area.

If no other site is available and the helicopter must land on a grade, you must be

## FIGURE 27-11

Approach a helicopter in a crouched position

**Danger** – Main rotor blades can dip to as low as 4 feet off the ground

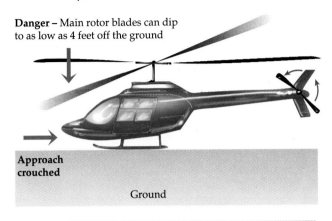

Approach crouched

Ground

## FIGURE 27-12

Approach a helicopter on a grade from the downhill side

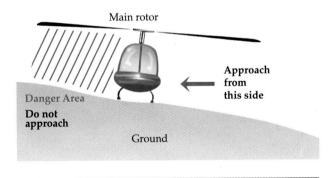

Main rotor

Danger Area
**Do not approach**

Approach from this side

Ground

even more careful. The main rotor blade will be closer to the ground on the uphill side (Figure 27-12). In this situation, approach the aircraft from the downhill side only. Do not move the patient to the helicopter until the crew has signaled that they are ready to receive you. A flight crew member will direct and assist you with loading the patient.

Although a helicopter can fly straight up and down, this is the most dangerous mode of operation. The safest and most effective way to land and take off is similar to that used by fixed-wing aircraft. Landing at a slight angle allows for safer operations. Takeoff is a reversal of this process, combining a gradual lift and forward motion to travel up and out on a slight angle.

Clearing a landing site is another important role you can play. Look for loose debris, electric or telephone wires, poles, or any other hazards that might interfere with the safe operation of the helicopter. If you note any hazards, inform the pilot by radio or other signal. The pilot will usually "overfly" or survey the site before final approach and landing to ensure that all potential dangers are identified. While the pilot actually chooses the landing site, you should designate suggested landing sites. If one of these sites is appropriate, the pilot will use it. Variables such as temperature, winds, and the helicopter's weight with cargo all play a part in the pilot's final selection of a landing site. Local protocols will determine whether flags, lights, or other signaling devices should be used to mark the proposed landing site.

Nighttime operations are considerably more hazardous than daytime operations due to the darkness. The pilot will fly often over the area with the helicopter's lights on, not only to show obstacles, but also to have the lights reveal the shadows of overhead wires. While wires may not be visible, the changing shadows are often noted.

Do not shine spotlights in the air to help the pilot. These lights may temporarily blind the pilot. Light beams should be directed toward the ground at the landing site. Even after the helicopter is on the ground, lights should not be aimed anywhere near it. Of course, smoking, open lights or flames, and flares are prohibited within 50' of the aircraft at all times.

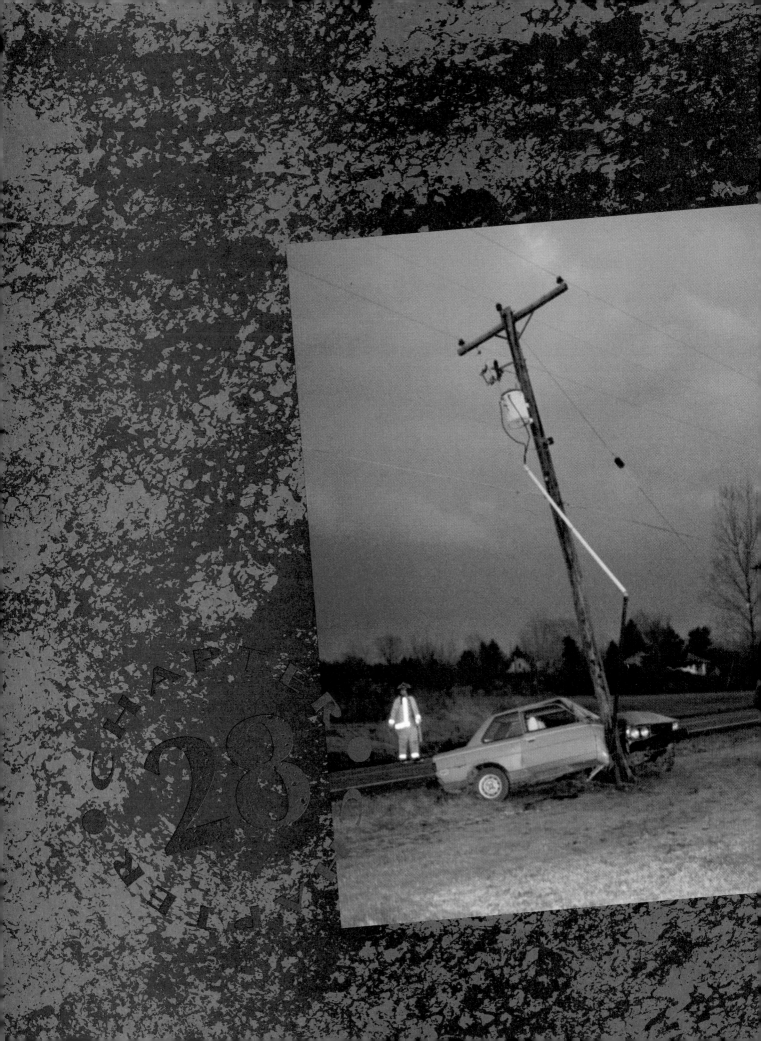

# CHAPTER 28

# Scene Techniques

## Objectives

After you have read this chapter, you should be able to:

- Describe the purpose and fundamental components of extrication.
- Discuss the role of the EMT-B in extrication.
- Identify personal safety equipment for the EMT-B in extrication.
- List the steps in protecting the patient during extrication.
- Evaluate various ways of gaining access to the patient.
- Distinguish simple access from complex access.
- Explain the role of the EMT-B during a hazardous materials incident, including what should be done while waiting for the HazMat team.
- Describe the actions that an EMT-B should take if there is a possible hazard at the scene, including steps to ensure bystander safety and the proper way to approach the scene.
- Discuss the various environmental hazards that affect EMS.
- Describe the criteria for a multiple-casualty situation.
- Discuss the role of the EMT-B in a multiple-casualty situation.
- Summarize the components of basic triage.
- Define the role of the EMT-B in a disaster operation.
- Describe basic concepts of incident management.

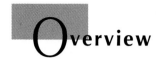

# Overview

As an EMT-B, you will not usually be responsible for rescue and extrication. Rescue involves many different processes and environments. It also requires training beyond the level of the EMT-B. Therefore, this chapter will simply introduce topics such as gaining access, and basic concepts involving hazardous materials and multiple-casualty situations. Appendix C provides an overview of basic fundamentals of extrication.

The first section of this chapter introduces basic principles of gaining access. Your main concern is reaching the patient so that you can begin providing care. In most instances, once you have reached the patient, extrication may occur "around" you and the patient.

The next section provides an overview of your responsibilities at a hazardous materials incident. When you are responding to this type of incident, you cannot rush in to provide patient care. Rather, you must take time to accurately assess the scene. That means identifying the size of the hazard area, finding a safe location to which patients can be removed, and taking self-protective measures. Safety is your prime consideration. If a hazardous materials incident is not carefully handled, a lot of people, including rescue personnel, can become casualties.

The final section of the chapter is a very basic introduction to incident management systems. The purpose of this section is to give you an idea of the larger structure at work during complex incidents. The role of the EMT-B within the system is explained. Concepts such as triage and multiple-casualty incidents are also discussed.

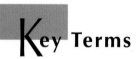

# Key Terms

**Chemical Transportation Emergency Center (CHEMTREC)** Assists emergency personnel in identifying and handling hazardous materials transport incidents.

**Extrication** Removal from entrapment or a dangerous situation or position. This is often used to mean removal of a patient from a wrecked vehicle.

**Incident management systems**
Organizational systems to help control, direct, and coordinate emergency responders and resources.

**Multiple-casualty situation (MCS)**
An event that places such a demand upon available equipment or personnel resources that the system is stretched to its limit.

**Protection level**    A measure of the amount of protective equip-ment that someone must have to avoid injury during contact with a hazardous material.

**Toxicity level**    A measure of the risk that anyone is subjected to by contact with a certain hazardous material.

**Triage**    The process of establishing treatment and transportation priorities according to the severity of injury and medical need.

# GAINING ACCESS

## THE EMT-B AND RESCUE

During all phases of rescue, your primary role is to provide emergency medical care and prevent further injury to the patient. You should provide care as extrication goes on around you, unless this proves too dangerous for you or the patient. **Extrication** is defined as removal from entrapment or a dangerous situation or position. In this chapter, it means removal of a patient from a wrecked automobile. However, the principles and concepts of automobile extrication can also apply to other situations.

It is important that you and members of the rescue team communicate throughout the process. Every rescue team should have a defined structure of leadership. You and the rescue team leader should be talking with one another as soon as you arrive at the scene. You will need to coordinate your efforts with that of the rescue team, and vice versa. Respect that the rescue team has a job to do, and they will do the same.

In some areas there may not be enough personnel for two separate units. In these areas, you and your team may have to "wear both hats." As stated above, it is critical that one person be in charge of the overall rescue operation. This person must be medically trained and qualified to judge the priorities of patient care. This person also has to be experienced in extrication. If there is no identifiable leadership at the scene, the rescue effort and patient care will suffer. Leaders should be identified as part of a larger incident management system. This system is described later in this chapter.

## EQUIPMENT AND SAFETY

You must always be prepared for any incident that requires rescue or extrication. Your first step is to prepare yourself physically and mentally. The most important part of this preparation is thinking about your safety and the safety of your team. Safety begins with the proper mind set and the proper protective equipment.

The equipment you use and the gear you wear depend on the situation (Figure 28-1). A complete discussion of basic protective gear is presented in chapter 2, The Well-Being of the EMT-B. Special protective gear for hazardous materials incidents is described in the next section. However, the importance of wearing latex or vinyl gloves at all times during patient contact cannot be emphasized enough. If you will be involved with extrication, you should wear a pair of leather gloves over your disposable gloves. Handling ropes, tools, broken glass, hot or cold objects, or sharp metal can result in injury if you are not wearing the proper gloves.

### Patient and Bystander Safety

As you are gaining access to the patient and during extrication, you must make sure that the patient remains safe. Be sure that you talk to the patient and describe what you are doing as you do it, even if you think

## FIGURE 28-1

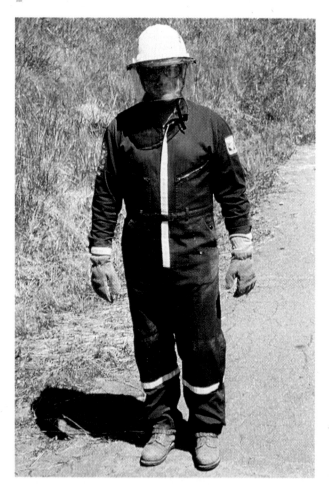

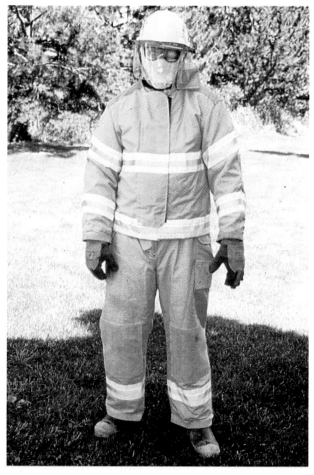

**A**  Minimum protective clothing

**B**  Full turnout gear

the patient is unconscious. This is the time when extrication tools and equipment are closest to the patient. You should cover the patient with a heavy, nonflammable blanket to protect against flying glass or other objects. In many instances, you or another member of the team will be providing immobilization of the cervical spine or other care during extrication. These personnel should be covered with a blanket during extrication as well. A short spine board may also be used as a protective shield. Try to keep heat, noise, and force to a minimum. Use only that needed to extricate the patient safely.

Bystanders and family members can be hazards themselves. If they are allowed to get too close, they are at risk of injury. They may also pose significant risk to the overall management of the incident. The rescue team will set up a danger zone in which bystanders cannot enter (Figure 28-2). Help the rescue team in setting up this zone. If you arrive before the rescue team, you should coordinate crowd control with law enforcement officials.

Occasionally, a bystander, especially one who claims to have medical credentials, may be difficult to manage. This situation is always challenging. Your EMS service should have a protocol for dealing with this potential problem. Many states provide wallet-sized copies of licensure to physicians for use as identification. However, not all physicians have training in emergency medical care. Thus, when this situation occurs, inform medical control immediately. Communication between medical control and the physician at the scene may eliminate some of these problems. You may also assign the individual duties that will allow him or her to become minimally involved at the scene. This will reduce the risk of a possible confrontation.

## GAINING ACCESS TO THE PATIENT

The exact way you gain access or reach the patient depends on the type of incident. During the size-up, you should identify the safest, most efficient way to access the patient (Figure 28-3). Frequently, patients are thrown as a result of explosions. Sometimes they are hard to find due to darkness, uneven terrain, tall grass, shrubbery, or the wreckage. As you size up the situation, you must remember these factors. Size-up is a continuing process, because the situation often changes. These changes often demand that you change your plans for gaining access and providing treatment. For example, you need to consider the exact location and position of the patient. You and your team should consider the following questions:

- Is the patient in a vehicle? In some other structure?

- Is the vehicle or structure severely damaged?

- In what position is the vehicle? On what type of surface?

You must also take into account the patient's injuries and their severity. You may have to change your course of action as you learn more about the patient's injuries. Do

## FIGURE 28-2

Keep bystanders out of marked danger zone

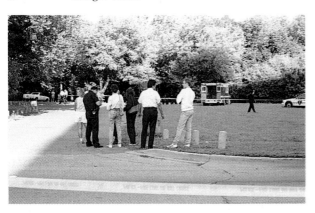

## FIGURE 28-3

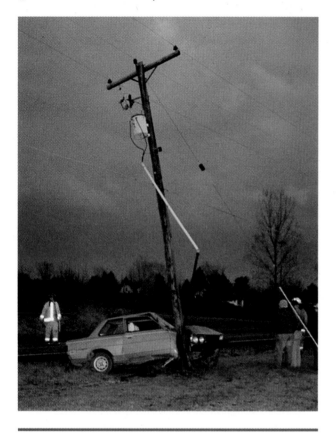

Scene size-up

not try to access the patient until you are sure that the vehicle is stable and that hazards have been identified and eliminated.

However, you may have to quickly remove a patient from a threatening environment. You may also need to move the patient quickly in order to do CPR. CPR is not effective when the patient is in a sitting position or lying on the soft seat of a vehicle. In these instances, you and your team may have to use the Rapid Extrication technique. This method is described in detail in chapter 6, Lifting and Moving Patients.

### Simple Access

Your first step is to try to get to the patient as quickly and simply as possible, without using any tools or breaking any glass. Automobiles are built to allow easy entry and exit. Always try to open the doors manually before using tools or other forcible entry methods. Whenever possible, try to unlock the doors (or ask the patient to unlock them) and use the door handles to gain access. When there is no danger to the patient, you should enter through the doors. However, if there is a medical emergency or other hazard, you should gain more direct access to the patient through one of the windows.

### Complex Access

Complex access requires the use of special tools and special training. Most of these skills are beyond the scope of this text. However, for a more detailed introduction to extrication, see appendix C, Fundamentals of Extrication.

## REMOVING THE PATIENT

Even though the patient is trapped in a vehicle, your steps in providing care are the same as for any other patient. However, you must first make sure that you and the patient are protected. Make sure that you and the patient(s) are covered with a thick, fireproof canvas or blanket (Figure 28-4). This will protect you from broken glass, sparks from tools, and other hazards during extrication.

Unless there is an immediate threat of fire or explosion, you should perform an initial assessment while the patient is still in the vehicle. Stabilize the patient's vital functions before extrication begins. Open the airway, control bleeding, support the cervical spine, and treat any critical injuries. Monitor the patient's vital signs as extrication proceeds.

As you prepare to remove the patient from the vehicle, make sure that the cervical spine is manually immobilized in a neutral position. Apply a cervical collar, if possible,

## FIGURE 28-4

Protect yourself and the patient with a fireproof canvas

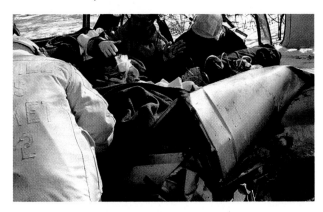

to support the spine and provide extra protection against glass fragments. Applying a splint inside a vehicle is difficult and often impossible. Thus, you can immobilize the extremities by securing the patient's arms to his or her body, and the legs to each other. This will be adequate until the patient is secured to a long spine board.

Remember that quick, smooth movements reduce the risk of further injury to the patient. Thus, if you and your team must remove the patient from the vehicle, plan the move carefully. At this point, you should also discuss whether the Rapid Extrication technique is needed. If not, secure the patient to a short spine board or other device before you remove him or her from the vehicle. This type of support is to make sure that possible spinal injuries are protected.

As you transfer the patient from the vehicle to the unit, choose the easiest route and continue to protect the patient from hazards.

## SPECIALIZED RESCUE

In some situations or disasters, special rescue teams are needed. Specialized rescue re-

## CHEMISTRY GONE CRAZY

Two college students decide to increase their meager incomes by manufacturing illegal drugs in the back of the house they rent. Inattention to details results in an explosion that blows out the back wall of the house, causing the roof to partially collapse. By the time you arrive, the fire department has put out the small fire and found most of the parts of one victim. They point you to the part of the house still standing, where they think the other "chemist" is trapped.

YOU ARE THE EMT

### For Discussion

1. Discuss some of the hazards and problems associated with extrication. What can you do to address these obstacles?

2. Describe the role of the EMT-B during extrication.

quires many skills not taught in the EMT-B training program. If you see that a special rescue team is needed, inform the dispatcher. You should assist these teams as necessary. Remember that members of special rescue teams are likely to be trained in emergency medical care as well as in their rescue specialty. If so, they can assist you in providing basic emergency medical care. If you are interested in specialized rescue, you should speak with the head of your EMS service or contact the rescue team in your area.

# INTRODUCTION TO HAZARDOUS MATERIALS

Your training has taught you that rapid response to the scene of an accident can save lives. You and your team can make quick decisions and act on them. Even so, sometimes you are criticized for taking too much time at the scene of an accident. When you arrive at the scene of a possible hazardous materials accident, you must first step back and assess the situation.

A hazardous materials scene is usually obvious, but other times, it is not. Sometimes, many people are injured or killed before the danger is identified. This often happens when odorless, poisonous gases or vapors have been released (Figure 28-5). Thus, it is important that you understand the potential dangers of hazardous materials. If you do not follow the proper safety measures, you and/or your team could end up dead.

Safety—for you, the patient, and the public—is your most important concern. There will be times when you are the first to arrive at the scene of a possible hazardous materials incident. Your first step is to assess the situation, making certain that you protect yourself, and then call for a trained HazMat team. Try to provide as much information

to dispatch about the scene as you can. Try to read labels and identification numbers from a distance. Use binoculars if necessary. Do not go into the area unless you are absolutely sure that no hazardous spill has occurred. If you are not sure and go in anyway, you risk exposure. Relay any information to your dispatch center where it can be used to identify the hazardous material.

## IDENTIFYING HAZARDOUS MATERIALS

The single most important step in any hazardous materials incident is to identify the substance(s) involved. Accurate identification of the materials is critical. You should be able to easily find this information on all of the following:

- boxes or cartons that contain a hazardous material (Figure 28-6a)
- vehicles that transport hazardous materials (Figure 28-6b)
- factories that produce hazardous materials

The law requires manufacturers and transport vehicles to display a four-digit identification number on the ends of a tank, vehicle, or railroad car that is used to carry hazardous materials (Figure 28-7). Sometimes the letters UN or NA come before this

## FIGURE 28-5

Scene of a hazardous materials incident

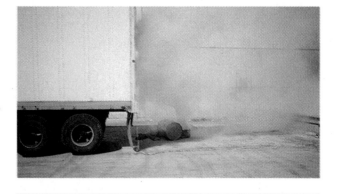

FIGURE 28-6

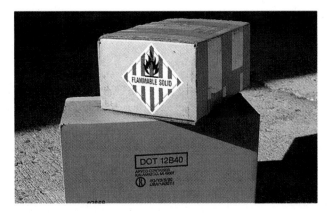

**A** Box identifying hazardous material

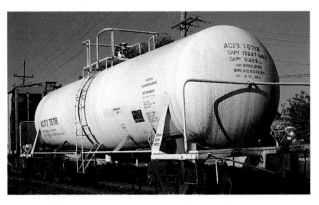

**B** Railroad car identifying transport of hazardous material

FIGURE 28-7

4-digit number identifying the type of hazardous material

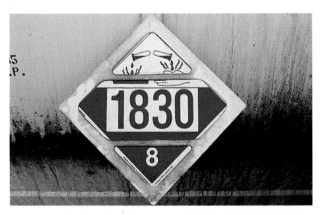

number. The name of the material is also commonly displayed along with the number. This same number can also be found on the shipping papers or packaging of the material (Figure 28-8). Different kinds of hazardous materials have different colored and shaped labels to help in identification (Figure 28-9).

Unfortunately, due to the lack of consistency in labels and placards, identifying materials can be difficult. The laws and regulations that cover labeling of packages and transport vehicles can also be misleading. In most cases, the package or tank must contain a certain amount of a hazardous material before a placard is required.

For example, a truck is carrying 99 lb of HazMat #1 and 99 lb of both HazMat #2 and HazMat #3. Because of the small quantities, the truck is not required by law to have any labels or placards. In fact the truck has only a "Please Drive Carefully" placard. Other motorists are not aware that the truck is carrying a combination of hazardous materials. However, an experienced HazMat technician knows that this is the most dangerous placard. The implication is that the truck carries no hazardous materials when in fact it could be loaded with them. Thus, an accident involving this truck is a serious situation—one you would not be aware of if you relied on labels and placards.

The driver of a commercial truck and the conductor of a train must carry papers that identify what is being transported in their care. These papers may be available to you depending upon the nature of the incident. Looking at these papers may be your first clue that there is a possible HazMat problem.

Finally, pay attention to your own senses. Strange-looking fumes or funny odors coming from a wrecked vehicle are also clues. You may have a major problem on your hands.

Only people trained to handle these incidents should enter the area, or hazard zone. As an EMT-B, you are not one of these people. Your job is to provide patient care once the patient can be safely moved out of the area. In most cases when a patient has been exposed to a hazardous material, it will be quite a while before he or she will come to you for care. The patient must be decontaminated or "clean" first. However, while you are waiting, you can help the hazardous materials team by providing medical backup to them.

Take special care when toxic fumes are present. The safe area is upwind from the site of the spill. You should park your unit upwind from the site at a safe distance, usually 100', from the site. If the area is hilly, you, your team, and the unit should be uphill as well as upwind. Remember that wind direction can change quickly. Someone at the site should be responsible for monitoring the wind and general weather conditions.

## Classification of Hazardous Materials

Hazardous materials are classified according to both toxicity levels and protection levels. Many of the publications dealing

## FIGURE 28-8

A shipping bill for transport of hazardous material

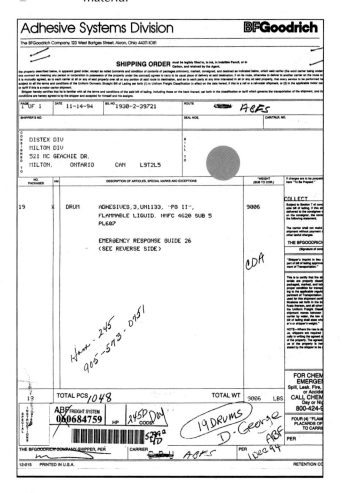

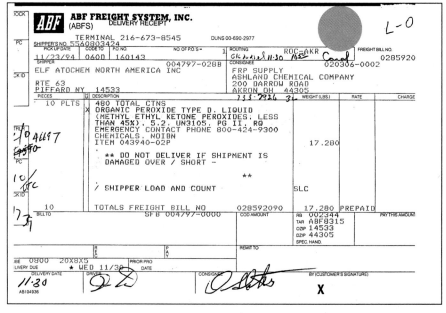

## FIGURE 28-9

Hazardous materials warning labels

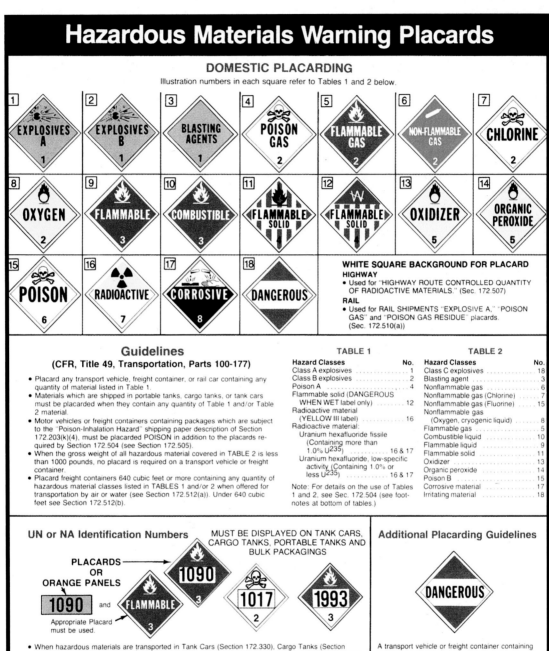

FIGURE 28-9 *continued*

Hazardous materials warning labels

# Hazardous Materials Warning Labels

## DOMESTIC LABELING

EXPLOSIVE A — 1 | EXPLOSIVE B — 1 | EXPLOSIVE C — 1 | BLASTING AGENT — 1 | POISON GAS | FLAMMABLE GAS | NON-FLAMMABLE GAS — 2

CHLORINE — 2 | OXYGEN — 2 | FLAMMABLE LIQUID — 3 | FLAMMABLE SOLID | DANGEROUS WHEN WET — 4 | OXIDIZER — 5.1 | ORGANIC PEROXIDE — 5.2

POISON — 6 | IRRITANT — 6 | (Infectious Substance) | RADIOACTIVE I — 7 | RADIOACTIVE II — 7 | RADIOACTIVE III — 7 | CORROSIVE — 8

## General Guidelines on Use of Labels
### (CFR, Title 49, Transportation, Parts 100-177)

- Labels illustrated above are normally for *domestic shipments.* However, some air carriers *may* require the use of International Civil Aviation Organization (ICAO) labels.

- Domestic Warning Labels *may* display UN Class Number, Division Number (and Compatibility Group for Explosives only) [Sec. 172.407(g)].

- Any person who offers a hazardous material for transportation MUST label the package, if required [Sec. 172.400(a)].

- The Hazardous Materials Tables, Sec. 172.101 and 172.102, identify the proper label(s) for the hazardous materials listed.

- Label(s), when required, must be printed on or affixed to the surface of the package near the proper shipping name [Sec. 172.406(a)].

- When two or more different labels are required, display them next to each other [Sec. 172.406(c)].

- Labels may be affixed to packages (even when not required by regulations) provided each label represents a hazard of the material in the package [Sec. 172.401].

**Check the Appropriate Regulations
Domestic or International Shipment**

## Additional Markings and Labels

**HANDLING LABELS**

Cargo Aircraft Only
172.402(b)

CAUTION

Bung Label
172.402(e)

ORM-E
172.316

INNER PACKAGES
COMPLY WITH
PRESCRIBED
SPECIFICATIONS
173.25(a)(4)

Package
Orientation
Markings
172.312(a)(c)

Fumigation
173.9

 EMPTY
173.427

Here are a few additional markings and labels pertaining to the transport of hazardous materials. The section number shown with each item refers to the appropriate section in the HMR. The Hazardous Materials Tables, Section 172.101 and 172.102, identify the proper shipping name, hazard class, identification number, required label(s) and packaging sections.

## Poisonous Materials

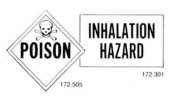

POISON
172.505

INHALATION
HAZARD
172.301

Materials which meet the inhalation toxicity criteria specified in Section 173.3a(b)(2), have additional "communication standards" prescribed by the HMR. First, the words "Poison-Inhalation Hazard" must be entered on the shipping paper, as required by Section 172.203(k)(4), for any primary capacity units with a capacity greater than one liter. Second, packages of 110 gallons or less capacity must be marked "Inhalation Hazard" in accordance with Section 172.301(a). Lastly, transport vehicles, freight containers and portable tanks subject to the shipping paper requirements contained in Section 172.203(k)(4) must be placarded with POISON placards in addition to the placards required by Section 172.504. For additional information and exceptions to these communication requirements, see the referenced sections in the HMR.

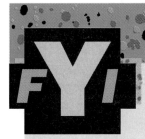

## HazMat Rule of Thumb

Some incidents involve small quantities of toxic materials. However, others involve barrels, boxes, tanks, or even carloads of harmful substances. If you are first to arrive at the scene, an important first step is to identify a danger zone. This is the area where exposure to the toxic substances may occur. The HazMat Rule of Thumb is one way to determine the size of the danger zone. To use this method, hold your arm straight out, with your thumb pointing up. Center your thumb over the hazardous area. Your thumb should completely cover the hazardous area from your view. If it does not, move back, try it again. Keep doing so until your thumb completely blocks the area from view.

Remember, do not enter a hazardous materials area without the proper training and proper equipment. Your use of the HazMat Rule of Thumb should be to estimate the size of the area and report it to the HazMat team or the incident commander.

with the handling of hazardous materials refer to these levels.

**Toxicity Level**   Toxicity levels are identified as 0, 1, 2, 3, or 4. **Toxicity levels** are a measure of the risk that the substance poses to anyone coming in contact with it. The higher the number, the greater the toxicity (Table 28-1). Level 0 includes materials that would cause little if any health hazard if you came into contact with them. Levels 1 and 2 include materials that are only slightly hazardous. However, if you are going to come into contact with them, you must wear a self-contained breathing apparatus (SCBA). Level 3 includes materials that are extremely hazardous to health. Before you come into contact with these, you must wear full protective gear, with none of your skin surface exposed. Level 4 includes mate-

rials that are so hazardous that minimal contact will cause death. For Level 4 substances, you need specialized gear designed for protection against that particular hazard.

**Protection Level**   Protection levels are identified as A, B, C, or D. **Protection levels** indicate the amount and type of protective gear that you need to prevent injury from a particular substance (Table 28-2). Level A is the most hazardous. It requires encapsulated protective clothing and offers full body protection as well as special sealed equipment.

Level B requires nonencapsulated protective clothing. This means clothing designed against a particular hazard. Usually this clothing is made of material that will let only limited amounts of moisture and vapor pass through (nonpermeable). Level B

**TABLE 28-1**     TOXICITY LEVELS OF HAZARDOUS MATERIALS

| Level | Health Hazard | Protection Needed |
|---|---|---|
| 0 | Little to no hazard | None |
| 1 | Slightly hazardous | SCBA only |
| 2 | Slightly hazardous | SCBA only |
| 3 | Extremely hazardous | Full protection, with no exposed skin |
| 4 | Minimal exposure causes death | Special HazMat gear |

also requires breathing devices that contain their own air supply, such as an SCBA, and eye protection.

Level C, like Level B, requires the use of nonpermeable clothing and eye protection. Face masks that filter all inhaled outside air must be used.

Level D requires structural fire-fighting clothing. All levels of protection require the use of gloves. You should wear two pairs of rubber gloves, so that you can remove one pair if it becomes heavily contaminated, and still be protected.

## ESTABLISHING A HAZARD ZONE

While the hazardous material is being identified, a hazard zone should be created. Using the HazMat Rule of Thumb, identify and isolate the danger area. Remain upwind of the area and avoid low areas where toxic fumes may tend to settle. Keep bystanders away. Often, well-meaning people try to help. However, unless they are trained for these types of incidents, they should be moved from the area. Remember, though,

**TABLE 28-2**     COMMON CLASSES OF HAZARDOUS MATERIALS

| Class Number | Nature of Materials |
|---|---|
| 1 | Explosives |
| 2 | Gases |
| 3 | Flammable liquids |
| 4 | Flammable solids |
| 5 | Oxidizers and organic peroxides |
| 6 | Poisons and etiological agents |
| 7 | Radioactive materials |
| 8 | Corrosives |
| 9 | Other regulated materials |

experienced, knowledgeable people such as industrial safety officers may be valuable.

## CARING FOR PATIENTS AT A HAZARDOUS MATERIALS INCIDENT

Never enter a possible hazardous materials area unless you are adequately protected. This is a job for trained and equipped Haz-Mat teams. If you do not have the necessary equipment with you, your best course of action is to notify dispatch that a HazMat team is needed. The level of protection needed depends on the toxicity level and protection level of the substance or substances involved.

Your care of injured patients and/or rescuers should focus mainly on supportive care. There are very few specific antidotes or treatments for most hazardous materials injuries. Also remember that people may respond differently to contact with the same hazardous material. Most serious injuries and deaths from hazardous materials result from airway and breathing problems. Thus, the patient must first be removed from the hazardous area by trained and properly protected personnel. Once the patient is clear of the area and "clean," monitor respirations and other vital signs closely. Maintain the airway and give oxygen at 10 to 15 L/min with a nonrebreathing mask if the patient appears to be in distress. If respiratory problems continue, you may need to assist ventilations.

## RESOURCES

The U.S. Department of Transportation (DOT) has developed and published *Hazardous Materials: The Emergency Response Guidebook* (DOT P 5800.4, 1993) (Figure 28-10). This publication lists most hazardous materials and describes the proper emergency action to control the scene and provide emergency

## FIGURE 28-10

1993 *Emergency Response Guidebook*

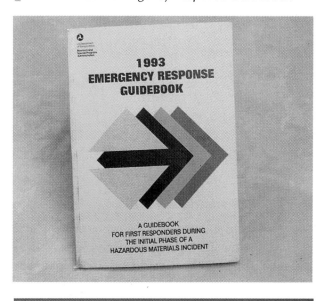

medical care. Several similar publications are also available. Some state and local government agencies may also have information about hazardous materials commonly found in their areas. A copy of the *Guidebook* and other information relevant to your local area should be in every unit and in the dispatch center. These resources are important so that you will know what the proper procedures are as soon as the material is identified.

Another valuable resource is the **Chemical Transportation Emergency Center (CHEMTREC).** CHEMTREC was established by the Chemical Manufacturers Association and is located in Washington, DC. CHEMTREC assists emergency personnel in identifying and handling hazardous materials transport incidents. The center operates 24 hours a day, 7 days a week. Its toll-free number is 1-800-424-9300 from anywhere within the continental United States except the District of Columbia. In the District of Columbia, the number is 483-7616. In Alaska, call that number collect: 0-202-483-7616.

CHEMTREC provides information, warnings, and guidance for proper emergency management and treatment. However, you must provide CHEMTREC with the correct DOT identification number, the chemical name, or the product name of the material. CHEMTREC cannot identify an unknown substance.

If you are interested in learning more about hazardous materials incidents and rescue requirements, you can look to the following:

- National Fire Protection Association (NFPA) standard #479
- OSHA standard #1910.120
- Federal Emergency Management Agency (FEMA) guidelines for coping with hazardous material incidents

## INCIDENT MANAGEMENT SYSTEMS

In recent years, a number of leadership and command systems have been developed to improve the on-scene management of emergency situations. Law enforcement, fire, and EMS have each come up with similar programs, called **incident management systems,** to help control, direct, and coordinate emergency responders and resources. Incident management systems are also called incident command.

### COMPONENTS OF AN INCIDENT MANAGEMENT SYSTEM

On a call with only one patient and no need for fire fighters or any other special rescue units, it may seem that an incident management system is not needed. However, there will be times when your unit becomes part of a larger situation in which personnel from different agencies and political jurisdictions need to work together. In these situations, a pre-established system that identifies who is in charge and who reports to whom is obviously necessary. In major incidents, it is common for this planning to take another step, known as unified command. With unified command, there is a single command post for EMS, police, fire, and political leadership (Figure 28-11). At the command post, data are gathered and decisions are made by the leadership. Agency commanders can then put these decisions into action within their own systems. For example, law enforcement actions are implemented through the police system. Medical actions are implemented through the EMS system.

## FIGURE 28-11

Unified command at work

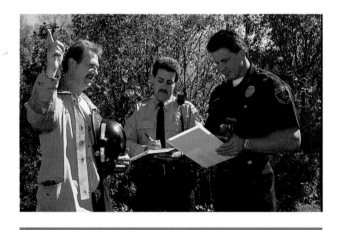

How these systems work and fit together depends on the nature of the event. For example, with a major airplane crash, the leading agency is typically the fire department. In this situation, EMS is usually one aspect of the overall fire incident command system. Within their own system,

EMS personnel establish and carry out their tasks. However, ultimate control of the incident will rest with the fire commander. Another example, such as widespread injuries at a rock concert, is primarily medical. In this situation, the EMS incident management plan would be established. Thus, fire and law enforcement personnel acting as

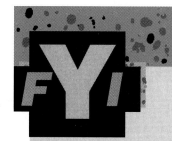

## Decontamination

Many people involved in a hazardous materials incident will need to undergo decontamination. This is the process of removing and properly disposing of hazardous materials from the patient, equipment, and rescue personnel. Failure to decontaminate adequately and promptly will result in prolonged exposure. This may cause even more serious injury to the patient. It may expose other EMT-Bs, rescue, and hospital personnel to the hazardous materials as well.

However, there will be times (such as blunt abdominal trauma or a crushed chest) when the patient's traumatic injuries may be more life threatening than the contamination. You will have to determine whether it is more important to decontaminate the patient or provide prompt transport. Consult medical control in these situations. In some cases, decontamination and emergency care of injuries may go on at the same time. However, if you must make a choice, consider the following: A patient is better blistered and living than decontaminated and dead. In such cases, inform the hospital that you are bringing in a critically injured patient and that the patient is contaminated. The hospital

will need to set up a decontamination zone for this patient.

Decontamination begins as soon as you know you are going to a scene that may involve hazardous materials. Before transporting a contaminated patient in your unit, you should tape the cabinet doors shut, and cover the floor and side walls with plastic sheeting. This will save you time later when you must decontaminate the unit. Leave openings in the plastic for windows, the power vent ceiling fan, and air conditioning unit. This prevents creating a "closed box" in the patient compartment. It also limits your exposure while transporting the patient.

You may be asked to help establish a decontamination zone at the scene. All contaminated personnel, patients, clothing, and equipment should be kept in this zone until it is decontaminated. The Haz-Mat team should lay out the decontamination zone and take charge of it. Help the team as best you can. Remember that your primary mission is to provide emergency care. The decontamination zone should be well marked with plastic, tape, or other warning devices to control traffic. Special containers for contaminated clothing should be available at the scene.

First Responders would follow the EMS commander's decisions.

A good incident management system provides an orderly means of communication. This allows for a good two-way flow of information. Information flows to the commanders so that proper decisions can be made. Then, information flows to personnel who must carry out the decisions. Because a single commander for each agency (fire, law enforcement, EMS) is in place, interactions between all the different agencies at the scene are much smoother.

At one time or another, your unit is likely to be the first to respond to an incident that will involve more than one EMS unit, or one or more non-EMS agencies. In this situation, the senior EMT should establish command and identify himself or herself to the dispatcher. For example this EMT could say, "Dispatch, this is Squad 71, establishing 'Route 43' command." From that point on, all communications from the dispatcher to the scene will be directed to "Route 43 Command." If you arrive after command has been established, advise the dispatcher that you are on scene and "reporting to command." Then, find the command post and report for assignment.

## STRUCTURE OF AN INCIDENT MANAGEMENT SYSTEM

Incident management systems vary from town to town and jurisdiction to jurisdiction. Terms change, and very little is exactly identical from one place to another. You may hear terms such as "sectors," "divisions," "task forces," or "platoons." The possibilities are endless, although the intent and general design are similar. Thus, you must learn your system's plan thoroughly. You must also be familiar with the terms and concepts used by your local law enforcement and fire incident command systems. You will be working closely with them.

As an example of how responsibilities may be assigned at a major EMS incident, consider the following typical assignments:

- *Extrication sector.* This is for disentangling and removing patients from the scene and moving them to the triage area.

- *Triage sector.* This is a sorting point at which patients are prioritized according to the severity of their injuries. They are directed to specific areas of the treatment sector.

- *Treatment sector.* This is where thorough assessments can be made and prioritized on-scene treatment begun until transport can be arranged.

- *Transportation sector.* This is where ambulances and crews are organized to transport patients from the treatment sector to area hospitals.

- *Staging sector.* This is a holding area for arriving ambulances and crews, until they can be assigned a particular task.

- *Supply sector.* This is an area in which to assemble extra equipment and supplies, such as blankets, oxygen bottles, bandages, and backboards, so that they can be dispersed to the other sectors as needed.

- *Mobile command center.* This is typically a vehicle or building at the scene where the EMS commander establishes an "office." This is where the commander oversees the activities of the various sectors and coordinates with the commanders of other involved agencies.

As you respond to an incident, you will be assigned to a sector and sector officer (or

FIGURE 28-12

Mass-casualty incident

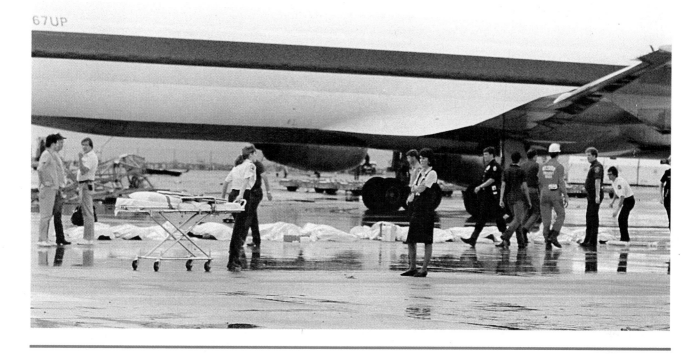

may be assigned *as* the sector officer). Once you are assigned, report to your sector officer for your assignment. When you have finished your assigned task, report back to that same sector officer for another assignment. If your sector's duties are complete, you will be assigned to the staging area for reassignment to another sector.

It is crucial to the success of any incident management system that everyone perform their assigned tasks and work within the system. For example, an EMS team is assigned to extrication, but decides to transport patients from the scene. This team bypasses the triage, treatment, and transport sectors. Thus, all hope for discipline and coordination is lost, and chaos will prevail. The cost of "doing your own thing" is high. Lives may be needlessly lost.

## MULTIPLE-CASUALTY SITUATIONS

A **multiple-casualty situation (MCS)** or mass-casualty incident (MCI) is an event that places such a demand upon available equipment or personnel resources that the system is stretched to its limit (Figure 28-12). Airplane crashes or earthquakes typically come to mind as multiple-casualty situations. The truth is that MCSs and MCIs are far more common and usually much smaller in scope. Ask yourself the following questions:

- How many seriously injured patients can you care for effectively and transport in your ambulance? One? Two?

## DECISIONS, DECISIONS

You and your partner are dispatched to a remote location for a car accident. A tanker truck has driven into the side of a small sports car. The driver of the car is unconscious and unresponsive to any stimuli. He has obvious head trauma and extensive injuries to the left side of the chest, pelvis, and the lower extremities. The driver is trapped. Rescue will require extensive extrication. You report your findings to your partner. He says the driver of the tanker is also trapped—one foot is jammed under the pedals. The tanker driver appears to have a broken ankle and a broken left arm. He is alert and oriented, but in a lot of pain.

### For Discussion

1. Describe the general procedure for responding to a potentially hazardous scene in your area.

2. How does the availability of people or equipment affect the classification of patients during triage?

---

- What happens when you have three patients to deal with?
- What do you do when two cars each carrying four people crash head-on at high speed?

Obviously, you and your team cannot treat and transport all of them at the same time. Within the confines of your team and unit, you have just encountered a multiple-casualty situation. It may not be an earthquake, but you will remember and talk about it for months.

### TRIAGE

To manage such calls and to ensure that as many patients as possible survive, you need to think and act somewhat differently than if you had only one patient. An essential feature of such calls is triage, a French word that means sorting. Triage is a technique of establishing treatment and transport priorities in situations with more than one patient. With triage, you quickly assess and sort patients into categories. The category you assign depends on the severity and survivability of their injuries. It is important to note that triage is a continuing process.

Usually, the most highly trained medical person at the scene directs triage. If you are the first EMT at the scene, you should begin triage after you contact dispatch for additional resources. *If you assume the initial duties of triage officer, you should not be-*

*come involved in patient care.* You are responsible for assigning patient care to other EMS personnel.

Precisely how and where triage will be carried out varies, depending on the event and your local protocol. Although it was taught for many years, it is difficult for one or two EMTs to wade through a field of victims. Whenever possible, it is better to establish one central triage clearinghouse. All patients are then brought to this clearinghouse on their way to the treatment areas. In major incidents, separate triage areas may have to be established to accommodate the size and geography of the area.

### Triage Priorities

Patients are sorted into four triage levels or groups. Each level may be identified by a certain color or number (Table 28-3). Treatment areas are usually identified by colored flags or markers (Figure 28-13). The highest priority for treatment is given to patients whose injuries are critical, but probably survivable with prompt resuscitation. The lowest priority is given to patients with very minor injuries or those who are not injured. Individuals who are obviously dead or whose injuries are so catastrophic that certain death is very near are also low priority.

It may seem cruel to assign the lowest priority to those who are obviously dead or unlikely to survive devastating injuries. Although it seems uncaring, you must focus on patients who can benefit from your care. This is especially true if you have limited resources. *The cardinal rule of triage is to do the greatest good for the greatest number.* Patients whose injuries are not an immediate threat to their airway, breathing, or circulation should also be placed in lower priority categories.

### Triage Procedures

Triage is a dynamic, on-going process. The triage officer assigns a triage priority and then the patient is taken to the appropriate treatment area. Once there, other EMS personnel will begin treatment and conduct a more thorough assessment. The patient's condition then is re-evaluated routinely. EMS personnel at the treatment area consider the following:

- Is the patient improving? Can he or she be moved to a lower level of care?

- Is the patient becoming worse? Does he or she need more immediate transport?

A patient may be assigned a high priority (Red) due to severe bleeding. However, once the bleeding is controlled, the triage priority may change. Changing the patient's assigned category is the responsibility of the treatment sector officer. This officer is also responsible for communicating with the transportation sector officer to arrange transport for patients to the hospital.

Treatment and triage continue until all patients have been treated and transported. The transport officer should try to allocate patients, based on number and severity, among local medical facilities. This should minimize overload on any one facility. These record keeping and allocation duties may be delegated, but the ultimate responsibility belongs to the transport officer. If the incident is large scale, this officer may designate a communications operator. A communications operator controls and directs radio traffic between the hospitals and the transport point.

### Special Triage Situations

There is a separate category of triage for patients who have been contaminated by radiation and are carrying radiation particles. This category is higher than all others. Contaminated patients must be moved away from all other patients. They must not be allowed to contaminate other patients, EMS personnel, ambulances, or hospitals.

**TABLE 28-3**     **TRIAGE PRIORITIES**

| Triage Category | Typical Injuries |
|---|---|
| Highest priority (Red)<br>Patients who need immediate care and transport. Treat these patients first and transport as soon as possible. | Airway and breathing difficulties<br>Uncontrolled or severe bleeding<br>Decreased level of consciousness<br>Severe medical problems<br>Shock (hypoperfusion)<br>Severe burns |
| Second priority (Yellow)<br>Patients whose treatment and transportation can be delayed temporarily. | Burns without airway problems<br>Major or multiple bone or joint injuries<br>Back injuries with or without spinal cord damage |
| Lowest priority (Green)<br>Patients whose treatment and transportation can be delayed until last. | Minor fractures<br>Minor soft tissue injuries |
| Lowest priority (Black)<br>These patients are already dead or have little chance for survival. If resources are limited, treat "salvageable" patients before these patients. | Obvious death<br>Obviously mortal wounds, such as major open brain trauma, full cardiac arrest |

**FIGURE 28-13**

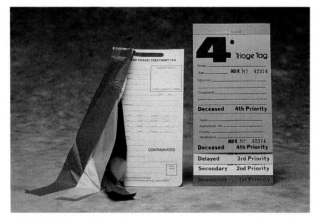

**A**  Triage tags

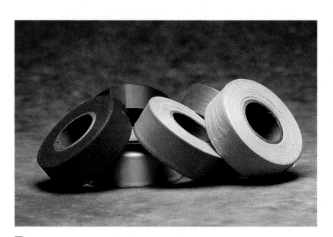

**B**  Triage tape

In certain large urban areas where regionalized care is provided, another concept of triage is used. Single patients with specific medical problems, such as burns, trauma, cardiac, or neonatal, are "triaged" to specialized regional centers for treatment. Making the decision to transport a patient to a special treatment center is difficult. This decision depends on many factors including, but not limited to, the following:

- the specific illness or injury
- the severity of the illness or injury
- the availability of local resources at the time of the event
- local rules and protocols

If there are special treatment centers in your area, you must know the specific triage protocols that apply. These decisions are often made only after on-line communication with medical control. Also note that in the event of a multiple-casualty incident, the usual specialized center triage plan is often not used. The center can easily be overloaded. A school bus accident in which all 30 or 40 patients are children can overwhelm a pediatric hospital. Similarly, 10 burn patients from a petroleum plant fire could immobilize a burn center. Good triage and communication with medical control are essential to providing each patient with the best available treatment.

Most urban areas have regional trauma care centers. The American College of Surgeons has developed specific guidelines that define the resources needed by a hospital to qualify as a certain type of trauma center. Severe, life-threatening injuries should be treated in facilities prepared to deal immediately and completely with the problem. Ideally, severely injured patients should be identified in the field and sent to a designated Level One Trauma Center.

You should learn about all triage methods used by your EMS system to identify patients who should be transported to specialized treatment facilities. As with the other skills you are learning, you must practice triage techniques as well. Your EMS system should conduct disaster drills yearly, preferably with the participation of local hospitals and other public safety and rescue units. Disaster plans must be developed and practiced in advance of need. The mass confusion of a disaster site is no time to experiment with organization.

# SECTION 8

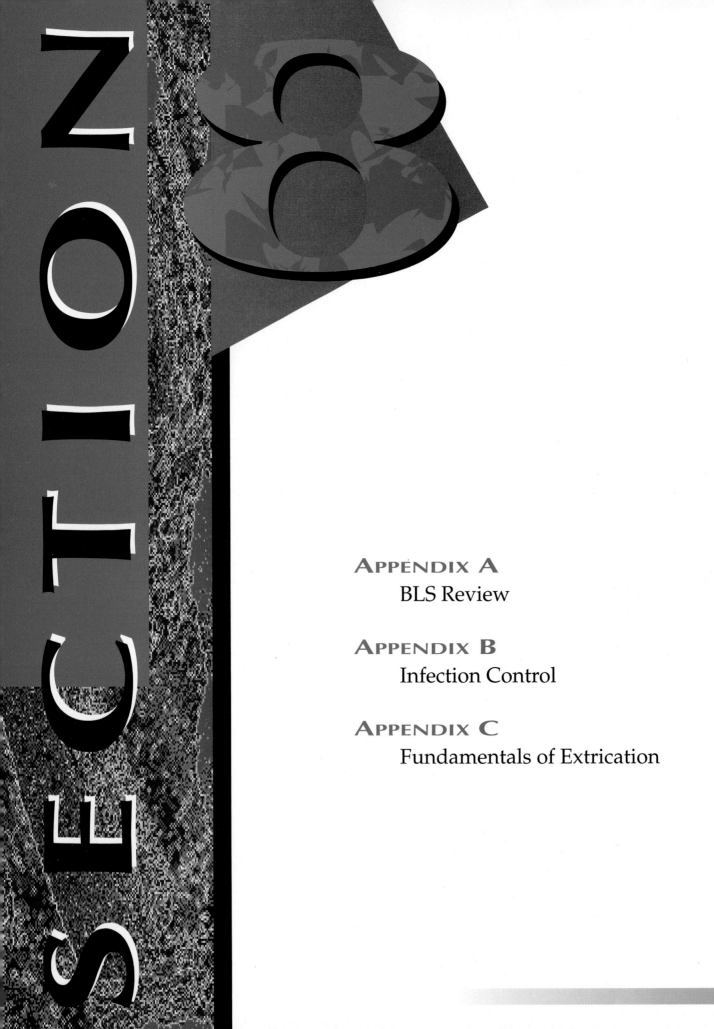

# Appendices

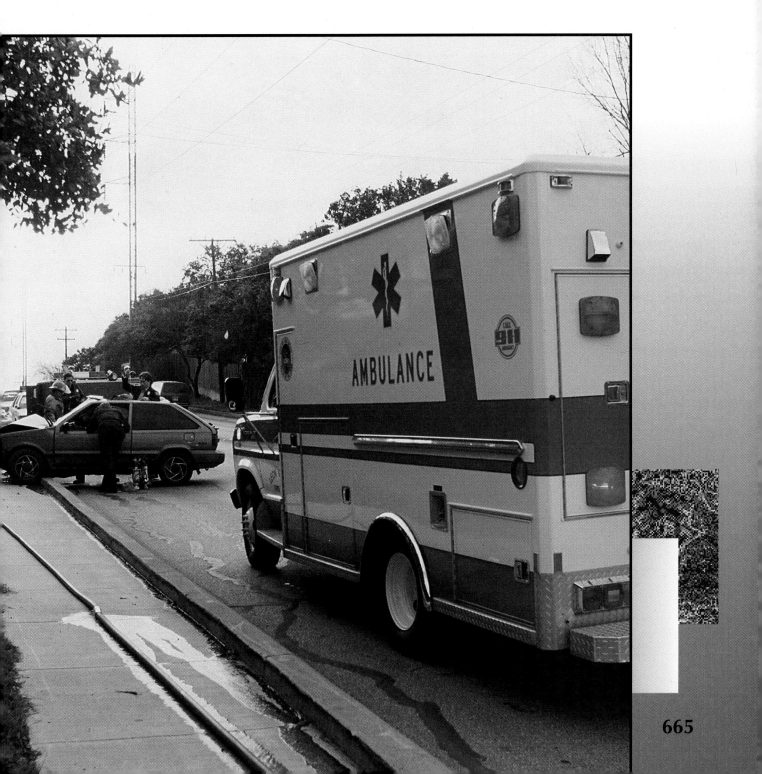

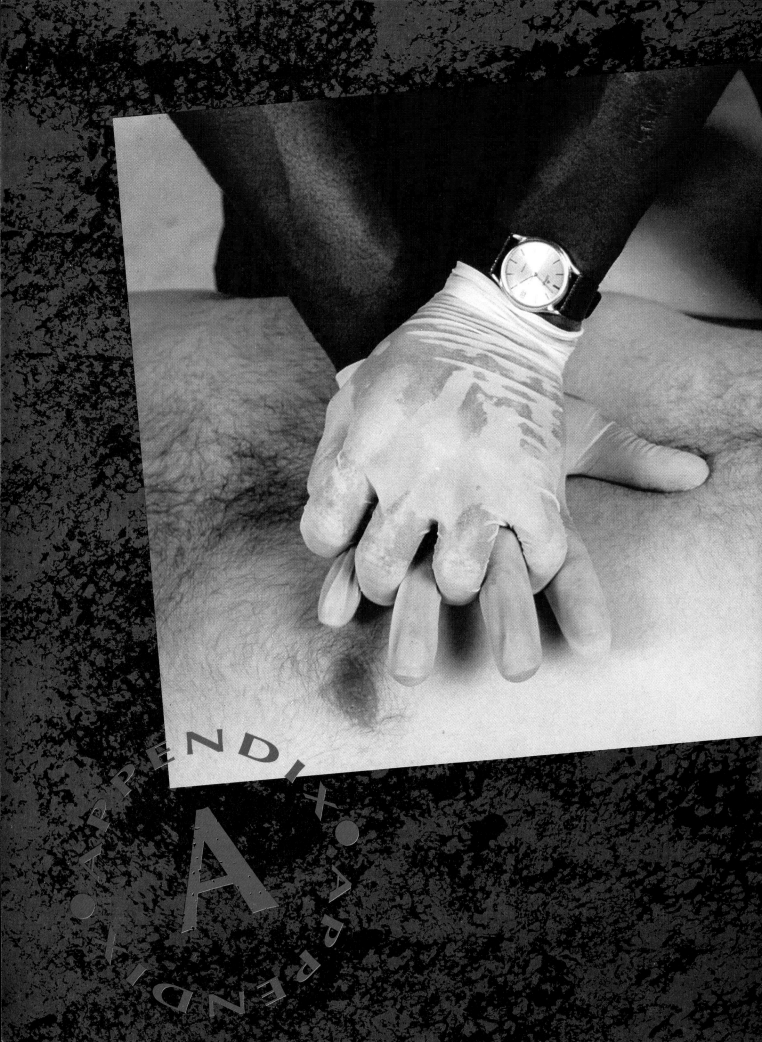

APPENDIX · APPENDIX · APPENDIX

A

# Appendix A
# BLS Review

## Objectives

After you have read this chapter, you should be able to:

- Explain the urgency for basic life support measures.
- Describe the EMT-B's responsibilities in starting and stopping CPR.
- Identify the proper way to position a patient to receive basic life support.
- Identify the four techniques for opening the airway in adults.
- Describe how to perform mouth-to-mask ventilation in adults and how to relieve gastric distention.
- Distinguish foreign body obstructions from other conditions that cause respiratory failure.
- Describe the techniques for dislodging foreign objects that are obstructing the airway.
- Explain how to adapt artificial ventilation procedures to infants and children.
- Describe techniques for providing artificial circulation to adults.
- Describe techniques for providing artificial circulation to children or infants.

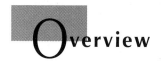

# Overview

While the principles of basic life support were first introduced in 1960, the specific techniques are reviewed and revised every 5 to 6 years. The revised guidelines are then published in the *Journal of the American Medical Association*. The most recent revision occurred as a result of the 1992 National Conference on Standards and Guidelines for Cardiopulmonary Resuscitation and Emergency Cardiac Care. The guidelines in this appendix follow those proposed at the 1992 conference and later adopted by the American Heart Association.

This appendix begins with a definition and general discussion of basic life support—why it is lifesaving and your responsibilities in providing it. The next section describes methods of opening the airway in adults, followed by steps for providing artificial ventilation and circulation. The third section focuses on BLS care for infants and children. The appendix concludes with a step-by-step description of how to relieve foreign body obstruction.

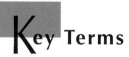

# Key Terms

**Abdominal-thrust maneuver**
A method of dislodging food or other material from the throat of a choking victim. Also known as the "Heimlich" maneuver.

**Advanced life support (ALS)**
Advanced lifesaving procedures, such as cardiac monitoring, starting IV fluids, giving medications, manual defibrillation, and using advanced airway adjuncts.

**Artificial circulation**   Provides blood circulation to the body by external chest compressions.

**Artificial ventilation**   Opening the airway and restoring breathing by mouth-to-mask ventilation and by the use of mechanical devices.

**Basic life support (BLS)**
Essential noninvasive emergency lifesaving care used for patients in respiratory or cardiac arrest.

**Cardiopulmonary resuscitation (CPR)**   Establishes artificial ventilation and circulation in a patient who is not breathing and has no pulse.

**Ischemia**   Lacking oxygen.

**Recovery position**   Position used to help maintain a clear airway in a patient with a decreased level of consciousness who has not had traumatic injuries and is breathing on his or her own.

# GENERAL CONSIDERATIONS

**Basic life support (BLS)** is noninvasive emergency lifesaving care used to treat respiratory or cardiac arrest. **Cardiopulmonary resuscitation (CPR)** is a series of steps used to establish artificial ventilation and circulation in a patient who is not breathing and has no pulse. **Artificial ventilation** is opening the airway and restoring breathing by mouth-to-mouth or mouth-to-nose ventilation and by the use of mechanical devices. **Artificial circulation** provides blood circulation to the body by external chest compressions. Identifying a patient in respiratory and/or cardiac arrest, followed by immediate treatment, is critical for CPR to be effective. You are expected to be able to recognize cardiac or respiratory arrest without difficulty and to quickly institute proper basic life support measures.

BLS care focuses on the following:

- A   Airway (obstruction)

- B   Breathing (respiratory arrest)

- C   Circulation (cardiac arrest or severe bleeding)

Thus, BLS must be started as soon as possible after respiratory or cardiac arrest has occurred. You do not need special equipment to perform BLS. BLS can be given by one or two EMT-Bs. It can also be provided by First Responders and alert and well-trained bystanders.

Even though you do not need equipment to perform BLS, you should use a barrier device to perform rescue breathing. Rescue breathing will deliver exhaled gas from you to the patient. This gas contains 16% oxygen, which is more than enough to maintain the patient's life. Once you identify that the patient needs BLS care, you should begin rescue breathing immediately and begin efforts to support the circulation and correct cardiac problems.

BLS is not the same as advanced life support. **Advanced life support (ALS)** involves advanced lifesaving procedures, such as cardiac monitoring, starting IV fluids, giving medications, manual defibrillation, and using advanced airway adjuncts. However, when done correctly, BLS can maintain life until ALS measures can be given. In some instances, such as choking, drowning, or lightning injuries, early BLS may be all that a patient needs to be resuscitated. Of course, these patients must also be transported to the hospital for evaluation.

BLS measures are only as effective as the person giving them. Competence in giving BLS is high immediately after training. However, it declines rapidly unless you are retrained periodically or you use the skills often. If you do not perform a certain technique very often, you do not tend to do it well. If you do not use these basic skills regularly, you must practice them under close supervision every 90 days. BLS measures must be started immediately and properly. Therefore, maintaining your skills is absolutely necessary.

# THE URGENT NEED FOR BLS CARE

Ideally, only seconds should pass between the time you recognize that a patient needs BLS care and the start of treatment. Time is critical, for every second that oxygen does not reach the brain, brain cells die. Thus, you must quickly assess the patient's airway, breathing, and circulation so that you can begin BLS measures, if they are needed. BLS permits the earliest possible treatment of airway obstruction, respiratory arrest, or cardiac arrest without the initial need for special equipment or material.

If a patient is not breathing well or at all, you may simply need to open the airway to get the patient breathing again. Very often, simply clearing the airway will help the patient to breathe normally again. However, if the patient has no pulse, you must combine rescue breathing with artificial circulation. If a patient stops breathing before the heart stops, he or she will have enough oxygen in the lungs to stay alive for several minutes. But, when a patient first goes into cardiac arrest, the heart and brain stop receiving oxygen right away. Permanent brain damage may occur if the brain is without oxygen for 4 to 6 minutes. After 6 minutes without oxygen, some brain damage is almost certain. Therefore, you must recognize the need for BLS measures as soon as possible.

## INITIAL ASSESSMENT

Because of the urgent need to start BLS, you must complete an initial assessment, as described in chapter 11, Scene Size-up and Initial Assessment, as quickly as possible. During the initial assessment, you quickly evaluate the patient's airway, breathing, circulation, and level of consciousness, or ABCD. Level of consciousness is a good guide to the extent of BLS the patient needs. A patient who is alert and oriented does not need BLS. However, patients who are not fully conscious often need some degree of BLS. Not all unconscious patients need all elements of BLS. Some unconscious patients may be breathing well on their own. However, all patients who need full BLS are unconscious.

If you must begin CPR on an unconscious patient, it is important that you learn if the patient has had a head or cervical spine injury. If a patient has had such an injury, you must protect the spinal cord from further injury as you perform CPR. The fact that a patient has had a head or spinal injury should not keep you from starting BLS. It simply means that you need to take special care with the spine as you perform BLS measures. If there is even a remote possibility of this type of injury, you should begin appropriate precautions during the initial assessment.

If you are alone with an adult patient in need of BLS, you should activate the EMS system first. This means calling for additional help and for ALS, if it is available. For the general public and when you are off duty, activating the EMS system is the highest priority after establishing unresponsiveness or the need for adult CPR. EMS should be activated before beginning CPR. If you are on duty, you should contact dispatch for more help while your partner begins one-rescuer CPR.

## WHEN TO START AND STOP BLS CARE

As an EMT-B, it is your responsibility to start CPR in virtually all patients who are in cardiac arrest. There are only two general exceptions to the rule, as follows:

1. You should not start CPR if the patient has obvious signs of irreversible death. Obvious signs of biological death are called dead on arrival (DOA) criteria. Two signs of "clinical" (or reversible) death are absence of the pulse and absence of breathing. Along with these two signs, one of the following signs of "biological" (or irreversible) death must also be present:

   • Rigor mortis—stiffening of the body after death

   • Dependent lividity (livor mortis)—a discoloration of the skin due to pooling of blood (Figure A-1)

   • Putrefaction or decomposition of the body

   • Separation or obvious destruction of major body organs, such as the brain or heart

## FIGURE A-1

Dependent lividity

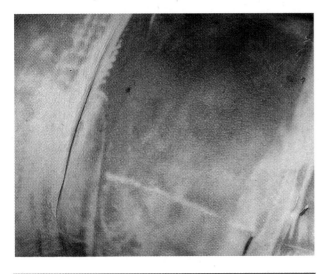

Rigor mortis and dependent lividity develop after a patient has been dead for a long period of time. Severe injuries, decapitation, incineration, and other conditions obviously incompatible with life are also reasons not to begin CPR.

2. You should not start CPR if the patient and his or her physician have previously agreed upon do-not-resuscitate or no-CPR orders. This may only apply to situations in which the patient is known to be in the terminal stage of an incurable disease. In this situation, CPR serves only to prolong the death of the patient. However, this can be a complicated issue. Advance directives, such as living wills, may express the patient's wishes. These documents are not usually binding for health care providers, especially outside of a hospital or nursing home. Learn your local protocols and the standards in your system before being called to treat terminally ill patients. Some EMS systems have computer notes of patients preregistered with the system. These notes usually specify the amount and extent of treatment desired at the time of the incident.

In all other instances, you should begin CPR on anyone in cardiac arrest. Because every situation has so many variables, it is impossible to know how long the patient has been without oxygen to the brain and vital organs. Factors such as ambient temperature or the hardiness of the patient's tissues and organs can affect the patient's ability to survive. Thus, most legal advisers recommend that when in doubt, you should always give "too much" care rather than too little. Therefore, you should always start CPR if any doubt exists.

If you begin CPR in the field, you must continue until one of the following events occurs:

- S  The patient **starts** breathing and has a pulse.

- T  The patient is **transferred** to a higher medical authority in accordance with accepted practice.

- O  You are **out** of strength or too fatigued to continue.

- P  A **physician** present assumes responsibility for the patient.

Do not stop CPR unless you can no longer physically perform it. You are not responsible for making the decision to stop CPR. CPR should always be continued until the patient's care is transferred to a physician at the hospital or higher medical authority in the field. In some cases, your medical director or a designated medical control physician may order you to stop CPR based on the patient's condition.

Every EMS system should have clear standing orders or protocols that provide guidelines for starting and stopping CPR. Your medical director and your system's legal adviser should be in general agreement with these protocols. These protocols should be closely administered and reviewed by your medical director.

# POSITIONING THE PATIENT

For CPR to be effective, the patient must be lying supine on a firm surface. There must be enough clear space around the patient to allow two EMT-Bs to perform CPR. If the patient is crumpled up or lying facedown, you will need to reposition the patient. The few seconds you spend to properly position the patient will greatly improve the delivery and effectiveness of CPR.

For a patient who is not a trauma victim, you can use the recovery position to facilitate airway management. The **recovery position** is used to help maintain a clear airway in a patient with a decreased level of consciousness who has not had traumatic injuries and is breathing on his or her own (Figure A-2). It also allows vomitus to drain from the mouth. Roll the patient onto his or her right or left side so that the head, shoulders, and torso move as a unit without twisting. You should then place the patient's hands under the cheek. The recovery position is also used once a patient begins breathing on his or her own after rescue breathing.

## FIGURE A-2

Recovery position

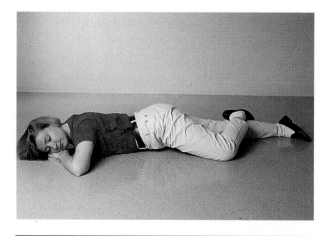

If you suspect that a patient has had a traumatic spinal or head injury, you and your partner must use considerable caution when repositioning. The patient's head, neck, and back must be log rolled as a single unit.

You should reposition an unconscious adult patient for airway management in the following way: *(Again, always be aware of the possibility of a cervical spine injury!)*

1. Kneel beside the patient. You and your partner must be far enough away so that when rolled toward you, the patient does not come to rest in your lap (Figure A-3a). For patients with no spinal injury, use of the recovery position is very important to prevent aspiration of vomitus.

2. Rapidly straighten the patient's legs and move the nearer arm above the head (Figure A-3b).

3. Place your hands behind the back of the head and neck of the patient to maintain the cervical spine. Your partner should place his or her hands on the distant shoulder and the hip (Figure A-3c).

4. Turn the patient toward you by pulling on the distant shoulder and the hip. The head and neck should be controlled so that they move as a unit with the rest of the torso. In this way, the head and neck stay in the same vertical plane as the back. This single motion will minimize aggravation of any spinal injury. At this point, apply a cervical collar.

5. Replace the patient's farther arm back at the side once the patient is supine.

The patient should be log rolled onto a long spine board, when possible (Figure A-3d). This device will provide support during transport and emergency department care. Once the patient is properly positioned, you can easily assess the patient's airway, breathing, and circulation, and BLS can be started if necessary.

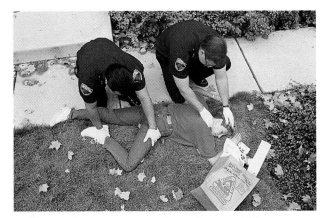

**A** Place the patient in the recovery position

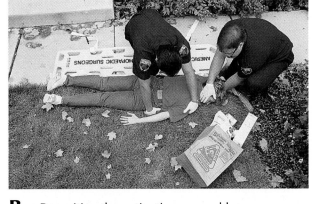

**B** Reposition the patient's arms and legs

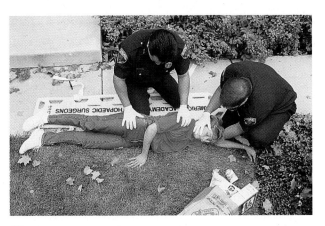

**C** Protect the head and neck as you log roll the patient onto the backboard

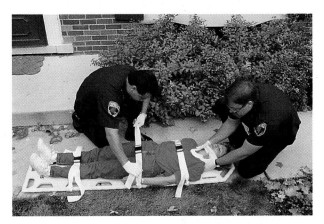

**D** Secure the patient to the backboard

## OPENING THE AIRWAY IN ADULTS

The most important element for successful CPR is immediate opening of the airway. An open airway is needed for artificial ventilation to be effective. Airway obstruction in an unconscious patient is most commonly due to relaxation of the muscles of the throat and tongue. The airway becomes blocked by its own tissues, as the tongue tends to fall back into the throat (Figure A-4). Four techniques for opening the airway are presented below.

Also note that dentures, blood clots, vomitus, mucus, food, or other foreign bodies may cause an obstruction. Airway obstruction due to an aspirated foreign body is discussed later in this appendix.

### HEAD-TILT/CHIN-LIFT MANEUVER

Opening the airway can often be done quickly and easily by simply tilting the patient's head backward. This procedure is known as the **head-tilt maneuver**. Sometimes this simple maneuver is all that is

The tongue obstructing the airway

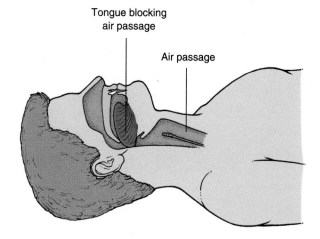

Tongue blocking
air passage

Air passage

The head-tilt maneuver

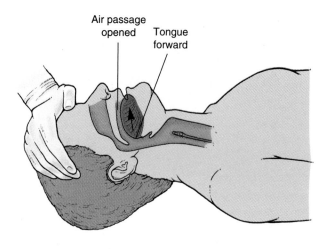

Air passage
opened    Tongue
forward

needed for the patient to begin breathing on his or her own. The head tilt is the first and most important general step in opening the airway.

You should perform the head-tilt maneuver in an adult in the following way:

1. Make sure the patient is supine. Kneel close beside the patient.

2. Place one hand on the patient's forehead, and apply firm backward pressure with your palm. Move the patient's head as far back as possible (Figure A-5).

This extension of the neck will move the tongue forward, away from the back of the throat. This movement will clear the airway, if the tongue is blocking it. However, you may have difficulty achieving an effective head tilt with only one hand on the forehead. You may need to perform a chin lift as well. The head-tilt/chin-lift maneuver combines two movements to open the airway. *Remember that neither the head-tilt maneuver nor the head-tilt/chin-lift maneuver should be used in cases of possible spinal injury.*

You should perform the head-tilt/chin-lift maneuver in an adult in the following way:

1. Perform the head-tilt maneuver, as described above, with one hand.

2. Place the tips of the fingers of your other hand under the bony part of the chin.

3. Lift the chin forward, bringing the entire lower jaw with it, helping to tilt the head back (Figure A-6).

You must be sure that your fingers do not compress the soft tissue under the chin. This would block the airway. Continue to hold the forehead to maintain the backward tilt of the head. You should lift the chin so that the teeth are nearly brought together. However, you should avoid closing the mouth completely.

Loose dentures can be held in place with the chin lift, making obstruction by the lips less likely. Performing mouth-to-mouth ventilation is much easier when dentures are in place. However, dentures that do not stay in place should be removed. Partial dentures (plates) may come loose following an accident or as you are providing care. Check patients with partial dentures periodically to make sure their plates are firmly in place. Performing mouth-to-mask ventilation is much easier if loose dentures are removed.

## FIGURE A-6

The head-tilt/chin-lift maneuver

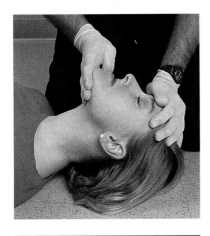

## FIGURE A-7

The jaw-thrust maneuver

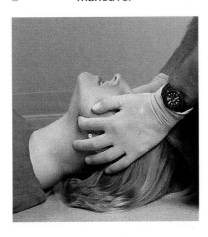

## FIGURE A-8

The modified jaw-thrust maneuver

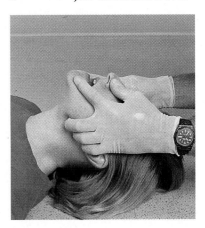

## JAW-THRUST MANEUVER

The two methods described above are effective for opening the airway of most patients. In some cases, forward movement of the lower jaw, the jaw-thrust maneuver, may be needed. The jaw-thrust maneuver is a technique to open the airway by placing the fingers behind the angle of the jaw and bringing the head forward.

You should perform the jaw-thrust maneuver in an adult in the following way:

1. Kneel above the patient's head. Place your index or middle fingers behind the angles of the patient's lower jaw and forcefully move the jaw forward.

2. Tilt the head backward without significantly extending the cervical spine.

3. Use your thumbs to pull the patient's lower jaw down, to allow breathing through the mouth as well as the nose (Figure A-7).

If you suspect a cervical spine injury, you can modify this maneuver to keep the head in a neutral position as you move the jaw forward and open the mouth. However, only an unconscious patient will tolerate the maneuver. A mask can be used easily with both hands doing the jaw thrust while at the same time you seal the mask around the mouth. The nose may also be sealed with your thumbs using the modified jaw-thrust maneuver. Use your index and long fingers to thrust the jaw anteriorly while the thumbs compress the nose (Figure A-8).

## ARTIFICIAL VENTILATION IN ADULTS

Once you open the airway, the patient may start to breathe on his or her own. To assess whether the patient is now breathing, place your ear about 1" above the patient's nose and mouth. Listen carefully for sounds of breathing (Figure A-9). Turn your head so that you can watch for movement of the patient's chest and abdomen. If you can feel and hear movement of air and can see the patient's chest and abdomen move with each breath, breathing has returned. Feeling and hearing the movement of air are far

## FIGURE A-9

Look, listen, and feel for respirations

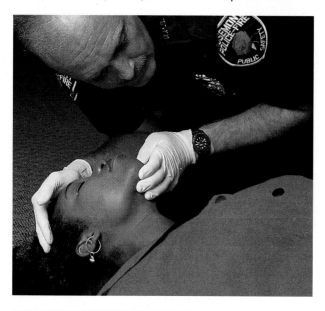

more important than seeing the chest and abdomen move.

With airway obstruction, there may be no movement of air, even though the chest and abdomen rise and fall as the patient tries to breathe. You may also have difficulty watching for movement of the chest and abdomen if the patient is fully clothed. Finally, in some patients, you may see very little or no chest movement at all. This is particularly true in patients with chronic lung disease. Thus, if you do not feel any air movement as you look, listen, and feel, you must begin artificial ventilation.

A patient will die from a lack of oxygen, along with too much carbon dioxide, in the blood. Without artificial ventilation, these changes cannot be corrected. Adequate artificial ventilation requires slow, deliberate inhalations that last 1½ to 2 seconds. This gentle, slow method of ventilating the patient prevents air being forced into the stomach.

## MOUTH-TO-MOUTH VENTILATION

Mouth-to-mouth ventilations are now done routinely with a barrier device, such as a mask. Barrier devices feature a plastic barrier placed on the patient's face and a one-way valve to prevent backflow of secretions and gases (Figure A-10). These devices provide good infection control. Providing mouth-to-mouth ventilations without such a device is appropriate only in extreme conditions. Mouth-to mouth ventilations are best done with a one-way valve mask to prevent possible disease transmission.

You should perform mouth-to-mouth ventilation with a simple barrier device in an adult in the following way:

1. Open the airway with the head-tilt/ chin-lift maneuver, as described earlier.

2. Press on the forehead to maintain the backward tilt of the head. Pinch the patient's nostrils together with your thumb and index finger.

3. Depress the lower lip with the thumb of the hand lifting the chin. This will help keep the mouth open during mouth-to-mouth ventilation.

## FIGURE A-10

A barrier device

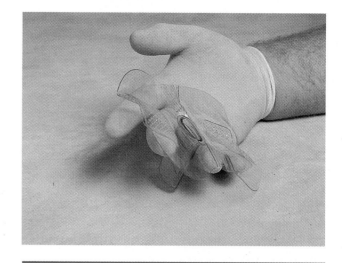

## FIGURE A-11

Slow, gentle method of ventilating

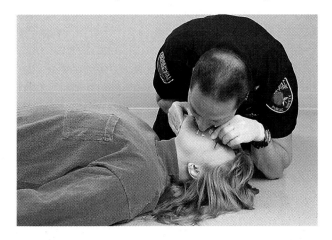

4. Open the patient's mouth widely and place the barrier device over the patient's mouth.

5. Take a deep breath, then make a tight seal with your mouth around the patient's mouth. Breathe slowly into the patient's mouth for 1½ to 2 seconds. This slow, gentle method of ventilating keeps from forcing air into the stomach (Figure A-11).

6. Remove your mouth and allow the patient to exhale passively. Turn your head slightly to watch for movement of the patient's chest.

If you use the jaw-thrust maneuver to open the airway, you must move to the patient's side. Keep the patient's mouth open with both thumbs, and seal the nose by placing your cheek against the patient's nostrils (Figure A-12).

## MOUTH-TO-NOSE VENTILATION

In some cases, mouth-to-nose ventilation is more effective than mouth-to-mouth ventilation. It is a good alternative to mouth-to-mouth ventilation. Mouth-to-nose ventilation is recommended in the following four situations:

1. It is impossible to open the patient's mouth.

2. It is impossible to ventilate a patient through the mouth because of severe facial injuries.

3. It is difficult to achieve a tight seal

## FIGURE A-12

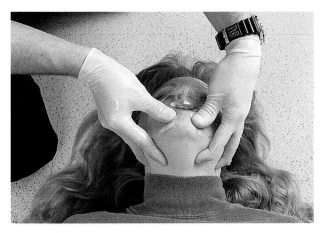

**A**   Keep patient's mouth open with both thumbs

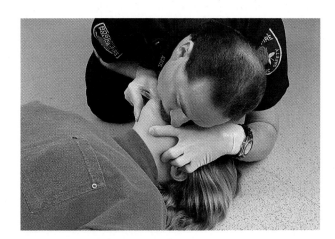

**B**   Seal nose by placing cheek against the patient's nostrils

around the mouth because the patient has no teeth.

4. You prefer the nasal route for some other reason.

## FIGURE A-13

Mouth-to-nose ventilation using the chin-lift maneuver

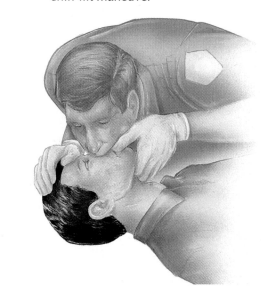

To perform mouth-to-nose ventilation, tilt the patient's head back with one of your hands on the forehead as you lift the patient's jaw with your other hand (Figure A-13). This will seal the lips. Then take a deep breath, seal your lips around the patient's nose, and blow in slowly until you feel the lungs expand. Remove your mouth and allow the patient to exhale on his or her own. You can see the chest fall when the patient exhales. You may need to open the patient's mouth or separate the lips to allow air to escape during exhalation. When you use the jaw-thrust maneuver to maintain the airway, use your cheek to seal the patient's mouth. Do not use your thumbs to pull back the lower lip when you give mouth-to-nose ventilation.

## MOUTH-TO-STOMA VENTILATION

Patients who have undergone surgical removal of the larynx often have a permanent tracheal stoma. A stoma is an opening in the neck that connects the trachea directly to the skin. The stoma may be an opening at the midline at the front base of the neck. Many patients will have other openings in the neck, depending on the type of operation done. Any opening other than a stoma should be ignored. Because the stoma is at the midline, it is the only opening that will move air into the patient's lungs (Figure A-14).

## FIGURE A-14

A tracheal stoma

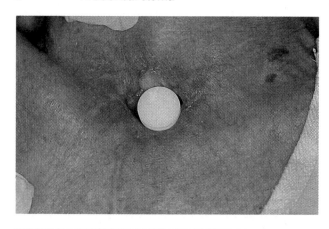

To perform direct mouth-to-stoma ventilation, you do not need to position the patient's head with the head-tilt/chin-lift or the jaw-thrust maneuvers. If the patient has a tube in the stoma, you should ventilate through the tube. Seal the patient's mouth and nose with one hand. This will prevent air from leaking up the trachea as you ventilate. Release the patient's nose and mouth for exhalation. This allows the air to exhale through the upper airway as well as the stoma.

## GASTRIC DISTENTION

Artificial ventilation often results in the stomach becoming filled with air. This condition is called gastric distention. While it most commonly happens in children, it also occurs in adults. Gastric distention is most likely to occur if you blow too hard as you ventilate, if you give several rapid breaths in a row, or if the patient's airway is obstructed. Thus, it is important for you to give slow, gentle breaths. Slow, gentle breaths are also more effective in ventilating the lungs. Serious inflation of the stomach is dangerous, as it causes the patient to vomit during CPR. It can also reduce lung volume by elevating the diaphragm.

Acute, massive gastric distention that interferes with adequate ventilation must be relieved promptly. You can often relieve this distention by applying moderate pressure on the patient's abdomen. First, turn the patient onto his or her side. Next, place the palm of your hand between the umbilicus and the rib cage and press. The patient is likely to vomit as you apply pressure. You must be careful to prevent aspiration of vomitus into the lungs as you relieve the distention. Therefore, you should turn the patient's entire body to the side before you apply pressure. Make sure a suctioning unit is available if you need to remove any vomitus or other material from the patient's mouth.

## ARTIFICIAL CIRCULATION IN ADULTS

Once you arrive at a scene in which a patient is unconscious, you must do the following:

- assess the patient's ABCD to determine responsiveness
- activate the EMS system
- position the patient

- open the airway
- assess the circulation
- start artificial ventilation
- start artificial circulation, if needed

An immediate initial assessment is needed to determine if the patient is breathing and has a pulse. A patient who has been in cardiac arrest for more that 10 seconds will be unconscious because the brain is not receiving enough oxygen. As described above, a patient who is not breathing, but has a pulse, should be positioned for artificial ventilations. Use one hand to tilt the head back to maintain the airway. Use your other hand to locate the carotid pulse. If the patient has a pulse, but is not breathing, give artificial ventilations as described earlier until the patient begins breathing again. If the pulse is absent, begin external chest compressions. This adds artificial circulation to artificial ventilation.

A patient in cardiac arrest will not have a palpable pulse in the large arteries. You can palpate the carotid artery in the neck. To find the carotid artery, lightly place two fingers on the larynx (Adam's apple) at the front of the neck. Then slide these fingers to one side. You can feel the pulse in the groove between the larynx and the sternocleidomastoid muscle. Make sure to hold the tips of your index and long fingers side by side (Figure A-15).

## FIGURE A-15

Location of the carotid pulse

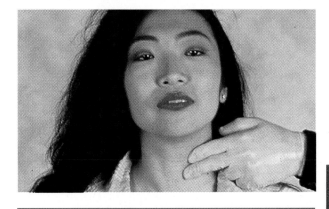

Do not apply excessive pressure on this artery, as it could obstruct the carotid circulation, dislodge blood clots, or produce marked slowing of heart activity.

## EXTERNAL CHEST COMPRESSIONS

The heart is located slightly to the left of the middle of the chest between the sternum and the spine (Figure A-16). You can provide artificial circulation by applying rhythmic pressure and relaxation to the lower half of the sternum.

### FIGURE A-16

Location of the heart and other structures

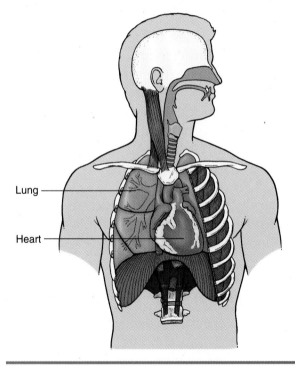

Lung

Heart

External chest compressions, even done without any mistakes, provide only 25% to 33% of the blood normally pumped by the heart. For this flow rate to be achieved, you must place the patient on a firm, flat surface. This surface may be the ground, the floor, or a spine board on a stretcher. A patient who is in bed must be placed on the

floor. Moving the patient to the floor is quicker than looking for some type of firm support. This also minimizes the delay in starting chest compressions. External chest compressions must always be accompanied by artificial ventilation.

## ONE-RESCUER ADULT CPR

If you are working alone, call dispatch for help, and then position the patient properly. Kneel close to the patient's side, with one knee at the level of the head and the other at the level of the upper chest. Place the heel of one hand on the lower half of the body of the sternum. Take great care not to place the hand on either the xiphoid process, or beside the sternum onto the ribs or costal cartilages (Figure A-17). The former could result in lacerated abdominal organs, and the latter results in fractured and dislocated ribs.

Slide the index and long fingers of the hand nearer the patient's feet along the costal margin (edge of the rib cage) until they reach the xiphoid notch in the center of the chest (Figure A-18a). Push the long finger as high as possible into the notch. Then place the

### FIGURE A-17

Location of the xiphoid process

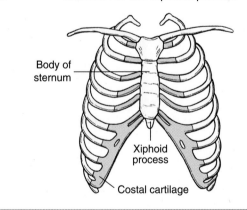

Body of sternum

Xiphoid process

Costal cartilage

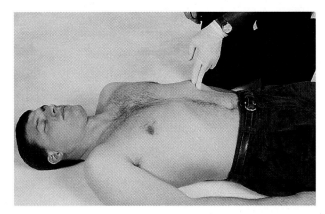

**A**  Locate the notch at the center of the chest

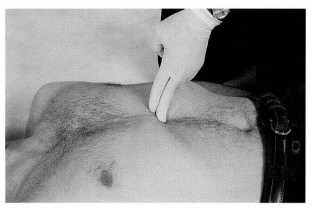

**B**  Place your long finger on the notch and your index finger on the lower part of the sternum

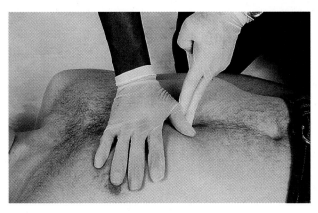

**C**  Place the heel of your hand on the lower part of the sternum

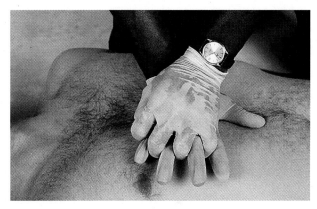

**D**  Place the other hand on top of the first and prepare to compress the chest

index finger on the lower part of the sternum with the two fingers touching (Figure A-18b). Next, place heel of the other hand on the lower half of the sternum (Figure A-18c) so that it touches the index finger of the first hand. Remove the first hand from the notch in the center of the rib cage, then place it over and parallel to the hand now resting on the patient's lower sternum (Figure A-18d). Only the heel of one hand is in contact with the lower half of the sternum. It may be more comfortable for you if the fingers of your lower hand are interlocked with the fingers

of your upper hand and pulled slightly away from the chest wall. This interlocking position may also improve technique.

Apply pressure vertically down through both arms to depress the sternum 1½" to 2". Use a rocking motion, then rise up gently. This motion allows you to apply pressure vertically down from your shoulders while your elbows are kept straight (Figure A-19). *After you apply this pressure, you must follow with an equal period of relaxation.* The ratio of compression to relaxation should be 1:1.

## FIGURE A-19

Use vertical downward pressure to apply external chest compression

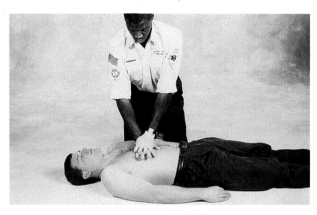

As you compress the chest, make sure your movements are smooth, rhythmic, and uninterrupted. Short, jabbing strokes are not effective in producing artificial circulation.

Do not remove the heel of your hand from the chest during the relaxation period. However, you must remember to completely release pressure on the sternum so it can return to its normal resting position between compressions. Compression and relaxation must be rhythmic. Do not bounce your hand or move it from the patient's chest during compression (Figure A-20).

You must use care as you give chest compressions, as even when well done, it carries some risk. Even with chest compressions done correctly, some patients have had fractured ribs, a lacerated liver, a ruptured spleen, or a fractured sternum. Although these injuries cannot always be avoided, you can help prevent them by using good, smooth technique and proper hand placement.

When you are doing CPR alone, you must give both artificial ventilations and chest compressions. After every 15 cardiac

## FIGURE A-20

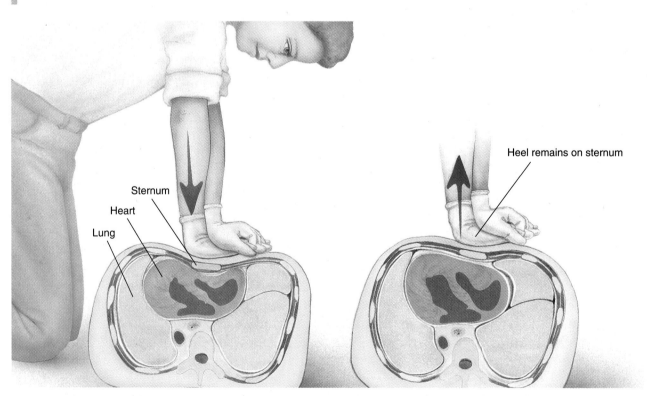

**A**   Compression of the heart during chest compression

**B**   Relaxation of the heart during chest compression

compressions you should deliver 2 ventilations. This is a ratio of compressions to ventilations of 15:2. The 15 compressions are delivered in approximately 10 seconds, for a rate of 80 to 100 per minute. You should give 2 full ventilations in the next 7 to 8 seconds, using at least 1½ to 2 seconds for each breath you deliver, and at least 3 seconds for exhalation of the first breath. Your second ventilation will be completely exhaled by the effects of the next chest compression. Check for the return of a spontaneous carotid pulse after 1 minute of CPR and then at least every 5 minutes after.

## TWO-RESCUER ADULT CPR

You and your team should be able to perform both one-rescuer and two-rescuer CPR with ease. Two-rescuer CPR is a coordinated effort that is less tiring to rescuers and is more effective for the patient. Thus, two-rescuer CPR should be used whenever possible.

When you and your partner arrive at the scene to give two-rescuer CPR, you must both act quickly and efficiently. You should immediately go to the head of the patient and perform the initial assessment. Your partner should immediately get into position to give chest compressions. You should assess the patient's ABCD by the look, listen, and feel technique and feel for the carotid pulse with one hand. If the patient is not breathing and has no pulse, you should give two artificial ventilations. Your partner should then begin chest compressions.

To perform two-rescuer CPR, you and your partner should be on opposite sides of the patient (Figure A-21) so that you can easily switch positions when necessary. To switch, you should move into position to begin chest compressions after giving a breath. Your partner should give the fifth

compression, then move to the patient's head. Your partner should then check the carotid pulse for 3 to 5 seconds. If the patient has no pulse, your partner should say, "No pulse. Continue CPR."

### FIGURE A-21

Positioning of two EMT-Bs during two-rescuer CPR

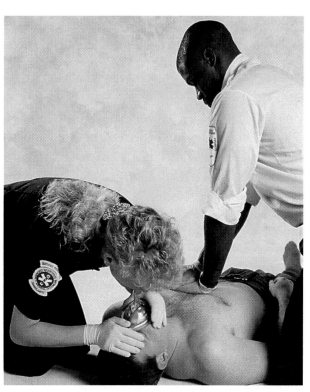

### ADDING A SECOND RESCUER TO ONE-RESCUER CPR

Once one-rescuer CPR is in progress, a second rescuer can be added very easily. Without stopping CPR, the first rescuer announces that he or she is ready to switch to two-rescuer CPR.

The second rescuer can most easily enter after a cycle of 15 compressions and

2 breaths. The second rescuer feels for the patient's carotid pulse as the first rescuer performs the set of 15 compressions. The second rescuer then evaluates the pulse generated by the first rescuer's compressions, along with the patient's color, the position, and the overall effectiveness of the CPR. The first rescuer then delivers 2 ventilations and feels for a spontaneous carotid pulse for 5 seconds while CPR is not being performed. The second rescuer should then place his or her hands in the proper location on the sternum and be ready to begin chest compressions. If the first rescuer finds no pulse, he or she should say, "Continue CPR."

The second rescuer then begins a series of five chest compressions at a rate of 80 to 100 per minute. With two-rescuer CPR, every 5 compressions should be followed by 1 ventilation. This is a ratio of compressions to ventilations of 5:1. After 1 minute of CPR, you should assess the carotid pulse for about 5 seconds. Pulse checks should then be done after every 5 minutes of CPR. The best time to switch positions is during the pulse checks. However, rescuers can switch positions any time one of the rescuers needs to change.

When EMTs are switching positions they follow the same sequence as described above. Following a ventilation by the EMT who has been delivering the ventilations, the EMT who has been performing chest compressions checks for a spontaneous carotid pulse while the EMT who has been ventilating moves to the chest and establishes his or her hand position on the sternum. Compressions start with the command, "Resume CPR."

## MONITORING THE EFFECTIVENESS OF TWO-RESCUER CPR

To determine whether two-rescuer CPR has been effective, the carotid pulse must be assessed for 3 to 5 seconds after the first four cycles of compressions and ventilations. Palpating the carotid pulse will allow you

to assess the return of a spontaneous, effective heartbeat. The rescuer giving artificial ventilations during two-rescuer CPR should palpate the pulse after the first minute of CPR and every 5 minutes after. The pulse should also be checked just before you and your partner switch positions during CPR.

You may also assess the pupils for responsiveness. Pupillary reaction to light is generally considered a good sign. However, normal pupillary reactions may be altered by eye operations and many types of prescription medications. These reactions are also drastically changed by heightened levels of adrenaline. Return of normal skin color or the resolution of cyanosis may also be a positive sign.

## INTERRUPTING OR STOPPING CPR

No matter how well it is performed, BLS measures are rarely enough to save a patient's life. Without ALS measures at the scene, you must provide immediate transport, continuing two-rescuer CPR en route. CPR is an important "holding action" that provides minimal circulation and ventilation until the patient can receive definitive care at the hospital.

In certain situations, you may need to move a patient, or conditions may make it impossible for you to continue effective CPR. In these instances, you will have to move the patient. *Try not to interrupt CPR for more than 5 seconds, except when it is absolutely necessary.* When a patient has to be moved up or down stairs, it is best to continue CPR to the head or foot of the stairs. You should then interrupt CPR at an agreed-upon signal and move quickly to the next level where you can continue CPR. At this next level, you can begin CPR again. Try to keep interruptions as short as possible. Do not move the patient until all transport arrangements are made. Thus, your interruption of CPR can be kept at a minimum.

CPR may also be stopped in certain situations. When a physician or higher medical authority assumes responsibility for the patient, he or she may order you to stop CPR. In this case, you may follow those orders. Local protocols should govern these situations. When ALS measures are to be performed, you may have to briefly interrupt CPR. You may have to stop CPR if you become exhausted and have no way to transport the patient, as could occur in a wilderness or rural setting. Of course, you should stop CPR if you can feel a pulse and the patient begins to breathe on his or her own.

## BLS CARE IN INFANTS AND CHILDREN

The basic principles of BLS are the same for infants, children, and adults. For the purposes of BLS, anyone under 1 year of age is considered an infant. A child is between the ages of 1 and 8 years. For children older than 8 years of age, techniques used for adults can generally be used. However, these definitions are to be considered guidelines only, as children vary in size. Some small children may well be treated best as infants, and larger children as adults. The differences in providing BLS care for infants and children are twofold:

1. The emergencies that require BLS care have different underlying causes for infants and children than those for adults.

2. The airways of infants and children are smaller in size than those in adults.

In most cases, full cardiac arrest in infants and children results from respiratory arrest. If uncorrected, respiratory arrest will lead to cardiac arrest and death. In adults, cardiac arrest usually occurs first. Respiratory arrest in infants and children has a variety of causes, as follows:

- aspiration of foreign bodies into the airway, such as parts of hot dogs, peanuts, candy, small toys
- poisonings and drug overdose
- airway infections, such as croup and epiglottitis
- near-drowning accidents or electrocution
- sudden infant death syndrome (SIDS)

Thus, in one-rescuer CPR of infants and children when you are off duty, you should give 1 minute of CPR before you activate the EMS system.

## OPENING THE AIRWAY IN INFANTS AND CHILDREN

Your first step in caring for any infant or child is to make sure that the airway is clear and that the patient is breathing. If the child is breathing or struggling to breathe, it is important to first activate the EMS system so that EMT-B and ALS care can be rapidly provided. In many instances, simply opening the airway and providing artificial ventilations are all that is needed to get the patient breathing again.

As a result of the initial assessment, you will know whether the patient is unresponsive, cyanotic, or in acute respiratory distress. Your next step is to secure an open airway. In children (1 to 8 years of age), the chin-lift maneuver alone is preferred (Figure A-22). Because a child's neck is so

The chin-lift maneuver on a child

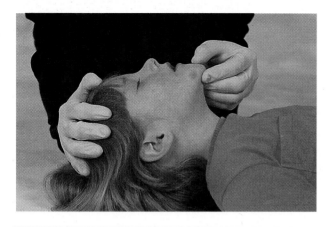

flexible, the head-tilt maneuver may result in excessive extension of the neck. Thus, the head-tilt maneuver itself may cause airway obstruction. Therefore, you should maintain the child's neck in a neutral position as you lift the chin to open the airway.

The jaw-thrust maneuver without a head tilt may also be used to open a child's airway. In fact, it is the best method to use if you suspect a spinal injury. The jaw-thrust maneuver should be performed in the same way as that for an adult.

As soon as you open the airway, assess the patient's breathing. Place your ear over the patient's nose and mouth and look for movement of the chest and abdomen. You know that the patient is breathing if you see the chest and abdomen rise and fall and if you feel and hear air move during exhalation.

## ARTIFICIAL VENTILATION IN INFANTS AND CHILDREN

If you and your partner arrive at the scene and find an infant or child is not breathing or

has cyanosis, you should call for additional help as your partner begins one-rescuer CPR.

Children in respiratory distress are usually struggling to breathe. As a result, they will usually stay in a position that will keep the airway open enough for air to move. Let them stay in that position as long as their partial airway obstruction does not become a complete airway obstruction.

For infants, the preferred technique of artificial ventilation is mouth-to-nose-and-mouth ventilation. With this technique, a seal must be made over the mouth and the nose. Various pocket masks or other barrier devices are recommended for this technique. If the child is large enough so that a tight seal cannot be made over both mouth and nose, you should perform mouth-to-mouth ventilation as you would in an adult.

Once you have made an airtight seal over the mouth, give two 1- to 1½-second gentle breaths. These initial breaths will help you to assess for airway obstruction as well as expand the lungs. Because the lungs of infants and children are much smaller than those of an adult, you do not need to blow in a great amount of air. Limit the amount of air to that needed to cause the chest to rise.

Remember, too, that a child's airway is smaller than that of an adult. Thus, there is greater resistance to airflow. As a result, you will need to use a bit more ventilatory pressure to inflate the lungs. Infants and children should be ventilated once every 3 seconds or 20 times per minute. As soon as you see the chest rise, you are giving the correct amount of air volume.

If air enters freely with your initial breaths and the chest rises, the airway is clear. You should then check the pulse. If air does not enter freely, you should check the airway for obstruction. Reposition the patient to open the airway and give another two breaths. If air still does not enter freely, you should suspect an airway obstruction. The airway must then be cleared.

## GASTRIC DISTENTION

Artificial ventilation can cause stomach distention, especially in infants and children. The amount of pressure used to give artificial ventilation to infants and children forces air into the stomach. Distention can elevate the diaphragm, decrease lung volume, and result in vomiting. You can minimize gastric distention by using slow, 1- to 1½-second breaths. This will limit the pressure of the air entering the stomach and lungs to the point at which the chest rises.

As you give artificial ventilation, watch the child's abdomen so that you can relieve the distention before the abdomen is so tense that ventilation is ineffective. To relieve gastric distention, turn the child's entire body to the left side, head down, and apply firm manual pressure to the abdomen. The child is likely to vomit, so make sure you have a suctioning unit ready before you press on the abdomen. It is important that you remove vomitus from the throat promptly.

## ARTIFICIAL CIRCULATION IN INFANTS AND CHILDREN

As discussed above, in most cases, cardiac arrest in infants and children begins with respiratory arrest. Children consume oxygen two to three times as rapidly as do adults. Secondary cardiac arrest results from hypoxia and ischemia (lacking oxygen) of the heart. Therefore, you must first focus on opening the airway and providing artificial ventilation. In many instances, simply opening the airway and providing artificial ventilations are all that is needed to get the patient breathing again.

Once the airway is open and ventilations have begun, you can focus on circulation.

As with an adult, you should first check for a palpable pulse. Absence of a palpable pulse in a major artery means that you must begin external chest compressions.

You can usually palpate the carotid pulse in a child, but it is difficult in an infant. The very short and, oftentimes, fat neck of an infant makes feeling the carotid pulse difficult. Thus, you should palpate the brachial artery in infants.

The brachial artery is located on the inner side of the arm, midway between the elbow and shoulder (Figure A-23). Place your thumb on the outer surface of the arm between the elbow and shoulder. Then place the tips of your index and long fingers on the medial side of the biceps and press lightly toward the bone.

### FIGURE A-23

Location of the brachial pulse in an infant

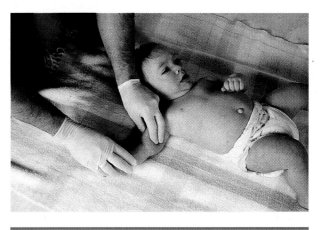

### EXTERNAL CHEST COMPRESSIONS

Most BLS techniques are the same for infants, small children, larger children, and adults. However, the technique for chest compressions in infants and children differs due to the following anatomic differences:

- position of the heart
- small size of the chest

- faster heart rate
- relative fragility of the surrounding organs

External chest compression on a child must be coordinated with ventilations, as in the adult. The rate of compression to ventilation is 5:1 for both one-rescuer CPR and two-rescuer CPR. When you are the only EMT-B present, you should open the airway and ventilate the patient once after each set of five compressions. If you and your partner are caring for the patient, the ventilation rate is the same. For infants, one ventilation (1- to 1½-seconds per breath) should be given after every fifth compression. One-rescuer infant CPR is usually practiced in the field, although two-rescuer CPR is possible in certain settings.

### Position of the Heart

As the chest grows, the proportion of space occupied by the heart decreases. The heart in the infant or child is located at about the same level as in adults. Imagine a line drawn between the nipples on a child. The proper area for compression is one finger's breadth below this line on the sternum. Place your index finger just below the line as it crosses the sternum. The adjacent long finger is the most superior point for compression (Figure A-24).

To locate the proper position for chest compressions, use the same technique as for an adult. Find the xiphoid notch in the center of the chest with your long finger. The area just under your index finger is the proper place for compression. The sternum of the child is only 6 to 7 cm long. The thickness of two fingers of an adult is 3 to 4 cm. Two fingers will easily cover the lower half of the sternum.

### Chest Size

The chest of an infant or child is smaller and more pliable than that of an adult. Thus, two hands are not necessary for effective compression. In an infant, two fingers are enough. With your fingers on the lower sternum, depress it ½" to 1". As with an adult, an infant or child must be lying on a hard surface for the best results. You may need to use more force with a child than with an infant, but the use of two or three fingers or the heel of one hand is usually adequate.

Make sure that the hand closest to the head remains on the child's forehead during chest compressions. Your other hand may remain on the chest as you give artificial ventilations. If the chest does not rise, remove the hand on the patient's chest, and then reposition the airway using the head-tilt/chin-lift maneuver. Return the compression hand to the chest. In this instance, you

### FIGURE A-24

Location for chest compressions in an infant

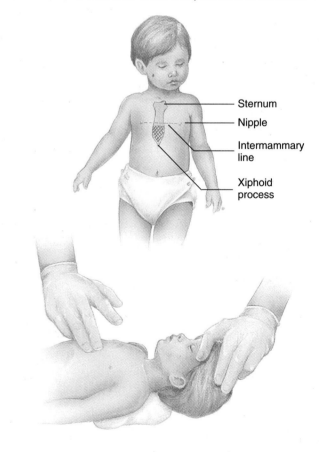

Sternum

Nipple

Intermammary line

Xiphoid process

do not need to physically relocate the exact position on the sternum. You can find the correct position visually in order to save time. Place only the heel of your hand on the sternum. Keep your fingers off the patient's chest. If the patient is large enough to require the heel of the hand, compress the sternum 1" to 1½ ".

### Heart Rate

Because of the faster heart rate in infants and children, the compression rate must also be faster. For infants and children, the minimum compression rate is 100 per minute.

### Fragility of Organs

The organs of infants and children are more fragile than those in adults. Thus, you must use extra care when performing chest compressions. The liver is relatively large, immediately under the right side of the diaphragm, and very fragile, especially in infants. The spleen on the left is much smaller and much more fragile than in adults. The liver and spleen are easily injured if you are not careful in performing chest compressions. Because these organs are so fragile and so easily injured, make sure that you place your fingers in the midline of the chest.

## AMERICAN HEART ASSOCIATION GUIDELINES

The American Heart Association (AHA) has developed CPR skill test sheets for One- and Two-Rescuer CPR on adults, children, and infants. The American Red Cross publishes skill sheets that are almost identical to those of the AHA. Consult your local protocols and state agencies for guidelines that may differ from these skill sheets.

## FOREIGN BODY AIRWAY OBSTRUCTION IN ADULTS

Airway obstruction may be caused by many things, as follows:

- relaxation of the throat muscles in an unconscious patient
- vomited or regurgitated stomach contents
- blood clot, bone fragments, or damaged tissue after an injury
- dentures
- foreign bodies in the airway

Ways in which to open an airway were discussed earlier in this appendix. Loose dentures and large pieces of vomited food, mucus, or blood clots in the mouth should be swept forward and out with your gloved index finger. You should use suctioning to maintain a clear airway. Occasionally, a large foreign body will be aspirated and block the upper airway.

### RECOGNIZING FOREIGN BODY OBSTRUCTION

Sudden airway obstruction by a foreign body in an adult usually occurs during a meal. In a child, it usually occurs during mealtime or at play. Children commonly choke on peanuts, large bits of hot dog, or small toys. It is important to identify an airway obstruction as soon as possible. Your treatment of airway obstruction will be based on the cause of the obstruction. Thus, you must learn to identify airway obstructions caused by a foreign body and those due to respiratory failure or arrest, such as fainting, stroke, or heart problems.

### Conscious Patient

A sudden airway obstruction is usually easily recognized in an individual who is eating or has just finished eating. The individual is suddenly unable to speak or cough, grasps the throat, turns cyanotic, and makes exaggerated efforts to breathe. Air is either not moving in and out of the airway, or it is so slight that it is not detectable. At first, the patient will be conscious and able to clearly indicate the nature of the problem. If you are at the scene, you should ask the patient, "Are you choking?" The patient will usually answer by nodding "yes." If the foreign body is not removed quickly, the lungs will use up their oxygen supply. Unconsciousness and death will follow.

### Unconscious Patient

When you discover an unconscious patient, your first step is to determine whether the patient is breathing and has a pulse. The unconsciousness may be due to airway obstruction, cardiac arrest, or a number of other problems. Thus, you should first treat any unconscious patient as if he or she has had a cardiac arrest. Then you can concentrate on possible airway obstructions.

You should suspect an airway obstruction if the standard maneuvers to open the airway and ventilation efforts do not effectively ventilate the patient's lungs. Once you open the airway, you should be able to ventilate the lungs effectively. However, if you feel resistance to blowing into the patient's lungs or pressure builds up in your mouth, the patient likely has some type of obstruction. You must then take steps to relieve the obstruction.

### Emergency Medical Care

Two manual maneuvers are recommended for relieving foreign body airway obstruction: 1) the abdominal-thrust maneuver (the Heimlich maneuver), and 2) finger sweeps and manual removal of the object.

### Abdominal-Thrust Maneuver

The **abdominal-thrust maneuver**, also called the Heimlich maneuver, is the best way to dislodge and force food or other material from the throat of a choking victim. Residual air, which is always present in the lungs, is compressed upward and used to expel the object.

You should give a series of five abdominal thrusts until the foreign body is dislodged. With the patient sitting or standing, follow these steps:

1. Stand behind the patient. Wrap your arms around the patient's waist.

2. Make a fist with one hand and grasp this fist with the other hand. Place the thumb side of the fist against the patient's abdomen, just above the umbilicus and well below the xiphoid.

3. Press your fist into the patient's abdomen with a quick inward and upward thrust (Figure A-25).

### FIGURE A-25

Applying the abdominal-thrust maneuver in a sitting or standing adult

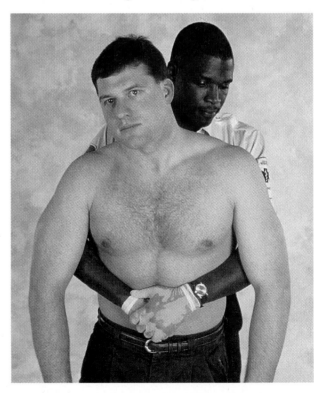

4. Repeat the thrusts in sets of five until the object is expelled from the airway, or the patient becomes unconscious.

With the patient supine, modify the technique as follows:

1. Place the patient in a supine position.
2. Kneel close to the patient's hips or straddle the patient's hips or legs.
3. Place the heel of one hand against the patient's abdomen above the umbilicus and well below the xiphoid process. Then place your other hand on top of the first.
4. Press the hand into the patient's abdomen with a quick inward and upward thrust and repeat five times (Figure A-26).

You can perform the abdominal-thrust maneuver safely in all adults and children. Pregnancy and obesity do not contraindicate its use. However, use a chest thrust for patients in advanced stages of pregnancy or for the markedly obese and for children younger than 1 year of age.

### Manual Removal

If the foreign body causing the obstruction appears in the mouth, or is believed to be in the mouth, you should remove it carefully with your gloved fingers. The abdominal-thrust maneuver may dislodge the foreign body, but not expel it. Use a tongue-jaw lift combined with a finger probe to remove the foreign material, as follows:

1. Keep the head in the neutral position.
2. Grasp the tongue and the lower jaw between your thumb and fingers and lift them forward. This pulls the tongue back away from the throat and away from the foreign body that may be lodged there.
3. Use the index finger of your opposite hand as a hook to sweep down inside the patient's cheek to the base of the tongue.
4. Dislodge any impacted foreign body up into the mouth.
5. When the foreign body comes up within reach, grasp and carefully remove it.

Make sure that you do not push the dislodged foreign body farther back into the airway. For this reason, "blind" finger sweeps are not advised in infants or small children. Instead, look first and then reach for the object with your index finger and thumb only after you see it.

## FIGURE A-26

Applying the abdominal-thrust maneuver in a supine adult

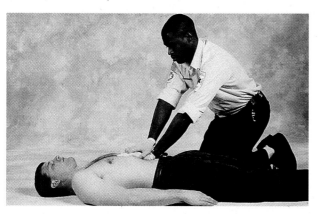

## PARTIAL AIRWAY OBSTRUCTION

Some patients may have only a partial airway obstruction. With a partial obstruction, the patient will be able to exchange some air, but will still have some degree of respiratory distress. Breathing is noisy and the patient may be coughing. *Your main concern is to prevent a partial airway obstruction from becoming a complete airway obstruction.* The abdominal-thrust maneuver is generally not effective in these situations. Manual removal is dangerous because you could force the object farther down the airway, causing a complete obstruction.

Therefore, for a patient with a partial airway obstruction, you should first try to open the airway using the head-tilt/chin-lift or jaw-thrust maneuvers. These maneuvers will support the airway in its most efficient position. You should then give 100% oxygen to the patient using a nonrebreathing mask and provide prompt transport. Of course, if the partial obstruction becomes a complete obstruction, you should immediately perform the abdominal-thrust maneuver.

## FOREIGN BODY AIRWAY OBSTRUCTION IN INFANTS AND CHILDREN

Airway obstruction is a common problem in infants and children. It is usually caused by a foreign body or an infection, such as croup or epiglottitis, resulting in swelling and narrowing of the airway. You should try to identify the cause of the obstruction as soon as possible. With an airway infection, the steps for dislodging a foreign body will not be helpful, can be dangerous, and will delay transport. See chapter 26, Infants and Children, for an explanation of croup and epiglottitis.

A previously healthy child who, while eating, playing with small toys, or crawling about the house, has sudden difficulty breathing has probably aspirated a foreign body. As in adults, foreign bodies may cause a partial or complete airway obstruction. With a partial airway obstruction, air exchange can be either good or poor. With good air exchange, the patient can cough forcefully, although there may be wheezing between coughs. As long as the patient can breathe, cough, or talk, you should not interfere with the patient's attempts to expel the foreign body. However, you should evaluate the child often, as good air exchange may progress to poor air exchange. You should give the patient oxygen and provide transport.

With poor air exchange, the patient will likely have an ineffective cough, stridor, increased respiratory difficulty, and cyanosis. You should give oxygen to a patient with poor air exchange. When oxygen does not convert poor air exchange into good air exchange, you must treat the patient as you would with a complete airway obstruction.

## EMERGENCY MEDICAL CARE

### Children

You should perform the abdominal-thrust maneuver on a child who has a complete foreign body obstruction. Deliver a series of five thrusts to an unconscious child. If the foreign body is not expelled, you should open the mouth. If you see the foreign body, perform the tongue-jaw lift and then use a finger sweep to remove it. In rare instances, when you cannot remove the foreign body, perform mouth-to-mask ventilation en route to the hospital.

The actual technique for delivering abdominal thrusts may vary with the size of the child. Ordinarily, you would deliver abdominal thrusts with the child supine. In children older than 8 years, you may be able to perform the maneuver in the same way as you would for an adult.

### Infants

The abdominal-thrust maneuver might injure the liver or other abdominal organs in an infant. Thus, you should deliver a series of five quick back blows, followed by a series of five chest thrusts to clear a foreign body airway obstruction.

# FIGURE A-27

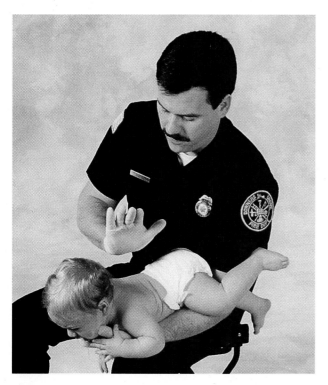

**A** Delivering back blows to an infant

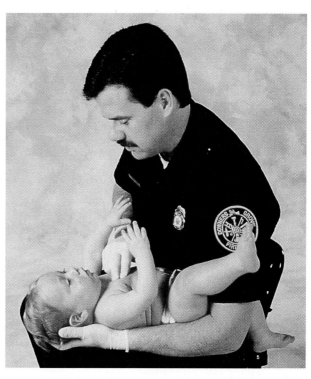

**B** Delivering chest compressions to an infant

To deliver chest thrusts or back blows, place one hand on the infant's back and neck and the other on the chest, jaws, and face. Remember to support the head by firmly holding the jaw. This "sandwiches" the infant between your hands and arms. Your forearm should rest on your thigh to support the infant. While you continue to provide support for the head and neck, hold the infant with the head lower than the trunk. Deliver five quick back blows between the shoulder blades using the heel of your hand (Figure A-27a).

Next, turn the infant over faceup, but make sure that you support the head and neck. Hold the infant in a supine position resting on your thigh with the head slightly lower than the trunk. Give five quick chest thrusts on the sternum in the same fashion

as for CPR, except at a slightly slower rate (Figure A-27b). If the infant is large, or your hands are small, you may need to place the infant on your lap to deliver the chest thrusts.

If the infant is unconscious, you should perform the tongue-jaw lift to open the mouth. Remove the object manually if you can see it in the mouth. As with adults, you should not perform blind finger sweeps, because the foreign body can easily be pushed farther back in the throat.

If the patient does not start breathing after these maneuvers, you should try to open the airway again and give artificial ventilation. If the chest does not rise, reposition the head and attempt ventilation again. If the chest still does not rise, continue giving back blows, followed by chest thrusts until the obstruction is cleared, or you reach the hospital.

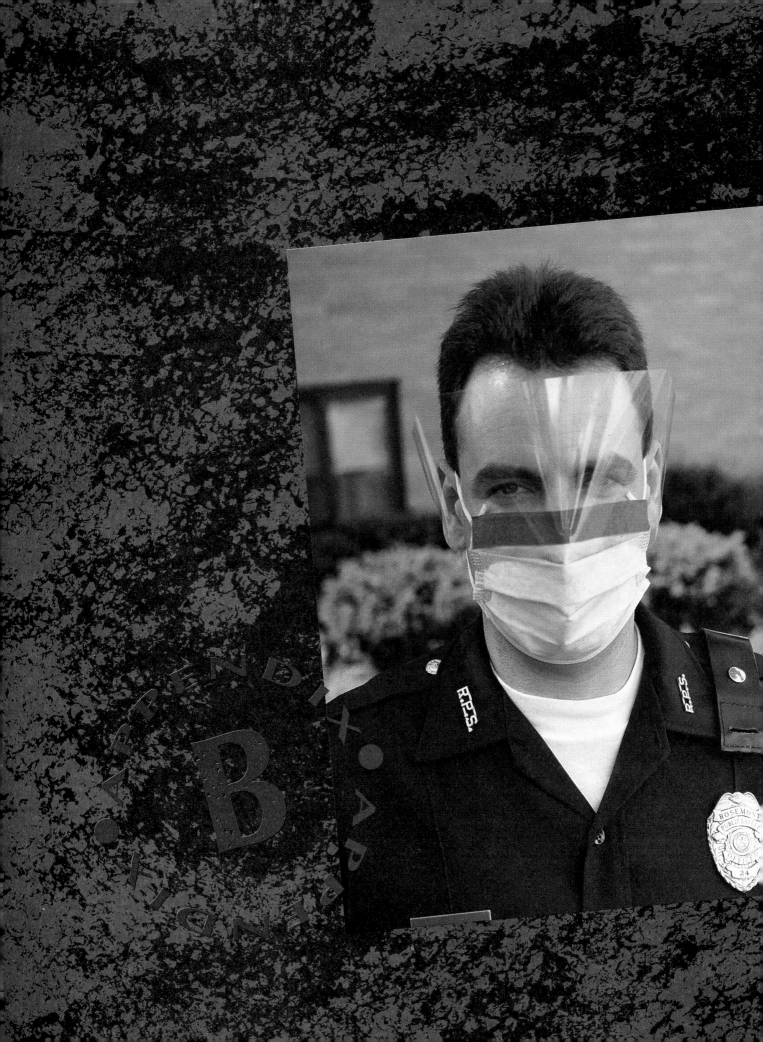

# Infection Control

## Objectives

After you have read this chapter, you should be able to:

- Explain the duty to care for patients with communicable diseases.
- List the principles of disease transmission.
- Identify appropriate task-specific personal protective equipment (PPE).
- Discuss the importance of obtaining a patient's history and assessment findings to identify possible communicable diseases.
- Identify possible occupational diseases and methods of risk assessment.
- Identify the benefits of an exposure control plan.
- List the components of postexposure management and reporting.

## Overview

Fear of "catching" a life-threatening communicable disease on the job has resulted in confusion and gross misunderstanding of the risks for transmission among care providers. One of the basic components of your training is that your safety comes first. You and your partner must judge the risks of approaching a violent or armed patient, or a dangerous situation. However, patients with a communicable disease do not fall into the same category. They do not pose a risk to your safety. Education and training about the actual risks for disease transmission are your best weapons against fear and overwhelming concern.

The purpose of this appendix is to clarify some basic infection control issues. Among the topics discussed are duty to care, the selection of personal protective equipment, risk assessment, and the exposure control plan. Several terms used in discussions of infection control issues are defined as well.

Education will reduce possible legal action against you and/or your service that stems from improper treatment or abandonment of patients with communicable diseases. This is a clear challenge for the 1990s.

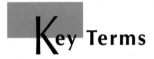 **Key Terms**

**Body Substance Isolation (BSI)** An infection control concept and practice that assumes all body fluids as being potentially infectious.

**Communicable disease** Any disease that can be spread from person to person.

**Designated officer** The individual in the department charged with the responsibility of managing exposures and infection control issues.

**Direct contact** Spread of a communicable disease from one person to another.

**Exposure** Contact with blood, body fluids, tissues, or airborne droplets by direct or indirect contact.

**Exposure control plan** Comprehensive plan that helps employees reduce their risk of exposure to or acquisition of communicable diseases.

**Host** The organism or person in which an infectious agent resides.

**Indirect contact** Transmission of disease from one person to another by contact with a contaminated object.

**Infection** The growth of an organism in a susceptible host with or without signs or symptoms of illness.

**Infection control** Procedures to reduce infection in patients and health care personnel.

**Pathogen** A microorganism that is capable of causing disease in a susceptible host.

**PPE** Personal protective equipment.

**Virulence** The strength or ability of a pathogen to produce disease.

**Universal precautions** A concept for infection control which considers blood and certain body fluids to pose a risk for transmission of bloodborne diseases.

# UNDERSTANDING DISEASE TRANSMISSION

A **communicable disease** is any disease that can be spread from person to person. A communicable disease can be caused by viruses (measles, hepatitis, HIV), by bacteria (tuberculosis), or by fungi and parasites.

Communicable diseases may be transmitted by either direct or indirect contact. **Direct contact** occurs when the disease is spread directly from one person to the other. A needlestick injury in which disease is spread from the needle to the person is an example of direct contact. **Indirect contact** occurs when disease is spread from one person to another by contact with a contaminated object. Handling a piece of bloody equipment without gloves on when you have a cut on your hand could result in indirect transmission of disease. **Exposure** occurs if you come into contact with blood, body fluids, tissues, or airborne droplets by direct or indirect contact.

Several factors must be in place in order for infection to occur. The presence of a pathogen is not enough to create a risk. A **pathogen** is a microorganism that is capable of causing disease in a susceptible person **(host). Infection** is the growth of an organism in a susceptible host with or without signs or symptoms of illness. Other factors include the following:

- dosage of the pathogen
- the strength or ability of the pathogen to cause disease **(virulence)**
- entry into the body
- host resistance

Another, often overlooked factor is your personal health (host resistance). The healthier you are, the less susceptible you are to infection. Staying healthy and making sure your immunizations are up to date make you less susceptible to various forms of disease. The Centers for Disease Control and Prevention (CDC) and NFPA Infection Control Standard 1581 list current recommendations for immunizations for EMS and fire service personnel (Table B-1).

## TABLE B-1 RECOMMENDED IMMUNIZATIONS FOR FIRE/EMS PERSONNEL

hepatitis B vaccine

measles, mumps, rubella vaccine

tuberculin skin testing (Mantoux method)— at least yearly

tetanus, diphtheria booster—every ten years

influenza vaccine—yearly

## DUTY TO CARE

You cannot deny care to a patient who you suspect has a communicable disease, even if you feel the patient poses a risk to your safety. To deny care to a patient in this situation is considered abandonment. It is also considered discrimination according to the Americans with Disabilities Act, especially if a public department or agency (such as an EMS service) is involved. Thus, it is important for you to understand the disease process and the factors necessary to put you at risk. You must understand these issues, as your response to them sometimes has legal consequences.

# RISK REDUCTION AND PREVENTION

## EMPLOYER RESPONSIBILITIES

Your employer, whether an independent EMS service, a hospital-based service, or a municipal service, cannot guarantee a 100% risk-free environment. The risk of exposure to or acquiring a communicable disease is a part of your job. You have a right to know about diseases that may pose a risk to you. Remember, though, that your risk for infection is *not* high. However, OSHA regulations require that all employees be offered a workplace environment that *reduces* the risk for exposure. OSHA regulations apply primarily to private and federal agencies. However, in states that have their own OSHA plans, state and municipal employees must be covered as well.

Other national guidelines and standards address reducing the risk for exposure to bloodborne pathogens and airborne diseases. In 1989, the CDC published guidelines for public safety personnel. NFPA Infection Control Standard 1581 also sets standards for risk reduction. The CDC guidelines and the NFPA standard establish a standard for care for all fire and EMS personnel. These standards apply to you no matter if you are a full-time paid EMT or a volunteer.

## PERSONAL PROTECTIVE EQUIPMENT

OSHA requires that the following **personal protective equipment (PPE)** be made available to you:

- vinyl and latex gloves
- heavy-duty gloves for cleaning
- protective eye wear
- masks, include the HEPA respirator
- cover gowns
- respiratory assist devices

PPE blocks entry of the organism into the body. Thus, the way to select the proper PPE for each task is based on the way in which a communicable disease is transmitted. While this may seem very simplistic, it is effective. For example, transmission of an airborne disease can be blocked if you wear a mask. Blood splatter into the eye can be stopped by wearing eye protection.

The most common type of PPE is gloves. The FDA, CDC, and OSHA have stated that *vinyl and latex gloves are equally protective.* Thus, it is your responsibility to evaluate the situation and then choose the glove that works best. Vinyl gloves may be best for routine procedures, and latex gloves may be best for invasive procedures. Heavy-duty utility gloves must be used for all cleaning and disinfecting procedures. Never use vinyl or latex gloves for cleaning.

You should wear protective eye wear when there is a possibility that blood or some other body fluid may splatter onto the surface of the eye. There is no requirement for goggles. If you wear prescription eyeglasses, add removable side shields to your eyeglasses when on duty.

Cover gowns are often not practical in the field. In fact, in some instances they might pose a risk for injury. For example, if you were to wear a cover gown while crawling into a vehicle to provide care, the neck of the gown may become caught and pull on your neck. Your department will decide if your uniform serves as PPE, or if cover gowns are needed. If your uniform serves as your PPE, then your department's exposure control plan should outline how and where contaminated uniforms are to be laundered. Meeting the requirement for PPE need not be expensive.

The use of masks has become a very complex area. This is especially true given the new OSHA and CDC requirements for protection from tuberculosis (TB). You should wear a standard surgical mask if blood or body fluid splatter is a possibility. If you believe that the patient has an airborne disease, then you should place a surgical mask on the patient. However, if you believe that the patient has TB, place a surgical mask on the patient and a HEPA respirator on yourself. Use of a HEPA respirator requires compliance with OSHA standards. OSHA respiratory standard 29 CFR part 1910.134 states that facial hair will prevent a proper fit. Therefore, you should not have long sideburns or a mustache if you are going to wear a HEPA respirator. In addition, never put a HEPA mask on the patient.

Respiratory assist or barrier devices are recommended for CPR. *Note that there are no documented cases of disease transmission to rescuers as a result of performing unprotected CPR on an infected patient.* You need to use a barrier device or mask because transmission is possible, even though there are no documented cases of disease transmission. If you use reusable BVM devices, be sure that the device is cleaned properly following the routine for high-level disinfection.

These recommendations for use of PPE are "on the books" and should be followed. However, there are times when these procedures cannot be performed. OSHA recognizes that this is a reality. Therefore, there is an "exception" statement in the OSHA regulation. It states that when you believe that taking the time to use PPE will delay the delivery of health care to the patient or will pose a risk to your personal safety, you may choose not to use PPE. Risk to personal safety means the likelihood of being attacked by a patient (with or without a weapon) or an animal. It does not refer to concern over acquiring a communicable disease. However, you will have to justify this action as an inquiry will follow, but it is your choice.

## EMPLOYEE RESPONSIBILITIES

In most cases, you can control your risk of exposure. You can greatly reduce your risk of exposure by wearing the proper PPE and following other simple procedures, as described below.

### Handwashing

The single most important measure for personal protection outside of wearing PPE is handwashing. In field situations where there is no running water available, waterless handwashing substitutes should be available. You should wash your hands before performing a procedure, after removing your gloves, and between patients when possible. If you use a waterless handwashing solution in the field, you should wash your hands when you arrive at the hospital. The proper procedure for handwashing is as follows:

- use soap and water
- work up a lather, rubbing your hands together for at least 10 to 15 seconds
- rinse your hands and dry them with a paper towel
- use a paper towel to turn off the faucet

### Body Substance Isolation

Another key way to reduce your risk of exposure is to follow **Body Substance Isolation (BSI)** techniques. These have been discussed throughout the textbook as part of your routine patient care. Any time you may come into contact with blood or any other body fluids, you should follow BSI techniques. BSI is the preferred infection control concept for fire and EMS personnel. **Infection control** is a set of procedures designed to reduce infection in patients and health care personnel.

The concept of BSI differs from universal precautions. When following **universal precautions**, you assume that blood and *certain* body fluids pose a risk for transmission of hepatitis B and HIV. In 1988, the CDC removed many body fluids from the risk category (Table B-2). Thus, the major difference between BSI and universal precautions is the presence of visible blood in the fluid. In most emergency situations, you may not be able to see blood in the fluid. It may be dark, or you may be reaching into an area and all you feel is wet. This is why EMS does not follow universal precautions. With BSI, you should consider all body fluids a possible risk.

If you believe you have been exposed to blood or any other body fluid, you must report to your department's designated officer. The **designated officer** is the person in your department responsible for managing exposures and infection control issues. Your risk of exposure will be assessed and the officer will make an initial decision about your need for medical follow-up. If so, you will be referred to the appropriate care provider.

OSHA recognizes and accepts the BSI concept in its standard 29 CPR Part 1910.1030. The role and need for a designated officer is defined in the Ryan White Law. The Ryan White Law (PL 101–381) is a federal law that requires that emergency care providers be provided notification and follow-up in exposure situations. This law went into effect April 20, 1994.

## EXPOSURE CONTROL PLANS

You and your team can also reduce your risk of exposure by following your department's exposure control plan. An **exposure control plan** is a comprehensive plan that helps employees reduce their risk of exposure to or acquisition of communicable diseases. This plan should incorporate CDC guidelines, OSHA regulations, NFPA Infection Control Standard 1581, and other applicable state and local regulations. The plan should also clearly reflect the reality of your daily workplace. The plan should address the following nine areas:

1. *Determination of exposure.* This area should define who is at risk for ongoing contact with blood and other body fluids. It also includes creating a list of tasks that pose a risk for contact with blood or other body fluids. This

**TABLE B-2**    **BODY FLUIDS WHICH POSE A RISK FOR TRANSMISSION OF HEPATITIS B AND HIV**

| Primary Risk | Secondary Risk | No Risk* |
|---|---|---|
| blood | synovial fluid | sweat |
| semen | cerebrospinal fluid | tears |
| vaginal secretions | pericardial fluid | saliva |
| | amniotic fluid | urine |
| | pleural fluid | feces |
| | | vomitus |
| | | nasal secretions |
| | | sputum |

*unless these fluids contain visible blood

list should also include the PPE needed to perform each task.

2. *Education and training.* This area should explain why a qualified individual to answer questions about communicable diseases and infection control is required. Your service or department cannot solely use packaged training materials. You must have a knowledgeable instructor present to answer questions. The training should cover the following bloodborne pathogens: hepatitis B and C, HIV, and syphilis. OSHA now also requires that tuberculosis be included. NFPA 1581 has a longer list, including childhood diseases, lice, and scabies. Education provides the best means for correcting many of the myths surrounding these issues (Table B-3).

3. *Hepatitis B vaccine program.* This area should spell out the vaccine you will be offered, its safety and efficacy, record keeping, and tracking. Your service or department should also address the need for post-vaccine antibody titers to identify individuals who do not respond to the initial three dose series.

4. *Personal Protective Equipment (PPE).* This area should list the PPE being offered to you and why it was selected. There should also be a list of how much equipment is available and where to obtain additional PPE. Training and department standard operating procedures should state when each type of PPE is to be used for each risk procedure.

5. *Cleaning and disinfection practices.* This area should describe how to care for and maintain vehicles and equipment. Where and when cleaning should be performed, how it is to be done, what PPE is to be used, and what solution is to be used should be identified. Medical waste collection, storage, and disposal should also be addressed.

**TABLE B-3    COMMON MYTHS**

Latex gloves offer more protection than vinyl gloves.

Exposure means infection.

HIV survives for a long time on surfaces, which are sources for exposure.

HIV poses the greatest risk to care providers.

You must use an antimicrobial for handwashing.

Blood can seep through your skin and infect you.

Bloodborne diseases can be transmitted through casual contact.

Mouth-to-mouth CPR poses a high risk for disease transmission.

All HIV infected persons will die of AIDS.

Pregnancy is a contraindication for taking hepatitis B vaccine.

TB is a highly communicable disease.

You need gloves to give an injection.

6. *Tuberculin skin testing/fit testing.* This area should address how often employees should undergo Mantoux skin testing and fit testing. Fit testing is done to determine the proper size mask you should wear to protect yourself from TB. All issues dealing with the new HEPA respirator masks should also be addressed.

7. *Postexposure management.* This area should identify who you notify when you believe you have been exposed, the forms you need to fill out, where to go for treatment, and what treatment should be given.

8. *Compliance monitoring.* This area should address how your service or department will be evaluating employee compliance with each aspect of the plan. The effectiveness of the plan depends on how well employees understand what they are to do and why it is important. Noncompliance should be documented, and the plan should state what disciplinary action might be taken for continued noncompliance.

9. *Record keeping.* This area should outline all the records that will be kept, how confidentiality will be maintained, and how records can be assessed and by whom.

Exposure control plans are very complex, but complete documents. The goal of the plan and approach is to reduce your risk of exposure by understanding the need for and using the following:

- proper PPE
- vaccines/immunizations and testing
- proper cleaning of equipment and vehicles
- procedures for postexposure medical care

Exposure control plans offer a win-win situation for both you and your service or department, as they offer risk reduction and cost reduction as well. All aspects of your department's plan should be incorporated into your education and training program.

## THE IMPORTANCE OF PATIENT INFORMATION

As you gather information about the patient during the initial assessment, the SAMPLE history, and your on-going assessment, you should keep infection control issues in mind. For example, the key to identifying the possibility of TB in a patient will be signs, symptoms, and history. You should ask about weight loss, night sweats, and coughing. If you suspect a patient has TB, place a surgical mask on the patient and a HEPA respirator on yourself.

You can ask patients about their HIV or hepatitis status, but they may not know that they are infected. However, there is no legal requirement for them to tell you. This is why you should follow BSI techniques. Thus, you should approach each and every body fluid as a possible risk and use PPE.

How you select the type of PPE to use in any given situation should be based on one of two things. First, select the proper PPE based on your knowledge of all the signs and symptoms and modes of transmission for all the communicable diseases. Second, you can select PPE based on the task you will be performing. Fire service and EMS training currently recommends that PPE decisions be based on the task to be performed (Table B-4). The information in this table was published by the CDC in 1989 and provides a basic, practical approach for field care providers. Some of the myths on use of PPE are also clarified in this table.

## TABLE B-4 EXAMPLES OF RECOMMENDED PPE FOR WORKER PROTECTION AGAINST HIV AND HBV TRANSMISSION[1] IN PREHOSPITAL[2] SETTINGS

| Task or Activity | Disposable Gloves | Gown | Mask[3] | Protective Eyewear |
|---|---|---|---|---|
| Bleeding control with spurting blood | Yes | Yes | Yes | Yes |
| Bleeding control with minimal bleeding | Yes | No | No | No |
| Emergency childbirth | Yes | Yes | Yes, if splashing is likely | Yes, if splashing is likely |
| Blood drawing | At certain times[4] | No | No | No |
| Starting an intravenous (IV) line | Yes | No | No | No |
| Endotracheal intubation, esophageal obturator use | Yes | No | No, unless splashing is likely | No, unless splashing is likely |
| Oral/nasal suctioning, manually clearing airway | Yes[5] | No | No, unless splashing is likely | No, unless splashing is likely |
| Handling and cleaning instruments with microbial contamination | Yes | No, unless soiling is likely | No | No |
| Measuring blood pressure | No | No | No | No |
| Measuring temperature | No | No | No | No |
| Giving an injection | No | No | No | No |

[1] The examples in this table are based on application of universal precautions. Universal precautions are intended to supplement rather than replace recommendations for routine infection control, such as handwashing and using gloves to prevent gross microbial contamination of hands (e.g., contact with urine or feces).

[2] Defined as setting where delivery of emergency health care takes place away from a hospital or other health-care facility.

[3] Refers to protective masks to prevent exposure of mucous membranes to blood or other potentially contaminated body fluids. The use of resuscitation devices, some of which are also referred to as "masks," is discussed on page 16 of *Guidelines for Prevention of Transmission of Human Immunodeficiency Virus and Hepatitis B Virus to Health-Care and Public Safety Workers*, Centers for Disease Control, January, 1989.

[4] For clarification see Appendix A, page 33, and Appendix B, page 38 of *Guidelines for Prevention of Transmission of Human Immunodeficiency Virus and Hepatitis B Virus to Health-Care and Public Safety Workers*, Centers for Disease Control, January, 1989.

[5] While not clearly necessary to prevent HIV or HBV transmission unless blood is present, gloves are recommended to prevent transmission of other agents (e.g., *Herpes simplex*).

# DISEASES THAT POSE A RISK

Diseases that have been identified as posing an occupational risk for health care providers include the following:

- HIV
- syphilis
- hepatitis B
- hepatitis C
- tuberculosis (TB)

While these are not the only diseases that pose a risk, they are the most significant.

## HEPATITIS B AND HEPATITIS C

Current figures on hepatitis B indicate that there are about 300,000 new cases of hepatitis B reported in this country alone each year. The current numbers for hepatitis C are about 150,000 new cases each year. Because transmission from patient to health care worker has been documented, it is clear that both diseases pose a potential risk.

Hepatitis B and C are caused by two different viruses, even though these conditions have a great deal in common. They both affect the liver, and both appear to share the same mode of transmission—contact with blood and sexual contact. Both can lead to long-term liver disease and/or liver cancer.

Hepatitis B has been studied for many years. However, hepatitis C was only identified in the 1980s. Both diseases have two phases. In the first phase, the patient may have fever, weakness, headache, pain in the right upper quadrant, nausea, and vomiting. Many persons infected with hepatitis B or C eventually develop the second phase of signs—jaundice, dark-colored urine, and clay-colored stools.

As an EMT-B, you should know that 50% to 60% of persons infected with hepatitis B do not know that they are infected. With hepatitis C, 75% of persons infected do not know that they are infected. They either do not become ill early, or they have mild symptoms during the first phase. Thus, many patients do not exhibit the more easily identified signs and symptoms of the second phase. Because such large numbers of infected patients do not know they have hepatitis, it is important for you to follow BSI techniques. Wearing gloves and washing your hands are important, yet simple, first steps to reduce your risk of exposure. Research has documented that the risk for hepatitis B from a contaminated needlestick injury in a nonvaccinated health care provider is between 6% and 30%.

You should participate in your department's free hepatitis B vaccine program. The OSHA regulation requires that this vaccine be offered to you free of charge and at a convenient time and place. This will reduce your risk of exposure to hepatitis B.

Currently, there is no vaccine or effective treatment to protect you from acquiring hepatitis C or for direct exposure. Therefore, it is important that you receive counseling and medical follow-up for any documented exposure. You may have to undergo a blood test up to 6 months after you have been exposed. The risk for hepatitis C following a needlestick injury is between 3% and 10%. Thus, the need to follow BSI techniques, especially using PPE, is essential.

## HIV INFECTION

Human immunodeficiency virus (HIV) is responsible for the greatest fear of infection among the public and health care providers. The HIV virus attacks and destroys certain white blood cells called T4 lymphocytes. The loss of these cells makes a patient with HIV infection more likely to develop infections. HIV virus does not survive outside the body in sufficient numbers to cause infection. It is easily killed by drying and most commonly used soaps and disinfectants.

*Note that statistics show that HIV is a low risk for occupational infection.* In fact, HIV is much less infectious than the hepatitis virus. To date, risk for exposure due to a contaminated needlestick injury is at 0.32%—far below that for hepatitis B. The risk of acquiring HIV from mucous membrane exposure is currently listed as 0.09%. The risk for blood contact with broken skin is between 0 and 0.11%.

HIV is transmitted through blood and sexual contact, not casual contact. Thus, HIV is not transmitted by shaking hands, kissing, toilet seats, telephones, hot tubs, swimming pools, or mosquito bites. In fact, there is no data to suggest any other mode of transmission except through contact with blood and sexual contact. Initial signs and symptoms of HIV infection are much like the flu. These include fever and heavy night sweats, swollen lymph glands, chronic diarrhea, and weight loss.

To date, there is no vaccine for protection from HIV infection. However, because you follow BSI techniques, there should be little fear of increased risk in caring for patients with HIV infection. Your department should provide on-going education and training about HIV infection. This will help you become more comfortable working with infected patients and co-workers. To date, there are no restrictions placed on infected prehospital care providers.

## SYPHILIS

Syphilis is most commonly thought of as a sexually transmitted disease. However, it is also a bloodborne disease. Thus, there is a small risk for transmission through a contaminated needlestick injury or direct blood-to-blood contact. The number of cases of syphilis in the United States is increasing.

This is one reason that OSHA added syphilis to the list of bloodborne pathogens.

## TUBERCULOSIS

Concern regarding occupational exposure to communicable diseases has usually focused on bloodborne diseases. However, due to the increasing number of tuberculosis (TB) cases, airborne diseases now receive just as much attention. TB is caused by bacteria that die when exposed to light and air. Thus, it is not as highly communicable as many people believe. In fact, only 10% of persons who test positive for TB ever develop symptoms of the disease. With proper diagnosis and treatment, TB has a high cure rate.

TB commonly affects persons who live in close, crowded conditions, such as shelters, nursing homes, and correctional facilities. It also commonly affects individuals who have an impaired immune system, either due to HIV or other chronic illness.

As an EMT-B, you can protect yourself against TB in the following ways:

- undergoing yearly skin testing (called the PPD)

- considering infection control issues as you assess patients

- wearing a HEPA respirator if you know or suspect a patient has TB

You can learn much by carefully listening to the patient's history and observing signs and symptoms. These signs and symptoms include coughing, weight loss, night sweats, and swollen lymph glands. Some patients may also cough up blood. If a patient has the signs and symptoms of TB, you should place a surgical mask on the patient and wear a HEPA respirator yourself. Report any possible exposure to your designated officer.

## BACTERIAL MENINGITIS

Meningitis is an inflammation of the meningeal coverings of the brain. It is an airborne disease that can be caused by bacteria or a virus. A patient with viral meningitis does not pose a risk to you. However, bacterial meningitis does carry a risk for transmission. It may be transmitted by direct contact with respiratory secretions, such as through suctioning, intubation, or possibly CPR. It is also transmitted by prolonged exposure to a patient in a confined space. Signs and symptoms include pink rash, fever, headache, nausea, vomiting, and stiff neck. Note that these signs and symptoms are present in other common childhood diseases. Thus, you should place a surgical mask on a patient if you suspect possible meningitis. If the patient will not wear a mask, put one on yourself.

## WHOOPING COUGH

Whooping cough, also called pertussis, is an airborne disease caused by bacteria. It most commonly affects children younger than 6 years of age. Signs and symptoms include fever and a "whoop" sound that occurs when a child tries to inhale after a coughing attack.

Cases of whooping cough have increased in recent years. In 1993, the CDC reported an 82% increase over 1992 in the number of reported cases. Whooping cough is preventable with administration of a routine childhood DPT (diphtheria, pertussis, tetanus) vaccination. However, many children have not received or completed their vaccine series and remain unprotected. Again, the best way to prevent exposure is to try to place a mask on the patient. If the patient will not wear the mask, put one on yourself.

## COMMON CHILDHOOD DISEASES

Measles, mumps, and chickenpox are childhood diseases that appear to present problems from time to time. The signs and symptoms for most of these diseases are very much the same. When caring for a child who has a fever, along with other signs and symptoms of these conditions, you should anticipate possible transmission. Place a mask on the child, if you can. It is also important to make sure that your immunizations are current. You should not be working in EMS without proof of measles, mumps, rubella vaccination (MMR), or a documented history of having had the disease.

## OTHER DISEASES OF CONCERN

Many new diseases, such as Hantavirus, *E. coli* 0157:H7, and drug-resistant bacteria are being reported and getting news coverage. These reports suggest problems of possible epidemics. However, these diseases are not problems of wide proportion. Most important is that these diseases are not transmitted from person to person. Thus, they are not communicable diseases and do not pose a risk to you during patient care.

# POSTEXPOSURE MANAGEMENT

## AIRBORNE DISEASE

In many instances, you will not know that a patient has an airborne disease. Thus, you could be exposed without knowing it. The Ryan White Law requires that the hospital notify your department's designated officer as soon as a patient with an airborne communicable disease is identified. Notification must take place within 48 hours of the time the hospital identifies the patient's disease. In the event of possible exposure, there should be a protocol in place to obtain information from your local hospital or other medical resource. You should also be screened and given information about the necessity of medical follow-up. Your designated officer will assist you with the necessary information. Treatment varies depending on the disease.

## BLOODBORNE DISEASE

If you experience a needlestick injury or some other unprotected exposure to blood, you must notify your department's designated officer as soon as possible. You must also complete an incident report. The designated officer can then contact the hospital for information. The hospital then has 48 hours to report back to your designated officer. Depending on your state laws and when possible, patient testing should be done, followed by baseline testing on you.

For exposure to a patient with HIV infection, or blood or body fluid exposure to a patient with unknown HIV status, you should do the following:

- complete an incident report form
- notify the designated officer
- get counseling before undergoing HIV testing
- sign an informed consent form and undergo HIV testing at the time of exposure
- retest for HIV at 6 weeks, 12 weeks, and possibly 6 months
- get counseling after HIV testing to review the results of each test

One of the most difficult aspects of caring for patients is that there are many dis-

eases for which there are no outward signs of infection. Thus, your protection lies in the use of personal protective equipment and/or prompt reporting of an exposure. Postexposure medical follow-up in the absence of the use of PPE will serve to offer protection from developing the disease to which you were exposed. Be familiar with the postexposure protocols outlined in your department's exposure control plan.

## ESTABLISHING AN INFECTION CONTROL ROUTINE

It is important that you and your team make infection control part of your daily routine. En route to any scene, make sure that all the necessary equipment is out and available. Upon arrival, make sure the scene is safe to enter, and then do a quick visual assessment of the patient. Note if there is blood present. Then select the proper PPE based on the tasks you are likely to perform. Remember that good handwashing is always necessary.

Remember to change gloves between patients, whenever possible, especially if there is a great deal of blood at the scene. However, do not delay care for the use of PPE if it puts the patient at risk. If there are multiple injuries and a great deal of blood at the scene, limit the number of persons involved in the care, when possible. If you or your partner are exposed as you are providing care, try to relieve one another as soon as possible so that you may seek care. The exposed person should call the designated officer and report the incident. This will also help maintain confidentiality.

## CLEANING

Routine cleaning of your unit is an essential part of the prevention and control of communicable diseases. Cleaning will remove surface organisms that may remain in the unit. Cleaning should be done following each run and on a daily basis. You do not need to spend a lot of time cleaning the entire unit each time. You need not "air out" your unit. Therefore, you can clean your unit rather quickly so that it may be returned to service. Address the high contact areas. These areas include surfaces that were in direct contact with the patient's blood and/or body fluids or surfaces you touched while caring for the patient after having contact with the patient's blood and/or body fluids.

Cleaning should be done at the hospital whenever possible. If you clean the unit back at the station, make sure you have a designated area with good ventilation and a floor drain. Medical waste should be bagged and disposed of at the hospital whenever possible. Any contaminated equipment left with the patient at the hospital should be cleaned by the hospital staff or bagged for transport and cleaning at the station. Follow your department's standard operating procedures for the PPE to be worn while cleaning in accordance with the Material Safety Data Sheet (MSDS) for the chemical agents being used.

Cleaning solutions need to be evaluated. The bleach and water solution is inexpensive and nontoxic at the 1:100 dilution. Also, any hospital-approved disinfectant solution that is effective against mycobacterium tuberculosis can be used. Alcohol is not a recommended cleaning solution, nor are aerosol spray products. A solution in a bucket or a pistol-handled spray container is advised.

Linen that has been contaminated with blood or body fluids should be removed and placed into an appropriate bag for handling. Each hospital may have a different system for handling of contaminated linen; therefore, you must learn hospital protocols.

The disposal of infectious waste, such as needles, sharps, and heavily soiled dressings, may also vary from hospital to hospital, as well as from state to state. Learn the regulations defining medical waste in your area.

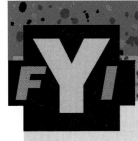

# Bibliography

29 CFR Part 1910.1030, Occupational Exposure to Bloodborne Pathogens; Final Rule, U.S. Department of Labor, Washington, DC, 1991

Enforcement Policy and Procedures for Occupational Exposure to Tuberculosis, Occupational Safety & Health Administration, Washington, DC, 1993

Guidelines for Prevention of Transmission of Human Immunodeficiency Virus and Hepatitis B Virus to Health-Care and Public Safety Workers, Centers for Disease Control, January 1989

National Fire Protection Association, NFPA 1581: Standard on Fire Department Infection Control, National Fire Protection Association, Quincy, MA, 1991

Ryan White Law (Public Law 101–381), Federal Register, March 20, 1994

Sande MA and Volberding PA: The Medical Management of AIDS, Third Edition, W.B. Saunders Company, 1992

Wenzel R: Handbook of Hospital Acquired Infections, CRC Press, Boca Raton, 1981

West KH: Infectious Disease Handbook for Emergency Care Personnel, Second Edition, ACGIH, Cincinnati, Ohio, 1994

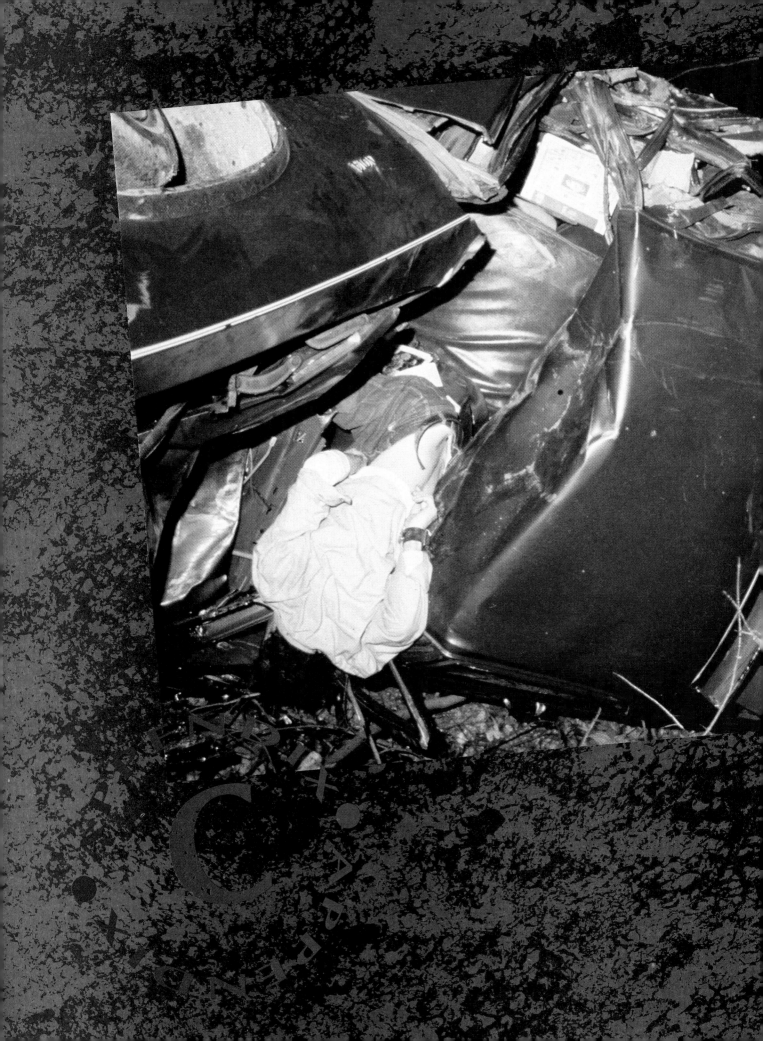

# Appendix C
# Fundamentals
## of Extrication

## Objectives

After you have read this chapter, you should be able to:

- Identify the four phases of an extrication operation.
- Identify potential risks and hazards to you and the patient at the scene.
- List the steps of the hazard survey.
- Explain the importance of personal protective equipment (PPE) during extrication.
- Describe various ways to stabilize a passenger vehicle.
- Identify the principal ways to gain initial access to a patient, including through windows and the windshield and by forcing and expanding doors.
- Describe how to incorporate patient assessment skills during extrication.
- Identify basic methods for releasing entrapped patients.
- Describe the impact of the local environment, terrain, highway conditions, and general traffic hazards as they affect an extrication operation.

# Overview

There are over 10 million vehicles on the highway today. Vehicles vary in size, weight, construction, speed, and the number of passengers they carry. Vehicles today also have many safety features that they did not have in the past. The most important safety feature developed in the past 25 years has been the safety belt. Today there are new or improved standards for braking systems, windshields, steering columns, door latches and hinges, rearview mirrors, air bags, and windshield wipers and defrosters.

As an EMT-B, you will be called to the scene of many accidents. During these incidents, you are a member of a team working under an organized incident management structure. Your responsibilities include patient assessment, care, packaging, and transport. This team approach improves scene safety, and ultimately patient safety.

You and your team must plan and prepare for incidents involving extrication. This preparation includes organized training programs and practice in simulated emergency situations. Vehicle extrications require that you have a basic knowledge of load/vehicle stabilization, simple machines, manual tools, rigging equipment, and power tools. With this information and with practice, you will be able to recognize and anticipate the elements of rescue. The true measure of an effective rescue operation is its outcome. A poorly planned, disorganized rescue operation will often result in injuries to the rescue team, additional injury to the patient, damaged equipment, or excessive extrication time.

Personal as well as patient and bystander safety factors must be the primary concern of every rescuer. Patient safety includes ensuring that further injury does not occur. Protecting the patient from flying debris and falling car parts, avoiding jolts and jerks from unstable vehicles, and attending to airway and bleeding problems result in a better outcome for the patient. Be sure to maintain proper barrier protection for you and the patient.

Rescuer safety includes using appropriate safety gear and adequate personnel when handling patients and equipment. Rescuer safety also includes sharing all pertinent data with the incident commander. The incident commander is dependent on the rescuers to provide any and all data needed to make decisions about the incident.

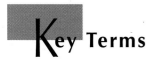

# Key Terms

**Base of support** Amount of vehicle surface that touches the ground.

**Chock** Use of wood blocks or other materials to stabilize a vehicle.

**Danger zone** An area at the scene that is immediately dangerous to health and life.

**Hazard survey** Process that allows the EMT-B to collect data about hazards at the scene.

**LAST sequence** Four phases of a rescue operation: Locate, Access, Stabilize, Transport.

**Maxi-Door method** Method de-signed to quickly remove both doors on one side of a four-door vehicle.

**Rigging** The use of chains, hooks and webbing to stabilize a vehicle, preventing unwanted movement during the extrication process.

**Safety zone** A 25' to 50' area around a vehicle marked with barrier tape or rope in which the rescue operation is performed.

**Strike zone** An area on the side of the vehicle next to the door that can be dangerous if the door "pops" as it is being forced open.

## FOUR PHASES OF VEHICLE EXTRICATION

All rescuer operations, including vehicle extrication, should follow the four-phase **LAST sequence,** as follows:

1. Locate the patient at risk or injured

2. Access the patient, ensuring scene safety

3. Stabilize the patient to prepare for transport

4. Transport the patient to the hospital

## LOCATE PHASE OF VEHICLE EXTRICATION

The rescue operation begins when the call to 9-1-1 is made. The dispatcher needs to know who, what, where, when, and how to begin the rescue response. Decisions about equipment and personnel are based on the information given by the caller and the existing protocols. Appropriate dispatch of equipment and personnel is critical.

As an EMT-B, you may be called upon to help locate patients. This requires a team approach, as many times you may find patients in hazardous, unlikely locations or positions (Figure C-1). It is important to function as a member of a team and to work under the direction of the incident commander. Your objective should be to make the Locate phase the shortest of the LAST sequence. Effective data collection about the incident is necessary so that this phase of the process can be completed quickly and efficiently.

## FIGURE C-1

Help to locate a patient

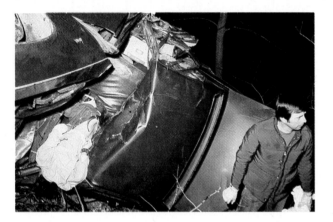

As described in chapter 11, scene size-up is the responsibility of every rescuer working at the incident. In some situations, you and other members of the team may be assigned to gather certain facts about the incident. However, the size-up should be completed in 2 to 4 minutes. The information should then be reported directly to the incident commander. The commander is responsible for informing all rescuers at the incident. Until all essential safety information is known, all rescue activities should be done with extreme care and in a limited manner.

### Hazard Survey

Two rescuers should circle around the vehicles, in opposite directions, from a distance of 25' to 50' to complete the hazard survey. The **hazard survey** helps you to collect data about hazards at the scene. Using two rescuers will allow the area to be checked twice in a very short time. If you are assigned to identify hazards, you should begin your survey in a place that allows a clear view of at least two sides of the incident. Check all sides of the incident when possible. Remember that this survey should be done quickly and systematically.

# ACCESS PHASE OF VEHICLE EXTRICATION

## ENSURING SCENE SAFETY

As you or the first rescue vehicle gets close to the scene, you should begin your scene size-up. Scan the area quickly to assess the need for other resources/equipment and to identify visible hazards (Figure C-2). Remember that as the extrication proceeds, the size-up and plan may change. Size-up is a dynamic process until the patient is freed, packaged, and en route to the hospital.

## FIGURE C-2

Scan the area for visible hazards

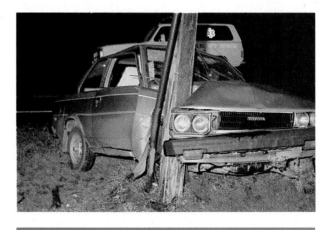

FUNDAMENTALS OF EXTRICATION

You are looking for the following hazards:

- traffic
- fire
- electrical hazards
- problems with vehicle stability
- location, number, and condition of patient(s)
- unusual sounds or odors

Once existing hazards have been identified and resolved, the 25' to 50' area around the vehicle should be marked with barrier tape or rope, when possible. This area is known as the safety zone. The safety zone should be cleared of all nonessential personnel and loose vehicle parts, although law enforcement may not want these parts moved. Your unit and other emergency vehicles should be moved from the safety zone.

Because size-up is an on-going process, you and your team should continue to look for developing hazards. Any new or changing hazards should be reported to the incident commander. The incident commander will keep all on-scene personnel informed of hazards and call for resources to resolve any new hazards.

### Use of PPE

You must not enter any scene without proper personal protective equipment (PPE). As described elsewhere in this text, your PPE must be appropriate for the task and the environment. Thus, you must learn what PPE is appropriate for your situation and understand the specific features of each. In selecting the PPE, you should consider the following factors: 1) protection from the weather, 2) trauma from the extrication process, 3) and protection from possible exposure to bloodborne or airborne pathogens. Firefighting bunker gear is often worn during extrication (Figure C-3). New

fabrics that have been certified to meet OSHA regulations for bloodborne pathogens are now used in some bunker gear.

## How to Control Hazards

### Parking Considerations

Do not park or position your unit on the initial approach to the incident closer than 50' from the emergency scene. Conditions may require that you park closer than 50', but whenever possible the 50-foot rule should be followed (Figure C-4). If there is a possible fuel spill, fire, or fire danger, you should park at least 100' from the incident. It is rare that any emergency vehicle will be parked within the 50-foot safety zone. As described in chapter 27, Ambulance Operations, you should park your unit uphill and upwind of the incident. Emergency vehicles should be parked to protect rescuers from traffic hazards, to warn approaching drivers, and to reduce possible interference from incoming emergency vehicles.

### Traffic Control

Law enforcement is generally in charge of traffic control. Any traffic control plan

### FIGURE C-3

Firefighting bunker gear is often worn during extrication

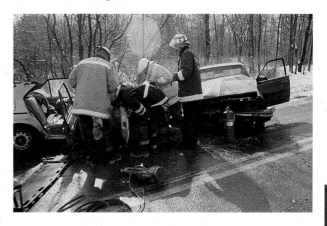

## FIGURE C-4

Follow the 50' parking rule if possible

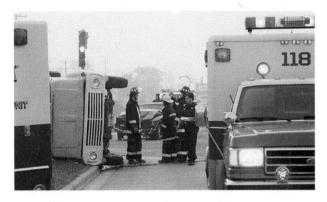

should ensure that both rescuers and patients are safe from on-coming traffic. At times, there will be heavy or fast-moving traffic at the scene. In these cases, the incident commander will decide, along with law enforcement, to stop or block, redirect, or reroute traffic. This decision should be based on prior experience, knowledge of other routes, and the anticipated scope of the rescue operations.

## TYPES OF HAZARDS

### Fuel Hazards

Diesel fuel, gasoline, and propane/natural gas are the most common fuels used in passenger vehicles. Because the fuel system is a real hazard throughout an extrication, fire fighters must be nearby with a charged hose line (Figure C-5). A 1½" hose line should be used, as it provides a minimum of 100 gallons per minute of water flow and allows the use of a foam additive such as "light water."

Fuel under the vehicle or leaking from the fuel system is a serious hazard. If you or anyone on the team sees leaking fuel, you should inform the incident commander immediately.

A danger zone should be established. A **danger zone** is an area at the scene that is immediately dangerous to health and life.

An active fuel leak may require that all rescuers move out of the area, and access to the danger zone be restricted. In this case, two charged 1½" hose lines with a continuous source of water are needed (a foam operation would be beneficial). Rescuers in the danger zone must wear full protective clothing, including a self-contained breathing apparatus (SCBA). The patient should be protected with a fire-resistant blanket. These precautions should continue until the fire fighters secure the fire hazard.

### Electrical Hazards

**Inside Hazards** Electrical hazards can be caused by a vehicle's electrical system or from an outside electrical source. Most vehicles have 12-volt electrical systems with one battery. However, many passenger vans and larger vehicles have two-battery systems. Diesel engine vehicles are also often equipped with two-battery systems for cold weather starting power. Therefore, you should not always assume that there is only one battery.

It is not always necessary to disconnect the battery on vehicles involved in an acci-

## FIGURE C-5

Fire fighters with a charged hose line

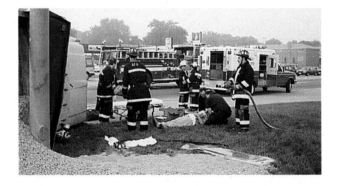

dent. Leaving the battery attached is especially helpful if the doors, windows, and the seat are power operated. Remember that you should try rolling down the windows and unlocking and opening the doors manually before using force to gain access. If you must disconnect the battery, disconnect the ground (negative side) first. This reduces the chances of a spark igniting the gases emitted from the battery or from spilled fuel. Once the battery cables are cut or removed from the battery post, make sure that cable ends are secured (fold the end back onto the cable) with electrical tape.

Newer model vehicles have more complex electrical systems and features. For example, some vehicles have radiator cooling fans that are controlled by a thermal control switch. These run independently of the ignition switch. The fan in these systems can be activated even though the engine is not running. You must use extra care when you work around the fan area of all cars. The electric fuel pump on many vehicles is now located inside the fuel tank. Electric fuel pumps will work as long as the ignition system is in the "on" position. All ignition systems should be put into the "off" position whenever possible to help reduce the possibility of activating the fuel pump.

**Outside Hazards**   When you identify an outside electrical hazard, such as a downed power line, you must inform the incident commander. The incident commander will then inform all on-scene personnel and designate a danger zone. If a downed power line comes in direct contact with a vehicle, tell the driver and any other passengers to stay in the car. A person trying to get in or out of a car that is in contact with an electrical source can become a conduit for the electrical energy to the ground. The result may be serious or fatal injuries. Leaping into or out of an "energized" vehicle does not guarantee safety.

**Catalytic Converter**   The catalytic converter is part of the exhaust system. It converts hot vehicle exhaust emissions into carbon dioxide and water. Carbon monoxide, hydrogen sulfide, and sulfur dioxide gases are also part of the vehicle's exhaust. The catalytic converter is a concern due to the high temperatures of the outer shell. When a car is running, the outer shell is often around 1,000°F. If the engine misfires, the outer shell can reach 2,000°F.

Thus, you should consider the catalytic converter a potential source of ignition. It can also start fires in dry grasses or leaves. The catalytic converter should be of concern when a vehicle is lying on its side or inverted. Rescue equipment, mainly air bags or air cushions, can easily be damaged if placed against or too close to the catalytic converter.

### Fire

As discussed throughout this text, fire fighters are trained to safely control and extinguish fires. Generally, this is not your job as an EMT-B. However, at the scene of a vehicle fire in which patients are involved, you may need to assist fire fighters or become involved in some way. If this is the case, follow the directions of the fire fighters.

Respiratory protection is necessary for fire fighters, rescuers, and the patient when there is any fire or smoke present at a vehicle accident. The smoke and gases from a fire in a vehicle are dangerous and may even be lethal (Figure C-6). An SCBA must be available for all fire fighters and rescuers at accidents with vehicle fires. Remember that you must be trained to use an SCBA.

It is also common practice to cover the interior rescuers and the patient with a fire-resistant blanket or a backboard during extrication (Figure C-7). This provides protection from a flash fire. However, the

## FIGURE C-6

Smoke and gases from a vehicle fire are dangerous

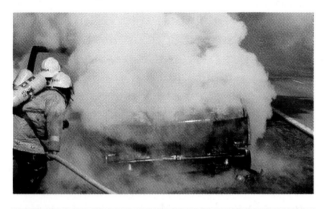

## FIGURE C-7

Cover inside rescuers and the patient with a fire-resistant blanket or a backboard

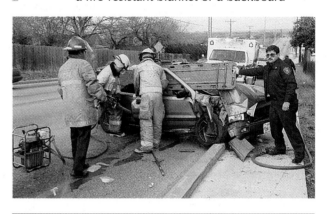

fire-resistant blanket will not provide sustained protection from fire. Fire fighters should stand by with charged lines during extrication, as this provides the most effective protection from potential serious injury.

## STABILIZING A PASSENGER VEHICLE

### UPRIGHT VEHICLE RESTING ON ALL TIRES

An upright vehicle (resting on all four tires) still needs to be stabilized. An unstable vehicle may move the patient and aggravate spinal injuries. Thus, once the safety zone is established, the extrication team will begin stabilizing the vehicle. The first step is to **chock** (stabilize) the wheels with wood cribbing (18" to 24" long) both in front of and behind the tires (Figure C-8). If wood chocks are not available, chock the wheels with other objects such as tires, rocks, and tree limbs. Do not try to open car doors or otherwise gain access until the wheels are chocked. As stated above, movement of the

## FIGURE C-8

Chock the wheels both in front of and behind the tires

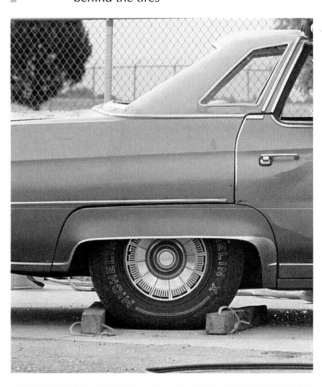

vehicle before the wheels are chocked can result in injury to the patient and to the rescue team.

Once the wheels are chocked, one rescuer should enter the vehicle. The "inside" rescuer can help to reduce the risk of rolling by putting the transmission in Park, turning the ignition off, and setting the parking brake.

The next step is to try to reduce the sway and bounce associated with the vehicle suspension system and the "give" in the sidewalls of the tires. This movement is significantly reduced when you place cribbing between the ground and the vehicle. Assess the vehicle for crossmembers or reinforcement points, such as the base of the pillars.

Pulling the tires' valve stems after the cribbing is in place will drop the vehicle down onto the cribbing. However, you will have to reinflate the tires or lift the vehicle to remove the cribbing at the end of the incident. Reinflating the tires may also help the towing contractor to clean up the accident site more quickly and restore traffic flow.

## UPRIGHT VEHICLE ON UNEVEN GROUND

### Facing Downhill on a Slope

An upright vehicle on uneven ground can easily move. Any direction in which the vehicle may move should be considered a danger zone. For example, the danger zone for a car that is facing downhill on a slope is the slope below the car. As you perform the hazard survey, you must not enter the danger zone. Estimate the center of gravity, assess the angle of incline, and then anticipate the potential direction of movement. To secure the car in the above example, you should approach and chock the tire from the side. Chock all four tires to increase the amount of resistance to rolling or sliding down the slope. Once the car has been secured, the incident commander can announce that the danger zone is clear.

If you think a vehicle may roll over the wheel chocks, you should add equipment such as chains, cables, come-alongs, and low-stretch rope to anchor the vehicle. Secure this equipment to strong attachment points, such as the frame, frame crossmembers, and T-hook slots in the frame. Do not use the bumper, as it is generally not strong enough to act as an attachment point on most cars. Next, look for anchor points such as guardrails, trees, emergency vehicles, or a tow truck located in line with the vehicle. Your anchor system may include ropes, cables, or chains that cross or enter a roadway. If this is the case, then traffic must be blocked so that it cannot move through or over the equipment.

### Facing Sideways on a Slope

If the vehicle is sideways on a slope, it may slide sideways or roll over. Estimate the center of gravity, determine the base of support, and assess the type of ground surface. Chock the wheels on the uphill side to minimize the rolling potential of the tires. Next, secure the vehicle using two solid attachments, one at either end of the vehicle on the uphill side. Once again, use the frame, frame crossmembers, or T-hook slots as attachment points. Follow the same guidelines listed above if the anchor system goes across the roadway or if a vehicle is used to provide the anchor point. Securing a vehicle in this manner will provide the best protection from sliding or rollover.

## OTHER CONSIDERATIONS FOR UPRIGHT VEHICLES

You should make stabilizing attachments to upright vehicles at their low points, as these are easier to access. There is also less potential movement during the rigging process. Rigging involves the use of chains, hooks, and webbing to stabilize a vehicle, preventing unwanted movement during the extrication process. Remember that knowing the estimated center of gravity of the vehicle is critical to proper rigging. If you can find only one anchor point, such as a guardrail, tree, or other vehicle, then locate that anchor point in line with the estimated center of gravity.

You must also know the estimated center of gravity before you attach any rigging equipment, such as chains, hooks, and webbing. Rigging equipment should be attached at two points, one located on either side of the estimated center of gravity. The webbing or chain is attached at either side of the vehicle and brought together to form a "V." The center of this V (also called the apex) should be in line with the estimated center of gravity and the single anchor point (when only one anchor point is used). Rigging that supports the estimated center of gravity reduces the potential of vehicle rotation. This type of rigging also distributes the weight of the vehicle more evenly on rigging equipment. An even distribution of weight means less chance of equipment failure and provides a safer working area for rescuers.

## FIGURE C-9

Use cribbing to widen the base of support

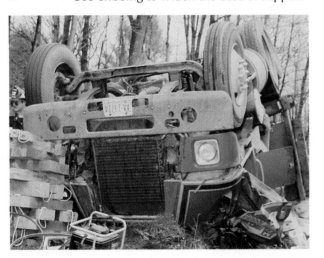

## VEHICLE ON ITS SIDE

A vehicle lying on its side can be very dangerous, as it can move with only a small amount of external force placed at or above the estimated center of gravity. For example, you can easily push over a 4,000-lb vehicle that is on its side by putting pressure high up on it.

Thus, your first step is to widen or extend the **base of support,** or the amount of vehicle surface that touches the ground. To do this, place cribbing between the ground and the vehicle (Figure C-9). Use a tool such as a pike pole to place the cribbing under the vehicle. The pike pole will extend your reach and keep you from crawling under the vehicle. However, extending the base of support with cribbing is not enough to make the vehicle completely stable. Mechanical struts, such as "Jimmy Jacks," provide excellent vehicle stability when used along with cribbing.

To provide the most stability to a vehicle on its side, attach rigging directly to the vehicle above and on either side of the estimated center of gravity. You will need a minimum of two attachment points and one anchor point. However, it is best to have four attachment points and two anchor points. As described above, this arrangement will form a V as the two attachment points come together to be secured to a single anchor. The point of the V is located between the estimated center of gravity and the anchor point.

A vehicle lying on its side on a slope may roll or break loose at the ground contact point. Select strong anchor points and attach cable, low-stretch rope, webbing, or chain directly to the vehicle. To keep the vehicle from rotating on the slope, secure both ends of the vehicle at the same time. First, secure the lower points of attachment and anchor(s). This helps minimize sliding of the base of support. Second, secure the two upper points of attachment at either end of the vehicle. This helps reduce the possibility that the vehicle will roll over down the slope.

As you and your team work to secure the vehicle, use extreme care. Avoid any vehicle movement as you make the attachments and secure the rigging to the anchors. Even slight movement may change the contact point on the ground. This may result in the vehicle slipping downhill or completely rolling over. As soon as the rigging is anchored and secured, add more cribbing to help broaden the base of support and reduce the possibility that the vehicle will rock or sway.

## GAINING ACCESS TO THE PATIENT

### INITIAL ACCESS

The next step in the process is accessing the victim. This concept was introduced in chapter 28, Scene Techniques. During your scene size-up, you identified the safest points to access the patient. Remember that before you or anyone on your team try to enter a vehicle, you must stabilize the vehicle and eliminate major hazards. You should try to enter the vehicle using the simplest, most direct methods. For instance, try to open the car doors first before you break windows or remove doors (Figure C-10).

Passenger vehicles are built to allow easy entry and exit. Always try to open the doors manually before using tools or any forcible method of entry. Check to see if the doors are locked. When there is no danger to the patient, you should try to access the patient through normal door openings. This will also result in minimal damage to the vehicle. However, if there is a medical emergency or a health hazard, you should

## FIGURE C-10

Open car doors first before breaking windows or removing doors

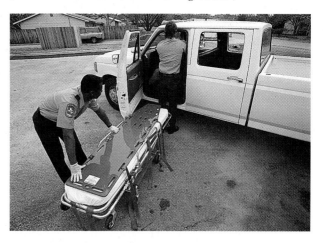

## FIGURE C-11

Obtain access through a window if you cannot open the doors

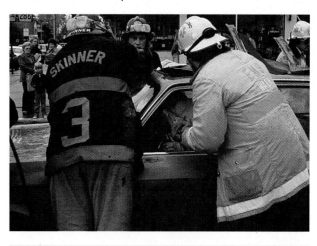

attempt more direct access through a window (Figure C-11).

There will be situations in which the doors are locked, and you need to remove an infant, child, or unconscious adult. You should manage these situations with a rapid door unlocking procedure. If the vehicle is still running, establish a danger zone in front of and behind the vehicle. Chock all four wheels to reduce the possibility that the vehicle will roll if it is slipped into gear. Remember that normally, the shift lever moves from park to reverse.

There are several excellent tools on the market that can open vehicle doors. However, none of these tools supports or uses the old style "Slim Jim" door tool. Rather, modern tools have small light probes so that you can see the lock linkage. These tool systems also include a set of prebent rods, wood wedges, and a current manual listing different ways to open vehicle doors. For more information, you should contact the American Automobile Association (AAA), the Associated Locksmiths of America, or the Towing and Recovery Association of America.

## ACCESS THROUGH A WINDOW

If you have tried to enter through all the doors without success, you should next try to enter through the rear window. If this is not possible, try the rear door windows. The glass in both of these locations is tempered safety glass. This type of glass is cooled very quickly in the manufacturing process. This quick cooling leaves a "tension" on the surface of the glass. Once the tension is released (by a sharp blow), the glass breaks into small round pieces (Figure C-12).

Many tools can be used to break tempered glass, including the following:

- spring-loaded center punches
- pneumatic chisels (flat blade)
- hand tools with a sharp point, such as a Halligan bar

You use all these tools in essentially the same way. Strike the window low in a corner to make sure that the tool does not enter the passenger compartment. Use both hands to hold and control the position of the spring-loaded center punch or the pneumatic chisel. Place your hands in a way that they will strike the car body when the window breaks. Hold long-handled tools, such as the Halligan bar, in such a way so that the handle strikes the car body as the window breaks.

### Use of Window Tape

You may wish to apply tape, self-adhesive paper, or a spray adhesive onto the window surface before you break it. This will hold the glass more or less together, which makes it easier to remove and it improves safety. When you use tape or self-adhesive paper, make sure that you cover only the glass. Do not cover the metal framework of the vehicle. Bonding the glass to the metal framework makes breaking the glass much more difficult. Remember that taping does take time and means additional work. In some situations, such as with excess moisture, cold temperatures, and oil or anti-freeze film, taping will not work, as it will not stick.

## FIGURE C-12

Gain access through the rear window

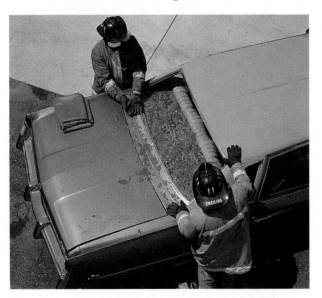

As one EMT-B gets inside the vehicle (the inside rescuer), he or she should try to open the doors, shift the vehicle into park, shut off the ignition, and lower the windows. If you have to force open a door, try to roll down or lower the window as you would normally. If you cannot, cover the exposed glass edge with a tarp, then break the glass with a spring-loaded center punch, a flat-headed ax, Halligan tool, or pneumatic flat chisel.

## ACCESSING A CHILD IN A CAR SEAT

Simply because a child is fastened into a car seat does not guarantee that the child will escape injury. You must perform a complete assessment as with any other patient involved in an automobile accident.

Most infant restraints are designed as a nonadjustable, partially reclining shell. Infants weighing up to 20 lb should always be restrained facing backward in the back-seat. Infant seats are secured to the seat with the vehicle's rear lap belt (Figure C-13). Normally, you can remove a car seat simply by unhooking the seat belt. However, after an accident, the lap belt may become jammed between the seats. Thus, you must cut the seat belt to lift the car seat, with the infant still secured in it, from the vehicle.

Convertible-type car seats are used for children between 6 months and 4 years old. Toddler seats and booster seats are similar to car seats but are larger in size. Children in larger car seats and booster seats face forward (Figure C-14). You may need to cut the seat belts in these instances also.

## ACCESSING VEHICLES FOR THE PHYSICALLY DISABLED

You may have to gain access to a vehicle that has been designed and retrofitted for an individual who is physically disabled.

### FIGURE C-13

Infant seat facing backward

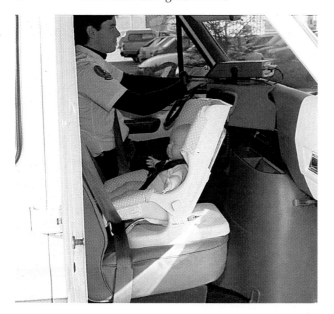

### FIGURE C-14

Children in larger car seats face forward

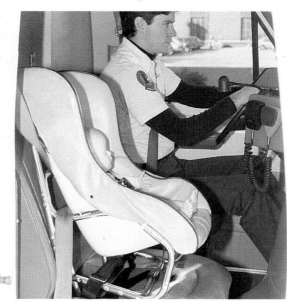

These vehicles may have lifts, ramps, hand controls, or be adapted for a wheelchair (Figure C-15). When used as a seat in a vehicle, a wheelchair should be securely anchored to the frame or other components capable of holding the wheelchair during impact. The anchor system must be attached to the frame, not the wheels, of the wheelchair to properly restrain the wheelchair. Restraints for the wheelchair passenger must also be anchored to the vehicle to provide effective protection. This means that the person should have trunk, shoulder, and head restraint protection. In the past, the wheelchair has been placed sideways in the back compartment of a van or bus, with the wheelchair backed up to the vehicle sidewall. This position does not provide adequate protection for the wheelchair passenger. Currently there are no laws that address how a wheelchair should be secured in a vehicle.

You may also see car restraints specially designed for physically disabled infants and children. There are even special adaptations that can be used with infants who weigh as little as 5 lb. These devices range from car beds to special straps that hook into car seats.

## FIGURE C-15

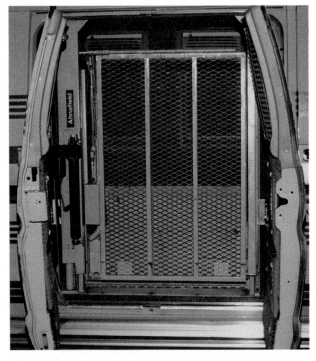

**A**  Vehicles may be specially adapted for the physically disabled

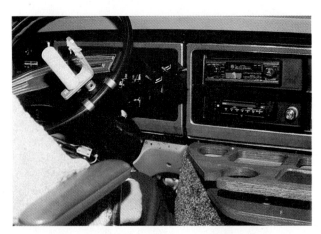

**B**  Special interior controls designed for the physically disabled

### Access Through a Window

Gaining access to these vehicles is the same as for any passenger car or van. Your first step is to communicate with the passenger or driver inside the vehicle, if possible. There is often a special unit that the driver or passenger can activate to unlock or open doors, windows, and lifts. However, if the driver cannot help you, you should try to open all doors and windows before forcing open the vehicle. As with other vehicles, the easiest point of entry will be through a window. The window you select depends on the following:

- where the passengers are sitting
- the damage to the vehicle
- the orientation of the vehicle

Remember that the side or rear doors may have a wheelchair platform that blocks the door opening. The rear area of a conversion van may be obstructed with couch seats.

Be sure to check for external power controls for the doors and lifts. These are usually located on the right side of the van at wheelchair height. The inside rescuer may be able to locate the remote controls that operate the windows, doors, lifts, ignition, and engine shut-off switches.

### Access Through a Door

You may also be able to gain access through one side of the van's doors. Use a power hydraulic spreader and a pneumatic hammer with the flat chisel. You can still force open power doors and special door locking systems using standard opening procedures. The power door closures on the automatic lift systems can be disabled or cut. The chain drive on the sliding doors is exposed and can be cut with a bolt cutter. The piston push rods on the double doors will normally have a cotter pin or a pull pin at the door end. You can remove the pin to allow the doors to operate independently.

# EXPANDING VEHICLE OPENINGS

The next step is to move and/or remove vehicle parts without putting the patient or inside rescuer(s) at unnecessary risk. A step-by-step approach is the safest for both you and the patient. You will not need to use excessive force, such as haphazard pounding, rocking, or cutting to move or remove part of a vehicle.

For some operations, you will only need a single tool. In others, you may need several tools in simultaneous operation. The incident commander will decide what equipment should be used during each step

of the operation. It is important that you know how extrication tools work and react if you are going to use them. This will minimize the possibility for injury to you and the patient.

## CUTTING AND REMOVING WINDSHIELD GLASS

The windshield on a passenger vehicle is laminated safety glass. The lamination process puts a layer of plastic between two layers of plate glass. In some newer models, another layer of lamination is placed on the interior of the windshield. This provides an additional protective barrier during a front-end collision. The windshields on passenger vehicles are held in place by an adhesive mastic material.

There are two general methods of dealing with the windshield. Before you begin, make sure you are wearing the proper protective gear, including heavy-duty gloves and protective eye wear. First, you can cut the bottom edge of the windshield using a saw or a flat-headed ax. You should then leave the windshield in place until the roof is rolled back. This first method is fast, but it presents added risk for the passengers and the inside rescuer because glass passes over their heads as the roof is rolled back. You can also force the roof flap with power hydraulic tools without cutting the windshield. This pulls the windshield from its adhesive. With this method, glass still passes over the passenger compartment. In addition, it is not an effective option when a third layer of lamination is present.

Second, you can cut and remove the windshield in a systematic, controlled way. This method requires at least two outside rescuers working on both sides of the windshield. Two more outside rescuers should be assigned to provide barrier protection for the patient and inside rescuer. The barrier should be placed inside the vehicle and should cover the entire area of the windshield. It should also be able to hold the glass fragments within the dashboard area.

At times, the patient may be close enough to the windshield to be struck by a windshield cutting tool. In these cases, you should add a barrier with a hard surface, such as a ¾" short backboard. You can use the following tools to cut the windshield:

- fire ax
- coarse-bladed handsaw
- pneumatic hammer with a flat chisel run at low pressure
- pneumatic hammer with special windshield cutting adapter
- reciprocating saw (Lenox 6" long, 18 tooth-per-inch blade)

Two rescuers, each with their own tool, can cut out a windshield in less than 2 minutes. A single rescuer can remove the windshield, or a single tool can be passed from one side of the vehicle to the other. However, this adds time to the operation.

### Cutting the Windshield

To cut and remove the windshield, you should make an opening in the center lower edge of the windshield, and then either chop or saw toward the outside edge. Next, you should make a cut on each upper side edge. Then saw or chop down the glass to the bottom, connecting the two cuts. In many passenger vehicles, you can pull the bottom edge of the windshield up and over the roof, then pull the top edge away from its set.

If the glass does not pull away from the vehicle, cut the top edge—working from the center to outside edge. A reciprocating saw with a Lenox 18 tooth-per-inch blade allows you to cut the top edge of the windshield and continue cutting through the A pillar. By cutting in this way, you can leave the windshield in place. However, you should cover the A pillar and the exposed windshield with a tarp to protect the interior rescuer and the patient. Remove the windshield (reciprocating saw cut is an exception) and move it out of the way. Oftentimes, you can place the windshield under the vehicle.

## FORCING HINGED VEHICLE DOORS

Not all damaged vehicle doors must be forced open. Carefully assess all the doors before you commit to forcing them open. Try to unlock and open the interior and/or exterior door latches on hinged doors. Next, try to determine why the door will not open. Check the location of the patient, the degree of impact, and the safety needs of the situation as you try to open the door. You can then determine the best approach and tools to use. Once you have evaluated the situation and discussed your recommendations with the incident commander, you can plan the operation. Share this information with the team, including those directly involved in patient care.

Safety is a great concern with these operations. You must make sure that effective barriers to flying glass or metal are in place before you begin. As stated above, a short or long wooden backboard is an effective initial barrier, along with a heavy aluminized blanket as secondary protection.

Your basic approach will be to force the latch/lock side of the door. A combination of power hydraulic, pneumatic cutting, cutting, and hand prying tools are excellent choices for forcing hinged vehicle doors in a timely manner (Figure C-16).

Forcing a door creates a **strike zone** on the side of the vehicle next to the door. Do not put your body in the arc of the swinging door. This is dangerous. Rather, use an indirect method, such as attaching a chain, webbing, wire rope, or low-stretch synthetic

## FIGURE C-16

Force hinged vehicle doors with hydraulic cutting or hand prying tools

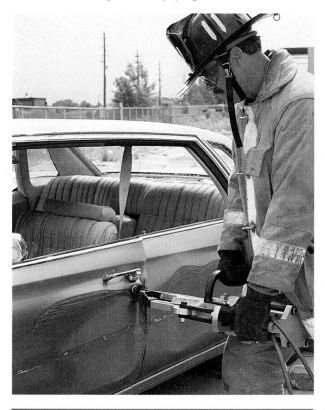

## FIGURE C-17

Use a chain or rope to control the arc of a swinging door

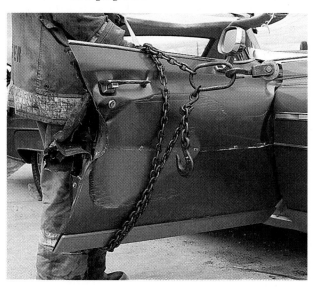

rope to the door (Figure C-17). This is safer for you, as it controls the force of the door opening.

### Forcing Cargo Doors

Many vans have two hinged doors that meet in the middle of the door's open space on the side or rear of the vehicle. You can force both doors open at the same time using the same basic techniques as those used on single doors on hinges. First, you must remove the glass and then expose the latch/lock. Once you expose the latch, spread and separate the latches with either a power hydraulic spreader or Porta-power spreader. The spreading action should be straight sideways. You should then force the doors outward in their normal arc. You can also force the hinged side of the cargo doors, breaking the hinges loose in the same way you would with single-sided vehicle doors.

### Forcing Side Van Sliding Doors

Sliding doors are more difficult to force open than are hinged doors. This is because the hinges on a sliding door are normally stronger and the door opening action more complex. The sliding door often slides in a track. The track must be free and intact for the door to work properly. Many sliding doors first move out and away from the vehicle body before moving back and open. To force open this type of door, you must separate the latch/pin, and then pull or push the door out toward the rear of the vehicle. For this operation, it may be best to have rescuers work on both the inside and outside of the vehicle. You may also wish to use a combination of spreaders, cutters, and pulling tools to force the side sliding door. Working from the inside alone is not always practical. You should also consider other options, such as forcing the rear doors or cutting a new opening on the opposite side wall panel.

## Forcing Rear Lift or Hatchback Gates

The rear gates on vans, hatchbacks, station wagons, and all-purpose vehicles can be dangerous as they are forced open. These gates move back and up and can strike you or a member of the team as they open. The lift is often assisted by gas or hydraulic cylinders. Thus, you must secure the gate open so that it does not fall as you are trying to remove the patient. Do not depend on the hydraulic cylinders to keep the gate open.

As you prepare to open the rear gate, tell the interior rescuer(s) so that appropriate barrier protection can be put into place. Once the window is taken out, place a J-hook chain (tow truck operators normally carry this type of chain assembly) over the window ledge. Then secure the loose end of the chain under the vehicle. This will keep the lift gate from swinging open too rapidly. Disable the lift cylinders by removing the piston attachment clip or screw. Remember that the cylinder is in the compression mode when the gate is shut. The piston/cylinder will move when released. Use a flat-bladed pry bar to open a space and find the latch mechanism. Use a hydraulic spreader to spread and separate the latch from the vehicle body. Two positive struts, such as pike poles, or 4 × 4s, should be used to keep the gate open. You can then secure the gate by rigging chain and a come-along, winch and wire rope, or low-stretch rope to the front of the vehicle. A fixed strut is more stable and takes less time to put in place than rigging to the front of the vehicle.

## EXPANDING DOOR OPENINGS

### Hinged Passenger Vehicle Doors

The purpose of expanding a door opening is to increase the space available for patient care, packaging, and removal. You can often move a hinged door out of the way to increase your working space as a continuation of forcing the door open with extrication tools. Do not use tow truck winches, apparatus winches, or manual force. Using such force can significantly increase the chance that the vehicle will move. This is particularly true when the vehicle is inverted or on a slippery surface.

A cable come-along with rigging chains and cribbing is one of the best ways to move vehicle doors in a controlled manner. You should use grade A (80) rigging chains for come-along operations. These chains should have a master link with an attached grab hook at one end, and a slip or grab hook at the other end. Unpainted hardwood cribbing generally supports the chain and cable at pressure points better than does the softer pine cribbing.

Most often you will move the door along a horizontal plane. Make sure to place cribbing at every place that the come-along, cable, or chain comes in contact with the body of the vehicle. This will distribute the weight of the pull over a wider area. Try to place rigging toward the center of the hood or down on the side of the vehicle so it is more in line with the natural arc of the door. This will decrease the tendency for the come-along to slide off the fender.

### Inverted Vehicle

The principles described above apply to expanding door openings when the vehicle is upright. When the vehicle is inverted, the rigging points are more accessible. This makes it easier to attach the come-along anchor chain. The direction of the pull should keep the door moving along a horizontal plane or at a slight upward angle. You must make sure that the master link on the chain wrapped around the door is in line with the come-along in order to pull the door evenly.

## Using a Power Hydraulic Spreader

You can use a power hydraulic spreader or hydraulic ram to expand the opening of a hinged door in either an upright or inverted vehicle. Once the door is open, place one spreader tip against the rocker panel and the other against the bottom edge of the door. The spreader tool is best positioned in a near vertical to 70° angle. Opening the tips will move the door out and away from the rocker panel. Move the spreader forward toward the hinge side of the door. In this way, you will maintain adequate contact between the spreader tip and the door panel.

## REMOVING HINGED DOORS

You must thoroughly assess the vehicle and the patient before you decide to remove a door. One reason to remove the door at the hinge side is your need for expanded access to the patient. Another reason is that with a side impact, the door often bends inward. The door guard beam or collision beam is located at about waist or lap height and is designed for impacts of low speed. Side impacts at highway speed often result in the collision beam bending into the passenger compartment.

Power hydraulic spreaders, door safety restraints (synthetic low-stretch rope, wire rope, or chain), and patient barrier protection are needed for breaking the hinge attachment points. Place patient barrier protection along with the door restraint, and then break any remaining door window glass. Remember to inform the interior rescuers of the window breaking before performing that task.

You may use one of two ways to remove the hinged doors on the vehicle passenger compartment. The first approach is from the hinge side of the door. Passenger vehicles usually have either stamped metal or cast metal hinges. The hinges are bolted or welded to the car body in two places—on the A pillar and to the door body—and pivot on a center pin. Bolt-on hinges sometimes have one bolt attached in a reverse direction (the bolt screws into the hinge from the interior wall of the A pillar). This makes it impossible to totally unbolt the door from the outside.

There are three basic ways to remove the hinges:

- breaking the hinge attachment point away from the door or car body
- unbolting the hinge
- cutting the hinge

### Breaking the Hinge Attachment

The most common approach is to break the top hinge first and then the bottom hinge with the power hydraulic spreader. Place the spreader tips above the top hinge with one tip against the A pillar side and the other against the door body (Figure C-18). The tool orientation is vertical, not horizontal, when the hinge is not readily visible. You can use either orientation, depending on the situation. As the spreader tips widen, the top hinge will generally fail. In some situations, the A pillar may collapse inward before the hinge fails. In these situations, you may wish to cut or disassemble the hinge.

Once the top hinge has failed, reposition the spreader just above the bottom hinge, and spread the tips until the bottom hinge fails. If the door is free of the latch/pin side after the top hinge is broken, take care to avoid forcing the bottom end of the door into the ground. Forcing the door down will likely lift the entire side of the vehicle off the ground. This creates an unstable situation, with possible unwanted movement of the patient. If the door is still connected to the latch/pin at the B pillar after the two hinges are broken, pull the hinge side out from the car and separate the latch/pin

## Figure C-18

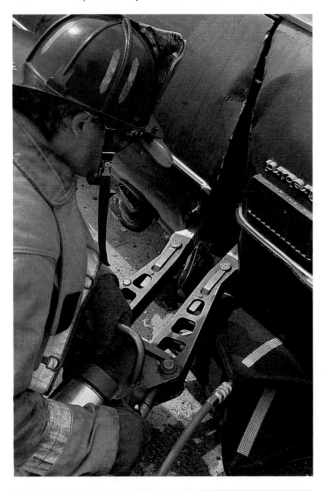

Break the hinge attachment with a power hydraulic spreader

using the spreader. Move the door so that it does not get in the way of other rescue and patient care activities.

### Unbolting the Hinge

Another way to remove the door is to unbolt the hinge from the A pillar or from the door body. This method is not always possible, as some hinges are spot welded, and others have one bolt on each hinge reversed so that it cannot be removed from outside the vehicle.

Before you try to unbolt a hinge, make sure that barrier protection is in place to shield the patient and inside rescuer(s). The door should be restrained as described above to control unwanted movement. Any remaining window glass in the affected door should be broken. To unbolt the door hinge, expose the hinge area, if it is not already, using a pneumatic chisel, flat-bladed pry bar, hydraulic spreader, or a combination of these tools. Remember that the position of the bolts will vary from vehicle to vehicle. Bolts may be either standard SAE or metric. Therefore, you should have both standard and metric sockets and wrenches. A breaker bar with an extension bar or a pneumatic impact wrench with an extension bar are also effective tools for removing the bolts. Of these, the pneumatic impact wrench is usually the fastest tool.

Remove the highest bolt in the top hinge last. Removing this bolt last helps support and make the door easier to control. Place box cribbing next to the door to help support and control the door, if necessary. This method works well for inverted vehicles also. If the vehicle is inverted or the situation demands total control over the door, build a box cribbing to support and keep the door from dropping as it is released. If the door is still attached to the latch/pin side of the door, pull the hinge side of the door away from the car, and use hydraulic spreaders to separate the latch from the pin.

### Cutting the Hinge

Cutting the hinges is another option. You can use a reciprocating electric or pneumatic saw or power hydraulic cutters. Again, you must gain access to the hinges and provide protection for the patient and inside rescuers before you begin.

### Maxi-Door Method

Another approach is called the **Maxi-Door method.** This method was developed to provide the quick removal of both doors on one side of a four-door vehicle. This approach provides full access to the front and the rear seat areas.

First, make sure that patient barrier protection and door restraints are in place. You should then advise the inside rescuer(s) that you are going to break out the remaining door window glass. To remove the doors, you may use power hydraulic cutters, power hydraulic spreaders, a pneumatic chisel (with a long flat blade), and a flat-bladed pry bar. Use the flat-bladed pry bar and the spreader to expose the bottom of the B pillar. Next, use the power hydraulic spreader to make the initial cuts in the bottom of the B pillar. Leave the top of the B pillar intact at this point. This will help support the pillar so that it does not drop down on the cutting tools. You may also use a wedge-shaped piece of cribbing to keep the cutting area open.

Use a long flat chisel to cut the back side of the B pillar as much as possible. Cut the B pillar next to the roof rail, and manually pull out and down on the B pillar. You may use a power hydraulic spreader between the cut B pillar and the roof rail to help push the two doors and the B pillar down. Additional cuts in the B pillar can be made at this point if necessary. Use the spreader on the rear door latch/pin to fully release the rear door. You can then swing both doors and the B pillar around to the front of the vehicle and out of the way.

## STABILIZE PHASE OF VEHICLE EXTRICATION

### HEAD THROUGH A WINDSHIELD

On rare occasions, you may arrive at the scene to find a patient with his or her head and neck lodged in a hole in the wind-

shield. As with all accident scenes, your first step is scene size-up, followed by establishing the safety zone. You must make sure the vehicle is stabilized before you access the patient. In the situation described above, stabilizing the vehicle is particularly important, as you or a member of your team must climb onto the car to stabilize the patient's upper torso, head, and neck. Once the car is stabilized, you must maintain the patient's head and neck in an in-line position. Apply a cervical collar, if possible, as this provides additional protection from the glass fragments. Be sure to assess the neck area for glass fragments before applying the collar. Remember that you can apply a cervical collar only if the patient's head and neck are in a neutral, in-line position.

Remove the windshield from around the patient by cutting the glass with some type of shear. Hydraulic shears work, but they are often too bulky and heavy. Large hand type shears such as those used on sheet metal may be a better option. The cutting action should enlarge the hole in the windshield, allowing for assessment and treatment. Secure the patient to a spinal immobilization device before you try to move the patient.

### SEVERE ENTRAPMENTS

With more severe crashes with entrapments involving the floor, dash, fire wall, and steering column, there is a more complex series of steps before you can package and remove the patient. One of the best options in these situations is to move the entire dash up and off of the patient. To do this, you must remember the following guidelines:

- If you must stop the raising and rolling process for rerigging or repositioning, use a second source of support to keep the vehicle components from coming back down on the patient. Cribbing and wood wedges are a good choice.

- Cut the A pillars first to allow the dash to move freely. At a minimum, you should cut the top edge of the windshield free of the roof or completely remove the windshield.

- Place proper cribbing between the ground and the vehicle (under the A and the B pillars). Also remember to distribute the forces exerted by the extrication tools and the chains equally on the vehicle. Failure to crib the tools and provide proper rigging will prevent maximum pushing/pulling potential.

## Raising and Rolling the Dash

**Patient Safety** Place a protective barrier between the people in the car (interior rescuer/patient), the dashboard, and the extrication tools. Next, make sure that fire protection is in place. It is important to maintain communications with the interior rescuer at all times. This is a noisy operation, so reassure the patient often.

**Laying the Roof Back** The next step is to lay the roof back or remove the roof. This makes the vehicle less rigid and the dash easier to raise. Use a pneumatic hammer with a long chisel to follow the power hydraulic cutter and clean up the cuts. Recycling the power hydraulic cutter to make simple cuts is very time consuming.

Use a power hydraulic cutter to cut either the rocker panel A pillar seam or the A pillar parallel and just above the rocker panel. Cutting the rocker panel allows the front part of the vehicle to move forward and the dash up. Cutting the A pillar allows the dash to roll up and pivot forward. Clean up the A pillar cut with a pneumatic hammer with a long flat chisel, if needed. Re-

member that the dash will roll in an arc. The straight pushing action of a hydraulic ram does not match the arc motion of the dash.

Place the power hydraulic or Porta-power rams (two 10-ton rams joined by a close nipple at the base are preferred) with the base of the ram against the rocker panel at the base of the B pillar. This push works best if a special metal jig is made to fit over the rocker panel and against the B pillar. Using a metal jig with multiple welded feet increases the strength of the B pillar and the rocker panel. This creates a good base from which the hydraulic ram can push.

Place the moving end of the hydraulic ram (for a single ram operation) against the A pillar just below the joint of the window or at the upper door hinge. These are both strong reinforced locations on the vehicle that will normally withstand the pushing force of the hydraulic ram.

If the hydraulic ram must be removed to facilitate patient care and removal, then make the dash push 6" to 12" further than needed. Crib the gap created at the base of the A pillar with wood wedges and release the ram. This should be far enough to keep the dash from coming back down and interfering with patient care.

**Raise the Dashboard** Consider using one set of equipment on each side of the vehicle. This will significantly reduce the extrication time. In addition, using one ram on either side of the vehicle at the same time gives a very controlled, uniform raise and roll across the entire dashboard. Using a second ram also allows one ram to be left in place on one side of the vehicle during patient removal.

Place a power hydraulic spreader with a minimum of a 28" spread with one tip on the rocker panel and one tip on the A pillar near the bottom of the dash. This should be done after all the cuts have been made in the A pillar and the roof laid back. Spreading the tips will lift one side of the dashboard, creating space in the passenger compartment. However, this lift is limited and is not as effective as the raise and roll maneuver, but it may be all that is needed to release the patient.

### Moving or Removing the Front Seats

**Remove the Seat Cushions**  Securing and effectively stabilizing a patient on a moving seat is very difficult. There are times that removing the seat back cushion will greatly simplify providing patient care. Seat back cushions have two points of attachment. The first is at the outer edges of the seat between the bottom cushion and the back cushion. The inside attachment point for some bucket seats on four-door vehicles is sometimes a vertical pin. This pin allows the seat back cushion to be lifted up and off once the outside bracket is cut.

**Remove/Displace the Front Seat**  The front bucket seats or the front bench seat may be moved forward or rearward to open more space in the front passenger area for patient management. If the decision is made to move the seat back, the rescuer must secure/block the seat to prevent forward slippage, which might cause further injury. The regular seat control should be tried before deciding to force the seat out of the way. Releasing the manual seat control lever will allow the seat to move forward unless a force is applied to counteract the spring action. Electric seat controls may also be used to move the seat backward. Remember that the seats in transfer vans used by handicapped drivers will have multiple direction capabilities, including the ability to rotate.

The front seat can be forced forward in two ways:

1.  Pulling with a come-along rigged to the front of the vehicle

2.  Pushing forward with a spreader or ram using the base of the B or C pillar as a pushing base

Pulling the seat backward is generally done with a come-along. The come-along usually has enough cable to reach from a solid anchor point at the rear of the vehicle to the chain attachment point at the base of the seat.

The initial pulling action will compress the seat cushion before the seat begins to move to the rear of the vehicle. The seat will have a tendency to move backward along the seat track, break through the rear seat stop, and then begin to rise in the direction of the pulling force of the come-along. The rigging for pulling the seat with a come-along requires careful placement of cribbing. This will ensure that the come-along cable or chain does not bind up or collapse other vehicle structures.

You can move both sides of a bench seat at the same time, as follows:

- rigging the chain at the center of the bench seat around the lower seat cushion and below the seat back

- combining a push back with a spreader or hydraulic ram on one side and the chain/come-along on the other side

- rigging two chains on either side to a central pull point of a single come-along

- rigging two chains and two come-alongs, one set up on either side of the bench seat

A hydraulic spreader or a hydraulic ram can be used to force the seat to the rear or forward. The ram tip or the spreader tips can be placed on the seat at the bottom perimeter frame. The bottom perimeter frame is a narrow piece of metal frame around the base of the seat. You must feel for this metal component at the bottom edge of the seat. Do not push against the seat cushion or the seat support bracket frame. The spreader tips tend to slip inward as you push. Thus, they must be monitored continuously to protect the patient. The angle of push by the spreader or the ram should follow the normal angle of seat movement.

You may remove the seat by cutting the seat supporting braces, unbolting the seat braces, or by lifting and breaking the seat away from its attachments. A pneumatic hammer with a long flat chisel or a power hydraulic cutter can often reach under the seat and cut the metal bracing. However, before you make any cut, you must place cribbing to support the seat at its current position.

Unbolting the seat braces requires adequate lighting and reach to release the seat from the floor. If you cannot see the bolt, it is not practical to try to remove it.

### Pulling Brake/Clutch Pedals

You may need to cut the pedals, such as if the brake pedal is impaled in the groin, but these cases are rare. To cut the pedal arm, you can use power hydraulic cutters, a reciprocating saw, or a hacksaw. Note that there are small hydraulic cutters on the market that can fit into small spaces. One safe way to remove brake pedals is to pull them out completely. To wrap and pull the pedal, use 1" nylon or polyester webbing that has a minimum strength rating of 4,000 lb. These materials are lightweight, strong, thin, and highly maneuverable in what is normally a tight situation.

## TRANSPORT PHASE OF A RESCUE OPERATION

As discussed throughout this textbook, transporting a patient is not "the end" of your job as an EMT-B. You must be sure to continue assessments, drive safely, and make accurate reports to hospital staff.

Each extrication operation has some element(s) upon which you and your team can improve. Review the operation after you have returned to your base or station. Auditing the time and activities will help you, your team, and your department to improve your performance the next time. This is not the time to discipline or criticize one person or an entire agency. When you evaluate performance and objectively assess the outcomes of patients, you and your team may find that you need to alter the protocols.

Rescue and extrication are relatively new as a science. They are part of a body of knowledge and skills that can potentially improve and change patient outcomes. As equipment improves and changes, you can build on previous experience to develop a more effective approach. To be a vital part of the growth process, you must be willing to learn from each experience and then change practices to accommodate the needs of the patients.

# Glossary

**abandonment**   Failure to continue treatment.

**abdominal-thrust maneuver**   A method of dislodging food or other material from the throat of a choking victim. Also known as the *Heimlich maneuver.*

**abrasion**   Loss or damage of the superficial layer of skin after a body part rubs or scrapes across a rough or hard surface.

**absorption**   The process by which medications travel through body tissues until they reach the bloodstream.

**actions**   The effects that a drug is expected to have on the patient's body.

**acute myocardial infarction (AMI)** (ă-kyūt mī ō-kar´dē-ăl in-fark´shŭn) Heart attack; specifically, death of the heart muscle from obstruction of its blood flow.

**addiction**   A state characterized by an overwhelming desire or need (compulsion) to continue the use of a drug or agent and to obtain it by any means, with a tendency to increase the dosage.

**adult-onset diabetes**   The form of the disease that develops as the patient ages. Characterized by a partial deficiency in insulin and does not usually require insulin for its treatment. This term is no longer used medically, but you may still hear it. Now called *type II diabetes.*

**advance directive**   Written documentation that a competent patient uses to specify medical treatment should he or she become unable to make decisions. Also called a *living will.*

**advanced life support (ALS)**   Advanced lifesaving procedures, such as cardiac monitoring, starting IV fluids, giving medications, manual defibrillation, and using advanced airway adjuncts.

**agonal respirations** (ag´on ăl)   Occasional, gasping breaths that occur after the heart has stopped. The respiratory center in the brain continues to send signals to the breathing muscles.

**airway**   Refers to the upper airway tract or the passage above the larynx (voice box).

**allergens** (al´er-jen)   Substances that cause allergic reactions.

**allergic reaction**   Reaction that occurs when the body has an immune response to an agent that is introduced either on the surface of or into the body.

**ambient temperature**   The temperature of the environment.

**ambulance**   Vehicle used for treating and transporting patients who need emergency medical care from the scene to a hospital.

**American Standard System**   A safety system for large oxygen cylinders to prevent the accidental attachment of a regulator to a wrong cylinder.

**Americans with Disabilities Act (ADA)** Comprehensive legislation designed to protect disabled individuals against discrimination.

**amniotic sac**   The fluid-filled, bag-like

membrane that grows around the developing fetus, inside the uterus.

**anaphylaxis** (an ă-fi-lak´sis)  An extreme allergic reaction.

**anatomic position**  Position of reference with the patient standing, facing you, arms at the side, with the palms of the hands forward.

**angina pectoris** (an-jī´nă pek-tō´ris)  Chest pain from heart disease that is brought on by excitement or exertion and relieved by rest and nitroglycerin tablets.

**anterior**  The front surface of the body, the side facing you.

**Apgar score**  A measure of a baby's condition at birth.

**appendicitis** (ă-pen di-sī´tis)  Inflammation of the appendix.

**arrhythmia** (ă-rith´mē-a)  An irregular or abnormal heart rhythm. Also called *dysrhythmia*.

**arteriosclerosis** (ar-tēr´-ē-ō-skler-ō´sis)  A disease characterized by a thickening and destruction of the arterial walls, caused by fatty deposits within them; the arteries lose the ability to dilate and carry oxygen-enriched blood.

**articular cartilage**  A thin layer of cartilage, covering the articular surface of bones in synovial joints.

**artificial circulation**  Provides blood circulation to the body by external chest compressions.

**artificial ventilation**  Opening the airway and restoring breathing by mouth-to-mask ventilation and by the use of mechanical devices.

**assault**  Unlawfully placing a patient in fear of bodily harm.

**asthma**  A disease of the lungs in which muscles spasm in the small air passageways and large amounts of mucus are produced, resulting in airway obstruction.

**asystole** (ă-sis´tō-lē)  Complete absence of electrical activity in the heart.

**auscultate** (aws´kŭl-tāt)  Listening to sounds within the body. This is usually done with a stethoscope.

**auscultation**  Listening to sounds within the organs, usually with a stethoscope; a method of taking a patient's blood pressure.

**autonomic (or involuntary) nervous system**  The part of the nervous system that regulates functions, such as digestion and sweating, that are not controlled by conscious will.

**AVPU scale**  Method of assessing the patient's level of consciousness.

**avulsion**  An injury in which a piece of skin is either torn completely loose or is hanging as a flap.

**B**

**backboard**  Device used to provide support to patients suspected of having a hip, pelvic, spinal, or lower extremity injury. Also called a *spine board*.

**backdraft**  An explosion of gases in the smoldering phase of a fire.

**bag-valve-mask (BVM) device**  Device with face mask attached to a bag with a reservoir and connected to oxygen. Delivers more than 90% supplemental oxygen to the patient.

**barrier device**  A protective item, such as a valved pocket mask, that limits your exposure to the patient's body fluids.

**base of support**  Amount of vehicle surface that touches the ground.

**base station**  Any radio hardware containing a transmitter and receiver that is located in a fixed place.

**basic life support (BLS)**  A series of emergency lifesaving procedures that focus on the patient's airway, breathing, and circulation.

**basket stretcher** Device commonly used in technical rescues and water rescues. Also called a *Stokes litter*.

**battery** Touching a patient or providing emergency care without consent.

**behavior** Manner in which a person acts. Pertains to any or all activities, including physical and mental.

**behavioral emergency** A situation in which the patient acts abnormally in a way that is unacceptable or intolerable to the patient, family, or community.

**beta agonists** Agents that act like epinephrine by relaxing the smooth muscles in the bronchial tubes, causing them to open up.

**birth canal** The vagina and lower part of the uterus.

**blood pressure** The pressure of the circulating blood against the walls of the arteries.

**bloody show** A small, bloody mucous plug from the cervix that comes out of the vagina, often signaling the beginning of labor.

**body substance isolation (BSI)** An infection control concept and practice that assumes all body fluids as being potentially infectious.

**bone marrow** The central portion of all bones that produces red blood cells.

**borderline diabetes** Jargon used to characterize the patient whose blood glucose may be elevated on occasion or in whose urine sugar may be detected. It has little meaning and does not indicate the presence of the disease.

**bradycardia** (brād ē-kar'dē-ă) Abnormal slowing, but regular heart rhythm or pulse.

**brain stem** The part of the central nervous system that controls virtually all the functions that are absolutely necessary for life, including the cardiac and respiratory systems.

**breath sounds** An indication of air movement in the lungs. Breath sounds are heard by listening to the lungs with a stethoscope.

**breech presentation** Delivery in which the baby's buttocks, rather than the head, appears first.

**burnout** A condition of chronic fatigue and frustration that results from mounting stress over time.

## C

**capillary refill** The ability of the circulatory system to restore blood to the capillaries after you squeeze the fingertip.

**cardiopulmonary resuscitation (CPR)** Establishes artificial ventilation and circulation in a patient who is not breathing and has no pulse.

**cellular telephone** A low-power portable radio that communicates through an interconnected series of repeater stations called "cells."

**central nervous system (CNS)** The brain and spinal cord.

**cerebellum** (ser e-bel'ŭm) The part of the brain that coordinates body movements.

**cerebral edema** Swelling of the brain.

**cerebrum** (ser'ě-brŭm) The largest part of the brain, containing about 75% of the brain's total volume.

**cervix** The opening or mouth of the uterus.

**channel** An assigned frequency or frequencies used to carry voice and/or data communications.

**chemical transportation emergency center (CHEMTREC)** Assists emergency personnel in identifying and handling hazardous materials transport incidents.

**chief complaint** The patient's response to a general question such as "What's wrong?" or "What happened?"

**chilblains** A form of cold exposure where exposed parts of the body become very cold but not frozen. It is characterized by redness and swelling.

**child abuse** Any improper or excessive action that injures or harms a child or infant.

**chock** Use of wood blocks or other materials to stabilize a vehicle.

**chronic obstructive pulmonary disease (COPD)** A slow process of dilation and disruption of the airways and alveoli, caused by chronic bronchial obstruction.

**circulatory system** Complex arrangement of connected tubes, including the arteries, arterioles, capillaries, venules, and veins. System moves blood, oxygen, nutrients, carbon dioxide, and cellular waste throughout the body.

**closed fracture** Any fracture in which the skin has not been broken by the bone ends, and there is no wound anywhere near the injury site.

**coagulation** Formation of clots to plug openings in injured blood vessels and arrest blood flow.

**communicable disease** Any disease that can be spread from person to person.

**competent** Able to make rational decisions about personal well-being.

**conduction** The loss of body heat by touching a colder object.

**congestive heart failure (CHF)** A disease in which the heart loses its ability to pump blood, usually as a result of damage to the heart muscle.

**connecting nerves** Nerves that connect the motor and sensory nerves.

**contamination** The presence of infective organisms.

**contraindications** (kon tră-in di-kā´shŭns) Situations in which a drug should not be given because it would either harm the patient or have no positive effect on the patient's condition.

**contusion** A bruise.

**convection** The loss of heat through moving air, from the body surface to a colder area.

**CPR board** Device that provides a firm surface under the patient's torso so that you can give effective chest compressions.

**crepitus** (krep´i-tŭs) A crackling sound often heard when two ends of a broken bone rub together. Also air bubbles under the skin, giving the skin a crinkly feeling.

**critical incident stress debriefing (CISD)** A confidential group discussion of a highly traumatic incident that usually occurs within 24 to 72 hours of the incident.

**croup** (kroop) An infectious disease of the upper respiratory system that may cause partial airway obstruction and is characterized by a barking cough.

**crowning** The appearance of the baby's head at the cervix during labor.

**danger zone** An area at the scene that is immediately dangerous to health and life.

**decontamination** The orderly process by which radiation or chemical hazards can be removed from clothing, equipment, vehicles, and personnel.

**dedicated line** A special telephone line used for specific point-to-point communications. Also known as a *hot line*.

**defibrillation** (dē´fib ri-lā´shŭn) Delivery of a direct current electric shock (or countershock) to the chest over the heart.

**dehydration** Loss of water from the tissues of the body.

**depression** A state in which the patient may not want to do anything, even move, and may not cooperate or answer questions.

**dermis** (der´mis) Inner layer of the skin containing hair follicles, sweat glands, nerve endings, and blood vessels.

**designated officer** The individual in the department charged with the responsibility of managing exposure and infection control issues.

**diabetes mellitus** Literally means "sweet diabetes." It refers to the presence of sugar in the urine and is the disease most people are referring to when the term "diabetes" is used.

**diabetes** Metabolic disorder in which the body cannot metabolize glucose, usually due to a lack of insulin.

**diffusion** A process in which molecules move from an area with higher concentration of molecules to an area of lower concentration.

**dilation** Widening of the blood vessels, such as the coronary arteries.

**direct contact** Spread of a communicable disease from one person to another.

**direct ground lift** Lifting technique used for patients with no suspected spinal injury who are found lying supine on the ground.

**displaced fracture** Any injury that makes the limb appear in an unnatural position. Also called a *deformity.*

**disruptive behavior** Behavior that puts the patient or others in danger or delays treatment.

**distal** Structures that are nearer to the free end of the extremity.

**distention** The act or state of being swollen or stretched.

**distraction** When the spine is pulled along its length.

**diving reflex** Slowing of the heart rate caused by submersion in cold water.

**DNR orders** Written documentation that gives medical personnel permission not to attempt resuscitation in the event of cardiac arrest.

**dose** The amount of the drug that is given.

**drowning** Death from suffocation by submersion in water.

**duplex** Transmitting and receiving radio signals simultaneously.

**dyspnea** (disp nē´-a) Shortness of breath or difficulty breathing.

# E

**ecchymosis** (ek i-mō´sis) Discoloration associated with a closed wound.

**emergency medical services (EMS)** System that represents the combined efforts of several professionals and agencies to provide prehospital emergency care to the sick and injured.

**emergency medical technician (EMT)** A member of the EMS system who is trained to provide prehospital medical care. EMTs are categorized into three levels of training: basic, intermediate, paramedic.

**end tidal carbon dioxide detector** Plastic disposable indicator that signals, by color change, that the ETT is in the proper place.

**endocrine system** Complex message and control system that integrates many body functions, including the release of hormones.

**endotracheal intubation** A method of intubation in which an endotracheal tube (ETT) is placed through a patient's mouth or nose and directly through the larynx between the vocal cords into the trachea to open and maintain an airway.

**envenomation** Deposit of venom into a wound.

**epidermis** Outer layer of skin that acts as a watertight protective covering.

**epiglottis** (ep i-glo´tis) A thin, leaf-shaped valve that allows air to pass into the trachea but prevents food or liquid from entering.

**epistaxis** (ep i-stak´sis) Nosebleed.

**esophageal gastric tube airway (EGTA)** An esophageal obturator airway with an added gastric decompression tube; it allows gas in the stomach to be vented to the outside, thereby decreasing gastric distention.

**esophageal obturator airway (EOA)** A plastic, semirigid tube that can be inserted in the esophagus; the upper third, which has holes in it, lies at the level of the pharynx and provides free passage of oxygen-enriched air to the lungs.

**evaporation** The loss of body heat as a result of water changing from a liquid to a gas.

**exhalation** Part of the breathing process in which the diaphragm and the intercostal muscles relax. As these muscles relax, all dimensions of the thorax decrease, and the ribs and muscles assume a normal resting position.

**exposure** Contact with blood, body fluids, tissues, or airborne droplets by direct or indirect contact.

**exposure control plan** Comprehensive plan that helps employees reduce their risk of exposure to or acquisition of communicable diseases.

**expressed consent** Type of consent in which a patient expressly authorizes you to provide care or transport.

**extremity lift** Lifting technique that may be used for patients with no suspected extremity or spinal injuries who are supine or in a sitting position.

**extrication** Removal from entrapment or a dangerous situation or position. This is often used to mean removal of a patient from a wrecked vehicle.

**eyes forward position** Position in which head is gently lifted until the patient's eyes are looking straight ahead and the head and torso are in line.

**Federal Communications Commission (FCC)** Federal agency with jurisdiction over interstate and international telephone and telegraph services and satellite communications—all of which may involve EMS activity.

**fetus** The developing baby in the uterus (womb).

**first responder** The first medically trained person to arrive at the scene of sudden illness or injury.

**flashover** Violent reaction similar to an explosion; lightning current that travels over the surface of the person on its way to the ground.

**flexible stretcher** Device that can be folded or rolled when not in use. A rigid carrying device when secured around a patient.

**fontanels** (fon tă-nels´) Two soft areas on the baby's head, one near the front and one near the back.

**four-person logroll** Procedure for moving a patient from the ground to a long spine board. Recommended if you suspect a spinal injury.

**frostbite** The most serious local cold injury because the tissues are actually frozen. The affected tissues are hard and cold to the touch. The skin is usually white, yellow-white, or blue-white.

**frostnip** A form of cold exposure that occurs after prolonged exposure to the cold. The skin may be frozen, but freezing of the deeper tissues has not occurred. The skin becomes pale (blanched). Exposed parts of the body such as the ears and nose are commonly affected.

**full-thickness burn**  All skin layers are burned; the subcutaneous layers, muscle, bone, or internal organs may also be burned. The area is dry, leathery, and may appear white, dark brown, or charred. Clotted blood vessels may be visible under the burned skin, or the subcutaneous fat may be visible.

# G

**gastric distention**  Condition in which air fills the stomach as a result of high volume and pressure during artificial ventilation.

**general impression**  Overall initial impression formed to determine the priority for patient care. Based on the patient's surroundings, the mechanism of injury, or the patient's chief complaint.

**generic name**  The name of a drug as listed in the *United States Pharmacopoeia*; also generally the simple chemical name.

**glucose**  A simple sugar essential for cell metabolism in humans.

**Golden Hour**  The period of time during which treatment of a patient in shock or with traumatic injuries is most critical. This period of time is generally thought to be the first 60 minutes after injury.

**Good Samaritan laws**  Laws that prevent an individual who voluntarily helps an injured or suddenly ill person from being legally liable for any error of omission in rendering good faith emergency medical care.

**guarding**  Tensing of the abdomen during palpation.

**hazard survey**  Process that allows the EMT-B to collect data about hazards at the scene.

**HazMat Rule of Thumb**  A guide to how close you can come to a hazardous material spill before you know what the hazardous material is.

**head-tilt maneuver**  Technique to open the airway by tilting the patient's head backward.

**head-tilt/chin-lift maneuver**  Combination of two movements to open the airway in which the forehead is tilted back and the chin lifted.

**heat cramps**  Painful muscle spasms that occur after vigorous activity. They usually occur in the leg or abdominal muscles. The exact cause of heat cramps is not well understood. A change in the body's electrolyte balance and dehydration may play a role in the development of muscle cramps.

**heat exhaustion**  The most serious illness caused by heat. Also called *heat prostration* or *heat collapse*. It occurs when the body loses so much water and electrolytes through very heavy sweating that fluid depletion occurs. Patients who develop heat exhaustion are in mild hypovolemic shock. The skin is usually cold and clammy and the face gray. The patient may also complain of feeling dizzy, weak, or faint, with accompanying nausea or headache. The vital signs may be normal, although the pulse is often rapid. The body temperature is usually normal or slightly elevated, but on rare occasions it may be as high as 104°F (40°C). If not treated, heat exhaustion can develop into heatstroke.

**heatstroke**  The least common but most serious illness caused by heat exposure.

Left untreated, heatstroke will always result in death. When the body is subjected to more heat than it can handle and the normal mechanisms for releasing excess heat are overwhelmed, the body temperature can rise rapidly up to 106°F (41°C) or more. The skin is usually hot, dry, and flushed because the sweating mechanism has been overwhelmed. However, early in the course of heatstroke, the patient may still be sweating and the skin may be moist or wet. As the body core temperature (the temperature of the heart, lungs, and vital organs) rises, the patient's level of consciousness falls. As the patient becomes unresponsive, the pulse becomes weaker and the blood pressure falls.

**hematoma**  Blood collected within the body's tissues or in a cavity, occasionally palpable as a discrete mass.

**hemophilia**  Condition of lacking one or more of the blood's normal clotting factors.

**hemorrhage**  Bleeding.

**host**  The organism or person in which an infectious agent resides.

**hot line**  Same as a *dedicated line.*

**hydroplaning**  Condition in which the tires of a vehicle may be lifted off the road surface as water "piles up" under it. As a result, the tires are not in direct contact with the road surface. The vehicle then feels as if it is floating on the road surface.

**hyperthermia**  A condition in which the body gains or retains more heat than it loses, usually 101°F or higher.

**hyperventilation**  Rapid, deep breathing.

**hypothermia**  A condition in which the body loses more heat than it produces, usually 95°F or lower.

**hypovolemic shock**  Condition in which low blood volume, due to massive internal or external bleeding, results in inadequate perfusion.

**hypoxia** (hī-pok′sē-ă)  Dangerous condition in which the body's tissues and cells do not have enough oxygen.

**immersion foot**  Condition which occurs after prolonged exposure to cold water. Also called *trench foot.* It is common in hikers or hunters who stand for a long time in cold water. The skin of the foot is wrinkled, pale, and cold to the touch.

**implied consent**  Type of consent in which a patient who needs immediate emergency medical care to prevent death or permanent physical impairment is given treatment under the legal assumption that he or she would want treatment.

**incident management systems**  Organizational systems to help control, direct, and coordinate emergency responders and resources.

**indications**  The most common uses of a drug in treating a specific illness.

**indirect contact**  Transmission of disease from one person to another by contact with a contaminated object.

**infection control**  Procedures designed to reduce infection in patients and health care personnel.

**infection**  The growth of an organism in a susceptible host with or without signs or symptoms of illness.

**inferior**  The part of the body, or any body part nearer to the feet.

**informed consent**  Permission to be treated given by a competent patient who has had the potential risks, benefits, and alternatives to treatment explained.

**ingestion**  Swallowing; taking a substance by mouth.

**inhalant**  A substance that is or may be taken into the body by way of the nose and trachea, or through the respiratory system.

**inhalation**   The active muscular part of breathing that occurs as we inhale.

**inspect**   Assessing the body by looking.

**insulin**   An essential hormone produced by the pancreas that enables glucose to enter the cells of the body. Also manufactured to treat diabetes.

**insulin-dependent diabetes**   The form of the disease in which insulin must be used.

**intervertebral disk**   Cushion that lies between the vertebrae.

**intramuscular (IM)**   The injection of medication into muscle tissue.

**intravenous (IV)**   The injection of medication into the blood through the wall of a vein.

**involuntary activity**   Those actions we do not control.

**ischemia** (is-kē′mē-ă)   Tissue deprived of its blood supply and therefore of its oxygen and nutrients.

**jaw-thrust maneuver**   Technique to open the airway by placing the fingers behind the angle of the jaw and bringing the jaw forward.

**joint**   The place where two bones come in contact.

**jump kit**   A lightweight, durable, waterproof portable kit containing items used in the initial care of the patient.

**juvenile-onset diabetes**   The form of diabetes that first develops in childhood. Characterized by an absolute lack of insulin, which must be replaced daily for effective treatment. This term is no longer used medically, but you may still hear it. Now called *type I diabetes.*

**K**

**kinetic energy**   Energy associated with motion.

**labor**   A three-stage process that begins with the first regular uterine contractions, includes delivery of the baby, and ends with delivery of the placenta.

**labored breathing**   Breathing that requires effort, in which the person may be breathing either much slower or much faster than normal.

**laceration**   A smooth or jagged open wound.

**laryngoscope** (lă-ring′gō-skōp)   An instrument used to give a direct view of the patient's vocal cords during endotracheal intubation.

**LAST sequence**   Four phases of a rescue operation: **L**ocate, **A**ccess, **S**tabilize, **T**ransport.

**lateral**   Parts of the body that lie at some distance from the midline. Also called *outer structures.*

**ligament**   A band of fibrous tissue that connects bones to bones. It supports and strengthens a joint.

**Look, Listen, and Feel technique**   Way of assessing the airway of an unconscious patient.

**mania**   A state in which the patient may be severely agitated (manic), moving around frantically and speaking rapidly, but never finishing a sentence or a complete thought.

**Maxi-Door method**   Method designed to quickly remove both doors on one side of a four-door vehicle.

**mechanism of injury**   The way in which traumatic injuries occur. With a traumatic injury, the body has been exposed to some force or energy that has resulted in permanent damage or even death.

**meconium** (mē´-kō-nē ŭm)  Sterile fecal material released from the baby's bowels before birth.

**MED channels**  VHF and UHF channels designated by the FCC exclusively for EMS use.

**medial**  Parts of the body that lie closer to the midline. Also called *inner structures.*

**medical control**  Physician instructions given directly by radio (on-line) or indirectly by protocol/ guidelines (off-line) to EMTs in the field.

**medical director**  Physician who authorizes or delegates the authority to perform medical care in the field.

**meninges** (mě-nin´jēz)  Three distinct layers of tissue that surround and protect the brain and the spinal cord within the skull and the spinal canal.

**meningitis** (men-in-ji´tis)  An inflammation of the meningeal coverings of the brain and spinal cord caused by either a virus or a bacterium.

**metabolism**  The sum of all the physical and chemical processes of living organisms; the process by which energy is made available for the uses of the organism.

**metered-dose inhaler**  A miniature spray can designed to deliver medications inhaled into the lungs. Each use delivers the same dose.

**midaxillary line**  Imaginary vertical line drawn through the middle of the axilla (armpit).

**midclavicular line**  Imaginary vertical line drawn through the middle portion of the clavicle and parallel to the midline.

**midline**  Imaginary vertical line drawn from the middle of the forehead through the nose and the umbilicus (navel) to the floor.

**miscarriage**  Delivery of the fetus and placenta before 20 weeks gestation, for any reason.

**motor nerves**  Nerves that carry information from the CNS to the muscles.

**mucous membrane**  The lining of body cavities and passages that are in direct contact with the outside environment.

**multiple-casualty situation (MCS)**  An event that places such a demand upon available equipment or personnel resources that the system is stretched to its limit.

**musculoskeletal**  Pertaining to or composing the skeleton and the muscles, as the musculoskeletal system.

**musculoskeletal system**  The bones and voluntary muscles of the body.

**myocardium** (mi ō-kar´dē-ŭm)  Heart muscle.

**nasal cannula**  Oxygen delivery device in which oxygen flows through two small, tube-like prongs that fit into the patient's nostrils.

**nasopharyngeal airway**  Airway adjunct inserted into the nostril of a conscious patient who is not able to maintain a natural airway.

**nasotracheal intubation**  The placement of a tube through the nose into the trachea to improve ventilation.

**near drowning**  Survival, at least temporarily, after suffocation in water.

**negligence**  Consists of four elements: duty, breach of that duty, physical or psychological injury, and cause.

**neonate**  A newborn infant.

**nervous system**  System that controls virtually all activities of the body, both voluntary and involuntary activities.

**nitroglycerin**  Medication used to treat chest pain. Works by dilating the blood vessel walls.

**non-insulin-dependent diabetes** The form of the disease that can be managed without using insulin. Measures such as weight loss, the use of oral medicines to stimulate insulin release, and diet are generally effective in its control.

**nonrebreathing mask** A mask and reservoir bag system that is the preferred way to give oxygen in the prehospital setting. With a good mask to mouth seal, it can provide up to 95% inspired oxygen.

**open fracture** Any break in the bone in which the overlying skin has been damaged as well.

**OPQRST** The six "pain questions." **O**nset, **P**rovoke, **Q**uality, **R**adiation, **S**everity, **T**ime.

**oropharyngeal airway** Airway adjunct inserted into the mouth to keep the tongue from blocking the upper airway and to make suctioning the airway easier.

**orotracheal intubation** The placement of a tube through the mouth into the trachea to improve ventilation.

**OSHA** Occupational Safety and Health Administration. Develops and publishes guidelines concerning safety in the workplace.

**osteoporosis** (os´tē-ō-pō-rō sis) Reduction in the amount of bone mass, leading to fractures after minimal trauma.

**pacemaker** A device generally implanted under a heavy muscle or fold of skin that maintains a regular cardiac rhythm and rate by delivering an electrical impulse through wires that are in direct contact with the myocardium.

**packaging** The positioning, covering, and securing of an ill or injured patient for transportation.

**paging** Involves the use of a radio signal and a voice or digital message that are transmitted to pagers ("beepers") or desktop monitor radios.

**palpation** Examination by touch.

**paradoxical motion** Chest movement that is in the opposite direction of the normal rise and fall of breathing. Paradoxical motion is occurring if part of the chest wall expands outward as the patient exhales and inward as the patient inhales.

**paramedic** An EMT who has completed an extensive course of training in ALS. Skills include IV therapy, advanced pharmacology, cardiac monitoring and defibrillation, and advanced airway management.

**paranoia** A state in which the patient may believe that people (including you) are plotting to harm or kill him or her.

**partial airway obstruction** Condition in which a patient is able to exchange air in the lungs, but has some degree of respiratory distress.

**partial-thickness burns** The epidermis and some portion of the dermis are burned. The subcutaneous tissue is not injured. Blisters form, and the skin is white to red, moist, and mottled.

**pathogen** A microorganism that is capable of causing disease in a susceptible host.

**pediatrics** Medical practice devoted to the care of children up to age 18.

**perfusion** Circulation of blood within an organ or tissue in adequate amounts to meet the cells' current needs.

**peripheral nervous system** 31 pairs of spinal nerves and 12 pairs of cranial nerves in the form of long fibers that link the nuclei and cell bodies of the CNS to the body's various organs.

**placenta** Afterbirth that develops on the wall of the uterus and is connected to the fetus by the umbilical cord.

**pleura** The serous membrane covering the lungs and lining of the thoracic cavity, completely enclosing a potential space known as the pleural space.

**pleural space** The potential space between the parietal pleura and the visceral pleura. It is described as "potential" because under normal conditions the lungs fill this space.

**point tenderness** Tenderness sharply localized at the site of the injury found by gently palpating along the bone with the tip of one finger.

**poison** Substance whose chemical action could damage structures or impair function when introduced into the body in a relatively small amount.

**portable stretcher** Lightweight folding device without undercarriage and wheels.

**posterior** The back surface of the body, the side away from you.

**power grip** Technique that allows you to get maximum force from your hands.

**power lift** Posture that is safe and helpful for EMT-Bs when they are lifting. Also called *squat lift*.

**PPE** Personal protective equipment.

**premature** Any baby that delivers before 8 months gestation or weighs less than $5\frac{1}{2}$ lb.

**premature ventricular contractions (PVCs)** Abnormal heartbeats that result from uncoordinated electrical impulses in the heart.

**protection level** A measure of the amount of protective equipment that someone must have to avoid injury during contact with a hazardous material.

**proximal** Structures that are closer to the trunk.

**pulmonary edema** Fluid building up in the lungs, a result of congestive heart failure.

**pulse** The pressure wave that is felt with the expansion and contraction of an artery, consistent with the beat of the heart. It may be felt with a finger.

**quality improvement** A system of internal and external reviews and audits of all aspects of an EMS system.

**rabies** An acute viral infection of the central nervous system, transmitted by the bite of a rabid animal.

**radiation** The loss of body heat as a result of being in a colder environment.

**rale** Cracking, rattling breath sound that occurs in patients with fluid in the lungs.

**Rapid Extrication** Technique developed to quickly move a patient from sitting in a vehicle to supine on a long spine board in less than 1 minute.

**rapid trauma assessment** A quick area by area examination of a trauma patient to identify life-threatening injuries.

**rapport** A trusting relationship that you build with your patient.

**recovery position** Position used to help maintain a clear airway in a patient with a decreased level of consciousness who has not had traumatic injuries and is breathing on his or her own.

**repeater** A special base station radio that receives messages and signals on one frequency and then automatically retransmits them on a second frequency.

**respiration** The process in which oxygen enters the blood as we inhale and carbon dioxide and waste products are removed as we exhale.

**respiratory system** All the structures of the body that contribute to the process of breathing, consisting of the upper and lower airways.

**rigging** The use of chains, hooks, and webbing to stabilize a vehicle, preventing unwanted movement during the extrication process.

## S

**safety zone** A 25' to 50' area around a vehicle marked with barrier tape or rope in which the rescue operation is performed.

**salmonellosis** (sal´mō-nel-ō sis) Any disease caused by a salmonellal infection, which may be manifested as food poisoning with acute gastroenteritis, vomiting, and diarrhea.

**SAMPLE history** A patient's history consisting of **S**igns/symptoms, **A**llergies, **M**edications, **P**ertinent past history, **L**ast oral intake, and **E**vents leading to the illness/injury.

**scanner** A radio receiver that searches or "scans" across several frequencies until the message is completed. The process is then repeated.

**scene size-up** A quick assessment of the scene and the surroundings that provides you and your partner with as much information as possible about the safety of the scene before you begin patient assessment.

**scoop stretcher** Designed to be split into two or four sections that can be fitted around a patient who is lying on the ground or other relatively flat surface. Also called a *split litter.*

**self-contained underwater breathing apparatus (SCUBA)** A system that delivers air to the mouth and lungs at various atmospheric pressures, increasing with the depth of the dive.

**Sellick maneuver** Technique in which pressure is applied on the cricoid cartilage to prevent aspiration. Involves pressing posteriorly on the cricoid cartilage to compress and shut off the esophagus behind it.

**sensory nerves** Nerves that carry information from the body to the CNS and transmit senses, such as touch, taste, heat, cold, or pain.

**shivering** An involuntary response to generate more body heat through muscular activity.

**shock** Condition in which the circulatory system fails to provide sufficient circulation so that every body part can perform its function. Also called *hypoperfusion.*

**side effects** Any actions of a drug other than the desired effect.

**sign** A condition displayed by the patient that you observe, such as bleeding or a contusion.

**simplex** Single-frequency radio; transmissions can occur in either direction but not simultaneously in both; when one party transmits the other can only receive, and when one party is transmitting it is unable to receive.

**skeletal muscle** Striated muscles that are attached to bones and usually cross at least one joint.

**skeleton** Framework for the attachment of muscles. Also designed to allow motion of the body and protection of vital organs.

**solution** A liquid containing dissolved medication, which generally passes through a filter and does not settle. Solutions do not need to be shaken.

**somatic (or voluntary) nervous system** The part of the nervous system that regulates our voluntary activities, such as walking, talking, and writing.

**splint** A rigid or flexible appliance used to keep in place and protect an injured part.

**spontaneous pneumothorax** The presence of air in the chest cavity from the rupture of a congenitally weak area on the surface of the lungs.

**sprain** A joint injury in which some of the supporting ligaments are damaged.

**stair chair** A lightweight folding device used to carry a seated patient, especially up or down stairs.

**standing orders** Written documents, signed by the EMS system's medical director, that outline specific directions, permissions, and sometimes prohibitions regarding patient care. Also called *protocols*.

**stoma** An opening in the neck that connects the trachea directly to the skin.

**stridor** Noisy respirations resulting from a large partial blockage of the upper airway.

**strike zone** An area on the side of the vehicle next to the door that can be dangerous if the door "pops" as it is being forced open.

**stylet** Plastic-coated wire that gives added rigidity and shape to the ETT.

**subcutaneous (SC)** The injection of a medication into the tissue between the skin and the muscle.

**sublingual (SL)** Medications that are placed under the tongue and absorbed through the mucous membranes.

**substance abuse** The knowing misuse of any substance to produce some desired effect.

**sudden infant death syndrome (SIDS)** Death from unknown cause occurring during sleep in an otherwise healthy infant. Also called "crib death."

**suicidal act** A situation in which a patient may be threatening to kill himself or herself or may have already made an attempt.

**superficial burns** Only the epidermis is burned. The skin turns red but does not blister or actually burn through.

**superior** The part of the body, or any body part nearer to the head.

**SURVIVE study technique** Composed of the following techniques: **S**kim, **U**nderline, **R**ead, **V**erbalize, **I**ntegrate, **V**ary, and **E**valuate.

**suspension** A liquid containing particles of medication, which will generally settle when left standing. Suspensions need to be shaken.

**sympathomimetic drugs** (sim´pă-thō-mi-met ik) Agents that mimic the hormone epinephrine (adrenaline).

**symptom** A condition that the patient tells you about, such as "I feel dizzy."

**tachycardia** (tak i-kar´dē-ă) Abnormally rapid but regular heart rhythm or pulse.

**telemetry** A process in which electronic signals are converted into coded, audible signals. These signals can then be transmitted by radio or telephone to a receiver at the hospital with a decoder.

**tendon** A tough, rope-like cord of fibrous tissue that attaches a skeletal muscle to a bone.

**tolerance** The ability to endure large doses without ill effect, such as the ability to endure the continued or increasing use of a drug.

**tonsil tip** Type of suction tip best for suctioning the pharynx. Tonsil tips have a large diameter and are somewhat rigid to prevent collapse.

**topographic anatomy** The superficial landmarks of the body that serve as guides to the structures that lie beneath them.

**toxicity level**  A measure of the risk that anyone is subjected to by contact with a certain hazardous material.

**toxin**  A poison or harmful substance, produced by bacteria, animals, or plants.

**traction**  The act of exerting a pulling force on a structure.

**trade name**  The brand name a manufacturer gives a drug.

**transdermal**  Medication absorbed through the skin (topically). With transdermal patches, the medication is in direct contact with the skin until it is absorbed into the blood.

**triage**  The process of establishing treatment and transportation priorities according to severity of injury and medical need.

**UHF**  Ultra High Frequency. Radio frequencies between 300 and 3,000 MHz.

**umbilical cord**  The tissue that connects the placenta with the fetus.

**universal precautions**  A concept for infection control which considers blood and certain body fluids to pose a risk for transmission of bloodborne diseases.

**urticaria (hives)** (er ti-kar´i-ă)  Small areas of generalized itching and burning that appear as multiple raised, reddened areas on the skin.

**uterus**  The womb. The hollow organ inside the female pelvis where the fetus grows.

**vagina**  The outermost part of a woman's reproductive system. Forms the lower part of the birth canal.

**vallecula** (vă-lek´yū-lă)  Space between the base of the tongue and the epiglottis.

**ventricular fibrillation (VF)**  Disorganized, ineffective quivering of the heart.

**ventricular tachycardia (VT)**  Rapid, regular heart rhythm that results when several PVCs occur together.

**VHF**  Very High Frequency. Radio frequencies between 30 and 300 MHz. The VHF spectrum is further divided into "high" and "low" bands.

**virulence** (vir´ū-lens)  The strength or ability of a pathogen to produce disease.

**voluntary activity**  Those actions we consciously perform in which sensory input determines the specific muscular activity.

**vomitus**  Vomited material.

**wheeled ambulance stretcher**  A specially designed stretcher that can be rolled along the ground. It has a collapsible undercarriage so that it can be loaded into an ambulance.

**wheezing**  An audible high-pitched breath sound usually resulting from a small airway blockage.

# Index

*Numbers in italic indicate graphic material.*

# I

Ice, compression, elevation, and splinting (ICES), 494
Ice and slippery surfaces, 630
Identical twins, 456
Iliac crest, 62
Ilium, 62
Immersion foot, 413
Immobilization devices, 581
    cervical collars, 158, 581–582, *581*, 647, 731
    long spine boards, 582–583, *582*
    short spine boards, 582, *582*
Immunity, Good Samaritan laws and, 51
Immunizations, 38, *697*
Implied consent, 42, 44
Incident management system, 643, 656
    components of, 656
    structure of, 658–659
Incubators, transporting newborns in, 615
Indications, 308
    for medications, 309
Indirect contact, 696, 697
Infant restraints, accessing child in, 723
Infants
    anatomy of, 146
    Apgar score for, 449
    artificial circulation in, 687–689
    artificial ventilation in, 686–687
    basic life support care in, 685
    breathing patterns in, 151–152
    delivering, 445–447
    developmental concerns for, 596
    examination tips for, 597
    foreign body airway obstruction in, 692–693
    initial care of, 448–450
    multiple, 456
    opening airway in, 685–686
    premature, 456–458
    pulse in, 244
    respiratory arrest in, 162–164
    transporting, 615
Infection, 696, 697
    from miscarriage, 441–442
    risk of, from bleeding patient, 467
Infection control, 695–696, 696
    body substance isolation, 18, 25–28, 235, *237*, 696, 699–700
    definition of, 699
    diseases that pose risk, 704
        bacterial meningitis, 706
        common childhood diseases, 706
        hepatitis B and hepatitis C, 704
        HIV infection, 704–705
        tuberculosis, 705
        whooping cough, 706

establishing infection control routine, 707, 708
importance of patient information, 702–703
postexposure management, 706
    airborne disease, 706–707
    bloodborne disease, 707
risk reduction and prevention, 698
    employee responsibilities, 699–700
    employer responsibilities, 698
    exposure control plans, 700–702
    personal protective equipment, 698–699
understanding disease transmission, 697
Infectious waste, disposal of, 708
Inferior portion, 54, 56
Inferior vena cava, 78, 348
Informed consent, 42
Ingested poisons, 390
Ingestion, 384
Inhalants, 400, 402
Inhalation, 70, 142, 144, 145, *145*, 310, 325, 513
Inhaled poisons, 390–392
Injection
    intramuscular (IM), 308, 309, 316
    intravenous (IV), 308, 309, 316
    subcutaneous (SC), 308, 309, 316, *316*
Insect bites and stings, 406
    allergic reaction to, 385
    treatment of, 420–421
Inspect, 250, 266
Inspections, daily, for ambulance, 627
InstaChar, 394
Insta-Glucose, 380
Insulin, 93, 374, *375*, 381
Insulin-dependent diabetics, 375–376
Intercostal muscles, 70
Internal bleeding, 478–479
    emergency medical care for, 480
    mechanism of injury, 479
    signs and symptoms, 479–480
International Society of Fire Service Instructors, 7
Interpersonal communications, 298
    with children, 301–302
    with elderly patients, 300–301
    with learning-impaired, 302–303
    with non-English-speaking patients, 303
    skills in, 299–300
    with visually impaired, 303
Intervertebral disk, 60, 561, 564
Intoxication, 398
Intracerebral hematoma, 575, *577*
Intracranial bleeding, 575
Intracranial hematoma, 575
Intramuscular (IM) injection, 308, 309, 316
Intravenous (IV) injection, 308, 309

Involuntary activities, 561, 563
Involuntary muscle, 82
Involuntary nervous system, 564
Ischemia, 345, 350, 668
Ischial tuberosities, 62
Ischium, 62
Isoetharine (Bronkosol, Bronkometer), 311, 330
Isoproterenol (Isuprel, Medihaler-Iso), 315

# J

Jaundice, 101, 247
Jaw-thrust maneuver, 156, 161–162, *162*, *169*, 177, 178, 675, *675*, 686
    basic steps of, 241–242, *241*
Jellyfish, 423
J-hook chain, 728
Jimmy Jacks, 720
Joint, 516, 518–519
    injuries to, 524, 529
    knee, *519*
    temporomandibular, 564
Jump kit, 621, 626
Juvenile-onset diabetes, 376

# K

Kinetic energy, 259
Knee, 63–64, 554–555
    injuries to, 554–555, *554, 555*
Knee ligament, 554
    treatment of injuries to, 554

# L

Labor, stages of, 439–440. *See also* Obstetrics and gynecology
Labored breathing, 142, 150, 324
Laceration, 490, 494, *495*, 520
    scalp, 577–578, *577, 578*
Landing sites for helicopter, 639
Laryngectomy, 176
Laryngoscope, 198, 206–207, *206, 207, 208, 213*
    inserting, 212–213, *212, 213*
Larynx, 68, 143, 202
LAST sequence, 713
Lateral (outer) structures, 54, 56
Left ventricle, 345
Leg, 64, *64, 65*
    injuries to, 555–556, *556*
Leukocytes, 80
Lifestyle changes, 22
    balancing work, family, and health in, 23
    body substance isolation in, 25–28
    exercise in, 23